MEDICAL RADIOLOGY

Diagnostic Imaging and Radiation Oncology

Interstitial and Intracavitary Thermoradiotherapy

Contributors

J.M. Ardiet · L.V. Baert · L.W. Brady · J.C. Camart · T.C. Cetas · M. Chive
K.L. Clibbon · T.A. Colacchio · P.M. Corry · J.M. Cosset · C.T. Coughlin
J. Crezee · C.J. Diederich · R.R. Dobelbower, Jr. · E.B. Douple · B. Emami
J.J. Fabre · R. Fietkau · B. Frankendal · P. Fritz · J.-P. Gerard · D. Gersten
G.G. Grabenbauer · P.W. Grigsby · E.W. Hahn · J.W. Hand · L. Handl-Zeller
W. Hürter · K.H. Hynynen · H. Iro · E.L. Jones · R.S.J.P. Kaatee
C. Koedooder · F. Koenis · I.K.K. Kolkman-Deurloo · J.J.W. Lagendijk
S. Langer · P.C. Levendag · W.J. Lorenz · K.H. Luk · M.A. Mackey
C. Marchal · A. Martinez · A. McCowen · C.A. Meeuwis · H.W. Merrick
A.J. Milligan · C. Miyamoto · J. Mooibroek · F. Morganti · J. Nadobny
G.J. Nieuwenhuys · K.S. Nikita · P. Peschke · Z. Petrovich · B. Prevost
F. Reinbold · D. Ross · T.P. Ryan · R. Sauer · W. Schlegel · P. Schraube
M. Seebass · M.H. Seegenschmiedt · D.S. Shimm · C. Smed-Sörensen
P.K. Sneed· B. Sorbe · B. Stea · A.C. Steger · J.W. Strohbehn · N.K. Uzunoglu
J.D.P. van Dijk · C.A.J.F. van Geel · C. van Hooye · G.C. van Rhoon
N. van Wieringen · C.C. Vernon · A.G. Visser · N.L. Vora · M. Wannenmacher
G. Wolber · P. Wust

Edited by

M.H. Seegenschmiedt and R. Sauer

Foreword by

L.W. Brady and H.-P. Heilmann

Springer-Verlag
Berlin Heidelberg New York
London Paris Tokyo
Hong Kong Barcelona
Budapest

Dr. M. HEINRICH SEEGENSCHMIEDT
Professor Dr. ROLF SAUER

Strahlentherapeutische Klinik
Universität Erlangen-Nürnberg
Universitätsstraße 27
W-8520 Erlangen
Germany

With 153 Figures and 108 Tables

MEDICAL RADIOLOGY · Diagnostic Imaging and Radiation Oncology

Continuation of
Handbuch der medizinischen Radiologie
Encyclopedia of Medical Radiology

ISBN-13:978-3-642-84803-2 e-ISBN-13:978-3-642-84801-8
DOI: 10.1007/978-3-642-84801-8

Library of Congress Cataloging-in-Publication Data
Interstitial and intracavitary thermoradiotherapy / contributors, J. M. Ardiet . . . [et al.]: edited by M. H. Seegenschmiedt and R. Sauer: foreword by L. W. Brady and H.-P. Heilmann. p. cm. - (Medical radiology) Includes bibliographical references and index.
ISBN-13:978-3-642-84803-2
1. Cancer - Thermotherapy - Congresses. 2. Cancer - Radiotherapy Congresses. 3. Cancer - Radioisotope brachytherapy - Congresses. I. Ardiet, J. M. II. Seegenschmiedt, M. H. (Michael Heinrich), 1955 . III. Sauer, Rolf, IV. Series. [DNLM: 1. Brachytherapy - methods - congresses. 2. Hyperthermia, Induced - methods - congresses. 3. Neoplasms - radiotherapy congresses. 4. Neoplasms - therapy congresses. QZ 269 I5845 1993] RC271.T5I577 1993 616.99'40632-dc20 93-13822

Softcover reprint of the hardcover 1st edition 1993

Typesetting: Macmillan India Ltd., Bangalore-25
21/3130/SPS-5 4 3 2 1 0 - Printed on acid-free paper

To our parents

Hedwig Sauer
Friedrich and Adelheid Seegenschmiedt

Foreword

The use of hyperthermia in radiation oncology is well established. Many publications cover the whole field of possibilities and problems of this therapeutic modality. The new development of interstitial and intracavitary hyperthermia, however, is not well known: there are only a few relevant publications in different journals. Therefore, it was appropriate that SAUER and SEEGENSCHMIEDT organized an international meeting on this topic, where experiences with this new and promising technique were compiled and discussed by experts. The papers of this symposium together with additional review papers and clinical studies are published in this volume.

The publication begins with the physical and biological background of interstitial and intracavitary hyperthermia continues with comprehensive review papers on clinical topics and then gives examples for a wide variety of clinical applications.

This volume will contribute to better understanding and application of the treatment possibilities of radiooncology in combination with this new treatment modality.

Hamburg/Philadelphia, June 1993

H.-P. HEILMANN
L.W. BRADY

Preface

Heat has been employed as an independent or adjunctive therapy for the treatment of cancer for almost 5000 years, its use probably first being recommended for the treatment of breast tumors in the famous Edwin Smith Surgical Papyrus. The more or less constant search throughout history for heating methods to cure malignant tumors led to the development of various types of external and internal heating devices. However, in most instances these devices can be simply regarded as cautery; certainly they cannot be compared with state-of-the-art "internal" hyperthermia, the foundations of which were laid by J. Doss during the first International Symposium on Cancer Therapy by Hyperthermia and Radiation in Washington D.C. in 1975. In contrast to *external* hyperthermia methods which are administered through the intact skin to tumors at the surface of or within the body, interstitial and intracavitary heating techniques are *internal* heating methods by which heat is directly delivered to the tumor tissue in situ. Whereas interstitial hyperthermia techniques use directly implanted probes within the tumor, intracavitary hyperthermia techniques approach the tumor volume by means of probes introduced into natural body cavities. These internal heating methods can be considered the best heating approach by virtue of: (1) the level of temperature which can be achieved, (2) the homogeneity of the temperature distribution, (3) the possibility of selectively heating a specified target volume with reduced heating to surrounding structures, (4) the option of individual power steering of all heat sources, and (5) the intrinsic option of invasive thermometry.

The basic biological and clinical rationale of hyperthermia is well established and calls for a main treatment strategy like radiotherapy and chemotherapy to be combined with hyperthermia to take advantage not only of the cytotoxic but also of the radio- and chemosensitizing potential of heat. Therefore it is essential not to neglect the importance of appropriate full-dose irradiation or chemotherapy when applying heat. Use of thermo-radiotherapy or thermo-chemotherapy, i.e., "piggy-backing" heat on standard radio- or chemotherapy, can provide decisive therapeutic enhancement which may result in reduced toxicity, increased local control, or improved survival as compared to the results achieved with the standard therapy alone. It is easy and reasonable to combine interstitial radiotherapy with interstitial or intracavitary hyperthermia, because the same indwelling probes and tubes as are employed for brachytherapy can be used for insertion of heat sources and thermometry probes. The geometric arrangement of the applicators permits a relatively uniform temperature distribution without deviation from traditional brachytherapy guidelines. Depending upon the specific clinical protocol, external radiation and/or chemotherapy can also be added without any special adjustments.

Within one decade various techniques for interstitial and intracavitary hyperthermia have been developed and implemented in clinical trials, generally in combination with radiotherapy. Nowadays several methods for producing interstitial and intracavitary hyperthermia can be distinguished. Radiofrequency (resistive and capacitive heating) and microwave (radiative heating) techniques are considered the "classical" heating methods and have been applied in most clinical trials. However, recently newer methods have become available, including hot source techniques which simply rely on thermal conduction and blood flow convection for heat transport (e.g., the hot water perfusion and ferromagnetic seed techniques). Moreover, advanced ultrasonic and laser hyperthermia, which are based on energy absorption in tissue, are technically sufficiently advanced to justify initial clinical trials. In addition, treatment planning, thermal monitoring techniques, and thermal modeling have been refined to allow improved concurrent treatment control and retro- and prospective thermal data evaluation. Another most significant step forward will be the clinical implementation of noninvasive thermal monitoring techniques such as impedance tomography and microwave radiometry, which are presented in this volume.

Special interstitial or intracavitary applicators specifically suited for tumors in different body sites have been used in a variety of phase 1 and phase 2 clinical studies and to develop technical and clinical quality assurance (QA) criteria. Preferably preirradiated tumor recurrences and in some instances advanced primary tumors in the head and neck and the pelvic region have been included in the initial trials. However, recent technologies have successfully approached tumors in many more anatomic sites, including brain and eye tumors, abdominal tumors (during the surgical procedure), and esophageal, broncheal, bile duct, vaginal and urethral malignancies. In this volume we provide evidence that most of the nonrandomized studies have indeed yielded very promising results, but presently we cannot demonstrate unequivocally an advantage of interstitial and intracavitary thermo-radiotherapy over standard therapy alone. Thus after these necessary pilot studies we need to design and carefully conduct multicenter randomized trials like those already being initiated by the American Radiation Therapy Oncology Group (RTOG) and the European Society of Hyperthermic Oncology (ESHO). The scientific tools and means to conduct these trials, together with future perspectives for clinical research, are set out in this book.

The current volume includes 41 contributions which illustrate the well-evolved state of this multidisciplinary field of oncologic research. We have structured the contents of the book into five sections: (1) biology, physiology, and physics of interstitial thermo-radiotherapy, (2) treatment control and treatment planning, (3) general review of clinical experience with interstitial thermo-radiotherapy, (4) special clinical experiences and applications, and (5) design and performance of multicenter clinical trials using interstitial thermo-radiotherapy. Each section contains both major review papers and special contributions dealing with ongoing intrainstitutional research activities. The logical order of all the contributions and a comprehensive subject index provide clear orientation in the field. The volume is designed in such a way as to allow both the specialist and the interested new researcher to start reading at any preferred area of interest and then to proceed to other selected topics.

The idea of compiling the present volume was conceived with the help of many contributing authors on the occasion of the international COMAC-BME Workshop on "Interstitial and Intracavitary Hyperthermia" held in the autumn of 1991 in Erlangen (Germany). The COMAC-BME project "Optimization of hyperthermia technology and assessment of clinical efficacy in the treatment of cancer," which was sponsored and supported by the European Community and chaired by Ron van Loon, Brussels (Belgium), fostered extensive exchange and many new initiatives for interinstitutional research into hyperthermia throughout Europe between 1989 and 1992. The international scientific faculty of the workshop in Erlangen and other renowned researchers from Europe and overseas have supplied selected contributions on the most attractive aspects and most frequent applications of interstitial and intracavitary hyperthermia in conjunction with radiotherapy.

Our aim in publishing this volume is to promote further scientific exchange between European and other researchers and institutions from overseas and to stimulate the diffusion of interstitial and intracavitary hyperthermia not only in the field of radiotherapy but also in all other specialized oncologic disciplines. Further biologic research, technical inventions, new clinical concepts, and novel therapeutic ideas even may give rise to a broad spectrum of non-oncologic applications of hyperthermia in the near future. Although it appears that interstitial hyperthermia should be included in the oncologist's armamentarium for palliation of disease, there is still a long way to go before thermo-radiotherapy moves from the experimental stage to become a truly established adjuvant treatment modality for various malignancies.

Although the techniques and applications of hyperthermia may further change in the future, the basic goal will remain the same, namely, *to cure our fellow human beings suffering from a fatal disease or to palliate their distressing, painful symptoms and improve their quality of life.* If our efforts are successful, we will advance a step further toward understanding the puzzling nature of cancer and will be able to offer more effective treatment of many malignant disorders.

Erlangen, June 1993

MICHAEL HEINRICH SEEGENSCHMIEDT
ROLF SAUER

Contents

Part I Biology, Physiology, and Physics

Part II Treatment Control and Treatment Planning

Part I
Biology, Physiology, and Physics

1 Biological Rationale of Interstitial Thermoradiotherapy

E.L. JONES

CONTENTS

1.1 Introduction

The biological rationale of interstitial thermoradiotherapy is based on the complementary actions of hyperthermia and radiation when combined for cancer therapy. As will be reviewed in following chapters, there is significant in vitro and in vivo evidence to suggest interstitial heat and radiation have synergistic interactions. Optimal clinical application of interstitial thermoradiotherapy depends on the essential biological interactions, the physics, and the practical implementation of interstitial thermoradiotherapy. To date, clinical studies using hyperthermia and radiation have yielded mixed results. This is related to variation between studies with regard to doses, timing of treatments, and technical differences. Defining consistent thermal dosimetry and uniform clinical endpoints has also complicated results.

Interstitial thermoradiotherapy using continuous lower temperature hyperthermia and brachytherapy offers several unique aspects. With this approach, it is technically feasible to administer simultaneous heat and radiation treatment. The use of lower temperature hyperthermia broadens the therapeutic window, since lower temperatures may be clinically effective and provide a greater safety margin for normal tissue tolerance. Radiobiological evidence strongly suggests that continuous lower temperature hyperthermia, which in itself is not cytotoxic and does not potentiate high dose rate radiation, does give significant interaction when combined with concurrent low dose rate radiation. This remarkable finding needs further exploration, and this chapter will review the fundamental radiobiological concepts which underline the use of radiation and hyperthermia. In addition, recent developments in understanding interstitial hyperthermia and radiation interactions will be summarized.

E.L. JONES, M.D., Ph.D., Harvard Joint Center for Radiation Therapy, 50 Binney Street, Boston, MA 02215, USA

1.2 Radiation

The effect of radiation on cells in vitro was first investigated by PUCK and MARCUS (1956). The cell survival curves were derived from measuring the colony-forming ability of HeLa cells exposed to orthovoltage x-rays at dose rates of 100–200 cGy/min. Survival curves represent a composite of two regions: the low dose shoulder region and the high dose exponential cell kill region. Important survival curve parameters include D_0, the dose needed to reduce survival by 37% in the exponential region; n (extrapolation number), the surviving fraction derived by extrapolating back from the exponential region to zero dose; and D_q (quasithreshold dose), the dose derived by extrapolating back from the exponential region to a surviving fraction of 1.0 (HALL 1978). From the shoulder region of these curves, the concept of sublethal damage (SLD) repair was developed in the classic experiments of ELKIND and SUTTON (1960). These experiments in Chinese hamster cells showed that the cell kill from two radiation doses separated in time was less than the effect of the same dose given in a single treatment. The magnitude of the recovery for fixed radiation fractions was related to the extrapolation number and D_0 derived from the survival curve of single radiation doses. For a given D_0, cells with a larger extrapolation number showed greater recovery between fractions. Recovery between fractions was essentially complete within approximately 2.5 h. Predictions of cell survival over a fractionated course of radiation were developed from single dose survival curves based on knowledge of SLD repair which occurs between fractions (ELKIND and SUTTON 1960).

While SLD is repaired under normal circumstances unless additional damage is added (i.e., further radiation or hyperthermia), the varying of postirradiation environmental conditions to modulate survival was described by PHILLIPS and TOLMACH (1966) as potentially lethal damage (PLD). By convention, the normal radiation response occurs under optimal growth conditions and PLD is studied under conditions which vary from this norm. Experiments have shown that postirradiation inhibition of DNA synthesis decreased PLD repair, while postirradiation inhibition of protein synthesis resulted in PLD repair. Kinetic studies indicated that PLD repair was completed within the first 5 h postirradiation (PHILLIPS and TOLMACH 1966). Later experiments showed that cells irradiated in density-inhibited state and allowed to remain for 6–12 h before subculturing showed increased survival, and postirradiation incubation with balanced salts rather than full growth medium also enhanced PLD repair (HAHN et al. 1973). PLD repair takes place under hypoxic conditions, with similar kinetics and magnitude to aerobic conditions (HAHN et al. 1973). In summary, PLD repair is enhanced when postirradiation conditions are suboptimal for growth.

1.3 Hyperthermia

Hyperthermia alone has been shown to have a cytotoxic effect (RAAPHORST et al. 1979b). The amount of cell killing depends on thermal dose, which is a function of temperature and time. Data from a broad variety of biological systems (in vivo and in vitro) exhibit an exponential relationship between time and temperature for a given hyperthermia isoeffect. In most cases, a 1°C increase in temperature requires a twofold decrease in time for the same effect above 43°C. Below 43°C, a 1°C change in temperature requires a three- to fourfold change in time for the same isoeffect (SAPARETO and DEWEY 1984). Another unique aspect of hyperthermia is the development of thermotolerance, or hyperthermia resistance, as a result of prior hyperthermia exposure. Thermotolerance can be induced by a short hyperthermia treatment at a higher temperature (> 43°C) followed by an incubation period at 37°C prior to a second hyperthermia dose (LAW et al. 1987), or by continuous heating at temperatures between 41.5° and 42.5°C (HENLE and DETHLEFSEN 1978). Continuous heating at 40°C for 7 h did not change the D_0 for subsequent 45°C hyperthermia test doses, but did increase the hyperthermic D_q by a factor of 3 (HENLE and DETHLEFSEN 1978). Thermotolerance has important implications for combined hyperthermia and radiation, since thermotolerant cells often show decreased radiosensitization to therapeutic heat treatments (HOLAHAN et al. 1986; HAVEMAN et al. 1987). However, studies using murine bone marrow progenitor cells show a lack of effect of thermotolerance on the radiation response and thermal radiosensitization (MICHVECHI and LI 1987). Hyperthermic sensitivity is also modified by pH, nutrient status, and cell cycle variation.

1.4 Repair

Hyperthermia used in conjunction with radiation has been shown to inhibit radiation-induced PLD and SLD repair (LI et al. 1976; MURTHY et al. 1977; RAAPHORST et al. 1979a, 1988; RAAPHORST and FEELEY 1990). Preheating plateau phase Chinese hamster cells at 43°C for up to 45 min before radiation had no impact on the magnitude of PLD repair, but did introduce a slow component of recovery which took up to 24 h to complete. Hyperthermia after radiation decreased the magnitude and slowed the kinetics of PLD repair, and 43°C 60-min hyperthermia after radiation completely inhibited PLD repair (LI et al. 1976).

Inhibition of SLD and PLD repair is dependent on hyperthermia dose. Studies investigated the effect of hyperthermia at 42.5°C and 45.5°C on recovery from radiation damage in Chinese hamster cells (RAAPHORST et al. 1979a). Small doses of hyperthermia (42.5°C 30 min, 45.5°C 4 min) prior to radiation did not inhibit SLD recovery, while recovery was inhibited by larger hyperthermia doses. The effects of 42.5°C versus 45.5°C hyperthermia on SLD recovery were similar when hyperthermia doses resulting in equal survival levels were used. PLD repair was assayed by incubating cells at 20°C after various hyperthermia/radiation combinations before subculturing. Results showed that

42.5°C 30-min hyperthermia before or after radiation did not have any great effect on PLD repair.

The sequence of hyperthermia and radiation treatment plays a role in repair. PLD repair in Chinese hamster V79 cells and normal and transformed C3H/10T1/2 cells verified that 42.5°C 30 min hyperthermia before radiation gave no PLD repair inhibition, while the same hyperthermia dose after radiation gave slight inhibition of PLD repair. Increasing the hyperthermia dose to 42.5°C for 75 min resulted in significant PLD repair inhibition for hyperthermia before radiation, and completely inhibited PLD repair when given after radiation (RAAPHORST et al. 1988).

In summary, hyperthermia-dependent inhibition of PLD and SLD repair are a function of hyperthermia dose (treatment duration and temperature) and treatment sequence. Furthermore, studies draw distinctions between radiation PLD and hyperthermia PLD, and recovery from each modality may be important in addition to the interaction of the two modalities (RAAPHORST and FEELEY 1990). The specific cell lines used for experiments are crucial, since intrinsic differences in hyperthermia and radiation sensitivity and sequence-dependent sensitivities for combined treatment have been noted (LI and KAL 1977; RAAPHORST et al. 1979b). Large differences in thermal response were observed for seven cell lines, and no correlation was found between differences in heat sensitivity and differences in radiosensitivity (RAAPHORST et al. 1979b). In experiments comparing Chinese hamster ovary cells (HA-1) and mouse mammary sarcoma cells (EMT-6) the sequence of heat and radiation yielding maximum thermal radiosensitization was opposite for the two cell lines when treated under identical conditions (LI and KAL 1977).

1.5 Oxygen Effect

Cells irradiated under hypoxic conditions are known to be radioresistant (KALLMAN 1972). Oxygen is a free radical scavenger which acts as a dose-modifying agent and must be present at the time of irradiation. The oxygen effect is expressed as the oxygen enhancement ratio (OER), the ratio of radiation dose with hypoxia to radiation dose with oxygen for the same biological effect. For sparsely ionizing radiation, the OER is typically 2.5–3. Some experiments using aerobic and hypoxic cells show a slight increase in heat sensitivity for hypoxic cells (GERWECK et al. 1974). However, this was likely related to concomitant changes in medium pH during the hypoxic episode. Later studies indicated that hypoxic cells buffered at pH 7.3–7.4 showed no change in heat sensitivity during hypoxia (GERWECK et al. 1981). For combined hyperthermia and radiation, some experiments have shown that hyperthermia causes a reduction in OER (ROBINSON et al. 1974; KIM et al. 1975), while other studies indicate that the OER is slightly increased or unchanged by hyperthermia (POWER and HARRIS 1977; BADANIDIYOR and HOPWOOD 1985).

The radioresistance of hypoxic cells has been postulated to be involved in local control failure, and cells greater than 150 µm from a capillary are prone to anoxic microenvironments (THOMLINSON and GRAY 1955). In addition to low oxygen tension, hypoxic microenvironments have concomitant poor nutrient supply and lowered pH secondary to increased anaerobic metabolism. Both pH and nutrient supply are important factors in potentiating the cytotoxic action of hyperthermia. Decreasing pH potentiates hyperthermia-induced cytotoxicity and hyperthermia-induced radiosensitivity (FREEMAN et al. 1981a, b; HOLAHAN et al. 1984). Poor nutrient supply also potentiates hyperthermia-induced cytotoxicity (GERWECK et al. 1984). While thermal radiosensitization increased at pH 6.8 compared to pH 7.2, glucose deprivation did not modify hyperthermic radiosensitization for cells in an acidic environment (FREEMAN and MALCOM 1985).

The role of radiation dose rate in OER is particularly important for interstitial radiotherapy (LING et al. 1985). One study measuring OER over a range of doses (276 Gy/h to 0.89 Gy/h) indicated that as dose rate decreased, OER initially increased to 3.7–4.0 for cells in full medium at dose rates between 20 and 60 Gy/h. As dose rate decreased further, OER decreased to 2.4 at the lowest dose rate. Interestingly, hypoxic cells under nutrient-deprived conditions showed complete lack of dose rate effect, and under these conditions OER decreased monotonically from 3.0 to 1.7 over the range of 276 to 0.89 Gy/h (LING et al. 1985). These results are shown in Fig. 1.1. This suggests that anoxic, nutrient-deprived cells have a diminished potential for SLD repair and implies that low dose rate irradiation may be advantageous if hypoxic cells are an important factor in tumor control.

In conclusion, some hypoxic cells appear to have a slightly increased hyperthermic sensitivity. However, the main advantage for using hyperthermia

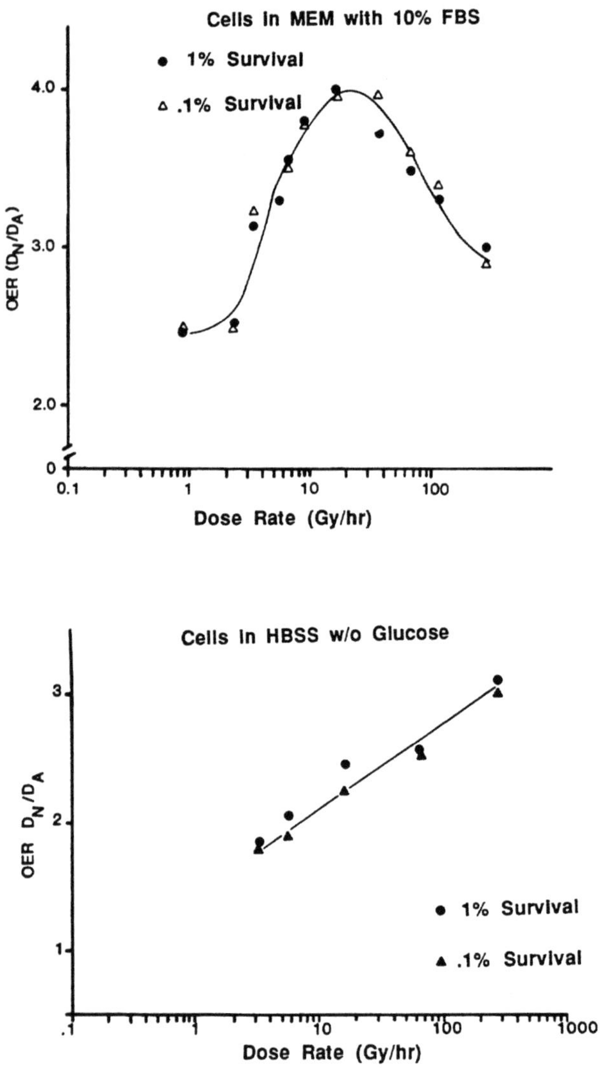

Fig. 1.1. Oxygen enhancement ratio (OER) as a function of dose rate. OER is taken as the ratio of doses needed in nitrogen and in air, respectively, to yield the same cellular survival. Upper panel: OER for V79 cells in MEM medium with 10% fetal bovine serum (FBS). Lower panel: OER for V79 cell in HBSS without glucose (nutrient deprived conditions). Both experiments performed at room temperature (23°C). LING et al., Int J Radiat Oncol Biol Phys 11: 1367–1373, 1985. Reproduced with permission of the publisher

with radiation in the treatment of hypoxic cells lies in the complementary nature of the two modalities. Radiation is most effective against well-oxygenated cells, while hyperthermia is most effective against hypoxic cells with concurrent localized acidity and poor nutrient supply. Moreover, hypoxic tumors with poor blood flow may show preferential heating due to reduced convection. The reduction of OER at low dose rates and increased hyperthermic sensitivity and radiosensitization of acidic, nutritionally depleted cells further magnifies the potential importance of interstitial thermoradiotherapy in the treatment of tumors with large hypoxic cell fractions.

1.6 Cell Cycle Effect

The sensitivity of cells to radiation varies during the cell cycle. Using HeLa cells exposed to 3 Gy at various times after mitotic harvest, peaks and troughs in the pattern of radiosensitivity were seen to correspond to phases in the cell cycle (TERASIMA and TOLMACH 1963). Further studies using a variety of cell lines confirmed these results (SINCLAIR and MORTON 1966; SINCLAIR 1968). Overall, cells are most radiosensitive during mitosis, and least sensitive during late S phase. G_1 has variable sensitivity depending on its duration. For mammalian cells S, G_2, and M phases have a relatively constant duration, and variation in G_1 dominates the overall cell cycle time. HeLa cells with a long G_1 exhibit a resistant phase during G_1, followed by decreasing survival as the cells approach S phase. Chinese hamster cells with a short G_1 do not show this variation in G_1 sensitivity, and have monotonically increasing radioresistance as cells progress from G_1 to S phase. G_2 tends to be a relatively sensitive phase (SINCLAIR and MORTON 1966). The increased radiosensitivity of mitotic and G_2 phase cells is reflected in almost complete absence of any shoulder in the survival curves. The OER, as described in the previous section, does not appear to vary during the cell cycle (HALL et al. 1968).

Radiation also causes division delay which is maximal for cells irradiated during S phase. This division delay is related to prolongation of S phase (only for cells irradiated during S phase) and causes a G_2 block for cells irradiated during all stages of the cell cycle. Maximal division delay induced by irradiation during S phase is on the order of 1–2 min/cGy and varies somewhat among cell lines (SINCLAIR 1968).

The sensitivity of cells to hyperthermia also varies during the cell cycle (WESTRA and DEWEY 1971; BHUYAN et al. 1977; RAAPHORST et al. 1985). For Chinese hamster cells heated at 45.5°C for various time intervals, maximal hyperthermia sensitivity was seen for S phase and mitotic cells. Cells were maximally heat resistant during late G_1 (WESTRA and DEWEY 1971). Later studies confirmed that Chinese hamster cells are most sensitive to hyperthermia during S phase when they are concomitantly least radiation sensitive (RAAPHORST et al. 1985). Analogous to radiation response, increased hyperthermic sensitivity of mitotic and S phase cells was associated with a decrease in the shoulder of the survival curves.

Hyperthermia also induced division delay which is proportional to thermal dose. For Chinese hamster cells, 45.5°C 6-min hyperthermia induced 11 h division delay, while 45.5°C 10 min hyperthermia induced 35 h division delay (WESTRA and DEWEY 1971). When studying the effect of hyperthermia at various stages of the cell cycle, tetraploidy was induced in 90% of cells heated during mitosis, indicating incomplete cytokinesis. Tetraploidy was not necessarily a lethal event, and 43% of cells sampled at 170 h following hyperthermia were tetraploid (WESTRA and DEWEY 1971).

Combined hyperthermia and radiation offers the advantage of complementary sensitivities in various phases of the cell cycle. In general, cells are most radiosensitive during mitosis and G_1, and most radioresistant during S phase. Conversely, cells are most heat sensitive during S phase and least heat sensitive during late G_1. Experiments using Chinese hamster cells treated with combined hyperthermia and radiation show enhanced cytotoxicity and decreased fluctuation in sensitivity over the cell cycle (RAAPHORST et al. 1985). Other groups have found greatest thermal radiosensitization in mid G_1 and S phase for rat 9L gliosarcoma cells as shown in Fig. 1.2 (HENDERSON et al. 1982). A similar result was demonstrated in HeLa cells, with maximal sensitivity to combined treatment in late S phase, and maximal resistance to combined treatment in early G_1, when cells are both heat and radiation resistant (KIM et al. 1976). In general, the fluctuation in response over the cell cycle to combined heat and radiation treatment tends to follow the pattern of heat sensitivity for most cell lines. Sensitivity varies two- to fourfold over the cell cycle for radiation or hyperthermia. These variations are of the same order of magnitude as the OER and have important consequences for combined hyperthermia and radiation.

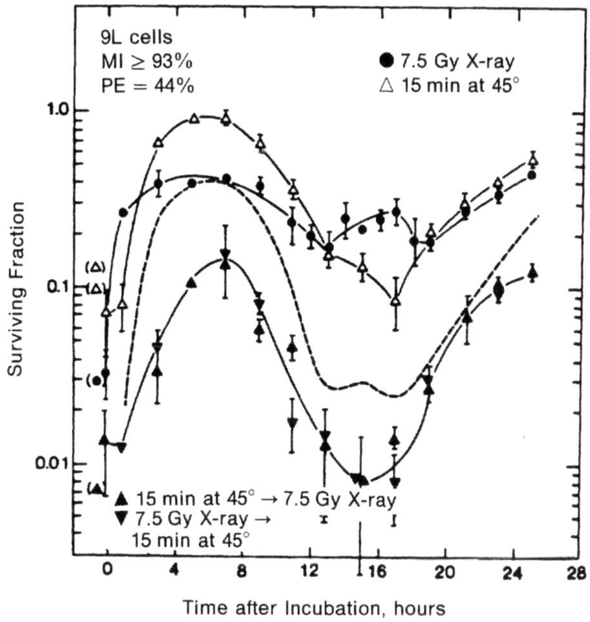

Fig. 1.2. Cell cycle variation of 9L cells selected in mitosis (≥ 93%) and treated with hyperthermia and/or radiation as a function of time after incubation. Cells are in S phase from 13–17 h after incubation. The dashed line represents the expected survival calculated as the product of the surviving fractions following single-agent treatment. HENDERSON et al., Radiat Res 92: 146–159, 1982. Reproduced with permission of the publisher

1.7 Dose Rate Effect

The dose rate effect is an important aspect of interstitial radiotherapy. As the dose rate decreases, the amount of cell kill is reduced, particularly for dose rates in the range of 1–100 cGy/min (HALL 1972). The reduction in cell killing is related to repair of sublethal damage during the protracted irradiation. This SLD repair changes the shape of the dose-response curve. While acute exposures give the classical shoulder and exponential region survival curves, as the dose rate is decreased the slope of the survival curves becomes more shallow and the extrapolation number approaches unity. Building on the concept of radiation fractionation (ELKIND and SUTTON 1960), continuous low dose rate irradiation can be modeled as multiple small fractions of acute radiation, with the net summation approximating a continuous irradiation (LAJTHA and OLIVER 1961).

Several studies examining low dose rate radiation and hyperthermia are outlined in Table 1.1. Important generalizations can be noted from these experiments. Protracted heating at lower temperatures results in minimal hyperthermia-induced cell kill or potentiation of high dose rate radiation, but it does provide significant radiosensitization of low dose rate radiation. Continuous low temperature hyperthermia abolishes the dose rate effect (HARISIADIS et al. 1978; ARMOUR et al. 1991; SPIRO et al. 1991). Simultaneous heat and low dose rate radiation usually resulted in maximal radiosensitization, although one study showed greatest radiosensitization for hyperthermia before radiation

(HARISIADIS et al. 1978). Another study showed no difference between heat before and heat during radiation (LING and ROBINSON 1988). Thermotolerance develops during continuous hyperthermia at lower temperatures. Thermotolerant cells have shown reduced hyperthermic radiosensitization in higher temperature, acute dose rate experiments (HOLAHAN et al. 1986; HAVERMAN et al. 1987). Despite thermotolerance, substantial radiosensitization does occur for cells treated with continuous low temperature hyperthermia and concomitant interstitial radiation.

Studies using in vivo models also demonstrate thermal enhancement of low dose rate radiation (BAKER et al. 1987; JONES et al. 1989; JONES and DOUPLE 1990a, b; MILLER et al. 1978; MOORTHY et al. 1984; SAPOZINK et al. 1983). Shifting from in vitro to in vivo experiments adds several layers of complexity, including variable intra- and intertumor blood flow with concomitant changes in

Table 1.1. Dose rate effect and hyperthermia

Authors	Radiation dose rates	Hyperthermia	Cell line	Results
BEN HUR et al. (1974)	360 cGy/min 12 cGy/min 3.3 cGy/min	Temperature: 39°, 40°, 41°, 42°C Duration: maximal irradiation interval at each dose Sequence: simultaneous heat and radiation	Chinese hamster V79	Thermal enhancement ratio (TER) calculated as ratio of D_0 at 37°C to D_0 at elevated temperature. Thermal enhancement increases with increasing temperature and varies inversely with dose rate. Cell cycle fluctuation in radiosensitivity of synchronized cells reduced by hyperthermia.
HARISIADIS et al. (1978)	93.95 cGy/min 3.33 cGy/min	Temperature: 41°C Duration: 6 h Sequence: heat before, during, and after radiation	Chinese hamster V79	TER calculated as ratio of radiation dose without/with heat required for same surviving fraction (SF). TER greater for low dose rate (LDR) when calculated at low (0.05) SF. TER greater for acute dose rate when calculated at high (0.5) SF. Hyperthermia before low dose rate radiation gave maximal TER. Dose rate effect abolished for simultaneous heat and low dose rate RT.
GERNER et al. (1983)	300 cGy/min 50 cGy/min 6.25 cGy/min 0.567 cGy/min	Temperature: 43°C Duration: 30 min Sequence: heat before radiation	Rat astrocytoma RT-9	TER calculated as ratio of radiation doses required for 0.1 SF. TER at 0.1 SF maximal for 300 cGy/min and 0.567 cGy/min. When TER formulated as ratio of D_0, TER maximal at lowest dose rate.
LING and ROBINSON (1988)	477 cGy/min 11.8 cGy/min	Temperature: 40°C Duration: 4 h Sequence: before, during, and after radiation	Chinese hamster V79	TER calculated as ratio of radiation doses required for 0.001 SF. No effect of sequence on acute dose rate irradiation. No difference for heat before or during low dose rate irradiation. Heat after low dose rate irradiation less effective than before or during.

Table 1.1. Contd.

Authors	Radiation dose rates	Hyperthermia	Cell line	Results
Armour et al. (1991)	110 cGy/min 0.83 cGy/min (given as 50-cGy fractions every 2 h)	41°C for 24 h or 43°C for 30 or 60 min before and/or after irradiation at 37°C or 41°C	Rat 9L gliosarcoma	TER calculated as ratio of radiation doses required for 0.01 SF and as ratio of D_0 at 37°C to D_0 with heat. Preheating cells at 41°C for 24 h did not affect slope of acute dose rate radiation curve, but did reduce shoulder. Dose rate effect abolished for simultaneous heat and low dose rate RT. Thermotolerance to continuous 41°C heating developed after 12 h. Magnitude of thermotolerance was comparable to thermotolerance with 43°C 30-min heat assayed 24 h after heat treatment.
Spiro et al. (1991)	1.43 cGy/min 500 cGy/min	Temperature: 39° or 40°C Duration: heat during radiation Sequence: simultaneous heat and radiation	Chinese hamster V79	Cells were not sensitized to high dose rate radiation for heating intervals up to 48 h at 40°C. For simultaneous heat and low dose rate irradiation, at 40°C the dose rate effect was abolished up to total doses of 15 Gy. Flow cytometry indicated no change in doubling time for low dose rate radiation at 37°C or 39°C. A decreased doubling time was seen after 18 h for low dose rate radiation and 40°C heat, and cell cycle distribution showed peaks in $G_2 + M$ phase fraction at 6 and 18 h.

oxygenation, pH, and nutrient supply, and tumor bed effects. Nonetheless, these studies all demonstrated significant interaction between hyperthermia and low dose rate radiation. Comparison of various treatment sequences in a murine tumor model indicated that maximal hyperthermic radiosensitization occurred for heat treatments given in the middle of brachytherapy treatment (Jones et al. 1989). All studies implicated inhibition of sublethal repair as a likely mechanism of action.

The question remains as to why concurrent low temperature hyperthermia and low dose rate radiation works. Clearly, the inhibition of SLD repair as reflected by reduction of the dose rate effect must play an important role. Flow cytometry studies indicate that cells build up at G_2 and M phases, likely caused by radiation-induced G_2 delay. During G_2 and M phases, cells are more radiosensitive, and cell cycle redistribution during protracted treatment may contribute to the overall response. The contribution of hyperthermia-induced division delay for cells treated with continuous low temperature hyperthermia remains unclear. In addition, cells are exposed to two continuous stresses, as compared to intermittent stresses with fractionated radiation and hyperthermia. This has implications for SLD and PLD repair and damage fixation during protracted treatment. Finally, hyperthermia treatments given within a low temperature range (39°–41°C) rather than a cytotoxic range of temperature (> 42°C) may have different mechanisms of interaction with radiation damage.

1.8 Summary

The effects of repair, oxygen status, cell cycle, and dose rate all play key roles in the response to combined heat and radiation. Several excellent reviews summarize the mechanisms involved (Roti Roti and Laszlo 1988; Dewey 1989). However, much less information is available concerning mechanisms of interaction of low dose rate radiation and hyperthermia as used for interstitial thermoradiotherapy. One universal theme found in all hyperthermia and low dose rate radiation studies is the inhibition of repair. Sublethal damage repair during protracted radiation dominates the overall dose rate response. Therefore, hyperthermic inhibition of SLD repair has a larger impact for low dose rate radiation since repair is a larger component of the response. Hyperthermia-induced inhibition of repair likely involves several processes. Hyperthermia modifies several enzymes responsible for radiation damage repair, particularly DNA polymerase β (Dikomey and Jung 1988). Hyperthermia may modify some of the x-ray-induced DNA lesions and convert them from repairable to non-repairable (Dewey et al. 1978). Hyperthermia alters cytosol, membrane, and microtubule function, which in turn could indirectly modify DNA repair.

Hyperthermia and radiation have complementary sensitivities for oxic and hypoxic cells. Oxic cells are most radiosensitive. Hypoxic cells are also nutrient deprived and subject to acidic microenvironments, both important factors in enhanced hyperthermic sensitivity. The OER decreases with decreasing dose rate, lending an advantage to interstitial thermoradiotherapy in treating cells with significant hypoxia. In addition, the dose rate effect is reduced for hypoxic nutrient-deprived cells, suggesting a diminished SLD repair capacity. Cells have complementary hyperthermia and radiation sensitivities at different phases of the cell cycle. Cells are most radiosensitive during mitosis and G_2, and are least radiosensitive during S phase. Cells are most heat sensitive during S phase, and least heat sensitive during late G_1. Interestingly, the shoulder portion of the survival curve is essentially absent in the phases of maximal heat or radiation sensitivity.

The development of thermotolerance during protracted hyperthermia treatments may serve to reduce the cumulative effect on cell survival. However, substantial thermoradiosensitization has been demonstrated for simultaneous hyperthermia and low dose rate irradiation at temperatures as low as 39°C–41°C. At these low hyperthermia temperatures, the development of thermotolerance may contribute less to the overall response. Thermotolerance induced by 40°C 7-h hyperthermia did not alter the D_0 of hyperthermic radiosensitization, but did tend to increase the shoulder of the survival curve (Henle and Dethlefsen 1978). In addition, the experiments of Harisidias et al. (1978) demonstrated that 41°C 6-h hyperthermia gave greatest thermal enhancement when given before low dose rate radiation as compared to simultaneous hyperthermia and radiation or hyperthermia after radiation. If thermotolerance reduced thermal radiosensitization, then hyperthermia before low dose rate irradiation would not be expected to yield the greatest thermal enhancement.

The simultaneous delivery of hyperthermia and radiation may be an important advantage of interstitial thermoradiotherapy. While the optimal sequence of heat and radiation varies among cell lines, the simultaneous application of heat and radiation consistently results in maximal thermoradiosensitization for acute radiation exposures (Dewey et al. 1977; Haveman and Wondergem 1988; Overgaard 1989). As noted above, thermal radiosensitization was maximal for the application of heat before low dose rate radiation, while another study showed no difference between heat before and heat during radiation.

Recent results offer promising indications that hyperthermia in the range of 39°C–41°C combined with simultaneous low dose rate irradiation results in enhanced cell killing (Ling and Robinson 1988; Spiro et al. 1991; Armour et al. 1991). Clinical techniques for interstitial thermoradiotherapy at temperatures between 39°C and 41°C are feasible given constraints in heating deep-seated tumors and practical limitations in patient tolerance. While much effort has focused on the interactions of acute dose rate radiation and hyperthermia, these encouraging results warrant further studies using low dose rate radiation and hyperthermia.

Acknowledgment. The author would like to thank Dr. Jack Hoopes, Dr. Evan Douple, and Dr. Julia O'Hara for their helpful recommendations.

References

Armour EP, Wang Z, Corry PM, Martinez A (1991) Sensitization of rat 9L gliosarcoma cells to low dose rate irradiation by long duration 41°C hyperthermia. Cancer Res 51: 3088–3095

Badanidiyor SR, Hopwood LE (1985) Effect of hypoxia on recovery from damage induced by heat and radiation in plateau-phase CHO cells. Radiat Res 101: 312–325
Baker DG, Sager HT, Constable WC (1987) The response of a solid tumor to x-irradiation as modified by dose rate, fractionation, and hyperthermia. Cancer Invest 5: 409–416
Ben-Hur E, Elkind MM, Bronk BV (1974) Thermally enhanced radioresponse of cultured Chinese hamster cells: inhibition of repair of sublethal damage and enhancement of lethal damage. Radiat Res 58: 38–51
Bhuyan BK, Day KJ, Edgerton CE, Ogunbase O (1977) Sensitivity of different cell lines and of different phases in the cell cycle to hyperthermia. Cancer Res 37: 3780–3784
Dewey WC (1989) Mechanism of thermal radiosensitization. In: Urano M, Douple E (eds) Hyperthermia and oncology, vol II. VSP BV, Netherlands, pp 1–16
Dewey WC, Hopwood LE, Sapareto SA, Gerweck LE (1977) Cellular responses to combinations of hyperthermia and radiation. Radiology 123: 463–474
Dewey WC, Sapareto SA, Betten DA (1978) Hyperthermic radiosensitization of synchronous Chinese hamster ovary cells: relationship between cell lethality and chromosomal aberrations. Radiat Res 76: 48–59
Dikomey E, Jung H (1988) Correlation between polymerase β activity and thermal radiosensitization in Chinese hamster cells. Recent Results Cancer Res 109: 35–41
Elkind MM, Sutton H (1960) Radiation response of mammalian cells grown in culture. I. Repair of x-ray damage in surviving Chinese hamster cells. Radiat Res 13: 556–593
Freeman ML, Malcom A (1985) Acid modification of thermal damage and its relationship to nutrient availability. Int J Radiat Oncol Biol Phys 11: 1823–1826
Freeman ML, Boone ML, Enseley BA, Gillette EL (1981a) The influence of environmental pH on the interaction and repair of heat and radiation damage. Int J Radiat Oncol Biol Phys 7: 761–764
Freeman ML, Holahan EV, Highfield DP, Raaphorst GP, Spiro IJ, Dewey WC (1981b) The effect of pH on hyperthermia and x-ray induced cell killing. Int J Radiat Oncol Biol Phys 7: 211–216
Gerner EW, Oval JH, Manning MR, Sim DA, Bowden GT, Hevezi JM (1983) Dose-rate dependence of heat radiosensitization. Int J Radiat Oncol Biol Phys 9: 1401–1404
Gerweck LE, Gillette EI, Dewey WC (1974) Killing of Chinese hamster cells in vitro by heating under hypoxic and aerobic conditions. Eur J Cancer 10: 691–693
Gerweck LE, Richards B, Jennings M (1981) The influence of variable oxygen concentration on the response of cells to heat and/or x-irradiation. Radiat Res 85: 314–320
Gerweck LE, Dahlberg WK, Epstein LF, Shimm DS (1984) Influence of nutrient and energy deprivation on cellular response to single and fractionated heat treatments. Radiat Res 99: 573–581
Hahn GM, Bagshaw MA, Evans RG, Gordon LF (1973) Repair of potentially lethal lesions in x-irradiated, density-inhibited Chinese hamster cells: metabolic effects and hypoxia. Radiat Res 55: 280–290
Hall EJ (1972) Radiation dose rate: a factor of importance in radiobiology and radiotherapy. Br J Radiol 45: 81–97
Hall EJ (1978) Radiobiology for the radiologist, 2nd edn. Harper and Row, New York, pp 31–38
Hall EJ, Brown JM, Cavanaugh J (1968) Radiosensitivity and the oxygen effect measured at different phases of the mitotic cycle using synchronously dividing cells of the root meristem of *Vicia faba*. Radiat Res 35: 622–634
Harisiadis L, Sung DI, Kessaris N, Hall EJ (1978) Hyperthermia and low dose-rate irradiation. Radiology 129: 195–198
Haveman J, Wondergem J (1988) Thermal enhancement of cell killing effect of x-irradiation in mammalian cells in vitro and in a transplantable mouse tumor: influence of pH, thermotolerance, hypoxia, or misonidazole. Recent Results Cancer Res 109: 149–160
Haveman J, Hart AA, Wondergem J (1987) Thermal radiosensitization and thermotolerance in cultured cells from a murine mammary carcinoma. Int J Radiat Biol 51: 71–80
Henderson SD, Kimler BF, Scanlan MF (1982) Interaction of hyperthermia and radiation on the survival of synchronous 9L cells. Radiat Res 92: 146–159
Henle KJ, Dethlefsen LA (1978) Heat fractionation and thermotolerance: a review. Cancer Res 38: 1843–1851
Holahan EV, Highfield DP, Holahan PK, Dewey WC (1984) Hyperthermic killing and hyperthermic radiosensitization in Chinese hamster ovary cells: effect of pH and thermal tolerance. Radiat Res 97: 108–131
Holahan PK, Wong RSL, Thompson LL, Dewey WC (1986) Hyperthermic radiosensitization of thermotolerant Chinese hamster ovary cells. Radiat Res 107: 332–343
Jones EL, Douple EB (1990a) The effect of in vivo GSH depletion on thermosensitivity, radiosensitivity, and thermal radiosensitization. Int J Hyperthermia 6: 951–955
Jones EL, Douple EB (1990b) Effect of step down heating on brachytherapy in a murine tumor system. Radiat Res 124: 141–146
Jones EL, Douple EB, Lyons BE (1989) Thermal enhancement of low dose rate irradiation in a murine tumor system. Int J Hyperthermia 5: 509–523
Kallman RJ (1972) The phenomenon of reoxygenation and its complications for fractionated radiotherapy. Radiology 105: 135–142
Kim SH, Kim JH, Hahn EW (1975) The radiosensitization of hypoxic tumor cells by hyperthermia. Radiology 114: 727–728
Kim SH, Kim JH, Hahn EW (1976) The enhanced killing of irradiated HeLa cells in synchronous culture by hyperthermia. Radiat Res 66: 337–345
Lajtha LG, Oliver R (1961) Some radiobiological considerations in radiotherapy. Br J Radiol 34: 252–257
Law MP, Ahier RG, Somaia S (1987) Thermotolerance induced by fractionated hyperthermia: dependence of the interval between fractions. Int J Hyperthermia 3: 433–439
Li GC, Kal HB (1977) Effect of hyperthermia on radiation response of two mammalian cell lines. Eur J Cancer 13: 65–69
Li GC, Evans RG, Hahn GM (1976) Modification and inhibition of repair of potentially lethal x-ray damage by hyperthermia. Radiat Res 67: 491–501
Ling CC, Robinson E (1988) Moderate hyperthermia and low dose rate irradiation. Radiat Res 11: 379–384
Ling CC, Spiro IJ, Mitchell J, Stickler R (1985) The variation in OER with dose rate. Int J Radiat Oncol Biol Phys 11: 1367–1373
Miller RC, Leith JT, Veomett RC, Gerner EW (1978) Effects of interstitial irradiation alone, or in combination with localized hyperthermia in the response of a mouse mammary tumor. J Radiat Res 19: 175–180
Mivechi NF, Li GC (1987) Lack of effect of thermotolerance on radiation response and thermal radiosensitization of murine bone marrow progenitors. Cancer Res 47: 1538–1541
Moorthy CR, Hahn EW, Kim JH, Feingold SM, Alfieri AA, Hilaris BS (1984) Improved response of a murine fibrosarcoma (METH-A) to interstitial radiation when combined

with hyperthermia. Int J Radiat Oncol Biol Phys 10: 2145–2148
Murthy AK, Harris JR, Belli JA (1977) Hyperthermia and radiation response of plateau phase cells. Radiat Res 70: 241–247
Overgaard J (1989) The current and potential role of hyperthermia in radiotherapy. Int J Radiat Oncol Biol Phys 16: 535–549
Phillips RA, Tolmach LJ (1966) Repair of potentially lethal damage in x-irradiated HeLa cells. Radiat Res 29: 413–432
Power JA, Harris JW (1977) Response of extremely hypoxic cells to hyperthermia: survival and oxygen enhancement ratios. Radiology 123: 767–770
Puck TT, Marcus PI (1956) Action of x-rays on mammalian cells. J Exp Med 103: 653–666
Raaphorst GP, Feeley MM (1990) Comparison of recovery from potentially lethal damage after exposure to hyperthermia and radiation. Radiat Res 121: 107–110
Raaphorst GP, Freeman ML, Dewey WC (1979a) Radiosensitivity and recovery from radiation damage in cultured CHO cells exposed to hyperthermia at 42.5°C or 45.5°C. Radiat Res 79: 390–402
Raaphorst GP, Romano SL, Mitchell JB, Bedford JS, Dewey WC (1979b) Intrinsic differences in heat and/or x-ray sensitivity of seven mammalian cell lines cultured and treated under identical conditions. Cancer Res 39: 396–401
Raaphorst GP, Broski AP, Azzam EI (1985) Sensitivity to heat, radiation and heat plus radiation of Chinese hamster cells synchronized by mitotic selection, thymidine block, or hydroxyurea. J Thermal Biol 10: 177–181
Raaphorst GP, Azzam EI, Feeley MM (1988) Potentially lethal radiation damage repair and its inhibition by hyperthermia in normal hamster cells, mouse cells, and transformed mouse cells. Radiat Res 113: 171–182
Robinson JE, Wizenberg MJ, McCready WA (1974) Combined hyperthermia and radiation suggest an alternative to heavy particle therapy for reduced oxygen enhancement ratios. Nature 251: 421–422
Roti Roti JL, Laszlo A (1988) The effects of hyperthermia on cellular macromolecules. In: Urano M, Douple E (eds) Hyperthermia and oncology, vol I. VSP BV, Netherlands, pp 13–56
Sapareto SA, Dewey WC (1984) Thermal dose determination in cancer therapy. Int J Radiat Oncol Biol Phys 10: 787–800
Sapozink MD, Palos B, Goffinet DR, Hahn GM (1983) Combined continuous ultra low dose rate irradiation and radiofrequency hyperthermia in the C3H mouse. Int J Radiat Oncol Biol Phys 9: 1357–1365
Sinclair WK (1968) Cyclic x-ray responses in mammalian cells in vitro. Radiat Res 33: 620–643
Sinclair WK, Morton RA (1966) X-ray sensitivity during the cell generation cycle of cultured Chinese hamster cells. Radiat Res 29: 450–474
Spiro IJ, McPherson S, Cook JA, Ling CC, DeGraff W, Mitchell JB (1991) Sensitization of low dose rate irradiation by nonlethal hyperthermia. Radiat Res 127: 111–114
Terasima R, Tolmach LJ (1963) X-ray sensitivity and DNA synthesis in synchronous populations of HeLa cells. Science 140: 490–492
Thomlinson RH, Gray LH (1955) The histological structure of some human lung cancers and the possible implications for radiotherapy. Br J Cancer 9: 539–549
Westra A, Dewey WC (1971) Variation in sensitivity to heat shock during the cell-cycle of Chinese hamster cells in vitro. Int J Radiat Biol 19: 467–477

2 In Vivo Experiments Using Interstitial Radiation and Hyperthermia

P. PESCHKE, E.W. HAHN, and G. WOLBER

CONTENTS

2.1 Introduction

Various strategies are employed to improve the efficiency of radiation and thereby increase its effect within tumors without transgressing the limits of normal tissue tolerance. The use of interstitial radiotherapy (IR) represents such a strategy. IR not only provides the physical advantage of a tailored dose distribution to the tumor volume but also has significant underlying radiobiological advantages.

Low dose rate continuous radiation in the range of 40 cGy/h for removable iridium-192 or cesium-137 implants and down to the range of 8–10 cGy/h with permanent iodine-125 implants to the periphery of the tumor, appears to be more effective than conventional teleradiation therapy because of:

1. reduction in the oxygen enhancement ratio (OER) for low dose irradiation, which has been attributed to the lack of repair of sublethal damage in hypoxic cells (HALL et al. 1966; HILL and BUSH 1973; SPIRO et al. 1985).
2. better tumor reoxygenation and cell reassortment during radiation to more sensitive cells, leading to a reduced net repair of damage in the tumor cells with a greater net repair and recovery potential in normal tissues (HILL and BUSH 1973; FU et al. 1975; KAL 1979; HALL and LAM 1978).

Lowering the dose rate while keeping the overall dose constant leads to increasing cell survival owing to ongoing repair of sublethal damage during protracted irradiation (MITCHELL et al. 1979). This dose effect could be clearly demonstrated with cells in vitro. The variance found with the different cell lines studied was attributed to the varying repair capacities.

Cells which are exposed to low dose rate irradiation accumulate in G_2 (BEDFORD and MITCHELL 1973) due to a block in the cell cycle. The accumulation in G_2 could be demonstrated in exponentially growing HeLa cells between 0.20 and 0.70 Gy/h. With a further reduction of dose rate the amount of radiation-induced cell mortality is compensated by proliferation. G_2 blocks following acute doses of x-rays in rodent tumors have also been observed in normal tissues (QUASTLER et al. 1959) and experimental tumors (KAL and BARENDSEN 1972; MCNALLY and WILSON 1986). Although the underlying mechanisms are not quite clear, one should keep in mind the fact that cells in G_2 are in general sensitive to radiation.

Preliminary results, obtained with the human cervical carcinoma ME-180 xenografted to nude athymic mice, demonstrated that 20 Gy of low dose rate irradiation (cesium-137 afterloading technique) induced an important redistribution of cells in the cell cycle. The G_2 block was evidenced in that the proportion of cells in the G_2 phase increased from 14.4% to 44.2% at 140 h after irradiation (RUTGERS 1988).

2.2 Low Dose Rate Irradiation and Hyperthermia

While we have presented evidence that ionizing radiation delivered at a low dose rate can increase the biological effectiveness of a given dose by reducing OER and the overall repair capacity, there is also evidence showing that low dose rate radiation may actually allow repair of sublethal damage in some cell lines and permit repopulation

P. PESCHKE, Ph.D.; E.W. HAHN, Ph.D.; G. WOLBER Ph.D.; Forschungsschwerpunkt Radiologische Diagnostik und Therapie, Deutsches Krebsforschungszentrum, Im Neuenheimer Feld 280 690009 Heidelberg, Germany to take place during the protracted treatment time (Fu et al. 1975). Therefore, the use of an adjunct therapy which inhibits or greatly reduces the cells' capacity to repair radiation damage might improve the effectiveness of interstitial low dose irradiation (Szechter et al. 1980; Moorthy et al. 1984). Hyperthermia as an adjuvant with conventional low LET radiation would be such a strategy.

Work done with animal tumors and cells in culture has provided the biological rationale for using heat and conventional teleradiation in clinical practice. For instance, cells in late S phase, usually the most radioresistant, are the most heat sensitive (Dewey et al. 1971) and become radiosensitive when treated with heat (Kim et al. 1976). There is no doubt that the fact that heat decreases the capacity of cells to repair radiation induced sublethal and potentially lethal damage contributes to this sensitizing effect (Ben-Hur et al. 1974; Rao and Hopwood 1985). When one also considers the unique microenvironment of the tumor with its poor and sluggish vasculature (Reinhold and Endrich 1986; Vaupel and Kallinowski 1987) in which the tumor cells are subjected to further heat-sensitizing factors such as chronic deficiencies of oxygen (Kim et al. 1975a, b) and nutritional substrata (Hahn 1974; Kim et al. 1980, 1982) under conditions of low pH (Gerweck and Richards 1981), a compelling rationale is provided for the use of heat and radiation in the treatment of cancer (Streffer and van Beuningen 1987).

In addition, there is an increasing understanding of the underlying molecular changes that lead to the cellular effects of hyperthermia. Heat as an entropic disordering agent is expected to disrupt highly ordered structures and processes in cells (Hahn 1982; Laszlo 1992). There is evidence that heat induces protein denaturation in membranes as well as in the tertiary structure of proteins within multimolecular complexes involved in energy metabolism (e.g., mitochondrial electron transport chain) and in transcription/translation (Lepock 1982; Bowler 1981; Didomenico et al. 1982). Additionally, the intermediate filament network, a part of the cytoplasmic matrix, is disrupted by heat (Welch et al. 1985).

In view of this, we have continued our earlier investigations (Moorthy et al. 1984; Nag et al. 1981; Alfieri et al. 1982) in order to achieve a better understanding of the interaction of interstitial radiation with localized hyperthermia. The basic aim of these studies is to clarify the underlying mechanisms involved and to determine the most effective means by which to apply the combined treatments.

2.3 In Vivo Experiments Using Interstitial Radiation and Hyperthermia

There is sufficient evidence from experiments with cells in vitro (Ben-Hur et al. 1974; Harisiadis et al. 1978; Szechter et al. 1980; Gerner et al. 1983) to suggest that interstitial low dose rate radiation combined with hyperthermia is a reasonably effective means of treating malignant tissues.

There are surprisingly few in vivo animal experiments with low dose rate radiation applied either by shielded protracted whole-body techniques with cesium-137 or cobalt-60, or by radioactive radium needles or iridium-192 seeds and iodine-125 seeds implanted into the tumor. In the present review we limit the expression "low dose rate interstitial radiotherapy" to that applied to the tumor tissue via radioactive sources inserted in the tissue as opposed to "external low dose rate brachytherapy", where the radioactive sources are placed near the tissue.

Miller et al. (1978) used interstitial irradiation from radium-226 and localized hyperthermia, either alone or in combination, on a transplantable mammary sarcoma (EMT-6) in the mouse. Localized hyperthermia combined with IR led to a greater than 60% reduction in tumor volume after 4 days of continuous treatment, compared to only a 20% reduction in tumor volume when either agent was given alone.

Concomitant localized tumor hyperthermia and interstitial implants of high intensity iridium-192 or iodine-125 were evaluated on the murine methylcholanthrene-induced fibrosarcoma and the spontaneous mammary adenocarcinoma (Alfieri et al. 1982). Dependent upon the biological systems and endpoints evaluated, the thermal enhancement ratio (TER), defined as the ratio of the doses producing the same effect at the physiological normal temperature and at the hyperthermic treatment temperature, ranged from 1.6 to 4.9.

A study by Sapozink et al. (1983) described the interaction of radiofrequency hyperthermia (44°C, 30 min) with iodine-125 continuous ultra low dose rate irradiation (initial dose rates: 1.06–2.65 Gy/day) in the RIF fibrosarcoma tumor growing on the C3H mouse. Single- and multiple-dose experiments indicated that heating of RIF tumors in the range of 41°–45°C achieved at best a transient partial tumor response. High dose rate irradiation required single doses in excess of 40 Gy to achieve a 50% cure rate.

MOORTHY et al. (1984) used removable iridium-192 implants which provided a dose of 10 Gy/day (approx. 41.5 cGy/h) to total doses of 20, 40 or 60 Gy, representing 2, 4, or 6 days of continuous radiation. For comparison doses of 10, 20, or 30 Gy were used in combination with local tumor hyperthermia (LTH) at 43.6°C for 35 min in a waterbath. LTH was administered once for each 10 Gy delivered. The local tumor control rates were 67% and 89% for the 20 Gy + LTH and 30 Gy + LTH groups, respectively, and a TER of 3.4–3.9 was calculated. Results are comparable to those achieved with total doses of fractionated external beam radiation. The combined treatment effect appears to be less dose rate dependent and more dependent upon total dose accumulation.

JONES et al. (1989) demonstrated in a murine mammary adenocarcinoma that localized hyperthermia (44°C, 15 min) before brachytherapy (iodine-125, dose rates from 15 to 40 cGy/h) was more efficacious (TER 1.33) than hyperthermia after brachytherapy (TER 1.07). In their experiments a single heat treatment given in the middle of an interrupted course of brachytherapy resulted in the greatest thermal enhancement (TER 1.64). Two heat treatments, one given before and one after brachytherapy (TER 1.38), had no greater effect than a single heat treatment given before brachytherapy. This indicated that the second heat treatment contributed little toward thermal enhancement of the brachytherapy, possibly due to the development of thermotolerance. However, this protocol was tested only at 44°C with 48 h irradiation. Longer intervals of irradiation might span the time of thermotolerance decay. Their analysis of the results was complicated by the fact that the mammary tumor showed a significant regrowth delay in response to both the hyperthermia treatment alone and the technical treatment set-up necessary to carry out the brachytherapy.

PAPADOPOULOS et al. (1989) investigated the efficacy of interstitial hyperthermia and/or brachytherapy on the rat mammary AC33 solid tumor model. Subcutaneous flank tumors were heated with an interstitial microwave (915 MHz) antenna to a temperature of 43° ± 0.5°C for 45 min for two treatments, 3 days apart, and/or implanted with iridium-192 seeds for 3 days (25 Gy tumor dose). Hyperthermia alone produced a modest delay in tumor volume regrowth, while interstitial radiation was substantially more effective. A further improvement in tumor regrowth delay was observed after the combined treatment.

In our study (HAHN et al. 1988) we used the Dunning prostate tumor system which arose spontaneously and is syngeneic and therefore weakly antigenic in the Copenhagen rat. It is a versatile tumor system (Table 2.1) as there are tumor sublines which have doubling times varying from 1.5 days to approximately 20 days with differing histologies, hormonal dependency, and metastatic potential (ISAACS and COFFEY 1983).

The R3327-AT1 anaplastic tumor subline (Fig. 2.1) which has a volume doubling time of 5.2 days appears to be quite radioresistant when irradiated with either single doses (HAHN et al. 1989) or fractionated doses of 60-Co (PESCHKE et al. 1992).

For our first studies we inserted one iridium-192 seed (40 cGy/h) into the center of the tumor. Radiographs confirmed the seed position within the tumor at the beginning of treatment (Fig. 2.2). The hyperthermia treatments were performed at 43.5°C for 30 min + 5 min equilibration time, using a circulating constant temperature water bath (Fig. 2.3). The dose of IR was limited to 30 Gy, which resulted in a treatment time of about 72 h. Figure 2.4 shows the influence of dose rate on growth delay in the Dunning prostate tumor subline R3327-AT1. For comparison with external irradiation the tumors were treated either with one single dose of 30 Gy or with ten equal daily fractions (3 Gy) of photons 5 days a week for 2 weeks at a dose rate of approximately 45 cGy/min (cobalt-60 housed in a Siemens Gammatron S). The tumor volume was calculated by the formula $4/3\pi r3$, r being the arithmetic mean of two orthogonal radii.

A single dose of 30 Gy photons yielded a larger growth delay than low dose irradiation, probably due to the greater recovery from sublethal and potentially lethal damage which occurs during

Table 2.1. General Characteristics of the Dunning Prostate Tumor System (from ISAACS and COFFEY 1983)

Arose spontaneously in an aging Copenhagen rat (1961)
Tumor sublines are available with:
Doubling times ranging from 2 to 20 days.
Histologies that range from anaplastic to well-differentiated adenocarcinomas
Low to high metastatic potentials
Hormone dependency and independency
Histologies and enzyme patterns comparable to human prostate
Ease of transplantation

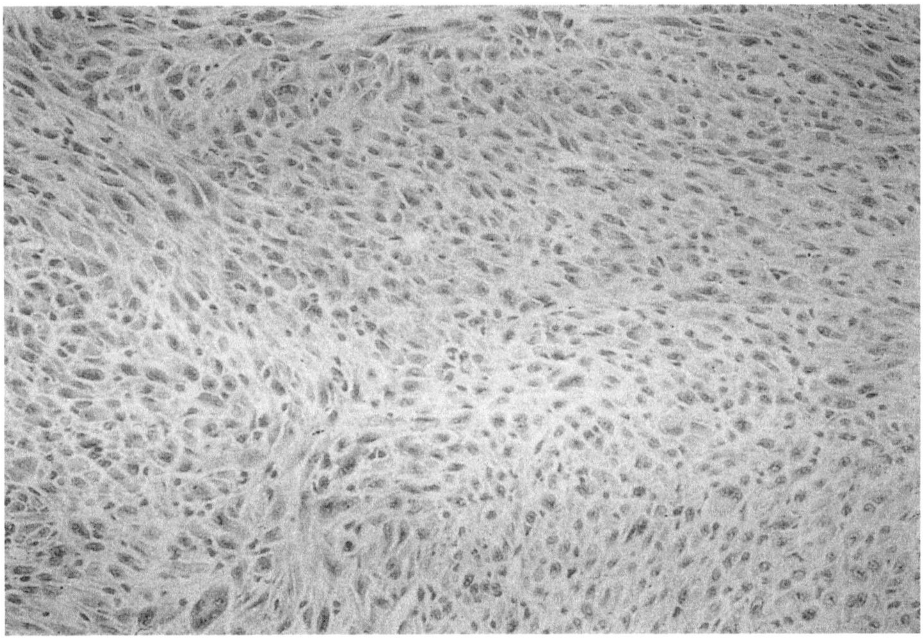

Fig. 2.1. Dunning prostate tumor subline R3327-AT1. Note undifferentiated and polymorphic tumor cells. The nuclei are cigar shaped and the cytoplasm elongated. The tumor cells grow in sheets. Occasionally small foci of necrosis can be seen with no large central necrosis. (H&E, X 160)

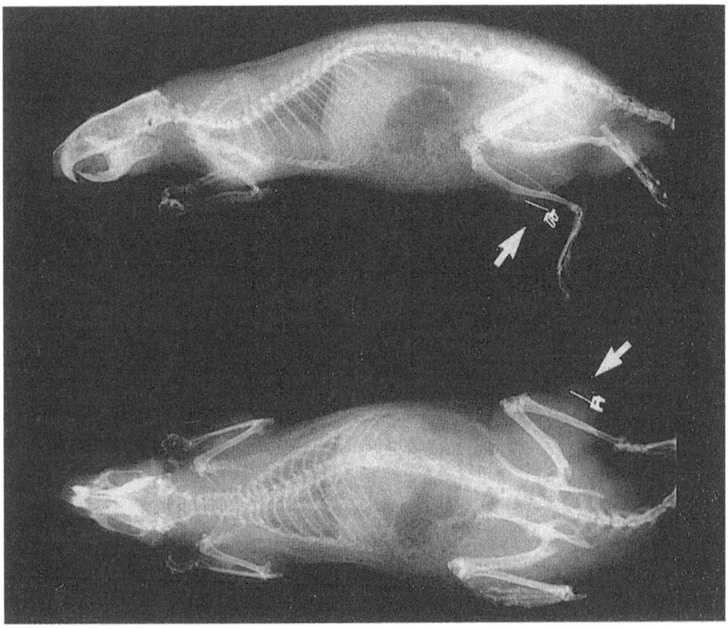

Fig. 2.2. Radiograph taken of a rat with one high-intensity iridium-192 seed inserted into a Dunning prostate R3327-AT1 tumor (see arrow)

protracted irradiation. Furthermore, these results show that low dose rate irradiation and fractionation have comparable consequences for radiation-induced repair and reoxygenation.

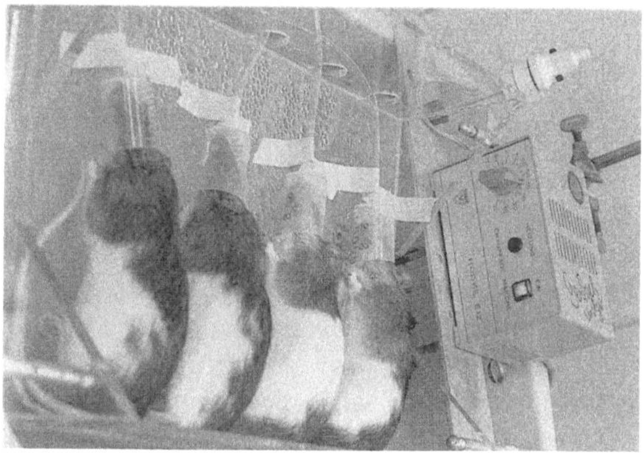

▲

Fig. 2.3. Local tumor hyperthermia. The rats are deeply anaesthetized with a mixture of halothane, oxygen and nitrous oxide. Thigh tumors are suspended in a circulating water bath

The basic design of the sequence study was such that the tumors received 30 Gy and one heat treatment given at the beginning, in the middle, or at the end of the radiation treatment. The results of these studies indicated that the subline R3327-AT1 is heat resistant inasmuch as LTH treatment without IR or with the insertion of a phantom seed did not produce any measurable change in tumor growth compared to untreated tumors. With regard to the sequence of heating, our results clearly showed that at least at the level of 30 Gy (= 72 h treatment time), one heat treatment given at the beginning of IR was the most effective treatment. In contrast one LTH given immediately after IR was the least effective treatment (Fig. 2.5).

In conclusion, all in vivo experiments studying the interaction of low dose rate irradiation and hyperthermia clearly show thermoradiosensitization, and these experiments have exhibited a wide

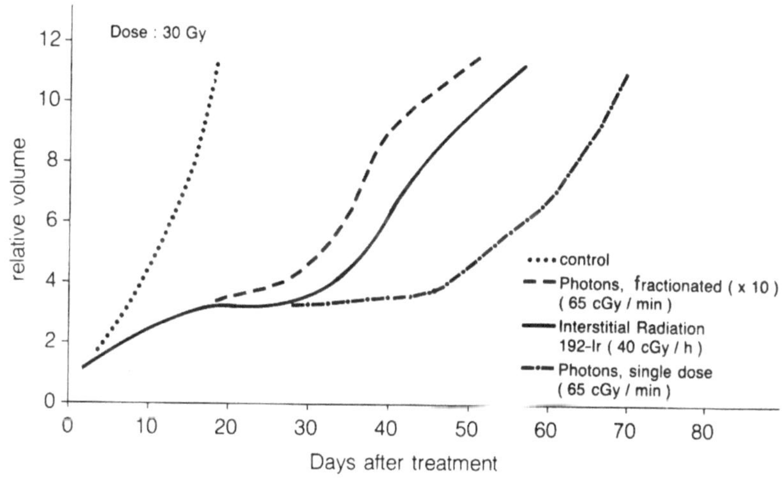

Fig. 2.4. Regrowth curves for the Dunning prostate tumor subline R3327-AT1 receiving 30 Gy either as a single dose, with ten equal daily fractions (3 Gy) of photons, or with low dose IR (iridium-192, dose rate 40 cGy/h)

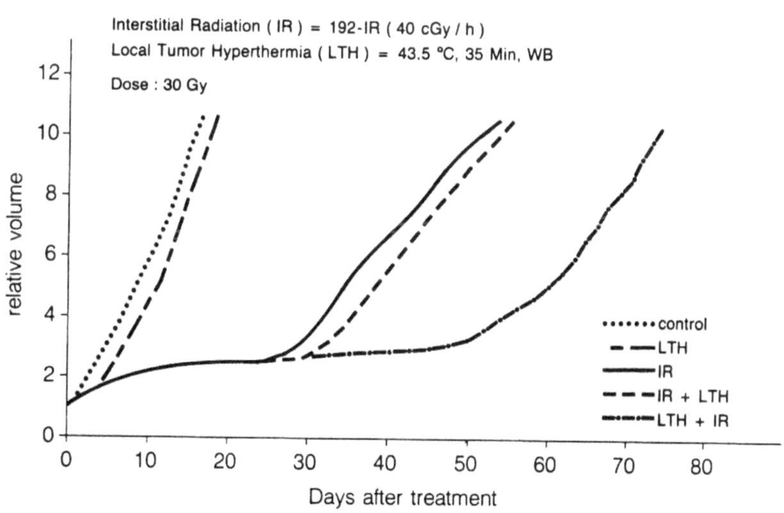

Fig. 2.5. Regrowth curves for the Dunning prostate tumor receiving a dose of 30 Gy IR with one iridium-192 seed (dose rate 40 cGy/h) over a period of 3 days and LTH

range of TER values which depend on dose rate, biological endpoint and treatment protocol. TER does not appear to increase significantly with decreasing dose rate. Therefore, TER seems to be less dependent on dose rate in the range of 40–600 cGy/h and more dependent on total dose (MOORTHY et al. 1984). At a low dose rate, the amount of dose per cell cycle seems to be more important than dose rate, since cell kill is enhanced by irradiating each cell through all phases of the cell cycle. At a sufficiently low total dose per cell cycle, cell division may equal or be greater than cell death and the total population may reach equilibrium. Determination of the optimum dose rate effect thus may be dependent on knowing the cell cycle time of the target tissue, which can become complicated because of the lengthening of cell cycle time at low dose rates.

With respect to the time sequence of IR and hyperthermia, in nearly all studies published so far, whether in vitro or in vivo, one treatment with hyperthermia given immediately after the cessation of IR seemed to be the least effective treatment. Nevertheless, it is important to keep in mind the fact that the optimal sequencing of hyperthermia before and during low dose rate IR remains to be determined.

Fractionation of hyperthermia may cause thermotolerance which is expressed as a transient increase in resistance in cells and tissues due to prior heating. The kinetics of thermotolerance are characterized by its development within 12–48 h after heat exposure and a much slower decay from 72 h up to more than 5 days in vivo (OVERGAARD and NIELSEN 1983). If heat is combined with irradiation, the central question is whether thermal resistance is as important for hyperthermic sensitization of radiation damage as for hyperthermia alone. This subject is still controversial (HENLE and DETHLEFSEN 1978; JUNG et al. 1986; DEWEY and HOLAHAN 1987) and the discrepancies might be due to differences in heating times, temperatures, sequencing, and cell type. Furthermore, environmental conditions in the tumor such as pH, nutrient media, oxygen status, cell cycle phase, and cell growth rate no doubt all play an important role (MAHER et al. 1981; GERWECK and DELANEY 1984).

HAHN (1982) pointed out the importance of cell proliferation kinetics in connection with fractionated studies and concluded that thermotolerance generally does not interfere with radiosensitization by radiation doses in the shoulder region but reduces the sensitizing effect in the higher dose range. Therefore, the role of radiosensitization during protracted irradiation should be carefully evaluated. While radiosensitization disappeared within a few hours after high dose rate irradiation (OVERGAARD 1980), a much longer and more pronounced sensitization was found with low dose irradiation (SZECHTER et al. 1980). Recent studies by LING and ROBINSON (1988) have shown that the effect of low dose rate irradiation can be enhanced by prolonged nonlethal modest hyperthermia exposures between 39° and 41°C.

For future studies, selection of the appropriate tumor model will be most important with regard to radiation sensitivity, antigenicity, heat response, repair capacity, and cell cycle time. What is needed on the radiobiological level are controlled studies with special emphasis on treatment-induced changes associated with proliferation kinetics, structural and cell interactions, blood flow, and vascularity.

In summary, low dose rate IR can in itself be effective in the treatment of cancer. The overwhelming majority of data available on the combined treatment of IR with hyperthermia clearly indicates that heat can be an important adjunctive therapy. But it is also clear that much more research is required in order to establish how best to apply the heat during IR treatment.

Acknowledgment. The authors gratefully acknowledge Prof. W.J. Lorenz (Chairman, Dept. of Radiology) for his enthusiastic support and helpful guidance.

References

Alfieri A, Nag S, Horowitz BS, Hahn EW, Kim JH, Hilaris BS (1982) Experimental application of hyperthermia and brachytherapy. In: Hilaris BS et al. (eds) Brachytherapy oncology 1982. Advances in lung and other cancers. Memorial Sloan-Kettering Cancer Center, pp 91–92

Bedford JS, Mitchell JB (1973) Dose-rate effects in synchronous mammalian cells in culture. Radiat Res 54 : 316–327

Ben-Hur E, Elkind MM, Bronk BV (1974) Thermally enhanced radioresponse of cultured Chinese hamster cells: inhibition of repair of sublethal damage and enhancement of lethal damage. Radiat Res 58 : 38–51

Bowler K (1981) Heat death and cellular heat injury. J Thermal Biol 8 : 426–430

Dewey WC, Holahan PK (1987) Thermotolerance as a modifier of radiation toxicity. In: Henle KJ (ed) Thermotolerance and thermophily, vol 1. CRC Press, Boca Raton, pp 113–125

Dewey WC, Westra A, Miller HH (1971) Heat induced lethality and chromosome damage in synchronized

Chinese hamster cells treated with 5-bromodeoxyuridine. Int J Radiat Biol 20: 505–520
Didomenico BJ, Bugaisky GE, Lindquist S (1982) The heat shock response is self regulated at both transcriptional and posttranslational levels. Cell 31: 593–603
Fu KK, Phillips TL, Kane LJ, Smith V (1975) Tumor and normal tissue response to irradiation. In vivo: variation with decreasing dose rates. Radiology 114: 709–716
Gerner EW, Oval JH, Manning MR, Sim DA, Bowden GD, Hevezi JM (1983) Dose-rate dependence of heat radiosensitation. Int J Radiat Oncol Biol Phys 9: 1401–1404
Gerweck LE, Delaney TF (1984) Persistence of thermotolerance in slowly proliferating plateau-phase cells. Radiat Res 97: 365–372
Gerweck LE, Richards B (1981) Influence of pH on the thermal sensitivity of cultured human glioblastoma cells. Cancer Res 41: 845–849
Hahn EW, Hildenbrand D, Peschke P, Wolber G, Zuna I, Lorenz WJ (1988) Hyperthermia and interstitial radiation (IR) on the rat Dunning prostate tumor (R3327-AT1): radiation dose and sequence of treatment (abstract). In: ESTRO 1988. Den Haag
Hahn EW, Wolber G, Bak M, Höver KH, Gerlach L, Volm M, Lorenz WJ (1989) Response of a Dunning prostate tumor to fast neutrons. Strahlentherapie 165: 283–285
Hahn GM (1974) Metabolic aspects of the role of hyperthermia in mammalian cell inactivation and their possible relevance to cancer treatment. Cancer Res 34: 3117–3123
Hahn GM (1982) Hyperthermia in Cancer. Plenum, New York
Hall EJ, Lam YM (1978) Renaissance in low dose rate interstitial implants. Radiobiological considerations. Front Radiat Ther Oncol 12: 21–34
Hall EJ, Bedford JS, Oliver R (1966) Extreme hypoxia: Its effect on the survival of mammalian cells irradiated at high and low dose rates. Br J Radiol 39: 302–307
Harisiadis L, Sung DI, Kessaris N, Hall EJ (1978) Hyperthermia and low dose irradiation. Radiology 129: 195–198
Henle KJ, Dethlefsen LA (1978) Heat fractionation and thermotolerance: a review. Cancer Res 38: 1843–1851
Hill RP, Bush RS (1973) Effect of continuous or fractionated irradiation on a murine sarcoma. Br J Radiol 46: 167–174
Isaacs JT, Coffey DS (1983) Model systems for the study of prostate cancer. Clin Oncol 2: 479–498
Jones EL, Lyons BE, Douple EB, Dain BJ (1989) Thermal enhancement of low dose rate irradiation in a murine tumor system. Int J Hyperthermia 5: 509–523
Jung H, Dikomey E, Zywietz F (1986) Ausmaß und zeitliche Entwicklung der Thermoresistenz und deren Einfluß auf die Strahlenempfindlichkeit von soliden Transplantationstumoren. In: Streffer C, Herbst M, Schwabe H: Lokale Hyperthermie. Deutscher Ärzte-Verlag, Cologne, pp 23–38
Kal HB (1979) Relationship between dose rate and oxygen enhancement ratio. Strahlentherapie 155: 774–775
Kal HB, Barendsen GW (1972) Effects of continuous irradiation at low dose rate on a rat rhabdomyosarcoma. Br J Radiol 45: 279–283
Kim SH, Kim JH, Hahn EW (1975a) The radiosensitization of tumor cells by hyperthermia. Br J Radiol 48: 727–728
Kim SH, Kim JH, Hahn EW (1975b) Enhanced killing of hypoxic tumor cells by hyperthermia. Br J Radiol 48: 872–874
Kim SH, Kim JH, Hahn EW (1976) The enhanced killing of irradiated HeLa cells in synchronous culture by hyperthermia. Radiat Res 66: 337–345
Kim SH, Kim JH, Hahn EW, Ensign NA (1980) Selective killing of glucose and oxygen deprived HeLa cells by hyperthermia. Cancer Res 40: 3459–3469
Kim JH, Hahn EW, Ahmed S (1982) Combination hyperthermia and radiation therapy for malignant melanoma. Cancer 50: 478–482
Lazlo A (1992) The effects of hyperthermia on mammalian cell structure and function. Cell Prolif 25: 59–87
Lepock JR (1982) Involvement of membranes in cellular responses to hyperthermia. Radiat Res 92: 433–438
Ling CC, Robinson E (1988) Moderate hyperthermia and low dose irradiation. Radiat Res 114: 379–384
Maher J, Urano M, Rice L, Suit HD (1981) Thermal resistance in a spontaneous murine tumor. Br J Radiol 54: 1086–1090
McNally NJ, Wilson GD (1986) Cell kinetics of normal and perturbed populations measured by incorporation of bromodeoxyuridine and flow cytometry. Br J Radiol 59: 1015–1022
Miller RC, Leith JT, Voemett RC, Gerner EW (1978) Effects of interstitial irradiation alone or in combination with localized hyperthermia on the response of a mouse mammary tumor. J Radiat Res 19: 175–180
Mitchell JB, Bedford JS, Bailey SM (1979) Dose rate effects in plateau-phase cultures of S3 HeLa and V79 cells. Radiat Res 79: 552–567
Moorthy CR, Hahn EW, Kim JH, Feingold SM, Alfieri AA, Hilaris BS (1984) Improved response of a murine fibrosarcoma (Meth-A) to interstitial radiation when combined with hyperthermia. Int J Radiat Oncol Biol Phys 10: 2145–2148
Nag S, Hahn EW, Alfieri AA, Kim JH, Hilaris BS (1981) High intensity I-125 brachytherapy (BRT) combined with hyperthermia: improved results in a murine fibrosarcoma (Meth A) when compared to I-125 alone (abstract). Int J Radiat Oncol Biol Phys 7: 1304
Overgaard J (1980) Simultaneous and sequential hyperthermia and radiation treatment of an experimental tumor and its surrounding normal tissue in vivo. Int J Radiat Oncol Biol Phys 6: 1507–1517
Overgaard J, Nielsen OS (1983) The importance of thermotolerance for the clinical treatment with hyperthermia. Radiother Oncol 1: 167–178
Papadopoulos D, Kimler BF, Estes NC, Durham FJ (1989) Growth delay effect of combined interstitial hyperthermia and brachytherapy in a rat solid tumor model. Anticancer Res 9: 45–47
Peschke P, Lohr F, Hahn EW, Wolber G, Hoever K-H, Wenz F, Lorenz WJ (1992) Response of the rat Dunning R3327-AT1 prostate tumor to fractionated fast neutron (N) treatment. Radiat Res 129: 112–114
Quastler H, Bensted JRM, Lamerton LF, Simpson SM (1959) Adaptation to continuous irradiation: observations on the rat intestine. Br J Radiol 32: 501–512
Rao B, Hopwood LE (1985) Effect of hypoxia on recovery from damage induced by heat and radiation in plateau-phase cells. Radiat Res 101: 312–325
Reinhold HS, Endrich B (1986) Tumor microcirculation as a target for hyperthermia. Invited review. Int J Hyperthermia 2: 111–138
Rutgers DH (1988) A Cs-137 afterloading device. Preliminary results of cell kinetic effects of low dose-rate irradiation in an experimental tumour. Strahlenther Onkol 164: 105–107
Sapozink MD, Palos B, Goffinet DR, Hahn GM (1983) Combined continuous ultra low dose rate irradiation and radiofrequency hyperthermia in the C3H mouse. Int J Radiat Oncol Biol Phys 9: 1357–1365

Spiro IJ, Ling CC, Stickler R, Gaskill J (1985) Oxygen radiosensitisation at low dose rate. Br J Radiol 58: 357–363
Streffer C, van Beuningen D (1987) The biological basis for tumor therapy by hyperthermia and radiation. Recent Results Cancer Res 104: 24–70
Szechter A, Kowalsky W, Schwarz G (1980) Modification of radiation-dose rate effects by mild hyperthermia in vitro. Radiat Res 83: 394
Vaupel P, Kallinowski F (1987) Physiological effects of hyperthermia. Recent Results Cancer Res 104: 71–109
Welch WJ, Feramesco JR, Blose SH (1985) The mammalian stress response and the cytoskeleton: alterations in intermediate filaments. Ann NY Acad Sci 455: 57–67

3 In Vitro Effects and Biological Potential of Long Duration, Moderate Hyperthermia

M.A. MACKEY

CONTENTS

3.1 Introduction

The response of cells to elevated temperatures has been studied at many levels of organization in the cell. Studies of the effects of heat exposure on gene regulation, membrane structure and function, cytoskeletal organization, and metabolic processes have provided a large body of literature describing the response of biological systems to temperature perturbation (LASZLO 1992; NOVER 1991; ROTI ROTI and LASZLO 1988). From a basic science viewpoint, the heat shock response is important as it allows examination of the genetic regulation of a certain class of proteins that are hypothesized to ameliorate the detrimental effects of stress exposure in living systems (GEORGOPOULOS et al. 1990). Furthermore, the response of other cellular processes to relatively mild temperature perturbations yields insight as to the importance of steady-state phenomena in a biological context (MACKEY and ROTI ROTI 1992). From a practical standpoint, the use of hyperthermia as a cancer treatment modality has stimulated interest in determining the mechanism of cell killing by heat, as such clinical use might benefit from explicit knowledge of critical lethal events (STEWART 1988).

M.A. MACKEY, Ph.D., Section of Cancer Biology, Division of Radiation Oncology, Mallinckrodt Institute of Radiology, Washington University School of Medicine, 4511 Forest Park Blvd., St. Louis, MO 63108, USA

Although heat kills cells in a reproducible manner, which is a factor in its clinical usefulness, no general mechanism of heat-induced cell killing has been elucidated. It is generally accepted that heated cells incur reproductive death in at least two distinctly different ways, dying either during interphase or through a process that appears to be linked with mitosis (HENLE and ROTI ROTI 1988). The majority of studies examining the mechanism of cell killing by heat have used short exposures in the higher temperature range (e.g., 44°–46°C). At temperatures below 43°C, however, the development of chronic thermotolerance (HENLE et al. 1978), defined as a transient resistance to further cell killing that develops during a heating interval, complicates the interpretation of experimental results. In contrast, chronic thermotolerance is not always observed in human cell lines (RAAPHORST et al. 1983). Because of the possibility of chronic thermotolerance expression, as well as for ease in administration, the goal of clinical hyperthermia has generally been to provide a brief (e.g., 1 h) treatment in excess of 43°C whenever possible.

Recently, clinical successes using hyperthermia in the moderate temperature range (e.g., 41.5°–42.5°C) employing treatment protocols involving up to 72 h of heating suggest that some human tumors may not be expressing chronic thermotolerance (MARCHOSKY et al. 1988; GARCIA et al. 1992). This report is a summary of recent developments in the study of the response of cells heated for long durations in the moderate range of hyperthermic temperatures (41.5°–42.5°C).

3.2 Transit of Cells Through S Phase of the Cell Cycle and Heat-Induced Cell Killing

Current evidence suggests a pivotal role for cell proliferation kinetics in the response of cells heated for long durations at temperatures in the moderate range of hyperthermic exposures (ROTI ROTI et al.

1992). When synchronized S phase Chinese hamster ovary (CHO) cells were heated at 41.5° or 42°C for up to 12 h, cell killing was not a simple monotonic function of exposure time (MACKEY and DEWEY 1988). A series of experiments demonstrated that cells were able to progress out of S phase and into more resistant cell cycle phases during a protracted heat treatment (MACKEY and DEWEY 1989), accounting in part for the observed change in the rate of cell killing. The extent of retardation of cells' passage through S phase correlated with increasing temperature and cell killing, and cells that were able to progress out of S phase, through division, and into G_1 during treatment at 41.5°C eventually expressed chronic thermotolerance. Cell cycle progression during long duration heat exposure of S phase cells was in contrast to that observed in G_1 phase CHO cells heated for up to 60 h at 42°C (READ et al. 1984), where a significant heat-induced G_1 block in cell cycle progression was observed. During the period of G_1 arrest, chronic thermotolerance was expressed, with tolerance decaying as cells overcame the block and progressed into S phase. In accord with these findings, human glioma cell lines heated at 42°C were more sensitive in exponential growth than when heated as confluent monolayers (RAAPHORST et al. 1989), with greater chronic thermotolerance expression under the density inhibited conditions.

Concomitant with progression of cells through S phase during the heat treatment, spontaneous premature chromosome condensation (SPCC) was observed. Thus, cells possessing abnormally condensed chromatin appeared, and such damage was associated with extensive nuclear fragmentation in a manner that correlated with cell killing, thus suggesting a causal role for heat-induced SPCC in the cytotoxic response (MACKEY et al. 1988). These studies implicated the prolongation of S phase in the induction of abnormal mitotic events. As such, this spectrum of damage was considered to be attributable to S phase-specific modes of lethality.

HeLa S3 cells heated for up to 56 h at 41.5°–42.5°C demonstrated no chronic thermotolerance (MACKEY et al. 1989; Fig. 3.1). This observation is in apparent contrast to results demonstrating that a transient resistance to higher (e.g., 45°C) temperature treatments did in fact develop and decay during the long duration treatments (MACKEY et al. 1992a; Fig. 3.2). Note that the shape of the 45°C survival curves (Fig. 3.2) obtained during long duration 41.5°C treatments exhibit chronic thermotolerance, suggesting that although

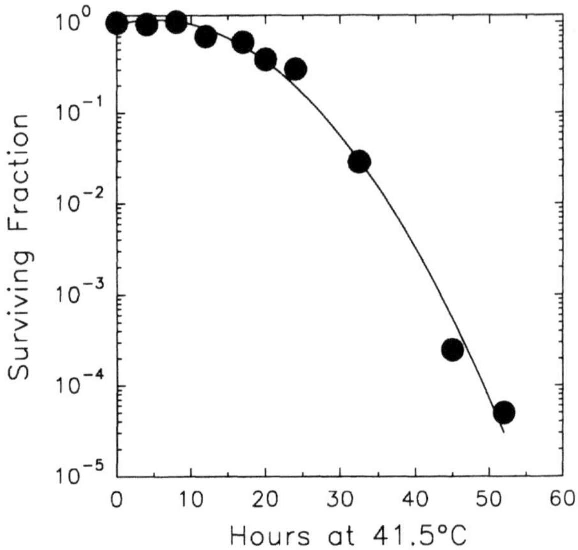

Fig. 3.1. Survival of HeLa cells heated at 41.5°C in suspension culture. Cells heated for varying durations were plated at a density sufficient to yield 50–100 colonies per culture dish. Cell density was held constant at 4000 cells/cm² using lethally irradiated feeder cells. Following colony formation (~ 10 days), colonies were fixed and stained using crystal violet. Survivors were scored as those colonies of 50 or more cells. Cellular multiplicity at the time of plating was 1.0

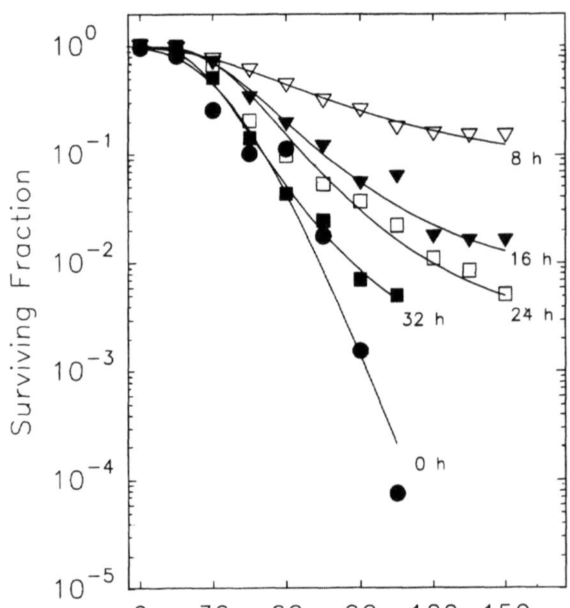

Fig. 3.2. Expression of chronic thermotolerance at 45°C. Cells were heated at 41.5°C for up to 32 h. At the indicated times, cells were shifted immediately to 45°C for various treatment durations, and plated for colony formation as described in the legend to Fig. 3.1. (From MACKEY et al. 1992a)

chronic thermotolerance develops during the lower temperature treatment, its expression is limited to conditions of higher temperature exposure. This is in contrast to previous reports of experiments using CHO cells where resistance to higher temperature treatment appeared to be coupled to chronic thermotolerance expression at the lower temperature (HENLE et al. 1978). These results allow a distinction to be made between chronic thermotolerance development and its expression. Chronic thermotolerance appears to develop during a long duration heat exposure of HeLa cells at 41.5°C, as demonstrated by the step-up heating experiments described above. Nevertheless, chronic thermotolerance expression at 41.5°C is not observed during the long duration heat exposure. Therefore, these studies suggest that the expression of chronic thermotolerance is a G_1-specific phenomenon, while its development does not have any cell cycle specificity. In light of these conclusions, it may be predicted that when cells are arrested in G_1 during a long duration 41.5°C exposure, chronic thermotolerance expression will be observed.

To verify that differences in sensitivity to G_1 arrest in CHO and HeLa cells could account for differences in survival response to 41.5°C, a series of experiments was conducted to directly compare the response of both cell lines under identical experimental conditions (MACKEY et al. 1992b). CHO cells were found to express chronic thermotolerance, whereas HeLa cells were continuously killed (Fig. 3.3). Correspondingly, CHO cells exhibited a G_1 block in cell cycle progression throughout the 32-h heating interval, while HeLa cells accumulated in S phase (Fig. 3.4). Subsequent to the accumulation of HeLa cells in S phase, SPCC was observed to occur, followed by nuclear fragmentation (MACKEY et al. 1992a, b). The incidence of both SPCC and nuclear fragmentation was correlated with cell killing in HeLa cells, while CHO cells presented insignificant amounts of SPCC and fragmentation in these experiments (Fig. 3.5). Note that, as previously mentioned, the SPCC-fragmentation effect does not appear to be restricted to HeLa cells, as CHO cells synchronized in S phase exhibited similar effects at this temperature (MACKEY et al. 1988). CHO cells were more readily blocked in G_1 during the heat treatment, as compared to HeLa cells, suggesting the paradox that it is the resistance of HeLa cells to heat-induced blocks to S phase entry that contributes to the cells' enhanced sensitivity to cell killing at these temperatures.

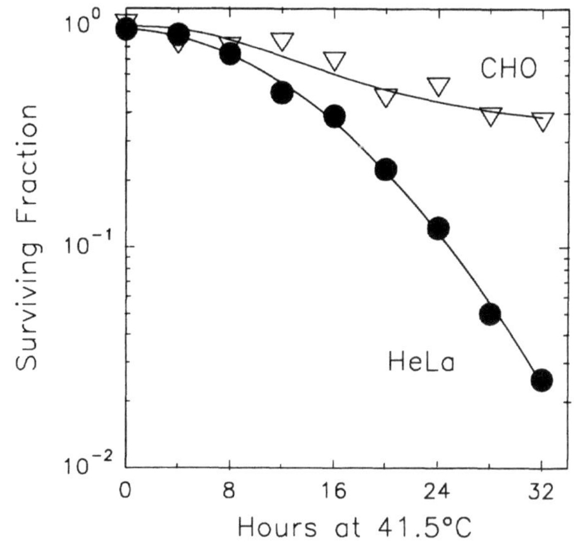

Fig. 3.3. A comparison of the 41.5°C survival response of CHO and HeLa cells treated under identical conditions. HeLa S3 and CHO cells were heated in suspensions and survival was assayed as described in Fig. 3.1. (From MACKEY et al. 1992b)

Since S phase cells are the most sensitive to heat-induced cell killing, the difference in cell cycle blocks observed in the comparison of exponentially growing CHO and HeLa cells at 41.5°C appears to explain the difference in cell killing between the two lines under the conditions tested. To test this hypothesis further, HeLa cells were heated in the presence of 4 mM caffeine, an agent that prolongs G_1 phase (HIGASHIKUBO et al. 1989), in order to delay entry into S phase. These experiments (MACKEY et al., manuscript in preparation) indicated that prevention of heat-induced accumulation of cells in S phase conferred protection from cell killing, suggesting a causal relationship between the accumulation of cells in S phase during a long duration, moderate heat treatment and cell killing (Fig. 3.6). Both the inhibition of progression into S phase and cell killing were accompanied by a decrease in SPCC induction (Fig. 3.7), again implicating SPCC induction in lethality under such conditions of accumulation of cells in S phase.

3.3 Molecular Mechanisms of Killing of S Phase Cells Heated for Long Durations at 41.5°C

The foregoing considerations suggest that cell killing at 41.5°C may involve heat effects on DNA replication. Although moderate hyperthermia exposure has been known for some time to cause a

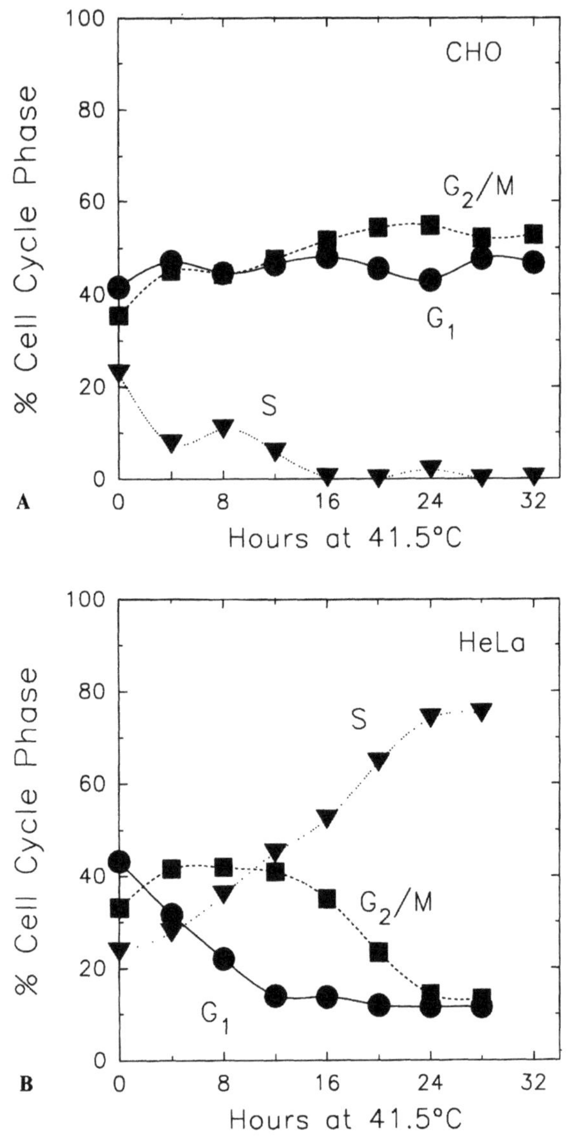

Fig. 3.4 A, B. Cell cycle rearrangement during 41.5°C exposure of HeLa and CHO cells. Cell cycle phase percentages were determined as described in the reference below. **A** CHO cells; **B** HeLa S3 cells. (From Mackey et al. 1992b)

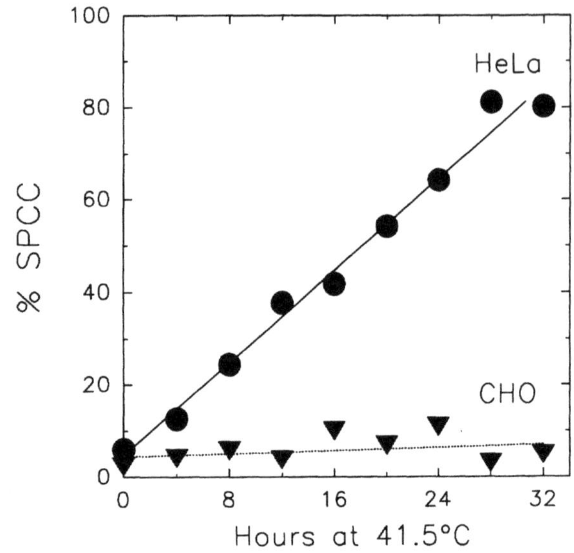

Fig. 3.5. SPCC induced by long duration heating at 41.5°C. SPCC was quantified flow cytometrically, as described in reference below. (From Mackey et al. 1992b)

decrease in ^{3}H-thymidine incorporation (e.g., Palzer and Heidelberger 1973), no detailed study of the mechanism of DNA synthesis inhibition in the temperature range 41.5°–42.5°C has been performed. In contrast, 45.5°C exposure has been found to lead to a transient inhibition of DNA synthesis (Wong and Dewey 1982; Warters and Stone 1983). After 45.5°C exposure, replicon initiation is inhibited to a greater extent than elongation, with ligation of replicons into clusters possessing an intermediate sensitivity (Wong and Dewey 1982). Heat-induced inhibition of replication is considered to be responsible for the increased sensitivity of S phase cells to cell killing, as compared to those in G_1 phase (Wong and Dewey 1986). Since previous studies demonstrated that SPCC induction is associated with both the accumulation of cells in S phase during the heat treatment and cell killing (Mackey et al. 1988, 1992b), the question arises of whether SPCC induction is causally linked to inhibition of replication. Accordingly, details of the regulation of the timing of the onset of mitosis, in the context of the completion of DNA replication, must be considered.

For many years it has been accepted that the onset of mitosis is regulated by a biochemical oscillator (Bradbury et al. 1974; Kauffman and Wille 1975; Tyson and Sachsenmaier 1978). Explicit details of the molecular regulation of mitosis have emerged only recently, due to the development of both genetic and biochemical approaches to the study of cell cycle control (for reviews, see Lewin 1990; Nurse 1990). It is now clear that there exists at least one specific M phase protein kinase that is implicated in phosphorylation-triggered nuclear envelope breakdown, chromosome condensation, and reorganization of the mitotic apparatus (Lohka and Maller 1985; Heald and McKeon 1990). M phase kinase was first identified in fission yeast cell division cycle cdc2 mutants (Draetta et al. 1987) and budding yeast cdc28 mutants (Reed et al. 1985). Since its discovery, homologous proteins with identical kinase function have been identified in human and lower vertebrate organisms

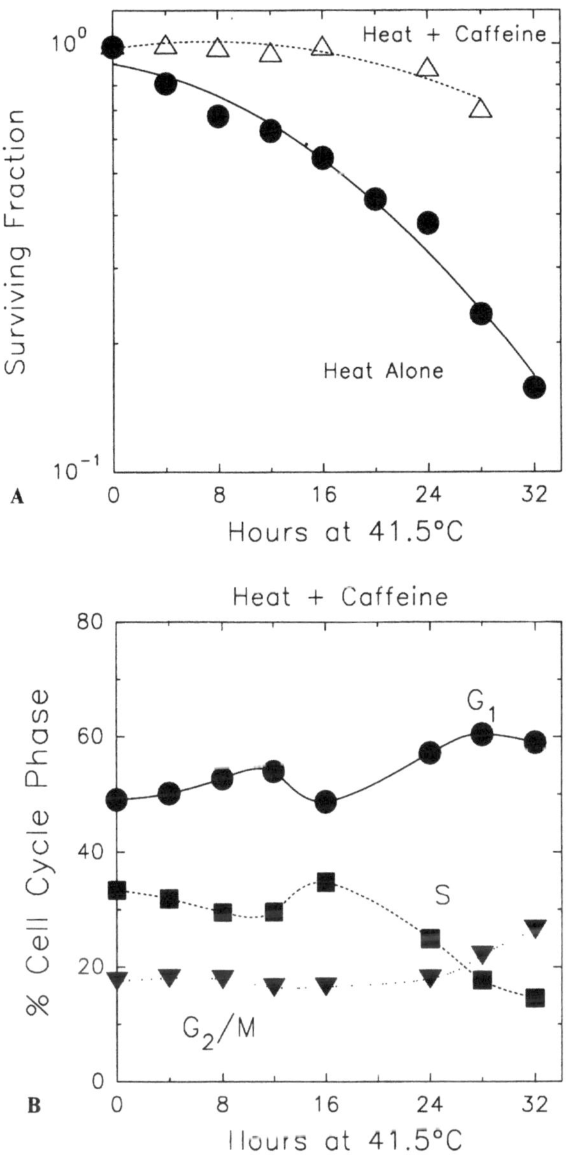

Fig. 3.6 A, B. Inhibition of cell cycle progression by 4 mM caffeine treatment during heating is associated with chronic thermotolerance expression in HeLa cells heated at 41.5°C. Cell survival was determined as for Fig. 3.1; cell cycle progression was monitored using anti-BrdUrd–propidium iodide bivariate flow cytometric analysis as described in MACKEY et al. (1992a). **A** survival; **B** cell cycle progression

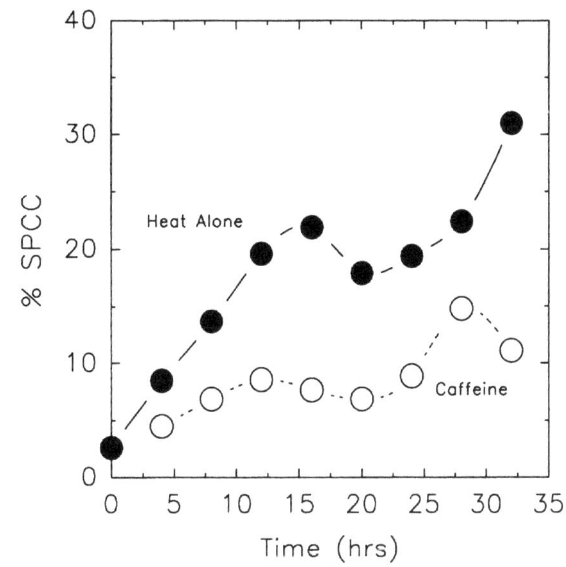

Fig. 3.7. Induction of SPCC during exposure of cells to 41.5°C alone or in the presence of 4 mM caffeine. SPCC was determined as described in MACKEY et al. (1992b)

(DRAETTA et al. 1987; ARION et al. 1988; LABBE et al. 1989). In human cells, this kinase activity is associated with a protein of M_r 34000, termed p34. The genetically based studies using the yeast cdc mutants were paralleled by the studies of maturation promotion factor (MPF) (NEWPORT and SPANN 1987; MURRAY et al. 1989; MURRAY and KIRSCHNER 1989; LOHKA et al. 1988), where it was demonstrated that a 34-kDa protein is one of only two proteins required for mitosis in *Xenopus laevis* oocytes (LOHKA et al. 1988; DUNPHY et al. 1988) or for mitotic-like events in cell-free systems (GAUTIER et al. 1988). The role of M phase kinase activation in the regulation of mitosis has been conserved throughout evolution and is thought to be part of a universal control scheme for mitosis in all eukaryotes (NURSE 1991).

At issue to the theme developed subsequently in this report lies the fact that the onset of mitosis is normally coupled to the completion of DNA replication (BLOW and LASKEY 1988). When G_2 phase cells are fused with S phase cells, mitosis is delayed in the heterokaryon until replication is complete in the S phase nuclei (RAO and JOHNSON 1970). In *Xenopus* cell-free systems, events associated with mitosis, such as M phase kinase activation, exhibit oscillatory behavior, even in the absence of DNA (LOHKA and MALLER 1985; DASSO and NEWPORT 1990). Addition of unreplicated DNA above a certain threshold amount delays these oscillations in a dose-dependent manner, suggesting a role for unreplicated DNA in the negative feedback regulation of M phase kinase activation (DASSO and NEWPORT 1990). Uncoupling of the onset of mitosis from the completion of DNA replication has been observed in organisms under two different circumstances: (a) fusion yeast cdc25 mutants, where cells deficient in cdc25 gene function undergo premature events prior to leaving S phase (REED et al. 1985), and (b) baby hamster kidney cells arrested in S phase using DNA synthesis inhibitiors in the presence of caffeine (SCHLEGEL and PARDEE 1986, 1987; SCHLEGEL et al. 1987). The cdc25 gene product has since been identified as the enzyme responsible for the dephosphorylation-mediated activation of $p34^{cdc2}$ kinase (MORLA et al. 1989). A study conducted using *Xenopus* cell-free systems containing unreplicated DNA established that caffeine-induced premature mitotic events were associated with activation of the cyclin–$p34^{cdc2}$ complex, not with aberrant cyclin or p34 synthesis or accumulation (DASSO and NEWPORT 1990). This finding led the authors to suggest that caffeine acts by interfering either specifically or nonspecifically with phosphatases or kinases that, among other functions, act to regulate M phase kinase activation. Contrary to this scheme, other workers have implicated elevated levels of cyclin A, due to reduced degradation in the presence of unreplicated DNA, as being involved in the inhibition of M phase kinase activation in the presence of unreplicated DNA (WALKER and MALLER 1991). Presumably, cell division prior to the completion of DNA replication would represent a lethal event, thus requiring strict regulation in cellular organisms (NURSE 1990). In this context, recent experiments have demonstrated that activation of M phase kinase occurs prior to heat-induced SPCC in HeLa cells heated at 41.5°C (MACKEY, LASZLO, and ROTI ROTI, manuscript in preparation), thus representing the first demonstration of the uncoupling of mitosis from the completion of DNA replication by an agent that induces a classic stress response. It therefore becomes instructive to consider what possible effects heat exposure may have upon the cell that would lead to such uncoupling.

A general effect of heat exposure on cells is the increase in protein coisolating with the nucleus (ROTI ROTI et al. 1979, 1986). This effect is believed to be due to either a heat-induced change in the solubility of nonhistone chromosomal proteins that are usually removed during the extraction procedure, or an actual translocation of cytoplasmic proteins into the nucleus. Hsp70 has been found to redistribute into the nucleus of heated cells in a time-temperature-dependent manner (OHTSUKA and LASZLO 1992), yet heat-induced translocation of other specific proteins has not been reported. Three possibilities for the observed heat-induced activation of M phase kinase can be distinguished. First, cytoplasmic cyclin B, normally translocating into the nucleus in late G_2 just prior to activation of M phase kinase (PINES and HUNTER 1991), might be prematurely redistributed into the nucleus as a result of the heat exposure, thus leading to SPCC, via premature activation of M phase kinase. Second, since it is known that heat causes a change in the activity of cellular protein kinases (LEGAGNEUX et al. 1990; LASZLO et al. 1992), it is possible that M phase kinase is prematurely activated prior to the completion of DNA replication by nonspecific, heat-induced dephosphorylation of $p34^{cdc2}$ kinase or via its effect upon the specific phosphatases or kinases responsible for the usual regulation of M phase kinase activity (RUSSELL and NURSE 1987). Third, nonspecific interactions between heat-induced excess nuclear proteins and unreplicated DNA may mimic the caffeine effect noted above, such that M phase kinase activation occurs prior to the completion of DNA synthesis. Deduction of the molecular basis of heat-induced SPCC will contribute to our general knowledge of the coordinate regulation of mitotic events with the completion of DNA replication.

Due to the foregoing considerations, a hypothetical scheme for the killing of cells during long duration, moderate hyperthermia emerges. The cells' growth cycle, from a biophysical viewpoint, consists of a sequence of biosynthetic or metabolic events that have historically been classified as related to either transcription, translation, or replication, with the sequence of events being punctuated by mitosis. Of course, there are other biosynthetic processes taking place as well as the repair of constantly occurring DNA damage due to background radiation and naturally occurring oxidative processes. Nevertheless, in proliferating cells, it is probable that the majority of cellular energetic resources are expended in the manufacture of RNA, DNA, and protein. In this regard, it is interesting that our experiments demonstrated that 41.5°C preferentially inhibits DNA synthesis, with little or no inhibition of RNA or protein synthesis (Fig. 3.8). It is possible that when such a metabolic imbalance is maintained for long periods, normal cellular regulation of the onset of mitosis is obviated, mediated by premature activation of $p34^{cdc2}$, resulting in premature mitotic events prior to the completion of DNA replication. Following the ensuing spontaneous premature chromosome condensation, the structural stability of the nucleus is compromised, resulting in nuclear fragmentation, a process that leads to permanent loss of coordination of macromolecular synthetic events and eventually to the loss of clonogenicity.

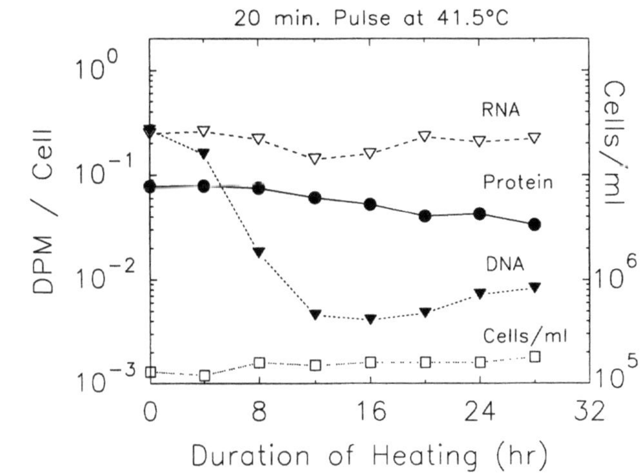

Fig. 3.8. ^{3}H incorporation into macromolecules during 41.5°C hyperthermia in HeLa cells. Replicate samples were pulse labeled for 20 min at 41.5°C with ^{3}H-labeled thymidine (DNA), uridine (RNA), or a lysine–leucine mixture (protein) at various times after the start of heating. Subsequently, aliquants of cells were precipitated in 5% trichloroacetic acid. Acid-insoluble material was collected on filters and solubilized. Radioactivity was determined using liquid scintillation counting

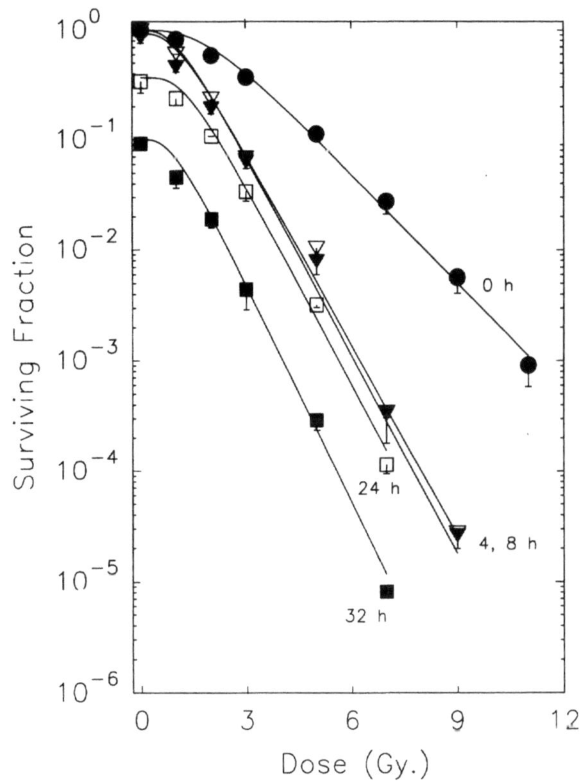

Fig. 3.9. Thermal radiosensitization during a long duration 41.5°C exposure in HeLa cells. Cells were heated for the indicated times at 41.5°C, followed by 10 min incubation at 37°C and irradiation (220 kVp x-rays) at 37°C. Survival was determined as described in Fig. 3.1. (From Mackey et al. 1992a)

3.4 Effects of Irradiation Delivered During a Long Duration, Moderate Hyperthermia Treatment

One rationale for combining radiation with hyperthermia lies in the complementarity of the cell cycle specificity of the two agents (Dewey et al. 1977), as relatively radioresistant S phase cells are very heat sensitive. In addition, heat combined with radiation is synergistic with respect to cell killing (Belli and Bonte 1963; Ben Hur et al. 1972). Previous studies have shown that in CHO cells the extent of thermal radiosensitization is dependent upon the surviving fraction from the preirradiation heat treatment alone (Holahan et al. 1984). However, when HeLa cells are irradiated at various times during a chronic exposure to 41.5°C, maximum thermal radiosensitization is achieved at 4 h heat exposure prior to the onset of heat-induced cell killing (Mackey et al. 1992a; Fig. 3.9). Subsequent cell killing at 41.5°C was additive to radiation-induced cytotoxicity. Since cells are accumulating in the radioresistant S phase during the heat treatment, it is unlikely that such changes in cell cycle distribution are responsible for this effect. Furthermore, maximum radiosensitization, quantifiable as a doubling of the D_0 of the radiation survival curve, occurs prior to any appreciable cell cycle redistribution or cell killing. Therefore, under these conditions, there does not seem to be a direct relationship between the extent of thermal radiosensitization and surviving fraction from heat alone, as was observed in the rodent cell lines. Clearly more studies using other human cell lines heated under different conditions are needed in order to generalize these effects.

3.5 Clinical Ramifications of In Vitro Studies

Understanding the molecular mechanisms underlying long duration, moderate hyperthermia-induced cell killing may be of considerable clinical importance. Whereas the modest temperature requirements of such hyperthermia can be achieved clinically (DeFord et al. 1990), previous goals of achieving uniform tumor temperatures in excess of 43°C for short (e.g., 1-h) treatments have presented technical problems associated with inadequate heating (Oleson et al. 1984; Dewhirst et al. 1984; Dewhirst 1989). If SPCC induction, in the absence of a heat-induced G_1 block, becomes established as a general mechanism of cell killing in cycling human tumor cells, this treatment modality would be indicated for tumors having a high growth fraction, determination of which could be accomplished clinically using flow cytometric techniques. SPCC induction and M phase kinase activation could be monitored from the analysis of tissue biopsies obtained during a course of long duration hyperthermia, in order to estimate the efficacy of the modality on a patient-by-patient basis. Furthermore, if lack of such indicators of cell killing is found in a particular patient during the course of treatment, hyperthermia administration could be stopped, thus avoiding needless treatment complications. While short duration, high temperature hyperthermic treatments appear to have less than optimal clinical utility (Perez et al. 1989), the rather modest temperature requirements of long duration hyperthermia, as well as definitive knowledge of its mechanism of cell killing, could combine to provide improved clinical efficacy.

Acknowledgments. The author is grateful to Dr. Joseph L. Roti Roti and Dr. Andrei Laszlo for critical reading of the manuscript and Nazan Türkel for expert technical assistance. This work was supported by grant CA 43198 awarded by the National Cancer Institute to Dr. Roti Roti.

References

Arion D, Meijer L, Brizuela L, Beach D (1988) cdc2 is a component of the M phase-specific histone H1 kinase: evidence for identity with MPF. Cell 55: 371–378

Belli JA, Bonte, FJ (1963) Influence of temperature on the radiation response of mammalian cells in tissue culture. Radiat Res 18: 272–276

Ben Hur E, Bronk VB, Elkind MM (1972) Thermally enhanced radiosensitivity of cultured Chinese hamster cells. Nature (New Biol) 238: 209–211

Blow JJ, Laskey RA (1988) A role for the nuclear envelope in controlling DNA replication within the cell cycle. Nature 332: 546–549

Bradbury EM, Inglis RJ, Matthews HR, Langan TA (1974) Molecular basis of control of mitotic cell division in eukaryotes. Nature 249: 553–556

Dasso M, Newport JW (1990) Completion of DNA replication is monitored by a feedback system that controls the initiation of mitosis in vitro: studies in *Xenopus*. Cell 61: 811–823

DeFord JA, Babbs CA, Patel UH, Fearnot NE, Marchosky JA, Moran CJ (1990) Accuracy and precision of computer-simulated tissue temperatures in individual human intracranial tumours treated with interstitial hyperthermia. Int J Hyperthermia 6: 755–770

Dewey WC, Hopwood LE, Sapareto SA, Gerweck LE (1977) Cellular responses to combinations of hyperthermia and radiation. Radiology 123: 463–474

Dewhirst MW (1989) A review of the University of Arizona experience in the treatment of spontaneous pet animal malignancies with hyperthermia alone/or radiotherapy. In: Urano M, Douple E (eds) Hyperthermia and Oncology, vol II. VSP, Utrecht, pp 1–12

Dewhirst MW, Sim DA, Sapareto S, Connor WG (1984) The importance of minimum tumor temperature in determining early and long term responses of spontaneous pet animal tumors to heat and radiation. Cancer Res 44: 43–50

Draetta G, Brizuela L, Potashkin J, Beach D (1987) Identification of p34 and p13, human homologs of the cell cycle regulators of fission yeast encoded by cdc2+ and suc1+. Cell 50: 319–325

Dunphy WG, Brizuela L, Beach D, Newport J (1988) The *Xenopus* cdc2 protein is a component of MPF, a cytoplasmic regulator of mitosis. Cell 54: 423–431

Garcia DM, Nussbaum GH, Fathman AE, Dryzmala RE, Bleyer M, DeFord JA, Welsh D (1992) Concurrent IR-92 interstitial brachytherapy and low temperature, long duration, conductive interstitial hyperthermia for treatment of recurrent carcinoma of the prostate. J Endocurietherapy 8(3)

Gautier J, Norbury C, Lohka M, Nurse P, Maller J (1988) Purified maturation-promotion factor contains the product of a *Xenopus* homolog of the fission yeast cell cycle control gene cdc2+. Cell 54: 433–439

Georgopoulos C, Tissieres A, Morimoto R (eds) (1990) Stress proteins in biology and medicine. Cold Spring Harbor Press, Cold Spring Harbor, NY

Heald R, McKeon F (1990) Mutations of phosphorylation sites in lamin A that prevent nuclear lamina disassembly in mitosis. Cell 61: 579–589

Henle KJ, Karamuz JE, Leeper DB (1978) Induction of thermotolerance in Chinese hamster ovary cells by high (45°C) or low (40°C) hyperthermia. Cancer Res 38: 570–574

Henle KJ, Roti Roti JL (1988) Response of cultured mammalian cells to hyperthermia. In: Urano M, Douple E (eds) Hyperthermia and oncology, vol I. VSP, Utrecht, pp 57–82

Higashikubo R, Holland JM, Roti Roti JL (1989) Comparative effects of caffeine on radiation- and heat-induced alterations in cell cycle progression, Radiat Res 119: 246–260

Holahan EV, Highfield DP, Holahan PK, Dewey WC (1984) Hyperthermic killing and hyperthermic radiosensitization in Chinese hamster ovary cells: effects of pH and thermal tolerance. Radiat Res 97: 108–131

Kauffman S, Wille JJ (1975) The mitotic oscillator in *Physarum polycephalum*. J Theor Biol 55: 47–93

Labbe JC, Picard A, Peaucellier G, Cavadore JC, Nurse P, Doree M (1989) Purification of MPF from starfish: identification as the H1 histone kinase p34cdc2 and a possible mechanism for its periodic activation. Cell 57: 253–263

Laszlo A (1992) The effects of hyperthermia on mammalian cell structure and function. Cell Prolif 25: 59–87

Laszlo A, Wright WD, Roti Roti JL (1992) Initial characterization of heat induced excess nuclear proteins. J Cell Physiol 151: 519–532

LeGagneux V, Morange M, Bensaude O (1990) Heat-shock and related stress enhance RNA polymerase II C-terminal-domain kinase activity in HeLa cell extracts. FEBS Lett 285: 122–127

Lewin B (1990) Driving the cell cycle: M phase kinase, its partners, and substrates. Cell 61: 743–752

Lohka MJ, Maller JL (1985) Induction of nuclear envelope breakdown, chromosome condensation, and spindle formation in cell-free extracts. J Cell Biol 101: 518–523

Lohka MJ, Hayes MK, Maller JL (1988) Purification of maturation-promoting factor, an intracellular regulator of early mitotic events. Proc Natl Acad Sci USA 85: 3009–3015
Mackey MA, Dewey WC (1988) Time-temperature analyses of cell killing of synchronous G1 and S phase CHO cells. Radiat Res 113: 318–333
Mackey MA, Dewey WC (1989) Cell cycle progression during chronic hyperthermia in S phase Chinese hamster ovary cells. Int J Hyperthermia 5: 405–415
Mackey MA, Roti Roti JL (1992) A model of clonogenic cell death after heat shock. J Theor Biol 156: 133–146
Mackey MA, Morgan WF, Dewey WC (1988) Nuclear fragmentation and premature chromosome condensation induced by heat shock in S-phase Chinese hamster ovary cells. Cancer Res 48: 6478–6483
Mackey MA, Türkel N, Roti Roti JL (1989) Evidence for the lack of chronic thermotolerance development in HeLa S3 cells heated from 41.5° to 42.5°C. In: Sugahara T, Saito M (eds) Proceedings of the Fifth International Symposium on Hyperthermic Oncology, Kyoto, Japan. Taylor and Francis, London, pp 97–99
Mackey MA, Anolik SL, Roti Roti JL (1992a) Changes in heat and radiation sensitivity during chronic low-temperature hyperthermia in HeLa S3 cells. Int J Radiat Oncol Biol Phys 24(3): 543–550
Mackey MA, Anolik SL, Roti Roti JL (1992b) Cellular mechanisms associated with the lack of chronic thermotolerance expression in HeLa S3 cells. Cancer Res 52: 1101–1106
Marchosky J, Moran C, Fearnot N (1988) 36th annual meeting of the Radiation Research Society (abstract Ch-7)
Morla AO, Draetta G, Beach D, Wang JYG (1989) Reversible tyrosine phosphorylation of cdc2: dephosphorylation accompanies activation during entry into mitosis. Cell 58: 193–203
Murray AW, Kirschner MW (1989) Cyclin synthesis drives the early embryonic cell cycle. Nature 339: 275–280
Murray AW, Solomon MJ, Kirschner MW (1989) The role of cyclin synthesis and degradation in the control of maturation promoting factor activity. Nature 339: 280–286
Newport J, Spann T (1987) Disassembly of the nucleus in mitotic extracts: membrane vascularization, lamin disassembly, and chromosome condensation are independent processes. Cell 48: 219–230
Nover L (1991) Heat shock response. CRC Press, Boca Raton
Nurse P (1990) Universal control mechanism regulating onset of M-phase. Nature 344: 503–508
Nurse P (1991) Cell cycle: checkpoints and spindles. Nature 354: 356–358
Ohtsuka K, Laszlo A (1992) The relationship between hsp70 localization and heat resistance. Exp Cell Res 202
Oleson JR, Sim DA, Manning MR (1984) Analysis of prognostic variables in hyperthermia treatment of 161 patients. Int J Radiat Oncol Biol Phys 10: 2231–2239
Palzer RJ, Heidelberger C (1973) Studies on the quantitative biology of hyperthermic killing of HeLa cells. Cancer Res 33: 415–421
Perez CA, Gillespie B, Pajak T, Hornback NB, Emami B, Rubin P (1989) Quality assurance problems in clinical hyperthermia and their impact on therapeutic outcome: a report by the Radiation Therapy Oncology Group. Int J Radiat Oncol Biol Phys 16: 537–558
Pines J, Hunter T (1991) Human cyclins A and B1 are differentially located in the cell and undergo cell cycle-dependent nuclear transport. J Cell Biol 115: 1–17
Raaphorst GP, Szekely J, Lobreau A, Azzam EI (1983) A comparison of cell killing by heat and/or X rays in Chinese hamster V79 cells, Friend erythroleukemia mouse cells, and human thymocyte MOLT-4 cells. Radiat Res 94: 340–349
Raaphorst GP, Feeley MM, DaSilva VF, Danjoux CE, Gerig LH (1989) A comparison of heat and radiation sensitivity of three human glioma cell lines. Int J Radiat Oncol Biol Phys 17: 615–622
Rao PN, Johnson RT (1970) Mammalian cell fusion: studies on the regulation of DNA synthesis and mitosis. Nature 225: 159–164
Read RA, Fox MH, Bedford JS (1984) The cell cycle dependence of thermotolerance: I. CHO cells heated at 42°C. Radiat Res 93: 93–106
Reed SJ, Hadwiger JA, Lorincz AT (1985) Protein kinase activity associated with the product of the yeast cell cycle gene cdc28. Proc Natl Acad Sci USA 82: 4055–4059
Roti Roti JL, Laszlo A (1988) The effects of hyperthermia on cellular macromolecules. In: Urano M, Douple E (eds) Hyperthermia and oncology, vol. I. VSP, Utrecht, pp 13–56
Roti Roti JL, Henle KJ, Winward RT (1979) The kinetics of increase in chromatin protein content in heated cells: a possible role in cell killing. Radiat Res 78: 522–531
Roti Roti JL, Uygur N, Higashikubo R (1986) Nuclear protein following heat shock: protein removal kinetics and cell cycle rearrangements. Radiat Res 107: 250–261
Roti Roti JL, Mackey MA, Higashikubo R (1992) The effects of heat shock on cell proliferation. Cell Prolif 25: 89–99
Russell P, Nurse P (1987) The mitotic inducer nim1 + functions in a regulatory network of protein kinase homologs controlling the initiation of mitosis. Cell 49: 569–576
Schlegel R, Pardee A (1986) Caffeine-induced uncoupling of mitosis from the completion of DNA replication in mammalian cells. Science 232: 1264–1266
Schlegel R, Pardee A (1987) Periodic mitotic events induced in the absence of DNA replication. Proc Natl Acad Sci USA 84: 9025–9029
Schlegel R, Croy R, Pardee A (1987) Exposure to caffeine and suppression of DNA replication combine to stabilize the proteins and RNA required for premature mitotic events. J Cell Physiol 131: 85–91
Stewart JR (1988) Prospects for hyperthermia in cancer therapy. In: Urano M, Douple E (eds) Hyperthermia and oncology, vol I. VSP, Utrecht, pp 1–12
Tyson JJ, Sachsenmaier W (1978) Is nuclear division in *Physarum* controlled by a continuous limit cycle oscillator? J Theor Biol 73: 723–737
Walker DH, Maller JL (1991) Role for cyclin A in the dependence of mitosis on completion of DNA replication. Nature 354: 314–317
Warters RL, Stone OL (1983) Macromolecular synthesis in HeLa cells after thermal shock. Radiat Res 96: 646–652
Wong RSL, Dewey WC (1982) Molecular studies on the hyperthermic inhibition of DNA synthesis in Chinese hamster ovary cells. Radiat Res 92: 370–395
Wong RSL, Dewey WC (1986) Effect of hyperthermia on DNA synthesis. In: Anghileri JL, Robert J (eds) Hyperthermia in cancer treatment. CRC Press, Boca Raton, pp 79–91

4 In Vivo Intraoperative Interstitial Hyperthermia in the Dog

A.J. MILLIGAN, H.W. MERRICK, and R.R. DOBELBOWER JR.

CONTENTS

4.1 Introduction

While it has become clear from research conducted in numerous laboratories that hyperthermia may be an effective adjuvant in the treatment of malignancy, many difficulties continue to be associated with delivery of heat to deep tissue (MEYER 1984; SAMULSKI et al. 1984). This investigation was designed to assess the feasibility of delivering interstitial hyperthermia to deep structures during a surgical procedure. We have investigated the feasibility of delivering hyperthermia in an intraoperative fashion. External heating of deep tumors of abdominal viscera necessitates heating skin, skeletal muscle, adipose tissue, and peritoneum to unwanted high temperatures, as well as making equal heat distribution to the target organ more difficult (CHEUNG and NEYZARI 1984). Advantages of intraoperative interstitial hyperthermia include: (a) better control of heat distribution within the tumor (LILLY et al. 1983), (b) sparing of normal tissue such as skin and skeletal muscle, and (c) possible combination of this technique with intraoperative radiation therapy or radioactive interstitial implantation (DOBELBOWER et al. 1989).

A.J. MILLIGAN, Ph.D., Department of Radiation Therapy and Nuclear Medicine, Thomas Jefferson University, 11th and Walnut Sts., Philadelphia, PA 19107, USA
H.W. MERRICK, M.D., Department of Surgery, Medical College of Ohio, C.S. # 10008, Toledo, OH 43699, USA
R.R. DOBELBOWER, JR., M.D., Ph.D., Department of Radiation Therapy, Medical College of Ohio, C.S. # 10008, Toledo, OH 43699, USA

4.2 Materials and Methods

The normal livers of 30 mongrel dogs were treated with intraoperative interstitial hyperthermia. All animals were treated to a temperature of 44°C for 40 min, with treatment times defined as commencing when central temperature in the heated volume reached 42°C.

Anesthesia for all animals was induced with sodium pentobarbital (50 mg/kg), administered intravenously. Employing sterile surgical technique, the liver was exposed via a midline anterior abdominal incision extending from the umbilicus to approximately 3 cm below the xiphoid process. A volume of the right lower lobe of approximately 4 × 2 × 2 cm was used as the volume of heating. A Plexiglas template was placed on the liver and four pairs of 16-gauge needle electrodes were inserted, allowing 1 cm spacing between pairs and 2 cm distance between the electrode planes. Electrodes were placed in the tissue through the entire depth of the liver parenchyma in direct contact with hepatic tissue. Three thermocouples with five sensors located axially on each thermocouple (0.5 mm spacing between sensors) were inserted through 16-gauge indwelling catheters at the center of the treatment field. A blood sample was obtained from each dog immediately after treatment, daily for 7 days, and weekly for the following 3 weeks for SMAC-20 and hematologic profile. After week 4, the animal was killed and samples of treated and untreated liver tissues were obtained.

In the normal lung and prostate, characterization of normal tissue response was accomplished by measuring blood flow at various times during the heating. Tissue blood flow was measured through the use of radioactive microspheres. The techniques for blood flow measurement with radioactive microspheres were identical to those reported by BRITTON et al. in 1979.

4.3 Results

The liver treatment volume was heated to a temperature of 44.0° ± 0.5°C. With the implantation of three multisensor thermocouples, each containing five sensors, temperature profiles were monitored in three dimensions. Additionally, systemic temperature measurements were made during the interstitial treatment, and no increase was noted throughout the procedure.

Analysis of the data from the SMAC-20 and CBC values showed a number of expected transient responses. While no difference was noted in many of the SMAC-20 values, several of the blood chemistry values peaked to very high levels immediately posttreatment (Table 4.1). These included alkaline phosphatase, serum glutamic-oxaloacetic transaminase (SGOT), serum glutamic-pyruvic transaminase (SGPT), creatine phosphokinase (CPK), and lactate dehydrogenase (LDH). Alkaline phosphatase increased from a control value of approximately 66 U/l to 208 U/l within 1 day posttreatment. The value remained significantly elevated for 6 days, but by 7 days posttreatment it had returned to within the normal range. CPK increased from a control value of 115 U/l for unoperated dogs to 2615 U/l within 1 day posttreatment. The value remained significantly elevated until the fourth day posttreatment, when it returned to within normal levels. SGOT increased from a control value of approximately 42 U/l to 305 U/l within 1 day posttreatment and returned to the normal range approximately 3 days posttreatment. SGPT also increased from a control value of 60 U/l to 740 U/l immediately after treatment. This value similarly decreased within 7 days to normal limits. LDH and, to a lesser extent, SGOT demonstrated an unexplained second rise in values during the second postoperative week. These values all indicated that damage of normal liver tissue had been inflicted by the interstitial hyperthermia. However, liver parenchyma injury appeared limited, given the return of clinical chemistry values to normal within 7 days posttreatment.

Biopsies were taken of normal and treated liver, both immediately after the treatment and upon necropsy of the animal either 7 or 28 days posttreatment. Physical examination of the liver showed scarring of the liver parenchyma in the center of the treated area, suggesting that interstitial hyperthermia destroyed normal liver parenchyma at temperatures of 44°C for 40 min. Histopathologic examination of the treated volumes indicated marked extramedullary hematophoresis occurring in the treated volume along with destruction of hepatocytes and replacement with fibrous tissue.

In the lung, blood perfusion rates were measured with radioactive microspheres at three points during the heating cycle described above (Table 4.2). Blood flow in the nonheated lung equaled 740 ml/min/100 g. After 12 min of 43°C interstitial hyperthermia, blood flow in the heated volume increased to 3430 ml/min/100 g, representing a 460% increase in the local perfusion. An increase in blood flow (by five- to tenfold) also may be observed in canine muscle following the identical hyperthermia treatment. To examine the effect of blood perfusion on heat removal, the right pulmonary artery was ligated after 12 min of heating and blood flow measured immediately after ligation. Blood flow at this point measured 30 ml/min/100 g, representing a 96% reduction in tissue perfusion rate from control values.

Blood flow values were also examined in the prostate of 20 normal dogs (Table 4.2). They were found to increase from a control value of 41.7 ml/min/100 g to 137.0 ml/min/100 g after 15 min of heating. This transient response was similar to that previously observed in canine muscle tissue by numerous investigators. Prostatic acid phosphatase increased from a control value of 0.4 U/l to 1.3 U/l within 24 h after heating. This value returned to normal within 3 days posttreatment. Histologically, early changes showed focal lesions at the site of the electrode with glandular

Table 4.1. Canine liver enzymes at 1 and 7 day posttreatment compared to control values

Enzyme	Control	1-day posttreatment	7-days posttreatment
Alk. Phos.	66 U/l	208 U/l	107 U/l
CPK	115 U/l	2615 U/l	160 U/l
SGOT	42 U/l	305 U/l	48 U/l
SGPT	57 U/l	740 U/l	108 U/l

Table 4.2. Blood flow values measured with radioactive microspheres in canine lung and prostate

Tissue	Control	Blood flow at 12–15 minutes of heating
Canine lung	740 ml/min/100 g	3430 ml/min/100 g
Canine prostate	41.7 ml/min/100 g	137.0 ml/min/100 g

regeneration in the normal tissues between the electrodes. Late effects included focal lesions at the implant site, including fibrosis with chronic inflammation at the location of the needle electrode.

4.4 Discussion

The above data indicate that interstitial intraoperative hyperthermia on normal tissues produces some limited tissue destruction. Elevations of liver transaminases, LDH, and alkaline phosphatase have also been shown to occur as a result of whole-body hyperthermia and isolated perfusion of the liver. Using whole-body hyperthermia, PETTIGREW et al. (1974) documented that the average serum activity of aspartate aminotransferase increased by 25-fold and that of alanine aminotransferase by eightfold. The return of these enzymes to normal pretreatment values within the first week postoperatively was not interpreted as an indication of cellular regeneration. OCHRAN et al. in 1992, reported on the use of an intraoperative ultrasound system for the delivery of heat to the canine spleen and kidney. Their studies investigated the temperature distributions at depths of 0.5 cm to 6.0 cm below the tissue surface. The date indicated that adequate power distribution were achievable using an appropriate water filled cone.

Little data have been published on the intraoperative application of hyperthermia to human tumors in vivo. In 1992, YAMASHITA et al. described the use of a 13.56 MHz capacitive system for the treatment of 12 patients with inoperable pancreatic cancer between 1986 and 1989. They reported that with this intraoperative technique, they were able to raise tumor temperature to 44°C. Clinical data indicated relief of pain in 86% of patients.

Histologic examination of the tissue specimens procured in the present study indicated that intraoperative hyperthermia was initially mildly toxic to the normal liver and prostate. Histologic sections of the liver revealed dilatation of sinusoids, red blood cells in the space of Disse, and an increase in the number of myelin figures. Mitochondria appeared to be unchanged, compared to the control specimen.

Two components suggested that lung tissue is an ideal organ for interstitial hyperthermia: (a) the high blood flow in the normal lung tissue, which cooled tissue when heat was delivered, and (b) the high air content of the lung tissue, which increased the electrical impedance of the tissue, making normal lung tissue difficult to heat with interstitial radiofrequency current fields. In summary, this study suggested that the heating of normal liver and prostate produces changes in response to injury with limited necrosis at 28 days posttreatment. In all tissues examined, most of the changes were reversible.

References

Britton SL, Lutherer LO, Davies OG (1979) Effect of cerebral extracellular fluid acidity on total and regional cerebral blood flow. Am Physiol Soc 818–826

Cheung AY, Neyzari A (1984) Deep local hyperthermia for cancer therapy: external electromagnetic and ultrasound techniques. Cancer Res 44 [Suppl]: 4736s–4744s

Dobelbower RR, Wagner SM, Fadell RJ, Howard JM, DiDio LJA (1989) Cancer of the pancreas. In: Dobelbower RR (ed) Gastrointestinal cancer. Springer, Berlin Heidelberg New York

Lilly MB, Brezovich IA, Atkinson W, Chakrobory D (1983) Hyperthermia with implanted electrodes: in vitro and in vivo correlations. Int J Radiat Oncol Biol Phys 9: 373–382

Meyer JL (1984) The clinical efficacy of localized hyperthermia. Cancer Res 44 [Suppl]: 4745–4751

Ochran TG, Rich TA, Boyer AL, Evans DB, Burdette EC, Johnson RL, Smith CW (1992) Intraoperative therapeutic ultrasound using an intraoperative electron beam cone system: phantom and canine studies. In: Gerner EW (ed) Hyperthermic Oncology. Arizona Board of Regents

Pettigrew RT, Galt JM, Ludgate CM, Horn DB, Smith AN (1974) Circulatory and biochemical effects of whole-body hyperthermia. Br J Surg 61: 727–730

Samulski TV, Lee ER, Hahn GM (1984) Hyperthermia as a clinical treatment modality. Cancer Treat Rep 68: 309–316

Yamashita T, Nakazama M, Sekiguchi K, Sunagawa Y, Hori M, Nishi M (1992) Intraoperative Hyperthermia by RF Wave for Unresectable Pancreatic Cancer. IBID

5 Radiofrequency Techniques for Interstitial Hyperthermia

A.G. VISSER, R.S.J.P. KAATEE, and P.C. LEVENDAG

CONTENTS

5.1 Introduction

In the following the term "radiofrequency techniques" is used to designate those electromagnetic heating methods using frequencies in the range of about 0.5–30 MHz. The use of radiofrequency currents at the lower end of this frequency range, to drive electrodes (e.g., implanted needles) which are in galvanic contact with the tissue volume to be heated, is conceptually the most simple technique for interstitial heating. Although this method of heating was the first to be applied and is therefore in a sense "established," several developments have taken place in recent years which appear worthy of discussion. The use of higher frequencies for interstitial heating is mainly motivated by utilization of capacitive coupling of electrodes inside nonconductive catheters instead of direct galvanic contact with the surrounding tissue. This different working principle of interstitial heating at the higher end of the frequency range and its consequences will also be discussed.

The first report of a radiofrequency (RF) interstitial hyperthermia technique was that by Doss (1975) although a similar idea had been proposed in 1970 by Robinson (cited by DEWEY 1989). Doss discussed several techniques, one of which involved applying a voltage at a frequency of 500 kHz between planar arrays of needle electrodes implanted into tissue on opposite sides of a tumor in an animal with the intention of elevating the temperature by ohmic heating due to conduction currents within the tissues. Doss referred to the technique as "localized current fields" (LCF); a detailed account is given in Doss and McCABE (1976).

5.2 Theory of LCF Technique

The frequency range which may be considered for LCF heating should satisfy the following requirements:

1. The resistive conduction current $\boldsymbol{J}_C$ $(=\sigma \boldsymbol{E})$ should dominate the capacitive displacement current $\boldsymbol{J}_D$ $(=\varepsilon\, \mathrm{d}\boldsymbol{E}/\mathrm{d}t)$; σ is the electrical conductivity (in S/m), ε denotes the (complex) permittivity (in F/m), and $\boldsymbol{E}$ is the electric field. This implies that

$$\frac{|\boldsymbol{J}_C|}{|\boldsymbol{J}_D|} = \frac{\sigma}{\omega \varepsilon_0 \varepsilon'} \gg 1 \ .$$

This condition is satisfied in tissues with high water content at frequencies up to a few tens of MHz and in tissues such as fat and bone at frequencies up to a few MHz.
2. The frequency should be sufficiently high to avoid direct electrical effects on nerve and muscle fibers; a few hundred kHz appears to be an acceptable lower limit.

Most LCF methods use a frequency in the range 500 kHz to 1 MHz. Typical impedance between two electrodes spaced 1–2 cm apart and implanted 5 cm into tissue is in the range $Z = 20\Omega - 20°$ to $15\Omega + 5°$ at operating frequencies in the range 0.5–15 MHz (STAUFFER 1990).

The electric fields within the tissue arise predominantly from the differences in (quasi)electrostatic potentials which are imposed on the implanted electrodes. In this frequency range the electric field can be viewed as a static field and can be calculated from a solution of the Laplace equation describing

A.G. VISSER, Ph.D.; R.S.J.P. KAATEE, M.Sc.; P.C. LEVENDAG, M.D., Ph.D.; Departments of Clinical Physics and Radiotherapy, Dr. Daniel den Hoed Cancer Center, Groene Hilledijk 301, P.O. Box 5201, NL-3008 AE Rotterdam, The Netherlands the distribution of the electric potential over the volume of interest.

In order to obtain a first idea about the electric field distribution and hence the absorbed power density distribution of an RF applicator implant it is useful to consider the electric field in the neighborhood of a single line applicator, e.g., a needle. If we assume, for reasons of simplicity, a single straight applicator (of infinite length in order to reduce the problem to a two-dimensional one) located at the axis of a second large, cylindrical applicator, the electric field $\boldsymbol{E}$ is in the radial direction and varies as $1/r$, with r the distance from the applicator. The absorbed power density, usually denoted as the specific absorption rate (SAR), is then found from

$$\mathrm{SAR} = \frac{1}{2}\frac{\sigma}{\rho}|\boldsymbol{E}|^2 ,$$

where ρ is the density of the medium. Thus the SAR is proportional to r^{-2} and falls off quite steeply with distance. Because RF applicators are often used in pairs, an illustrative example, given by HAND et al. (1991), is useful, namely two parallel straight electrodes with a separation small compared to the lengths of both electrodes. If a current I (A/m) is passed between these two electrodes, this will result in line charges $q = \pm I/j\omega$ (C/m). For a point located in the region between the electrodes at a distance r_A and r_B respectively from the two line sources, one can derive:

$$\phi(x, y) = \frac{q}{2\pi\varepsilon_0} \ln\frac{r_B}{r_A}.$$

The electric field $\boldsymbol{E}(x, y)$ at that point is found from:

$$\boldsymbol{E}(x, y) = -\nabla\phi = -\frac{\partial\phi}{\partial x}i + \frac{\partial\phi}{\partial y}j$$

and the SAR is found again from the expression given above. The SAR distribution for a pair of needle electrodes (of radius 0.5 mm and separated by 10 mm) in a homogeneous medium (HAND et al. 1991) is shown in Fig. 5.1. The rapid fall-off with increasing distance from the electrodes is evident. Indeed, the peak value of SAR along the midline between electrodes is only approximately 20% of that at the surface of the needles for this separation and is reduced to about 8% when the electrodes are 15 mm apart.

As in all hyperthermia applications, a temperature increase in most of the volume defined by the implant will depend strongly upon heat transport mechanisms and not only on local absorption of energy from the field. Although the SAR maxima close to the applicators seem large in relation to the shallow SAR values in the minima between the applicators, one should realize that the volumes receiving high SAR values are small and that heat transport mechanisms will have a considerable effect, resulting in more uniform temperature distributions.

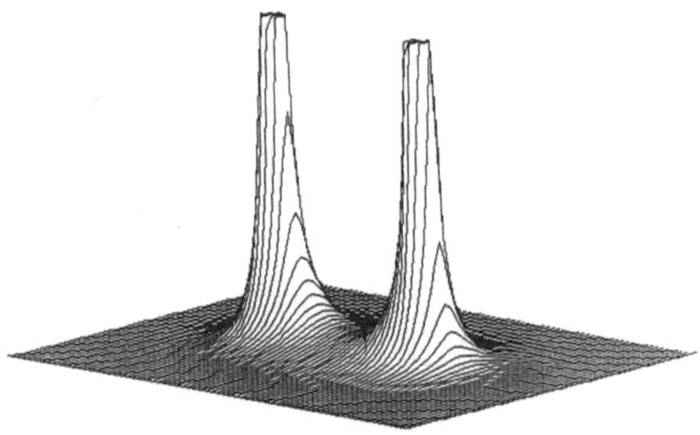

Fig. 5.1. SAR distribution associated with two needle electrodes in a homogeneous medium. The electrode separation is assumed to be ten times their diameter (HAND et al. 1991)

In practice, the SAR distribution is modified by the dielectric heterogeneity of the tissues and will also strongly depend on the geometry of the implant. Deviations from a strictly parallel geometry are expected to cause high SAR values in regions where the electrodes converge.

5.3 Practical Application of LCF Heating

A number of different methods are available to drive RF electrodes: a schematic illustration of these methods is given in Fig. 5.2.

The simplest method of implementing the LCF technique is to apply an RF voltage between two or more planes of electrodes (see Fig. 5.2A). This was the approach often adopted in early applications of RF interstitial hyperthermia but it offers very limited control over the treatment; only by disconnecting the electrodes can adjustments be made at selected locations within the implant. STROHBEHN (1983) modeled this approach and showed that the application of equal voltages on the electrodes in one plane results in an SAR distribution in which the SAR in the immediate region of an electrode is dependent upon the relative position of that electrode within the array.

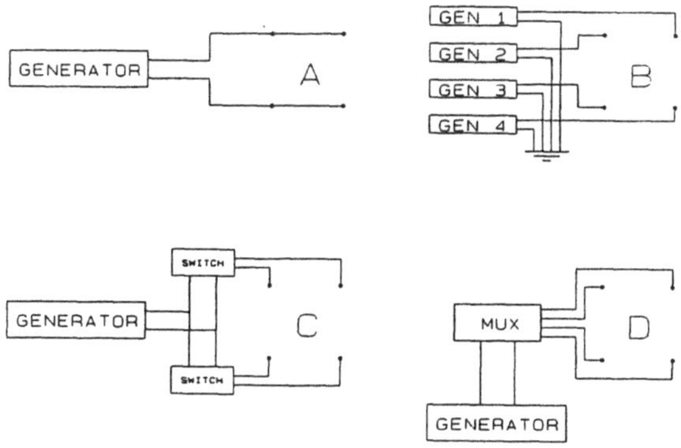

Fig. 5.2 A–D. Schematic illustration of different methods to drive RF electrodes for interstitial heating. **A** Two planes of electrodes directly connected to one generator. **B** Electrodes connected to individual generators which are operating in a "multifrequency mode" (hence incoherent). **C** One generator connected to preselected pairs of electrodes via (software-controlled) switches. **D** One generator can be connected to any pair of electrodes via a multiplexer (*MUX*) under software control. The choice of which pair of electrodes is activated and for what period of time depends on thermometry data from all applicators

Cosset et al. (1985) showed that better control can be achieved by driving preselected pairs of electrodes with separate generators operating either coherently (at 570 kHz) or incoherently at frequencies spaced at 20 kHz within the range 550–610 kHz. An advantage of this "multifrequency approach" is that to a certain extent the temperature at individual applicators can be controlled by connecting the different generators to single electrodes instead of to electrode pairs, as illustrated in Fig. 5.2B. Because incoherent generators are used, a "virtual ground plane" is created, allowing some control over individual applicators. The temperature at each applicator is measured by means of a thermistor positioned inside the applicator. However, a disadvantage is the small number (up to eight) of individually controlled electrodes available.

Astrahan and George (1980) switched power from a single generator between preselected pairs of electrodes, as illustrated in Fig. 5.2C. The pattern of sequencing and its overall cycle time, the time during which power is applied to each pair of electrodes, and the power level are adjustable. A feedback signal for control can be derived from the temperature at any of the locations of the thermocouple sensors (typically 32) used with the system.

Different authors (Kapp et al. 1988; Weisser and Kneschaurek 1987; Corry et al. 1990) have reported the application of systems in which it was possible to connect the generator to any two electrodes within an array via a multiplexer (Fig. 5.2D). In principle this method should offer the best possibility to obtain a relatively homogeneous temperature distribution. One condition is that each applicator contains at least one temperature sensor for control. A method of controlling such a system is to connect the generator to the coolest pair of electrodes each time the temperatures are sampled. The power level and dwell times can also be adjusted.

Prionas et al. (1989) developed electrodes consisting of several short segments, each electrically insulated from its neighbors. Each segment is connected to the multiplexer, providing control of power to individual segments. These electrodes are expected to achieve improved temperature distributions compared with single-segment electrodes since adjustments to account for a lack of parallelism of electrodes and/or the heterogeneity in the electrical and thermal properties of the tissues may be made.

5.4 Electrode Design in LCF Heating

The diameter of interstitial electrodes is typically in the range 1–2 mm. The upper limit is imposed by patient tolerance while the use of smaller electrodes would result in very high temperatures in regions close to them. Theoretical considerations suggested that spacing between electrodes should be no more than about ten times the electrode diameter in order to keep the SAR values at the minima between the electrodes at a reasonable level in comparison to the maxima at the electrodes. In practice, spacing of the implanted electrodes is likely to be determined by brachytherapy requirements: the separation between applicators is usually prescribed in so-called brachytherapy systems (e.g., the Manchester system or the Paris system), in which rules regarding the preferred geometries of implants are formulated and methods for dose specification are defined.

Rigid metallic needles were used in early applications of LCF but these caused discomfort to patients and, except at short insulated sections at the entrance and exit points in the tissue, heated intervening normal tissue as well as tumor. Flexible applicators (e.g., plastic afterloading catheters) are often to be preferred, certainly in less easily accessible implant locations, and also in terms of patient tolerance of the treatment.

The active length (i.e., that in direct galvanic contact with tissue) should be adaptable for individual treatments and to avoid unnecessary heating of normal tissue. If electrode pairs are hard-wired in pairs it may be important that the electrodes have the same active length (i.e., the length in direct galvanic contact with the tissues), to avoid unequal SAR distributions.

In order to avoid the problems associated with the use of rigid needles, alternative applicator designs have been proposed. COSSET et al. (1985) developed hollow electrodes formed from three sections: a central metallic section (of length compatible with tumor dimensions) and two flexible plastic sections glued to the ends of the central section. A metallic probe inserted through the lumen of one of the plastic sections provided the electrical contact with the central section.

The electrodes reported by KAPP et al. (1988) consisted of a hollow flexible plastic tube covered with fine-wire nickel braid which in turn was covered by a thin layer of electrical insulator. These electrodes could be customized for individual treatments by removing the outer insulation only in the target volume. The multiple-segment electrodes developed by PRIONAS et al. (1989) were constructed by successively depositing coaxial layers of electrically conducting (Cr/Al/Ni) and electrically insulating (SiO_2) materials on a rigid substrate (a hollow stainless steel trocar). Multiple-segment applicators of this type should give a better longitudinal control of the SAR distribution, especially in nonparallel geometries. A drawback is that to some extent the flexibility to adapt to the target volume during the implant procedure has been lost because nonstandard, prepared applicators have to be used.

5.5 Capacitive Coupling: Applicators as Current Sources

Local-current-field electrodes can be viewed as voltage sources. The current density at each electrode depends on the impedance with respect to neighboring electrodes with a different voltage level and thus on the geometry of the applicators. Deviations from true parallel geometries or the use of unequal active lengths is therefore expected to result in strong SAR variations, i.e., hot and/or cold spots.

As an alternative to LCF interstitial heating with electrodes in galvanic contact with the tissue, the use of interstitial hyperthermia systems at the frequency of 27 MHz has been reported (MARCHAL et al. 1989; VISSER et al. 1989; DEURLOO et al. 1991). These systems use applicators inside plastic (afterloading) catheters, i.e., the same catheters, used for brachytherapy with remote afterloading systems. This method is based on the same working principle as the LCF method, i.e., heating by low frequency currents passing through the target volume. However, the direct galvanic contact between needle (electrode) and tissue is replaced by a capacitive coupling between a conductor within a nonconducting catheter and the surrounding tissue. The working principle can be illustrated by the simple model shown in Fig. 5.3. The tissue impedance is indicated with the resistance R and the capacity C. The capacitive coupling between the applicator (inside the implanted catheter) and the surrounding tissue is represented by the capacity C(cath).

It can be argued (DEURLOO et al. 1991) that a capacitive coupling applicator can be viewed as a current source because of the rather large impedance associated with the capacity C(cath). Because of this large impedance the SAR distribution is expected to be less strongly dependent on variations in the separation between neighboring applicators. In LCF heating the impedance depends solely on the tissue impedance R and thus, for example, a geometry with converging or diverging electrodes is expected to result in strong hot or cold spots in the SAR distribution.

The type of applicator used for interstitial heating at 27 MHz by the Rotterdam group (DEURLOO et al. 1991) is illustrated in Fig. 5.4. The applicators should be thin enough to be inserted into commonly used brachytherapy catheters (ID = 1.5 mm,

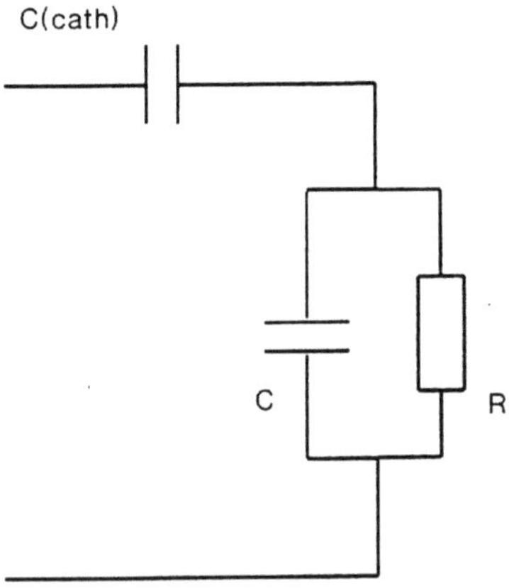

Fig. 5.3. Simple electrical model for 27 MHz interstitial heating. C(cath) represents the capacitive coupling, R the resistance of the tissue, and C the capacitance of the tissue

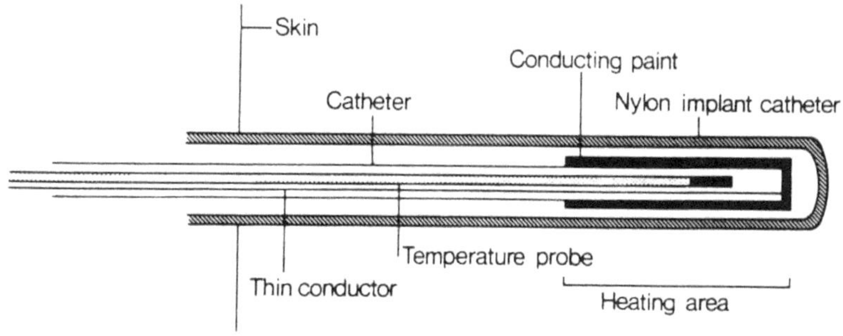

Fig. 5.4. Schematic diagram of an applicator of a capacitive-coupled interstitial heating system. Effective heating is limited to the length of the wide part of the applicator. A multipoint thermocouple probe is used for control

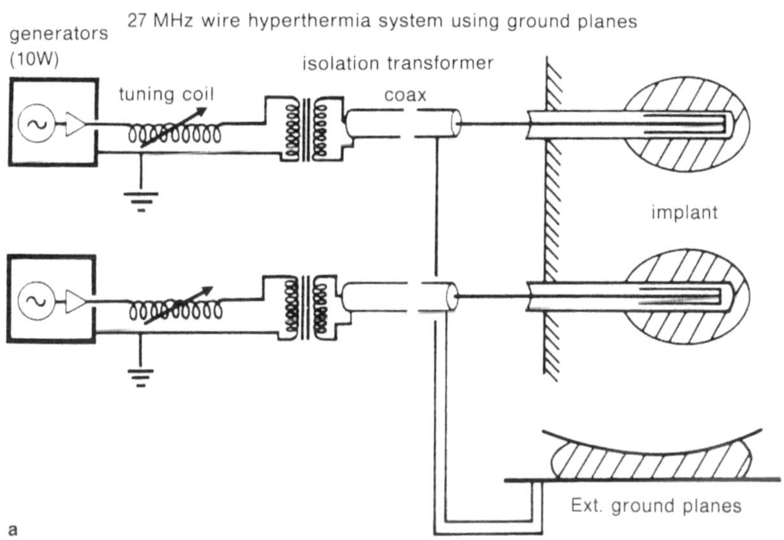

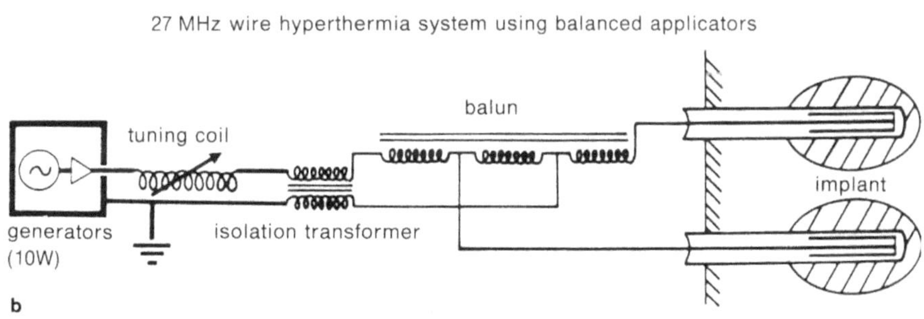

Fig. 5.5 a, b. Schematic view of two configurations of a capacitive-coupled interstitial hyperthermia system. **a** Configuration with individual applicators and external ground returns. **b** Configuration with balanced pairs of applicators; each pair of applicators is connected to a generator via a "balun", which transforms the signal from the generator into two balanced signals with a 180° phase difference

OD = 1.9 mm). This design enables temperature monitoring inside the applicator and heating over a limited length, avoiding heating of healthy tissue. It consists of a thin catheter (ID = 0.86 mm, OD = 1.27 mm) that is partially covered by a conducting paint. The paint is connected by a thin conductor inside the catheter to the coaxial cable connecting the applicator to the generator and matching network. The length of the catheter that has to be covered with the paint can be freely chosen. Due to the characteristics of capacitive

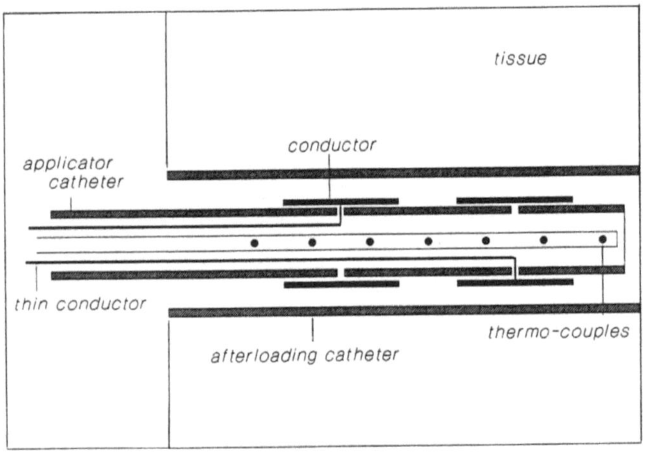

Fig. 5.6. Capacitive "dual electrode" applicator using two electrode segments within one catheter

coupling, energy transfer from applicator to tissue is only effective over the painted area.

Different applicator configurations can be used in capacitive-coupling interstitial hyperthermia:

1. Single applicators with external ground returns
2. Balanced pairs of applicators
3. Multiple electrode segments in the same catheter

In the first two configurations single-electrode, applicators are used and currents are either passed between applicators and external ground returns or between different applicators. These configurations have been studied by Deurloo et al. (1991) and are schematically illustrated in Fig. 5.5. The first configuration offers most individual control over applicators; with the second more applicators at a fixed number of generators can be used, but individual control is lost, which can result in unbalanced heating over a pair of electrodes.

The configuration with multiple electrode segments in the same catheter, as proposed by Lagendijk (1990), seems a promising method for interstitial heating. A "dual electrode" applicator consists of two capacitive-coupled segments in the same catheter between which a 180° phase difference is applied. The design of these electrodes is illustrated in Fig. 5.6. Similar to the interstitial microwave technique, the basic field distribution is created by a single catheter: the current flows between the two electrode segments. An external ground plate is used for defining the ground potential and to allow unbalanced operation of the two electrode segments. Catheter arrays can be operated coherently using constructive interference to maximize the absorbed power homogeneity and the maximum applicator separation allowed.

Model calculations and test measurements (Lagendijk 1990) indicate that relatively uniform SAR distributions can be obtained. Because the two segments can be separately controlled, the longitudinal control of the SAR distribution can also be improved.

The main problems encountered in designing a capacitive-coupled multielectrode system for interstitial hyperthermia concern, first, the impedance matching between electrodes and generators and, second, a strict control of power and phase of all individual electrodes. In a collaborative undertaking between the groups in Utrecht and Rotterdam a 64-channel system is being built and tested. In combination with sufficiently fast and extensive thermometry, this system should make possible improved spatial control of the SAR distribution.

References

Astrahan MA, George FW (1980) A temperature regulating circuit for experimental localized current field hyperthermia systems. Med Phys 7: 362–364

Corry PM, Martinez AA, Armour EP, Edmundson G (1990) Simultaneous hyperthermia and brachytherapy with remote afterloading. In: Martinez AA, Orton CG, Mould RF (eds) Brachytherapy HDR and LDR. (Proceedings of brachytherapy meeting. Remote afterloading: state of the art, 4–6 May 1989). Nucletron, Columbia

Cosset JM, Dutreix J, Haie C, Gerbaulet A, Janoray P, Dewar JA (1985) Interstitial thermoradiotherapy: a technical and clinical study of 29 implantations performed at the Institute Gustave-Roussy. Int J Hyperthermia 1: 3–13

Deurloo IKK, Visser AG, Morawska M, van Geel CAFJ, van Rhoon GC, Levendag PC (1991) Application of a capacitive-coupling interstitial hyperthermia system at 27 MHz: study of different applicator configurations. Phys Med Biol 36: 119–132

Dewey WC (1989) Dr Eugene Robinson (1925–1983) Int J Radiat Oncol Biol Phys 16: 531–532

Doss JD (1975) Use of RF fields to produce hyperthermia in animal tumors. In: Wizenberg MJ, Robinson JE (eds) Proceedings of an international symposium on cancer therapy by hyperthermia and radiation, Washington DC, April 1975. American College of Radiology, Bethesda, MD, pp 226–227

Doss JD, McCabe CW (1976) A technique for localized heating in tissue: an adjunct to tumor therapy. Medical Instrumentation 10: 16–21

Hand JW, Trembly BS, Prior MV (1991) Physics of interstitial hyperthermia: radiofrequency and hot water techniques. In: Urano M, Douple E (eds) Hyperthermia and oncology, vol 3. VSP, Zeist, pp 99–134

Kapp DS, Fessenden P, Samulski TV et al. (1988) Stanford University institutional report. Phase 1 evaluation of equipment for hyperthermia treatment of cancer. Int J Hyperthermia 4: 75–115

Lagendijk JJW (1990) A microwave-like LCF interstitial hyperthermia system. Strahlenther Onkol 166: 521

Lagendijk JJW (1990) A microwave-like LCF interstitial hyperthermia system. Strahlenther Onkol 166: 521

Marchal C, Hoffstetter S, Bey P, Permot M, Gaulard ML (1985) Development of a new interstitial method of heating which can be used with conventional afterloading brachytherapy using Ir-192 (abstract). Strahlentherapie 161: 543–544

Marchal C, Nadi M, Hoffstetter S, Bey P, Pernot M, Prieur G (1989) Practical interstitial method of heating operating at 27 MHz. Int J Hyperthermia 5: 451–466

Prionas SD, Fessenden P, Kapp DS, Goffinet DR, Hahn GM (1989) Interstitial electrodes allowing longitudinal control of SAR distributions. In: Sugahara T, Saito M (eds) Hyperthermic oncology 1988, vol 2. Taylor & Francis, London, pp 707–710

Stauffer P (1990) Techniques for interstitial hyperthermia. In: Field SB, Hand JW (eds) An introduction to the practical aspects of clinical hyperthermia. Taylor and Francis, London, pp 344–370

Strohbehn JW (1983) Temperature distributions from interstitial RF electrode hyperthermia systems: theoretical predictions. Int J Radiat Oncol Biol Phys 9: 1655–1667

Sugimachi K, Inokuchi K (1986) Hyperthermochemotherapy and esophageal carcinoma. Semin Surg Oncol 2: 38–44

Sugimachi K, Matsuda H (1990) Experimental and clinical studies of hyperthermia for carcinomas of the esophagus. In: Gautherie M (ed) Interstitial, endocavitary and perfusional hyperthermia. Springer, Berlin Heidelberg New York, pp 59–76

Visser AG, Deurloo IKK, Levendag PC, Ruifrok ACC, Cornet B, van Rhoon GC (1989) An interstitial hyperthermia system at 27 MHz. Int J Hyperthermia 5: 265–276

Weisser M, Kneschaurek P (1987) Kombination von interstitieller Hyperthermie mit Afterloadingtherapie hoher Dosisleistung. Strahlenther Onkol 163: 654–658

6 Microwave Techniques for Interstitial Hyperthermia

J.W. HAND

CONTENTS

6.1 Introduction

Microwave techniques for interstitial hyperthermia involve the use of needle-like antennas which, in most cases, operate at a frequency within the range 300–2450 MHz. The greatest experience appears to be with antennas driven at 915 MHz. Early studies of interstitial antennas include those described by TAYLOR (1978) and DE SIEYES et al. (1981), the latter showing the advantages of fully insulating the antenna from the tissue. Thus, antennas may be inserted into plastic catheters and the technique is readily compatible with brachytherapy methods.

At the frequencies used in these techniques, energy is transferred from the implanted antenna through a propagating electromagnetic wave which is subsequently attenuated in the tissue by dielectric losses. The method differs from other interstitial techniques in that significant levels of absorbed energy can be achieved away from the immediate environments of the implanted devices. Unlike radiofrequency localised current techniques in which current is passed between a pair of electrodes, heating is possible using a single microwave antenna.

A typical heating pattern associated with a single intersitial microwave antenna is an elongated ellipsoid of revolution with a very limited radial penetration (less than about 10 mm). Although this may be suitable for hyperthermia of brain tumours (e.g., SAMARAS 1984; RYAN et al. 1991), an array of implanted antennas is usually required for other clinical applications. The antennas in such arrays may be driven either coherently or incoherently. A characteristic of coherently driven arrays is that the specific (energy) absorption rate (SAR) at certain locations may be enhanced locally by constructive interference. For example, the SAR due to an array of N antennas can be increased N-fold (assuming that all antennas have the same polarisation, that each antenna contributes equal field strength with equal amplitude at the point in question and that the medium has uniform dielectric properties) when coherent, rather than incoherent operation is chosen. Although coherent operation has a clear theoretical advantage for some antennas (e.g., linear dipoles, particularly at 915 MHz), in practice complicating factors such as the dielectric inhomogeneity of tissues, the presence of phase differences between individual channels of coherent generators (which sometimes depend upon the power delivered) and the introduction of unwanted (and often unknown) phase shifts by impedance matching devices or networks, must also be considered.

The SAR distribution associated with an interstitial microwave antenna can be measured at a known radial distance (e.g., 5 mm) from the catheter and described by parameters such as the depth at which the peak SAR occurs, the length of the antenna over which the SAR is greater than or equal to 50% of the maximum value of SAR and the distance along the antenna from the tip to where SAR is 50% of the maximum (SATOH and STAUFFER 1988) (Fig. 6.1). The variation of these parameters with insertion depth should also be determined. Return loss as a function of frequency and insertion depth should also be known. Arrays of antennas can be characterised by similar parameters, although in this case the SAR in multiple planes transverse to the antennas should also be determined.

J.W. HAND, Ph.D., Hyperthermia Clinic, MRC Cyclotron Unit, Hammersmith Hospital, Du Cane Road, London W12 OHS, United Kingdom

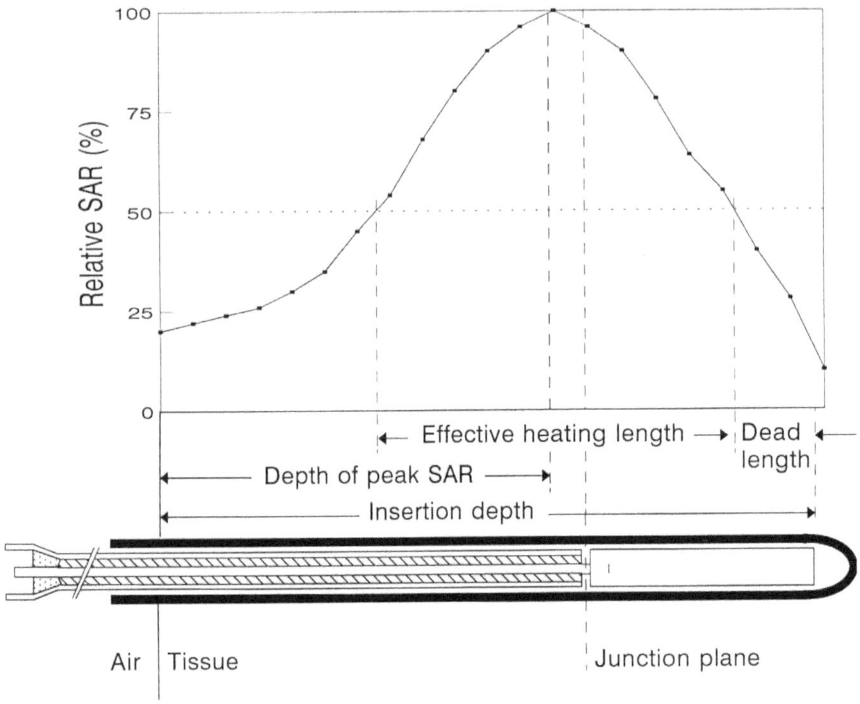

Fig. 6.1. Characteristics of an idealised SAR profile measured along an antenna/catheter at a fixed radial distance. The parameters shown, defined relative to 50% of the peak value of SAR, are discussed in the text

6.2 Dipole Antennas

A common form of interstitial applicator is a dipole antenna made from flexible miniature coaxial cable with an extension of the inner conductor at the distal end (Fig. 6.2). Characteristic dimensions of this type of antenna are the distances from the juction (i.e., where the extension to the inner conductor begins) to the tip (h_A) and to the tissue-air interface (h_B) and the radii of the antenna and of the catheter it is placed in. A voltage impressed at the junction results in currents which travel along the outside of the proximal and distal sections and it is these currents which induce the electromagnetic wave which propagates into the tissue. The behaviour of this type of antenna embedded in a lossy medium such as tissue has been described theoretically by KING et al. (1983). Subsequent

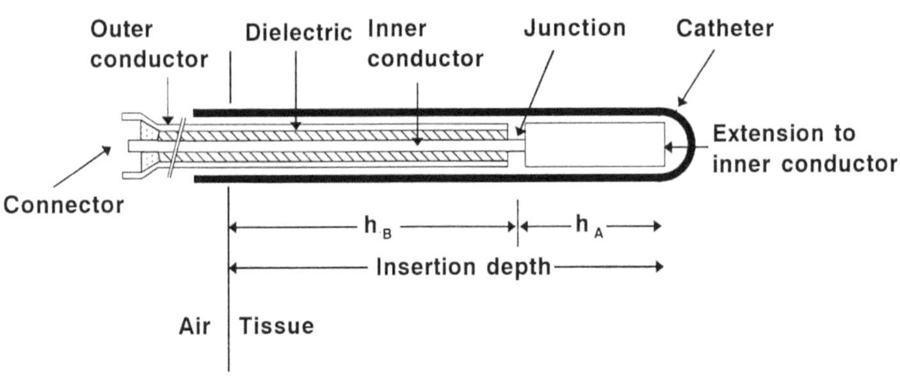

Fig. 6.2. Schematic diagram of a dipole antenna within a catheter (not to scale). For the antenna to be resonant when operating at 915 MHz in a nylon catheter (1.2 mm internal diameter, 2.2 mm outer diameter) inserted into muscle tissue, $h_A = h_B = 39$ mm (MECHLING et al. 1992). In practice, h_B is determined by the tumour geometry

theoretical studies include those by CASEY and BANSAL (1986), ISKANDER and TUMEH (1989) and ZHANG et al. (1988). There are benefits if the operating frequency and length of a dipole antenna are selected so that the antenna is near resonant (TREMBLY 1985; JONES et al. 1988, 1989). This occurs when the lengths of the sections (h_A, h_B) are approximately one-quarter of the wavelength, which is determined by the dielectric properties of the antenna, catheter and surrounding tissues as well as the operating frequency. One advantage of near-resonant antennas is that their impedance is close to 50Ω, negating the need for matching networks which can introduce phase shifts leading to unexpected SAR distributions in the case of coherently driven arrays. The importance of catheter size and wall thickness in determining SAR distributions has been demonstrated by JAMES et al. (1989) and RYAN et al. (1991).

In practice the insertion depth (the distance from the insertion point to the tip of the antenna) is determined by the size and location of the tumour to be treated, and so h_B can differ considerably from h_A (i.e., the dipole antenna becomes asymmetrical). Fields and SAR distributions around asymmetrical dipole antennas have been studied by ZHANG et al. (1988) and JONES et al. (1988, 1989). SAR distributions associated with dipole antennas are dependent upon insertion depth (KING et al. 1981; JONES et al. 1988). For example, in the case of a single antenna the longitudinal variation of SAR along the proximal section is dependent upon h_B although that along the distal section is approximately independent of h_B, as is the position of the maximum SAR, which remains close to the plane of the antenna junction. When h_B is somewhat greater than a quarter wavelength, the SAR distribution over both proximal and distal sections of the antenna is relatively insensitive to insertion depth. The behaviour of the SAR distribution associated with arrays of antennas is more complex and is discussed later.

Dipole antennas may be designed to minimise the dependence of the SAR distribution on insertion depth. For example, HÜRTER et al. (1991) incorporate a quarter wavelength sleeve on the feeding line proximal to the junction for this purpose. This also results in the impedance of the antenna remaining constant regardless of insertion depth when the choke and tip sections are completely within the lossy medium. RYAN et al. (1990) reported measurements of SAR produced by an array of dipoles with chokes along both proximal and distal sections (antenna C, Fig. 6.3) and showed a greatly decreased sensitivity on insertion depth for these antennas than for a similar array of conventional dipole antennas.

A disadvantage of conventional dipole antennas is that power deposition decreases towards the tip of the antenna, leading to inadequate heating in that area. Thus the antenna must be implanted beyond the target volume to ensure adequate heating within it. With this problem in mind, modified dipole antennas have been developed. For example, the diameter of the antenna may be increased towards the tip (antenna A, Fig. 6.3), providing increased coupling to the tissue in that region through the catheter (TURNER 1986; ROOS and HUGANDER 1988; TUMEH and ISKANDER 1989).

Cooling of the antenna–catheter combination to reduce temperatures close to the catheters has been investigated. EPPERT et al. (1991) considered open-ended catheters with air at 30°C forced through them and showed that a cooling rate of about 0.1 W/cm length of catheter is sufficient to improve the radial temperature uniformity associated with single antennas and some array configurations. Experimental verification of the predicted improvements were reported by TREMBLY et al. (1991). These authors suggest that air is a better cooling agent than water for this application since with the latter the antenna becomes bare rather than insulated, a configuration associated with poor radial penetration.

6.3 Arrays of Antennas

Several studies into coherent operation of linearly polarised applicators (e.g. dipole antennas) have shown that the SAR distribution within the implant may be controlled by suitable phase and amplitude modulation (TREMBLY et al. 1986; FURSE and ISKANDER 1989; ZHANG et al. 1990a, b, 1991a). Such modulation can produce relatively uniform SAR across a significant area of the array or a distribution in which the SAR in peripheral regions is greater than that in the central region of the array. Whilst theoretical studies demonstrate that control over SAR (at least in the region of the junction-plane of an array) is feasible, factors such as small differences between individual antennas and feed lines, antennas being inserted to different depths, and dielectric heterogeneities within the tissues must be accounted for in the implementation of this approach.

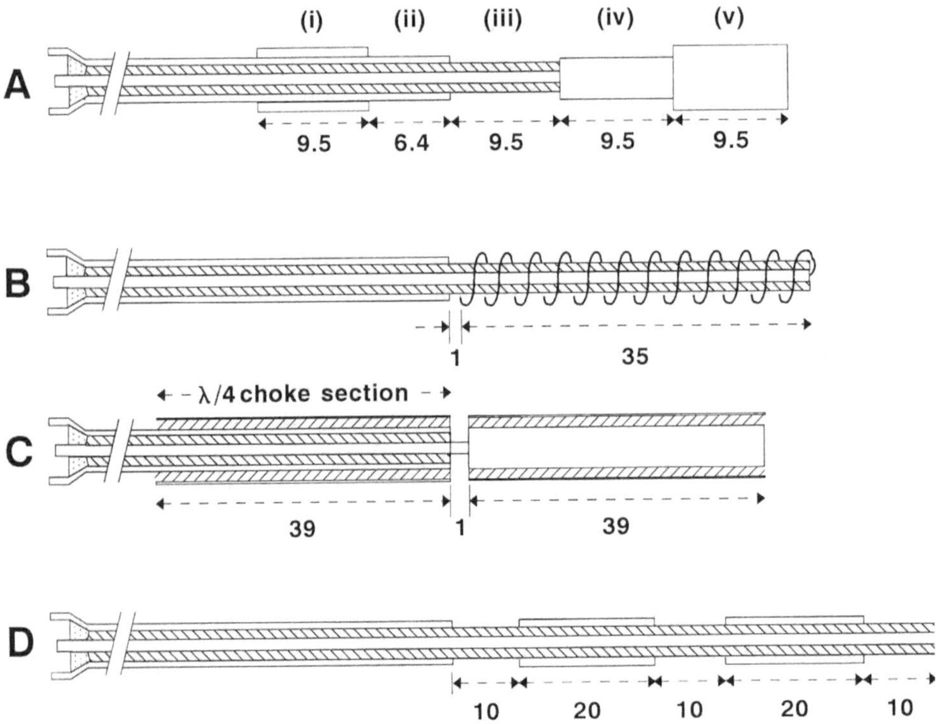

Fig. 6.3 A–D. Schematic diagrams of interstitial antenna structures (not to scale). Section lengths are in mm. **A** Multisection antenna based on 0.95 mm diameter coaxial cable in which sections (i) and (v) are collars of 1.07 mm diameter, (ii) and (iii) are, respectively, sections of the coaxial cable with and without the outer conductor, and (iv) is a metallic tube of 0.86 mm diameter (TURNER 1986). **B** Helical coil antenna designed for operation at 915 MHz (SATOH et al. 1988). The coaxial cable is 0.95 mm in diameter and the coil, wound from 0.32 mm diameter nichrome wire, has 35 turns with 1 mm pitch and is less than 1.2 mm in outer diameter. **C** Dipole antenna modified by the addition of quarter-wavelength choke sections over both proximal and distal sections (RYAN et al. 1990). **D** Three-node antenna (LEE et al. 1986) in which sections of the outer conductor of 0.95 mm diameter coaxial cable are removed, leaving the dielectric and inner conductor

The dependence of the SAR distribution on insertion depth for arrays of dipole antennas has been studied both experimentally and theoretically (CHAN et al. 1989; DENMAN et al. 1988; JAMES et al. 1989; ZHANG et al. 1991b; MECHLING et al. 1992). For example, in the case of 2 × 2 arrays of 915 MHz antennas with 2 cm spacing, a local region of high SAR on the central axis of the array can be expected to move and elongate, then break into two separate hot spots and finally return to a single hot spot near the junction plane as the insertion depth is increased. This behaviour can be explained in terms of basic transmission line models. The current on the antennas is zero at the antenna tips and at multiples of the resonant half-wavelength along the antennas whilst the charge distribution has maxima at these positions. Current maxima and charge minima will occur at positions one-quarter of the resonant wavelength away from these positions. Reflection occurs at the insertion point due to the large impedance change across the tissue-air interface and leads to heating in this area when the insertion depth is small. For large insertion depths the current is approximately zero at the insertion points of the antennas. When h_B is much greater than a quarter wavelength, the current near to the insertion point decreases, leading to a reduction in the hot spot in that area. SAR maxima at the surface of the antennas are associated with charge maxima whilst SAR maxima in the central region of the array arise predominantly from the current maxima. As the antenna is inserted deeper into tissue and h_B is increased, additional current and charge maxima occur on the proximal section and so corresponding SAR maxima are to be expected in this region; the current and charge distribution on the distal part of the antennas (h_A) remain essentially unchanged. The relative impedances of the proximal and distal sections of the antenna change with insertion depth, resulting in different currents on the antenna sections and consequently changes in SAR distribution.

Table 6.1. Characteristics of microwave interstitial hyperthermia (IHT) techniques

Advantages	Disadvantages
- May be used with plastic catheters - Strict parallelism between implanted antennas not required - Control of individual antennas - Significant power deposition at greater radial distances than other IHT techniques (leading to a more robust performance in the presence of high perfusion or the possibility of using a lower density of heat sources) - Coherently driven arrays offer SAR steering through phase/amplitude control - Several types of antenna available as part of commercial hyperthermia systems (although some antenna/catheter combinations are not necessarily optimised)	- SAR distribution along antennas difficult to adjust (for constant insertion depth) - SAR distribution is dependent upon insertion depth (but in a predictable manner) for some antennas - Recommended thermometry is by relatively expensive fibre-optic based systems

6.4 Other Types of Antenna

In view of some perceived disadvantages of dipole antennas (such as reduced heating at the tip and dependence of SAR distribution upon insertion depth), other antenna designs such as multinode antennas (antenna D, Fig. 6.3) (Lee et al. 1986), sleeved antennas (Lin and Wang 1987) and several types of helical coil antenna (Wu et al. 1987; Satoh and Stauffer 1988) have been proposed. Comparative measurements of antenna types have been reported by Ryan (1991) and Sathiaseelan et al. (1991).

The helical coil antennas are based on a helical winding positioned over the distal section of a semi-rigid coaxial cable along which the outer conductor has been removed (antenna B, Fig. 6.3). Performance is dependent upon the operating frequency, pitch of the helix and the manner in which the helix is connected to the coaxial cable. Satoh and Stauffer (1988) and Satoh et al. (1988) describe antennas operating at 2450 MHz and 915 MHz, respectively; a construction in which the helical coil was connected to the central conductor at the antenna tip and with a gap of approximately 1 mm between the proximal end of the coil and the outer conductor of the co-axial cable resulted in a marked shift of the heated volume toward the antenna tip and independence of the heating pattern from the insertion depth. These authors' results also suggested that the heating patterns for helical coil antennas were more cylindrical than the ellipsoidal patterns associated with conventional dipole antennas.

Sathiaseelan et al. (1991) and Ryan (1991) also describe SAR distributions associated with 915-MHz helical coil applicators. For single applicators, the peak SAR occurs close to the tip and the distance along the antenna over which SAR is equal to or greater than 50% of the peak value is slightly less than the length of the distal section. The distribution is fairly insensitive to insertion depth. Ryan (1991) observed heating beyond the tip when the antenna was placed in a close-fitting catheter. In the case of a 2×2 array with 2 cm spacing, the SAR distribution along the central axis of the array shows a peak at approximately midway between the junction and the tip. Although the position of the peak relative to the antennas changes little, the SAR distribution tends to elongate with increasing depth. The SAR in the central region of transverse planes relative to that near antennas is less for helical coil applicators than for dipole applicators. Sathiaseelan et al. (1991) claim that a "satisfactory heating length" of approximately 60%–70% of the insertion length may be expected along the axial direction of the array.

6.5 Summary

Some advantages and disadvantages of microwave interstitial hyperthermia are summarised in Table 6.1. A similar summary in which all interstitial hyperthermia techniques are compared has been compiled by Stauffer (1990).

References

Casey JP, Bansal R (1986) The near field of an insulated dipole in a dissipative dielectric medium. IEEE Trans Microwave Theory Tech 34: 459–463

Chan KW, Chou CK, McDougall JA, Luk KH, Vora NL, Forell BW (1989) Changes in heating patterns of interstitial microwave antenna arrays at different insertion depths. Int J Hyperthermia 5: 499–507

Denman DL, Foster AE, Cooper Lewis G et al. (1988) The distribution of power and heat produced by interstitial microwave antenna arrays: II. The role of antenna spacing and insertion depth. Int J Radiat Oncol Biol Phys 14: 537–545

de Sieyes DC, Douple EB, Strohbehn JW, Trembly BS (1981) Some aspects of optimization of an invasive microwave antenna for local hyperthermia treatment of cancer. Med Phys 8: 174–183

Eppert V, Trembly BS, Richter HJ (1991) Air cooling for an interstitial microwave array hyperthermia antenna: theory and experiment. IEEE Trans Biomed Eng 38: 450–460

Furse CM, Iskander MF (1989) Three-dimensional electromagnetic power deposition in tumors using interstitial antenna arrays. IEEE Trans Biomed Eng 36: 977–986

Hürter W, Reinbold F, Lorenz WJ (1991) A dipole antenna for interstitial microwave hyperthermia. IEEE Trans Microwave Theory Tech 39: 1048–1054

Iskander MF, Tumeh AM (1989) Design optimization of interstitial antennas. IEEE Trans Biomed Eng 36: 238–246

James BJ, Strohbehn JW, Mechling JA, Trembly BS (1989) The effect of insertion depth on the theoretical SAR patterns of 915 MHz dipole antenna arrays for hyperthermia. Int J Hyperthermia 5: 733–747

Jones KM, Mechling JA, Trembly BS, Strohbehn JW (1988) SAR distributions for 915 MHz interstitial microwave antennas used in hyperthermia for cancer therapy. IEEE Trans Biomed Eng 35: 851–857

Jones KM, Mechling JA, Strohbehn JW, Trembly BS (1989) Theoretical and experimental SAR distributions for interstitial dipole arrays used in hyperthermia. IEEE Trans Microwave Theory Tech 37: 1200–1209

King RWP, Shen LC, Wu TT (1981) Embedded insulated antennas for communication and heating. Electromagnetics 1: 115–117

King RWP, Trembly BS, Strohbehn JW (1983) Electromagnetic field of an insulated antenna in a conducting or dielectric medium. IEEE Trans Microwave Theory Tech 31: 574–583

Lee DJ, O'Neill MJ, Lam KS, Rostock R, Lam WC (1986) A new design of microwave interstitial applicators for hyperthermia with improved treatment volume. Int J Radiat Oncol Biol Phys 12: 2003–2008

Lin JC, Wang YJ (1987) Interstitial microwave antennas for thermal therapy. Int J Hyperthermia 3: 37–47

Mechling JA, Strohbehn JW, Ryan TP (1992) Three-dimensional theoretical temperature distributions produced by 915 MHz dipole antenna arrays with varying insertion depths in muscle tissue. Int J Radiat Oncol Biol Phys 22: 131–138

Roos D, Hugander A (1988) Microwave interstitial applicators with improved longitudinal heating patterns. Int J Hyperthermia 4: 609–615

Ryan TP (1991) Comparison of six microwave antennas for hyperthermia treatment of cancer: SAR results for single antennas and arrays. Int J Radiat Oncol Biol Phys 21: 403–413

Ryan TP, Mechling JA, Strohbehn JW (1990) Absorbed power deposition for various insertion depths for 915 MHz interstitial dipole antenna arrays: experiment versus theory. Int J Radiat Oncol Biol Phys 19: 377–387

Ryan TP, Hoopes PJ, Taylor JH, Strohbehn JW, Roberts DW, Douple EB, Coughlin CT (1991) Experimental brain hyperthermia: techniques for heat delivery and thermometry. Int J Radiat Oncol Biol Phys 20: 739–750

Samaras GM (1984) Intracranial microwave hyperthermia: heat induction and temperature control. IEEE Trans Biomed Eng 31: 63–69

Sathiaseelan V, Leybovich L, Emami MS, Stauffer P, Straube W (1991) Characteristics of improved microwave interstitial antennas for local hyperthermia. Int J Radiat Oncol Biol Phys 20: 531–539

Satoh T, Stauffer PR (1988) Implantable helical coil microwave antenna for interstitial hyperthermia. Int J Hyperthermia 4: 497–512

Satoh T, Stauffer PR, Fike JR (1988) Thermal distribution studies of helical coil microwave antennas for interstitial hyperthermia. Int J Radiat Oncol Biol Phys 15: 1209–1218

Stauffer PR (1990) Techniques for interstitial hyperthermia. In: Field SB, Hand JW (eds) An introduction to the practical aspects of clinical hyperthermia. Taylor & Francis, London, p 344

Taylor LS (1978) Electromagnetic syringe. IEEE Trans Biomed Eng 25: 303–304

Trembly BS (1985) The effects of driving frequency and antenna length on power deposition within a microwave antenna array used for hyperthermia. IEEE Trans Biomed Eng 32: 152–157

Trembly BS, Wilson AH, Sullivan MJ, Stein AD, Wong TZ, Strohbehn JW (1986) Control of the SAR pattern within an interstitial microwave array through variation of antenna driving phase. IEEE Trans Microwave Theory Tech 34: 568–571

Trembly BS, Douple EB, Hoopes PJ (1991) The effect of air cooling on the radial temperature distribution of a single microwave hyperthermia antenna in vivo. Int J Hyperthermia 7: 343–354

Tumeh AM, Iskander MF (1989) Performance comparison of available interstitial antennas for microwave hyperthermia. IEEE Trans Microwave Theory Tech 37: 1126–1133

Turner PF (1986) Interstitial equal-phased arrays for EM hyperthermia. IEEE Trans Microwave Theory Tech 34: 572–578

Wu A, Watson ML, Sternick ES, Bielawa RJ, Carr KL (1987) Performance characteristics of a helical coil microwave interstitial antenna for local hyperthermia. Med Phys 14: 235–237

Zhang Y, Dubal NV, Takemoto-Hambleton R, Joines WT (1988) The determination of the electromagnetic field and SAR pattern of an interstitial applicator in a dissipative medium. IEEE Trans Microwave Theory Tech 36: 1438–1443

Zhang Y, Joines WT, Oleson JR (1990a) The calculated and measured temperature distribution of a phased interstitial antenna array. IEEE Trans Microwave Theory Tech 38: 69–77

Zhang Y, Joines WT, Oleson JR (1990b) Microwave hyperthermia induced by a phased interstitial antenna array. IEEE Trans Microwave Theory Tech 38: 217–221

Zhang Y, Joines WT, Oleson JR (1991a) Heating patterns generated by phase modulation of a hexagonal array of interstitial antennas. IEEE Trans Biomed Eng 38: 92–97

Zhang Y, Joines WT, Oleson JR (1991b) Prediction of heating patterns of a microwave interstitial array at various insertion depths. Int J Hyperthermia 7: 197–207

7 Ferromagnetic Techniques for Interstitial Hyperthermia

J.D.P VAN DIJK, N. VAN WIERINGEN, G.J. NIEUWENHUYS, F. KOENIS, and C. KOEDOODER

CONTENTS

7.1 Introduction

An interesting hot source technique without the need of external temperature regulation consists in the implantation of tissue by ferromagnetic needles in combination with the use of an externally applied radiofrequency magnetic field. This technique for inducing hyperthermia in tumors has been under investigation since about 1982 at several centers.

The principle that within an oscillating magnetic field a metallic implant will be heated by Eddy currents is well known. The special feature of this hyperthermia technique arises from the application of metallic implants made of ferromagnetic alloys. These alloys have the property that they change from the ferromagnetic to the nonmagnetic state at the Curie point. This point indicates a temperature, the Curie temperature (T_c), at which the Eddy current heating decreases drastically. This means that the temperature of the tissue surrounding such a ferromagnetic needle will increase until the alloy reaches its Curie point. Then the power production of the seeds stops and the temperatures will stabilize. In this way internal self-regulating temperature stabilization and temperature control are obtained. Furthermore, the independent self-regulation of the temperature in each seed opens up the possibility of delivering more heat in tissue regions with relatively strong cooling, e.g., by blood flow, thus improving the homogeneity of the temperature distribution.

J.D.P VAN DIJK, Ph.D.; N. VAN WIERINGEN, M.Sc.; F. KOENIS, M.Sc.; C. KOEDOODER, Ph.D.; Department of Radiotherapy, Amsterdam University Hospital, Academisch Medisch Centrum, Meibergdreef 9, NL-1105 AZ Amsterdam Z.O., The Netherlands.
G.J. NIEUWENHUYS, Ph.D., Kamerlingh Onnes Laboratory, Leiden State University, Nieuwsteeg 18, NL-2311 SB Leiden, The Netherlands.

7.2 Principles of Operation

7.2.1 *Selective Seed Heating*

Alternating magnetic fields will also heat tissues directly by inducing Eddy currents within the tissues. Since the goal is to localize the heating to the implanted region the power absorption by the implant material should be enhanced whereas direct tissue heating should be reduced. Expressions have been developed (STAUFFER et al. 1984) for the absorbed power density in tissues (Eq. 1) and in cylindrical ferromagnetic implants (Eq. 2) resulting from magnetic field induced Eddy current heating. Figure 7.1 shows a cross-section of a patient inside a coil with some of the parameters used in these expressions. In the case of Eddy current heating in tissue

$$P_T = (\omega^2 \mu_T^2 r^2 \sigma_T H_0^2/8) \times 10^{-6}\ \mathrm{W/cm^3} \qquad (1)$$

is the power absorbed in 1 cm^3 of tissue at an electrical conductivity σ_T and a permeability μ_T. It has been assumed that this volume of tissue is located at a distance r from the center of the dielectric tissue mass which has been placed in a magnetic field of strength H_0 and frequency ω. Similarly,

$$P_I = \pi a (\omega\mu/(2\sigma))^{1/2}\ H_0^2 \times 10^{-2}\ \mathrm{W/cm^3} \qquad (2)$$

represents the power absorbed by a 1-cm-long cylindrical implant of radius a, permeability μ, and

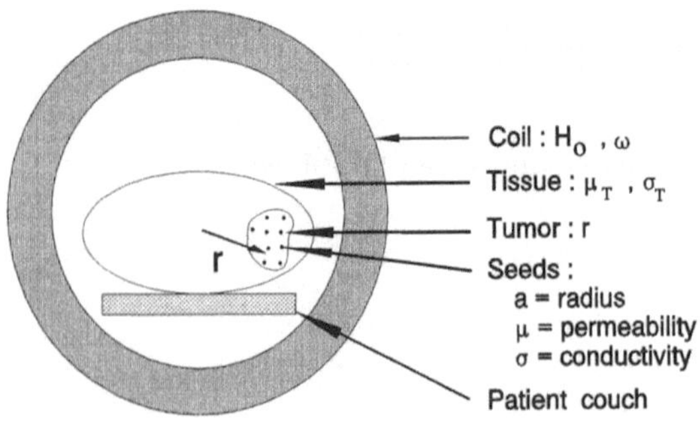

Fig. 7.1. Cross-section of a patient inside a coil. Some parameters of eqs 1 and 2 are explained

electrical conductivity σ, normalized to 1 cm^3 of tissue. If practical values are used for the different parameters in these equations it appears that heating of the implants predominates at frequencies below 2 MHz and direct tissue absorption predominates above 10 MHz (ATKINSON et al. 1984). In most of the recent studies on ferromagnetic seeds, a frequency in the range between 50 and 250 kHz has been used, which provides adequate heating of the seeds. The ferromagnetic seeds heat tissue by thermal conduction and by convection of heat radially from the implanted sources, which makes their use a typical "hot source" technique.

7.2.2 *Self-regulating Thermoseeds*

As stated above, a special feature of self-regulating seeds derives from the application of ferromagnetic materials, e.g., nickel and iron. In their pure form none of these metals have a Curie temperature in the hyperthermic temperature range. Lower values for T_c can be obtained by addition of alloy metals. The preparation of seeds using various combinations of two metallic elements has been investigated extensively. Reports on the preparation of seeds composed of Ni–Si (CHEN et al. 1988), Ni–Cu (BREZOVICH et al. 1984) or Ni–Pd (BURTON et al. 1971; KOBAYASHI et al. 1986; Meijer et al. 1993) have been presented. Variations in the Curie temperature of a seed can be obtained by adjusting the mass ratio of the two metals of which the seed is composed. For clinical applications the transition of the alloys from the ferromagnetic to the non-magnetic state should be as sharp as possible. Only a sharp transition will result in a temperature leveling at the correct temperature and proper self-regulation of each seed, which improves the homogeneity of the temperature distribution inside the tumor. Examples of the magnetic susceptibility as a function of temperature of cylindrical PdNi26.0 (26 atomic % Ni) and PdNi27.0 (27 atomic % Ni) seeds at a length of 1.0 cm are shown in Fig. 7.2.

7.2.3 *Power Absorption Efficiency*

In comparison with other hot source techniques ferromagnetic seeds do not require external connections. In addition they can be used at any length. The power production is maximal if the longitudinal axis of the seeds is aligned to the magnetic field. In clinical practice this alignment

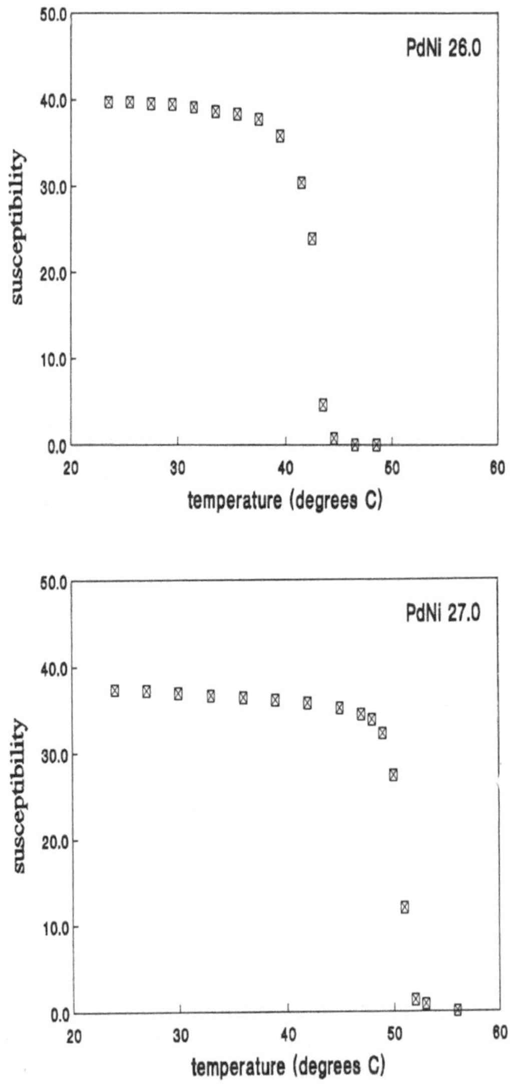

Fig. 7.2. The magnetic susceptibility as a function of temperature of cylindrical PdNi26.0 (upper graph) and PdNi27.0 (lower graph) seeds at a length of 1.0 cm

cannot always be accomplished completely. HAIDER et al. (1991) have shown that angles up to 20° are only slightly less effective and that orientations up to 45° can be compensated by increased field strength if more generator power is available. They also found that optimum power absorption of a cylindrical implant per unit volume occurs when the induction number (i.e., $\sqrt{2}*a/\delta$ with a = implant radius and δ = skin depth) is 2.5. This makes it possible to increase the power absorption in implants by using an appropriate number of implants with optimal diameter to fit into the same area as the original solid implant. As an example HAIDER showed that a four-filament (diameter of a filament = 0.46 mm) stranded implant absorbed 76% more heat than a solid implant (diameter = 1 mm) under similar conditions. Both implants were 96% Ni and 4% Si and came from the same batch.

7.3 Temperature Distribution

7.3.1 Some Aspects of Influence on the Temperature Distribution

As is typical for a hot source technique, the tissue is exclusively heated by thermal conduction. Therefore the temperature homogeneity and the minimum tumor temperature depend strongly on the seed spacing (MECHLING and STROHBEHN 1986; PALIWAL et al. 1989). MATLOUBIEH et al. (1984) showed, at various blood flow rates, that ferromagnetic seeds give a more homogeneous temperature distribution than constant power seeds. Constant power seeds have no transition point, but absorb a fixed amount of energy in a magnetic field with a given field strength regardless of the temperature of the seeds. Adjustment of the field strength will change the absorbed power of all seeds in an implant array at the same time. In both cases, however (i.e., for constant power seeds as well as ferromagnetic seeds), the temperature drops rapidly with increasing distance from the seed. This makes relatively dense implants necessary to obtain acceptable temperature homogeneity and sufficient minimum temperature in the center of an array of seeds. Furthermore, near the ends of a seed the heat is conducted from the seed axially as well as radially. This causes the temperature to decrease from the center of the seed to its end (CHIN et al. 1991). MATLOUBIEH et al. (1984) suggested that in order to compensate for this the ferromagnetic seed implant array should extend beyond the tumor boundary. BREZOVICH et al. (1984b) also showed the flexibility of the system by suggesting that seeds with a high Curie temperature be placed at the center of the tumor and seeds with a low Curie temperature at the periphery to assure destruction of the tumor core without damaging vital structures at the tumor margin. Another solution to this problem is to break the seed into smaller segments. By placing segments with a higher Curie temperature at the ends of the implant the steeper temperature gradient at these positions can be corrected.

7.3.2 Measurement and Calculation of the Temperature Distribution

Accurate knowledge of tissue temperature is necessary for effective delivery of clinical hyperthermia. To achieve this a pretreatment planning model and precise thermometry are needed. The conditions and requirements for thermometry are similar to those for other interstitial hyperthermia techniques. Some extra information is provided by the fact that the maximum temperature that can be reached inside the tumor is already known (the Curie temperature). As the described technique is a typical hot source technique (there is no direct energy absorption by tissue), there is no need to calculate the field penetration and power deposition in the tumor area in the pretreatment planning model. Temperature distributions calculated with two-dimensional models have been reported by various authors (BREZOVICH et al. 1984a; MATLOUBIEH et al. 1984; MECHLING and STROHBEHN 1986; PALIWAL et al. 1989). Figure 7.3 represents calculated isothermal contours in a plane perpendicular to a 2 × 2 implant array of seeds with T_c = 48°C and a diameter of 1 mm, implant spacing of 10 and 14.4 mm and a perfusion rate of $2.5 \cdot 10^{-6}$ m^3/kg·s. In these computations, which are based on the bioheat transfer equation using finite element techniques, the seed surface is maintained at its Curie temperature at steady state. The influence of the seed spacing on the temperature distribution is obvious. Increasing the distance between the seeds results in a decrease in temperature homogeneity and in the minimum tumor temperature. In the RTOG quality assurance guidelines for interstitial hyperthermia (EMAMI et al. 1991), an interseed spacing of 10–13 mm is recommended. These values agree with the spacings that have been used for

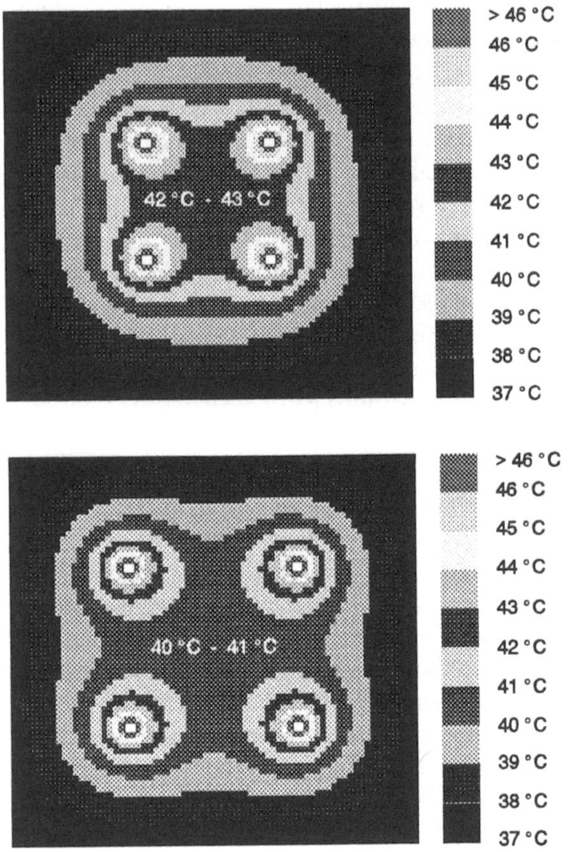

Fig. 7.3. Calculated steady-state isotherm contours in a plane perpendicular to a 2 × 2 implant array with $T_c = 48°C$ and perfusion rate $2.5 \cdot 10^{-6}$ m^3/kg·s in both cases. The seed spacing is 10 mm (upper plot) and 14.4 mm (lower plot), the seeds are indicated by white squares

patient treatments (Stea et al. 1990). Recently temperature distributions as calculated with three-dimensional models have been reported (Chen et al. 1991; Chin and Stauffer 1991). In their model Chen et al. included an empirical power absorption formula developed by Haider et al. (1991) to calculate the seed power absorption as a function of the seed temperature. A comparison of the results of two- and three-dimensional models shows that two-dimensional models overestimate the temperature distribution generated by finite length seeds, since the inherent assumption for two-dimensional models is that of an infinitely long seed. Two-dimensional models are found to be accurate in predicting the temperature distribution up to 1 cm from the ends of the seed.

7.4 Some Clinical Considerations

A schematic drawing of a clinical setup is shown in Fig. 7.4. In recent years, some clinical investigations and (phase I) trials have been reported by Au et al. (1989), Stea et al. (1990), Brezovich et al. (1990), Meredith et al. (1989) and Kobayashi et al. (1991). In these studies no major acute or long-term side-effects were encountered. Measurements during treatments have shown that the tumor temperature can be raised to a therapeutic level. It also appeared that the seed spacing indeed strongly influences the achieved temperatures.

In a phase I/II clinical trial, Stea et al. (1990) showed that 53% of the sensor points, which were located at the center as well as in the periphery of the tumor, reached a temperature ≥ 42°C when the seed spacing was in the range 1.0–1.2 cm. Only 13% of the sensor points reached this temperature if the seed spacing was 1.5 cm. They also analyzed the temperature distribution within the target volume. Only 39% of the sensors located at the

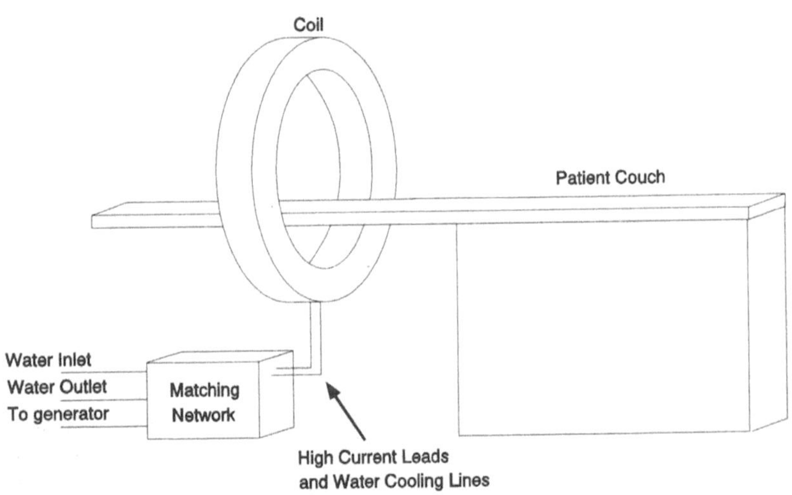

Fig. 7.4. Schematic drawing of a clinical setup (after example of setup as used in the University of Arizona, Tucson)

outermost 1 cm shell of the implant volume (highly perfused areas of the tumor) achieved a temperature $\geq 42\,°C$, whereas 89% of the sensors located in the center of the implant achieved this temperature.

Although clinical trials have been limited to removable implants until now, this technique offers the possibility of permanent implantation. BREZOVICH et al. (1990) studied the problem of seed migration and chemical toxicity in healthy rats and pet animals. They found that especially seed migration cannot yet be well controlled. These problems do not occur when the seeds are placed in removable catheters. This also allows convenient combination with interstitial radiation.

References

Atkinson JA, Brezovich IA, Chakraborty DP (1984) Usable frequencies in hyperthermia with thermal seeds. IEEE Trans Biomed Eng 31: 70–75

Au KS, Cetas TC, Shimm DS et al. (1989) Interstitial ferromagnetic hyperthermia and brachytherapy: preliminary report of a phase I clinical trial. Endocurie/Hyperthermia Oncol 5: 127–136

Brezovich IA, Atkinson WJ, Chakraborty DP (1984a) Temperature distributions in tumor models heated by selfregulating nickel-copper alloy thermoseeds. Med Phys 11: 145–152

Brezovich IA, Atkinson WJ, Lilly MB (1984b) Local hyperthermia with interstitial techniques. Cancer Res [suppl] 44: 4752s–4756s

Brezovich IA, Lilly MB, Meredith RF, Weppelmann B, Henderson RA, Brawner W, Salter MM (1990) Hyperthermia of pet animal tumours with self-regulating ferromagnetic thermoseeds. Int J Hyperthermia 6: 117–130

Burton C, Hill M, Walker AE (1971) The RF thermoseed – A thermally self-regulating implant for the production of brain lesions. IEEE Trans Biomed Eng 18: 104–109

Chen JS, Poirier DR, Damento MA, Demer LJ, Biancaniello F, Cetas TC (1988) Development of Ni-4 wt.% Si thermoseeds for hyperthermia cancer treatment. J. Biomed Mater Res 22: 303–319

Chen ZP, Roemer BB, Cetas TC (1991) Errors in the two-dimensional simulation of ferromagnetic implant hyperthermia. Int J Hyperthermia 7: 735–739

Chin RB, Stauffer PR (1991) Treatment planning for ferromagnetic seed heating. Int J Radiat Oncol Biol 21: 431–439

Emami B, Stauffer, P, Dewhirst MW et al. (1991) RTOG quality assurance guidelines for interstitial hyperthermia. Int J Radiat Oncol Biol Phys 20: 1117–1124

Haider SA, Chen JS, Wait JR, Cetas TC (1991) Power absorption in ferromagnetic implants from radio frequency magnetic fields and the problem of optimization. IEEE Trans Microwave Theory Tech 39: 1817–1827

Kobayashi T, Kida Y, Tanaka T, Kageyama N, Kobayashi H (1986) Magnetic induction hyperthermia for brain tumors using ferromagnetic implants with low Curie temperature. J Neurooncol 4: 175–181

Matloubieh AY, Roemer RB, Cetas TC (1984) Numerical simulation of magnetic induction heating of tumors with ferromagnetic seed implants. IEEE Trans Biomed Eng 31: 227–234

Mechling JA, Strohbehn JW (1986) A theoretical comparison of the temperature distributions produced by three interstitial hyperthermia systems. Int J Radiat Oncol Biol Phys 12: 2137–2149

Meijer JG, van Wieringen N, Koedooder C, Nieuwenhuys GJ, van Dijk JDP (1993) The development of thermoseeds for interstitial hyperthermia. Unpublished work.

Meredith RF, Brezovich IA, Weppelmann B et al. (1989) Ferromagnetic thermoseeds: suitable for an afterloading interstitial implant. Int J Radiat Oncol Biol Phys 17: 1341–1346

Paliwal BR, Wang GB, Wakai RT et al. (1989) A pretreatment planning model for ferromagnetic hyperthermia. Endocurie/Hyperthermia Oncol 5: 215–220

Stauffer PR, Cetas TC, Jones RC (1990) Magnetic induction heating of ferromagnetic implants for inducing localized hyperthermia in deep-seated tumors. IEEE Trans Biomed Eng 31: 235–251

Stea B, Cetas TC, Cassady R et al. (1989) Interstitial thermoradiotherapy of brain tumors: preliminary results of a phase I clinical trial. Int J Radiat Oncol Biol Phys 19: 1463–1471

8 Ultrasound Technology for Interstitial Hyperthermia

C.J. DIEDERICH and K.H. HYNYNEN

CONTENTS

8.1 Rationale for Ultrasound Interstitial Heating

Interstitial methods are most often used for treating bulky or unresectable deep-seated tumors or sites which are difficult to reach by external methods in the pelvis, intra-abdominal, and head and neck regions. Despite the invasive nature of the techniques, interstitial heating remains a treatment of choice for many tumors since the heating sources are inserted directly into the tumor, thereby localizing the heating to the target volume and sparing more of the surrounding normal tissue. Currently radiofrequency local current field (RF-LCF) electrodes, coaxial cable mounted microwave antennas, inductively heated ferromagnetic seeds, resistance wire, and hot water tubes are used for interstitial hyperthermia (STAUFFER 1990; SEEGENSCHMIEDT et al. 1991; COUGHLIN and STROHBEHN 1989). Although efficacious in many clinical situations, none of these methods (except hot sources) allows the power deposition to be easily varied along the length of the implant during the course of a treatment to account for heterogeneities in tumor structure and dynamic changes in blood perfusion. This is a critical problem, since in order to offer the best chances for a good clinical response, the whole tumor and tumor margins must be heated to therapeutic levels (GIBBS et al. 1981; DEWHIRST et al. 1984), with a steep transition to lower temperatures in the surrounding normal tissue region. In addition, these technologies require that the heating catheters be < 1–2 cm apart, and are often sensitive to the alignment and interaction of neighboring sources. This necessitates that a large number of catheters be implanted, and of these most will be used for heating purposes, leaving few for temperature monitoring and control of the treatment.

Ultrasound interstitial applicators, consisting of tubular radiators ≤ 2 mm OD (outer diameter), have the potential to be more effective for delivering interstitial hyperthermia than the above-mentioned techniques. The possible advantages of implantable ultrasound sources over other interstitial heating techniques can be summarized as follows:

1. Due to the better penetration of ultrasound energy in tissues, the catheters may be spaced further apart and require fewer needle insertions for a given implant volume.
2. Control of power to each individual tubular element of a multielement applicator will allow the tissue temperature to be controlled along the length of each catheter.
3. The power deposition pattern is not dependent on the length of insertion or placement with regard to other catheters in the implant.
4. The sources are amenable to the addition of a circulating system to control the temperature of the catheter/tissue interface, which would increase the radial depth of therapeutic heating from each source by forcing the maximum temperature away from the catheter surface.

Depending on the application, the length and/or number of transducer segments in each applicator can be varied to accommodate different size implant volumes and the required resolution of temperature control.

C.J. DIEDERICH, M.D., University of California, San Francisco, Radiation Oncology Department, San Francisco, CA 94143-0226, USA

K. H. HYNYNEN, M.D., University of Arizona Health Sciences Center, Radiation Oncology Department, 1501 North Campbell Avenue, Tucson, AZ 85724, USA

8.2 Interstitial Ultrasound Applicators

8.2.1 Cylindrical Transducers

Currently two types of interstitial ultrasound applicator are being developed: The first type consists of a multielement array of tubular piezoceramic transducers (≤ 2 mm OD, 4–9 MHz) (Diederich and Hynynen 1990a; Hynynen 1992), as depicted by a simplified diagram in Fig. 8.1a. The transducers are resonant across the wall thickness, radiating energy in the radial direction. The ultrasound field can be made fairly uniform along the longitudinal surface and collimated within the axial extent. The power level to each segment is controlled separately and can be varied during a treatment. The RF power lines (small diameter wire) to each element are within the lumen of the transducers and connected to microcoax cables at the exit of the catheter. For transmission of energy into the tissue, some type of coupling media must be inserted in between the applicator and the catheter wall. This is normally degassed water, which is either standing or circulated in order to control the temperature and provide a better heating distribution. This configuration (segmented tubular radiators and cooling) has evolved from previous work on intracavitary applicators using tubular radiators from 3 mm to 15 mm OD, which has illustrated the utility of this approach (Diederich and Hynynen 1989, 1990b).

The simplified schematic drawing of the segmented arrays underemphasizes the technical challenges required to develop these applicators. The most problematic design constraint imposed on these applicators is the OD. The device must be less than ≈ 1.8 mm OD to be compatible with current flexible brachytherapy afterloading catheters, which range in size from 1.5 to 1.8 mm ID and from 2.0 to 2.2 mm OD.

Another design constraint is on the wall thickness; the lumen must be sufficiently large that the RF power lines for all elements and cooling tubes (depending on cooling strategy) will fit inside. For thickness resonant cylinders, the wall thickness is $\lambda_T/2$, which is 0.4 mm at 5 MHz for PZT-4 material. λ_T is the wavelength in the transducer material at the fundamental frequency, which is 4 mm at 1 MHz for the PZT-4 material (3.78 mm for the PZT-5 material) and is inversely proportional to frequency. For a practical lumen size of 1 mm, the minimum OD of a cylinder resonant at 5 MHz is 1.8 mm. This dictates that the usable or practical frequency range starts at 4–5 MHz, depending on the OD and the number of elements (wiring limitations) in each applicator, with an upper limit imposed by decreased penetration of the higher frequencies and fragile nature of thin wall tubes.

The length of each individual segment is constrained to be $\geq 10\lambda_t$, where λ_t is the wavelength in tissue, to ensure that the beams are collimated (Diederich and Hynynen 1990b). ($\lambda_t \approx 1500\ \text{m s}^{-1}$/frequency for soft tissues, so for a 5-MHz tube the length must be 3 mm or greater.) Otherwise, the

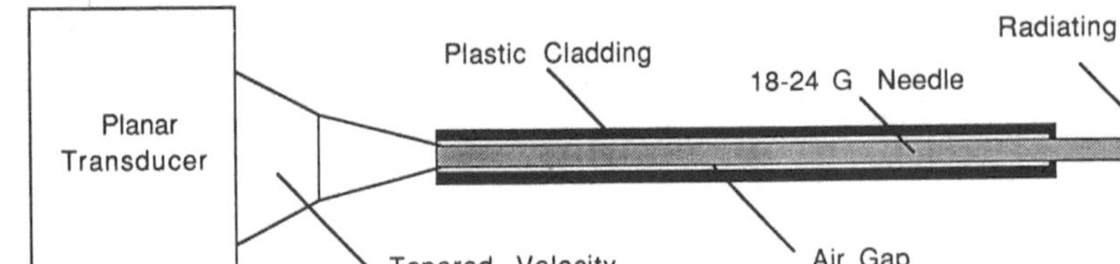

a

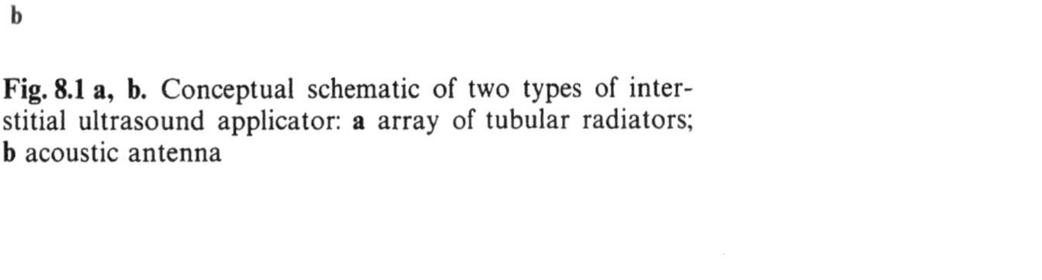

b

Fig. 8.1 a, b. Conceptual schematic of two types of interstitial ultrasound applicator: **a** array of tubular radiators; **b** acoustic antenna number of elements and lengths can be varied for each applicator to achieve the required adjustability of power deposition along the implant length (i.e., shorter elements provide a finer resolution in power control).

8.2.2 Acoustic Antennas

The second design utilizes an 18 to 24-G stainless-steel needle coupled to a small piezoelectric planar disk transducer (1.3 cm OD 1.024 MHz) by a variable-tapered conical velocity transformer (JAROSZ 1990, 1991), as shown in Fig. 8.1b. A plastic shroud over the proximal portion of the implant needle encapsulates an air gap to prevent the energy from being radiated except from the short unclad portion at the tip. The radiating portion can be adjusted in length by repositioning the plastic sleeve along the needle.

An advantage of this design is that applicators of less than 2 mm OD can be driven at lower frequencies (1 MHz), since the OD is determined by the air-backed plastic cladding, which is designed to conform tightly to the needle. A possible limitation on this design is the maximum output power of the driving piezoelectric element and the efficiency of energy transfer to the radiating tip. Due to the lower tissue absorption and increased radial penetration of energy at these lower frequencies, more acoustic output power will be required per length of radiator than for the higher frequency multielement devices. The maximum power level may also be limited by the mechanical properties of the applicator, where the stresses required for the large particle displacements could exceed the limits of elasticity of the needle or taper. A disadvantage is that there is no control of the power deposition along the length of the radiating portion, which is constrained to the tip.

8.3 Performance Characteristics

8.3.1 Experimental Studies

Experimental evaluations have been performed on a prototype applicator consisting of a single 1.0 mm OD piezoelectric tube, 25 mm long, resonating at 9.5 MHz (HYNYNEN 1992). The transducer was air backed, sealed with silicone adhesive, and electrically matched as previously described for multielement applicators. The ultrasound field measurements in degassed water (a non-attenuating medium) indicated that the beam energy was well collimated and fairly uniform within the axial extent of the cylinder (Fig. 8.2). The same characteristic pattern resulted when the applicator was inserted into an implant catheter with degassed water for coupling. This implies that these transducers can apply a well-defined energy pattern into the adjacent tissue region along the entire length, including the edges. Experiments using implant arrays with four single transducer applicators, spaced 2 cm apart in in vitro perfused dog liver and kidney preparations (HOLMES et al. 1984), have verified that enough acoustic power can be generated through a catheter wall to produce therapeutic temperature rises (Fig. 8.3) (HYNYNEN 1992). Tem-

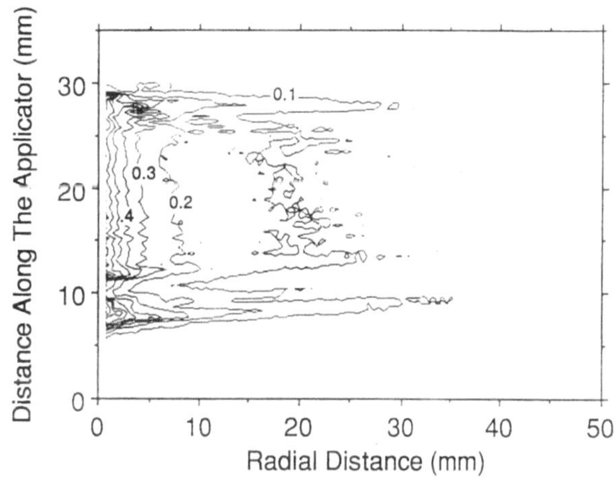

Fig. 8.2. Relative pressure squared distribution in water from a 1 mm OD, 25-mm-long piezoceramic tube at 9, 5 MHz

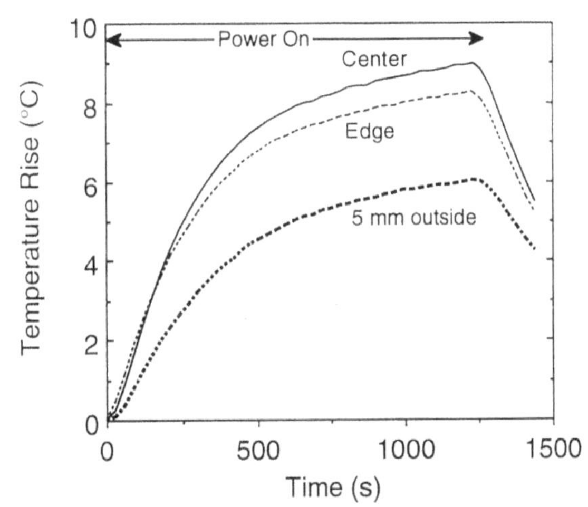

Fig. 8.3. Transient temperature rises measured within a 2 ×2, 2 cm spaced implant (single transducer ultrasound applicators within catheters) in a perfused liver preparation

peratures measured within the perfused liver preparation were maintained at 7°–8°C above ambient within the boundaries of the implant and 5°C above ambient at 5 mm outside the boundary, with an initial heating rate of 1.2°C/min.

The ultrasound field distributions from the acoustic antenna applicators have also been shown to be well collimated within the bounds of the active surface, but exhibited an axial standing wave pattern with a period of approximately 2.2 mm (JAROSZ 1991). These peaks are close enough together that in most cases thermal smearing will spatially average the effect of these variations to produce a uniform temperature distribution in the axial dimension. Peak heating rates (1.1°C/min) and transient curves, similar to those measured for the cylindrical transducer applicators, have been reported for single applicators in a static in vitro muscle tissue sample (JAROSZ 1990).

8.3.2 Theoretical Evaluation

The heating characteristics of these applicators can be evaluated by using computer simulation programs to calculate the acoustic fields and the corresponding thermal distributions of cylindrical ultrasound sources embedded in tissue (DIEDERICH and HYNYNEN 1989, 1990b). The acoustic intensity (I) distribution of these cylindrical sources can be approximated by the following expression:

$$I = \frac{I_0 r_0}{r} e^{-2\alpha f (r - r_0)}, \tag{1}$$

where I_0 is the intensity at the transducer surface, r_0 is the radius of the transducer, r is the radial distance from the center of the transducer, α is the amplitude attenuation coefficient, and f is the frequency. The intensity distribution of an applicator surrounded by a catheter wall can be calculated by assuming r_0 is the outer radius of the catheter. An attenuation coefficient of 5 Np $\mathrm{m^{-1}\,MHz^{-1}}$ (GOSS et al. 1978) is typically used to represent soft tissue. The power deposition term ($\langle q \rangle$) can be calculated as a function of the intensity via the following:

$$\langle q \rangle = \frac{-1}{r}\frac{\partial(Ir)}{\partial r} = 2\alpha f I. \tag{2}$$

The temperature distributions resulting from these power deposition patterns can be calculated using the bio-heat transfer equation (BHTE), a descriptive model of tissue thermal characteristics (PENNES 1948):

$$\rho c \frac{\partial T}{\partial t} = \nabla^2(kT) - \omega_b c_b (T - T_a) + \langle q \rangle, \tag{3}$$

where k is the tissue thermal conductivity, ω is the blood perfusion rate, c_b is the specific heat of blood, c is the specific heat of tissue, ρ is the tissue density, T is the tissue temperature, and T_a is the arterial temperature. The steady-state solution to this equation can be computed in one, two, or three dimensions using, among others, the finite difference technique with successive overrelaxation (ROEMER and CETAS 1984; CHATO 1990).

The improvement of radial depth of heating for ultrasound applicators over existing methods can be exemplified using the one-dimensional simulations, as shown in Fig. 8.4. The predicted radial temperature distributions from a 2.0 mm OD ultrasound radiator are shown for frequencies which bracket the usable range, and are compared to a thermal conduction and RF electrode source [$\langle q \rangle \propto 1/r^2$ (MECHLING and STROHBEHN 1986)] of the same dimensions. Simulated temperature distributions are also illustrated (for 5 MHz ultrasound sources and RF electrodes) with the temperature of the catheter/tissue interface maintained at 42.5°C, thereby moving the maximum temperature away from the catheter surface and increasing the radius of effective heating. This strategy of cooling the catheter has recently been investigated for RF (PRIOR 1991) and microwave (TREMBLY et al. 1991) sources. For example, the effective heating radius (> 42.5°C) of a 5 MHz interstitial ultrasound source was shown to be 18 mm using a cooling temperature at the catheter wall compared to 11 mm without cooling. The effective heating depths of the RF-LCF sources and conduction sources were considerably less, even when the RF electrode surface was cooled.

The heating capabilities of ultrasound applicators, RF-LCF electrodes, and thermal conduction techniques in a standard parallel implant configuration can be compared using two-dimensional simulations. Figure 8.5 shows the temperature contours for a 3 cm × 3 cm grid, across the middle of the four equally spaced parallel sources (2 mm OD sources, long implant). The perfusion of $\omega = 2.0\ \mathrm{kg\,m^{-3}\,s^{-1}}$ represents a moderately perfused tissue (resting muscle), which for most tumors ranges from 0.1 to 5.0 $\mathrm{kg\,m^{-3}\,s^{-1}}$ (JAIN and WARD-HARTLEY 1984). With the maximum tissue temperature constrained to 48°C at the applicator surface, the ultrasound devices maintain a therapy temperature of > 43°C beyond the outer boundaries of

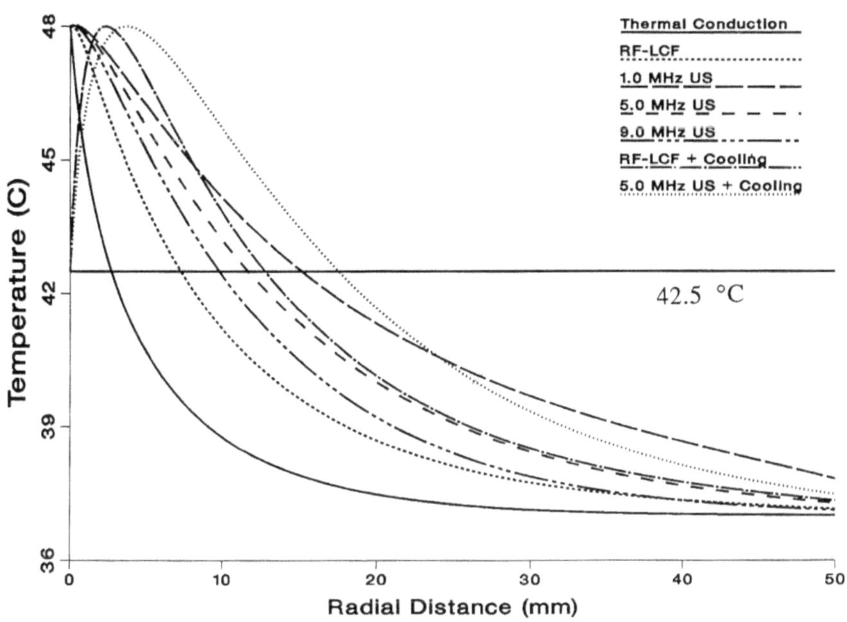

Fig. 8.4. Simulated radial temperature curves for 2 mm OD sources comparing ultrasound, RF-LCF, and thermal conduction applicators, including the effects of "catheter cooling" to 42.5°C

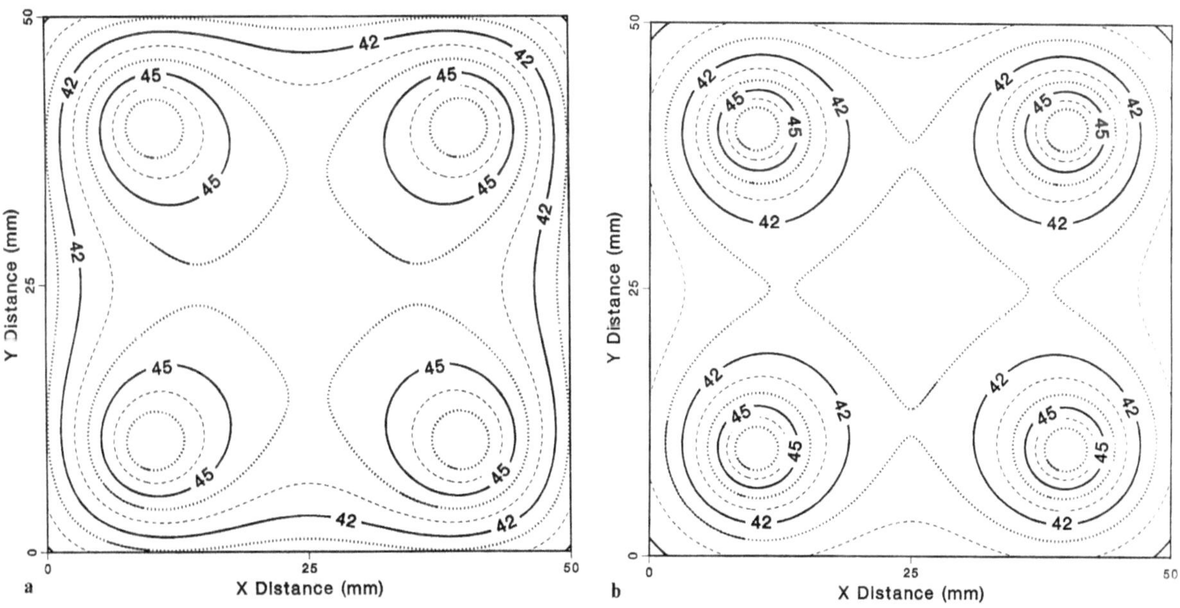

Fig. 8.5 a, b. Simulated two-dimensional temperature distributions across the center of an implant (2 ×2, 3 cm spacing) of 2 mm OD sources, for (a) 1 MHz ultrasound and (b) RF-LCF applicators

the implant, whereas the RF-LCF electrode and thermal conduction source (results not shown) arrays produced cold areas $< 41°C$ within the implant.

These differences between modalities can be quantified by comparing the cross-sectional area of effective heating, determined from the two-dimensional calculations as the region between 43°C and 48°C, as a function of frequency, implant spacing, and perfusion (Fig. 8.6). The acoustic output power levels varied from 0.2 to 1.5 $W\,cm^{-1}$ length for frequencies of 5 MHz and greater, and from 0.8 to 5 $W\,cm^{-1}$ length for a frequency of 1 MHz; as

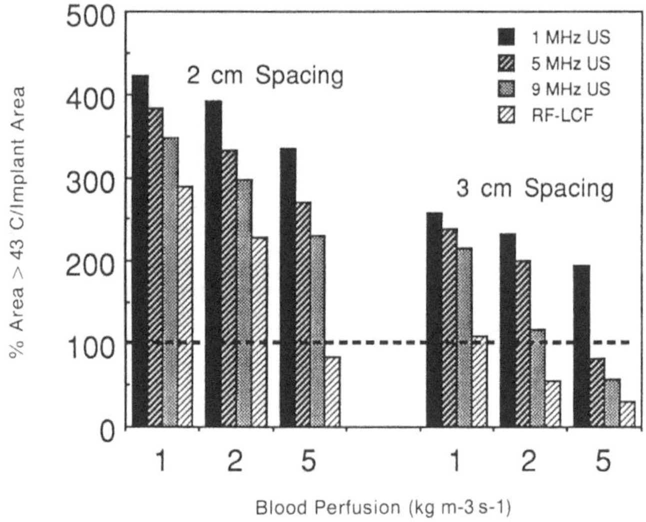

Fig. 8.6. Summary of heating effectiveness of ultrasound and RF-LCF applicators determined from the two-dimensional simulations as a function of implant spacing and blood perfusion. Cross-sectional heated area; 2 × 2 implant; 2 mm OD sources

expected, the larger powers were required for the larger implant spacing, higher perfusion levels, and lower frequencies. This clearly illustrates that ultrasound applicators can extend the implant spacing and perfusion limits imposed on existing interstitial heating modalities providing that adequate power can be delivered.

To illustrate the advantage of using multiple elements with uniform power deposition along each source, temperature distributions were calculated in a three-dimensional model with a 2 × 2 implant, and 3 cm spacing. Each ultrasound applicator was 3.4 cm long, consisting of three 1-cm-long transducers separated by a 2 mm dead space between adjoining elements. The temperature contours are shown in Fig. 8.7 for the longitudinal plane along (a) two of the applicators and (b) the central region between the four applicators for a peripherally enhanced power application pattern (100% outer elements, 75% center). For this case,

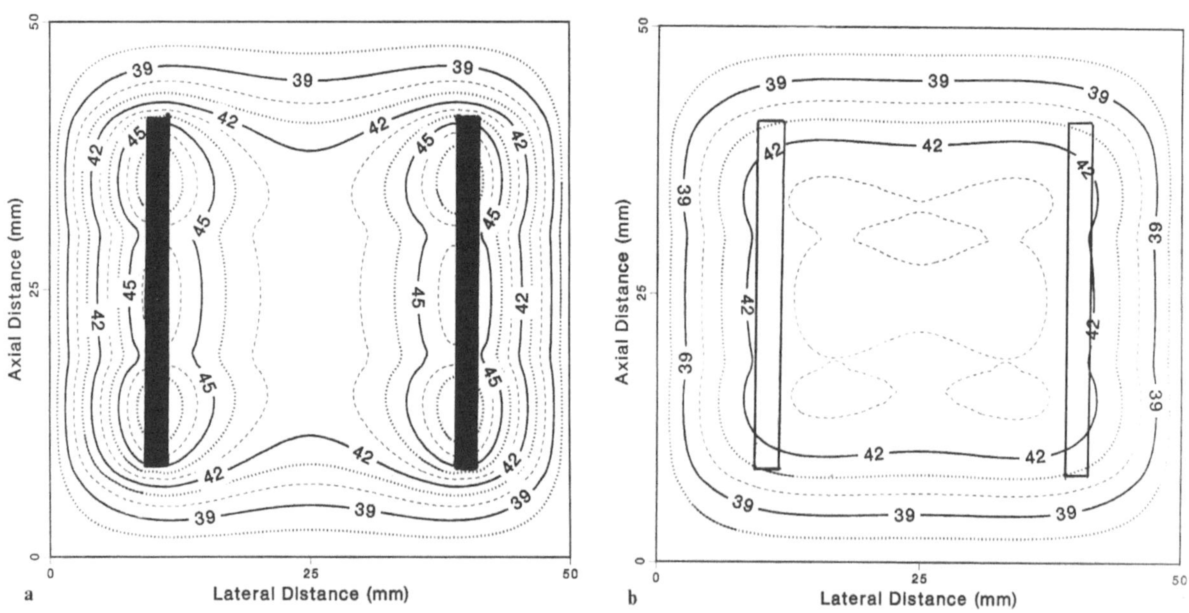

Fig. 8.7 a, b. Longitudinal temperature distributions from three-dimensional simulations of a peripherally enhanced, 5 MHz 2 × 2, 3 cm spaced implant using multielement ultrasound applicators (3.4 cm long, three elements, 2 mm OD) shown (**a**) along two applicators and (**b**) along the center of the implant

the outer boundaries of the three-dimensional model were constrained to 10 mm from the edges of the implant. By adjusting the power levels to a higher value at either end of the applicator, it is apparent that the temperature distribution can be elongated to include the tip of the implant.

8.4 Conclusions

The development of interstitial ultrasound applicators is an emerging technology that has the potential to be more effective for applying interstitial hyperthermia than the existing methods. Most notably, these devices exhibit an increased radial penetration of energy which is uniform along the length of the applicator, including the tip. In addition, applicators can be constructed from multiple transducer segments to form a linear array, allowing the power deposition to be varied along the length. This provides critical adjustability for accommodating irregular tumor geometry, heterogeneities of the tissue thermal properties, and dynamic changes in perfusion. In practice, the development of durable miniature applicators that perform in such a manner presents difficult technical challenges which will require a significant development effort. The characterizations of simple prototype applicators have demonstrated that the technology and devices are feasible. The next step of developing optimal designs will reach obstacles such as cost, availability, and manufacturability of miniature radiators, developing special catheters, compact controlling systems, etc.

Acknowledgments. This work was supported in part by a grant from the Whitaker Foundation and NIH Grant CA-09215.

References

Chato JC (1990) Fundamentals of bioheat transfer. In: Gautherie M (ed) Thermal dosimetry and treatment planning. Springer, Berlin Heidelberg New York, pp 1–56

Coughlin CT, Strohbehn JW (1989) Interstitial thermoradiotherapy. Radiol Clin North Am 27: 577–588

Dewhirst MW, Sim DA, Sapareto S, Conner WG (1984) Importance of minimum tumor temperature in determining early and long-term responses of spontaneous canine and feline tumors to heat and radiation. Cancer Res 44: 43–50

Diederich CJ, Hynynen K (1989) Induction of hyperthermia using an intracavitary multielement ultrasonic applicator. IEEE Trans Biomed Eng 36: 432–438

Diederich CJ, Hynynen K (1990a) The feasibility of interstitial ultrasound hyperthermia. Abstract presented at the North American Hyperthermia Group annual meeting, New Orleans, April 7–12 p 48

Diederich CJ, Hynynen K (1990b) The development of intracavitary ultrasonic applicators for hyperthermia: a design and experimental study. Med Phys 17: 626–634

Gibbs FA, Peck JW, Dethlefsen LA (1981) The importance of intratumor temperature uniformity in the study of radiosensitizing effects of hyperthermia in vivo. Radiat Res 87: 187–197

Goss SA, Johnston RL, Dunn F (1978) Comprehensive compilation of empirical ultrasonic properties of mammalian tissues. J Acoust Soc Am 64: 423–457

Holmes KR, Ryan W, Weinstein P, Chen MM (1984) A fixation technique for organs to be used as perfused tissue phantoms in bioheat transfer studies. In: Spiker RL (ed) 1984 Advances in bioengineering. American Society of Mechanical Engineers, New York, pp 9–10

Hynynen K (1992) The feasibility of interstitial ultrasound hyperthermia. Med Phys (in press)

Jain RK, Ward-Hartley K (1984) Tumor blood flow – characterization, modifications, and role in hyperthermia. IEEE Trans Sonics Ultrasonics 31: 504–526

Jarosz BJ (1990) Rate of heating in tissue in vitro by interstitial ultrasound. Proceedings of IEEE Engineering in Medicine and Biology Society Annual Meeting pp 274–275

Jarosz BJ (1991) Temperature distribution in interstitial ultrasonic hyperthermia. Proceedings of IEEE Engineering in Medicine and Biology Society Annual Meeting pp 179–180

Mechling JA, Strohbehn JW (1986) A theoretical comparison of the temperature distributions produced by three interstitial hyperthermia systems. Int J Radiat. Oncol Biol Phys 12: 2137–2149

Pennes HH (1948) Analysis of tissue and arterial blood temperatures in the resting human forearm. J Appl Physiol 1: 93–122

Prior MV (1991) A comparative study of RF-LCF and hot-source interstitial hyperthermia techniques. Int J Hyperthermia 7: 131–140

Roemer RB, Cetas TC (1984) Applications of bioheat transfer simulations in hyperthermia. Cancer Res. [Suppl] 44: 4788s–4798s

Seegenschmiedt MH, Sauer R, Brady LW, Karlsson UL (1991) Techniques and clinical experience of interstitial thermoradiotherapy. In: Sauer R (ed) Interventional radiation therapy, techniques – brachytherapy. Springer, Berlin Heidelberg New York, pp 343–355

Stauffer PR (1990) Techniques for interstitial hyperthermia. In: Field SB, Hand JW (eds) An introduction to the practical aspects of clinical hyperthermia. Taylor & Francis, New York, pp 344–370

Trembly BS, Douple EB, Hoopes PJ (1991) The effect of air cooling on the radial temperature distribution of a single microwave hyperthermia antenna in vivo. Int J Hyperthermia 7: 343–354

9 Laser Technology for Interstitial Hyperthermia

A.C. STEGER

CONTENTS

9.1 Introduction

Laser is an acronym for light amplification by the stimulated emission of radiation. The concept and the basic mathematics were derived by A. EINSTEIN in 1917. Spontaneous emission of radiation occurs when an atom moves down from one energy level to another in the course of which a photon is released. The frequency of this photon depends on the energy gap between the two levels. For this change to happen the atom has to attain a higher than resting energy state and does so by the absorption of radiation of the appropriate amount. This higher energy level is also referred to as excited as the atom is both at a higher level and less stable than at its normal resting level. EINSTEIN proposed that if an atom in its excited state were hit by a photon with the same energy as that emitted on the change from the excited to ground state, then two photons, the original and a second one at the same wavelength, would result. Hence the stimulated emission.

It was not until 1958 that TOWNES and SCHAWLOW outlined the theoretical conditions to overcome the problem of raising atoms to an excited state, population inversion, the first step necessary for the start of the laser process. MAIMAN in 1960 built the first working laser in which the material that "lased" was ruby. Since then there has been a vast expansion in the development of lasers, some of which has been in medicine. The basic construction of a laser is that there is a source that can produce excited atoms, population inversion; these atoms are pumped up to the excited level by a variety of means, usually a powerful flash lamp (xenon or krypton). The photons that result are contained within a chamber with mirrors at each end and therefore reflect backwards and forwards whilst increasing in number. The front mirror has a hole in it covered by a shutter and when this is lifted, light comes out and can be directed at a target or into a fibre. The lasing chamber is usually cooled by deionised water as the process is only about 2% efficient and a lot of energy goes directly into heat. This coolant is then further cooled.

The characteristics of laser light are that it is collimated, coherent and monochromatic. These mean that the light has a high power per unit cross-sectional area (irradiance) which may vary a little with beam shape. In the development of lasers in medicine a variety of different wavelengths have been investigated and the lasers can be liquid, solid state or gas with differing power supply requirements and cooling systems to allow for the energy lost as heat in the generation of the laser light beam. These design problems have become simpler in recent years, with less need for complex power supplies and cooling systems. As this has happened so the controls and reliability have improved and prices have started to come down.

Which laser is used for which medical purpose depends on the wavelength of that laser as there is a

A.C. STEGER, M.S., F.R.C.S., Department of Surgery, King's College School of Medicine and Dentistry, The Rayne Institute, 123 Coldharbour Lane, London, SE5 9NU, UK great difference in the response of different tissues to different wavelengths (NAKAMURA et al. 1990). The effect of laser light on biological tissue can be thermal, photoablative, electromechanical or photochemical.

9.2 Theoretical Laser–Tissue Interactions

The majority of uses of laser energy in medicine are thermal in nature, that is, the photon energy is converted into heat in the target tissue with an ensuing thermal biological response (WELCH 1984; SVAASAND 1984; MCKENZIE 1990). Once the energy is deposited, thermal conduction or diffusion occurs (SVAASAND et al. 1985). Because of the nature of laser light (coherent and collimated) and the precision possible in its control and delivery, attempts have been made to determine the fate of laser light in tissue. This is to try and understand the processes involved and then to predict the response of any tissue to the delivery into it of laser light and thus allow the development of therapeutic light dosages based on calculation rather than, as at present, on empirical observation. This is a complex matter depending on the wavelength of light involved, the way it reaches the tissue and tissue factors including optical and thermal characteristics. The fate of the light in the tissue has also to be taken into account, that is reflection from the surface (unless interstitial), forward penetration, scattering and absorption. There can be little or no comparison between different tissues and different wavelengths. Once all these variables are accounted for in any attempt to calculate or predict the behaviour of laser light in tissue, the immediate and continuing changes that the energy has on that tissue have to be allowed for, as does the fact that tissue is three-dimensional.

There have been a number of attempts to calculate and predict the size of lesions of thermal necrosis from optical and thermal formulae and to compare these with observed experimental lesions (WELCH 1984; VAN GEMERT and HENNING 1981; CUMMINS and NEUENBERG 1983; HALLDORSSON and LANGERHOLC 1978; LANGERHOLC 1979; NISHISAKA et al. 1983; YOON et al. 1987). To carry out these calculations, assumptions of the various tissue coefficients listed above have to be made, and it is on this basis that doubt exists over the validity of the results as the various formulae do not all take account of all optical and thermal properties and changes (WELCH 1984). Indeed, WILSON and PATTERSON (1986), in dealing only with the path and fate of light in tissue, and not any resultant thermal reaction, indicate the weakness of some of these calculations due in part to assumptions over tissue coefficients. A number of these are based on thin slab or layer geometry calculations (taking a very small, 10–100 μm thickness of tissue), vary in the number of dimensions that are included, and are based on Kubelka-Munk calculations (KUBELKA 1948) for the behaviour of light in a near totally reflecting isotropic medium, in fact paint (WILSON and PATTERSON 1986), which is not the same as tissue with its heterogeneous make-up. A better method of mathematical understanding is that provided by the Monte Carlo method, which traces the fate of photons in tissue and takes inhomogeneities into account (WILSON and PATTERSON 1986; PATTERSON et al. 1991a, b). The questions of interest are the fate of light entering tissue (scattering), the optical penetration, the rate of conversion of photon energy into heat (absorption), the effect that the latter has on the former, and, from a practical point of view, which predominates, optical penetration or thermal effects. The work described by Patterson et al. (1991a, b) is among the better and closer attempts to present mathematical modelling in a way that allows comparison with in vivo experimental work.

To attempt to measure tissue optical and thermal coefficients is difficult (WILSON and PATTERSON 1986) due to the problem of accurate placement of invasive accurate placement of invasive probes in three dimensions with as little disturbance as possible.

There has been some theoretical work that rather than just looking at the fate of light transmitted into tissue from outside, has looked at interstitial application for hyperthermia and compared calculated results with experimental observations. This has been done using the method of lines to solve the equation of heat conduction by computerised calculation (DAVIS et al. 1989; DOWDEN et al. 1987). The problem with this, as with other purely theoretical work on laser–tissue interactions, is that what happens once the light enters tissue is unclear. The amount of scattering or absorption is unknown, as are the optical and thermal characteristics of the tissue. Allowance is not made for changes in these in tissue that is being heated and how these changes affect further heating, in particular for the development of charring. There is, however, reasonable correlation (10%–15% variation) between the calculated lesion size in liver for both one and four fibres placed interstitially and that measured experimentally. The concept of calculating the amount of laser energy needed to heat and destroy a tumour based on its dimensions and delivered by preset computer control is attractive but it is apparent that we have some way to go to achieve this.

The sophisticated modelling developed in non-laser hyperthermia has yet to be well applied in combination with interstitial laser hyperthermia.

9.3 Laser and Fibreoptic Technology

The wavelengths of interest in laser-induced hyperthermia are between 800 and 1300 μm as in tissue containing blood, photons with this wavelength in theory scatter more. Because of surface reflection, interest in lasers for hyperthermia is in interstitial application. Laser light at the wavelengths above can be transmitted via a quartz (or silicon or sapphire) fibreoptic. This has a thin 20- to-40-μm cladding around it and the light is reflected along the fibreoptic quartz because of the change of refraction at the quartz–cladding interface, giving near total internal reflection. If the wavelength and entry angle allow refraction within the critical angle of refractive change at the quartz–cladding interface then light is transmitted along the fibreoptic with minimal loss.

A fibreoptic waveguide is thus an efficient way to transmit energy. Such fibreoptic waveguides are compact, flexible, insensitive to electromagnetic interference and of small diameter – in medicine 2–600 μm, which is thin enough to permit placement into solid internal organs, down a guiding hollow metal needle if need be, with little chance of mechanical damage from size alone. For these reasons the use of a fibreoptic to deliver laser light energy for interstitial hyperthermia is a very attractive idea, allowing efficient energy delivery by a method that should cause little tissue damage en route and not interfere with monitoring systems. The development of techniques of interstitial laser hyperthermia (ILH) has been fuelled by the possibility of using laser energy to destroy cancer tissue in situ rather than just using heat as an adjuvant therapy and with this the potential for treating difficult cancers such as those of the liver, pancreas or prostate.

Laser energy has in the past been used to destroy tumour by external application to the surface of the tumour. The disadvantages of this type of work are access, surface reflection and the severe tumour disruption with scattering of tumour cells (Mullins et al. 1967; Hoye et al. 1968). The first use of ILH to treat cancers was by Bown in 1983. There has been some theoretical modelling of ILH as discussed above, but relatively little phantom type modelling. There is an increasing amount of in vivo practical experimental work which has been aimed at determining the laser energy parameters that are most appropriate combined with modifications to the tips of the fibres to alter the pattern of light distribution through tissue, monitoring of the heating process and clinical application. These will be described and comparisons will be made where possible with more conventional hyperthermia work. It will be seen that the temperatures that result in ILH are much higher than 45°C taken as an upper limit of normal in most non-laser hyperthermia work. Despite this I think that the term hyperthermia is relevant to this work as there are overlaps and similarities between both approaches and the term describes the basic nature of the tissue damage being undertaken.

9.4 Experimental Interstitial Laser Hyperthermia – Biological Studies

It is worth describing some of the effects of external laser applications in the liver (the organ that has been most studied with regard to the biological effects of ILH and the monitoring thereof), as some of the findings are similar to those with ILH. The liver is relatively easy to use and has enough volume for the purposes of the studies carried out. External application of laser energy to the liver involves the emitted light falling on the liver surface, whence some is reflected back and the rest enters the tissue to be scattered, propagated or absorbed. Back-reflection results in loss of applied energy to the tissue under investigation and for this reason powers used have to be higher than in interstitial application, where this does not occur. The organ in which the fate of laser photons has been most studied is skin (Parrish and Deutsch 1984), which differs in its physical properties from liver, which has been little studied from this point of view and only a little more with regard to the gross biological response to laser irradiation.

The neodymium yttrium aluminium garnet laser (Nd-YAG, wavelength 1064 nm) has been used as its wavelength is within the 600- to 1200-nm window at which there is tissue attenuation of light rather than absorption by water (Svaasand et al. 1985). It is also a fairly readily available laser that can be used for other non-ILH laser therapies. There is developing interest in the use of other laser wavelengths including laser diodes (wavelength about 850 μm) and the erbium YAG laser (wavelength 2094 μm, Dickinson et al. 1991). It may well be that in the future these and other wavelengths will be more developed and appropriate for ILH.

In the primate (monkey) liver, Mullins et al. (1967) found that 25% of liver surface could be coagulated with resolution of the resulting abnormal liver function tests by 2 weeks. The lesions of thermal necrosis produced with a pulsed Nd glass laser (550–800 J) (this was before the development of fibreoptics) were punched out and well circumscribed, measuring 8–15 mm in width with a depth of 10 mm. Hoye et al. (1968), in similar work on the rabbit liver, described in detail the pathological response to surface irradiation. They noted a central vaporised area surrounded by firstly a zone of vacuolation and then a zone of inflammation and fibrosis. Resolution was taking place but not complete by 3 weeks. Mordon et al. (1983) showed that in the rat liver the maximum surface temperature of the area of liver undergoing irradiation was related linearly to energy density at high and low powers. Depth of necrosis was related to pulse duration and peak power density. The pulsed laser was more associated with greater control of surface temperature and lesion reproducibility than a CW laser, although for equal energies both gave similar lesions of thermal necrosis (Mordon et al. 1987). The emphasis in this work was on controlling the surface temperature and calculating the thermal diffusion, rather than maximising the size of lesion possible or looking beyond the immediate histology to the fate of any lesion of thermal necrosis.

In induced hepatic tumours in the monkey, Mullins et al. (1967) found that with high power pulses small (< 2 cm) tumours could be eradicated. There was, however, a risk of causing tumour emboli and distant implantation of tumour. The lesions made were punched out with surrounding vascular sealing. Hoye et al. (1968) found a similar response to that observed in normal liver when small (2–15 mm) tumour deposits were irradiated. An attempt has been made to use external beam Nd-YAG irradiation controlled by a thermocouple-linked computer to treat experimental murine liver tumours at "conventional" hyperthermic temperatures. 42°–45°C (Waldow et al. 1988). This produced some control of small (7–9 mm diameter) tumours, but not of larger ones (10–15 mm diameter). The observation was made that the higher the temperature, the more likely was tumour eradication.

Interstitial hyperthermia with lasers by the insertion of the light-conducting quartz fibre into tumour was first described by Bown (1983). Whilst this method of energy delivery is invasive, it has the advantages that there is little back-scattering and impact loss as light strikes tissue, and in order to reach a specific point within an organ, the surface does not have to be heated or used as a thermal conduit. Interstitial light delivery has been investigated in four ways.

9.4.1 Low Power Application: Energy–Dose Response; Single- and Multiple-Fibre Systems

Experimental work showed that with very low powers from a Nd-YAG laser (0.5–2 W) it was possible to produce areas of thermal necrosis of predictable extent in the rat liver (up to 1.6 cm in diameter) which healed by fibrosis and regeneration (Matthewson et al. 1987) (Fig. 9.1). This work established that there was a "dose response" between energy given and the size of necrotic lesion that resulted when powers of 1 and 1.5 W were used. At the site of the tip of the fibre (600 μm in diameter), charring was seen. There was a clear cut-off or boundary zone between the necrotic and surrounding normal liver. Post-mortem angiography showed that there was obstruction of small arteries up to 1.5 mm in diameter. Vascular obstruction is one of the methods by which this form of hyperthermia may work. With this technique there was no difference in the size of the necrotic lesion whether a continuous wave or pulsed laser was used to deliver an equivalent amount of energy for an average power of 1 W (Matthewson et al. 1986). This technique can be applied to tumours in the rat colon with eradication of dimethylhydrazine-induced polypoid tumours (Matthewson et al. 1988). A subcutaneous transplantable fibrosarcoma was treated similarly with eradication of some tumours and reduction in growth rate of others (Matthewson et al. 1989). There was a statistically significant increase in the median survival in those tumour-bearing animals so treated ($P > 0.05$).

The use of a single-fibre tip in the porcine liver (Bosman et al. 1991; Dachman et al. 1990) at

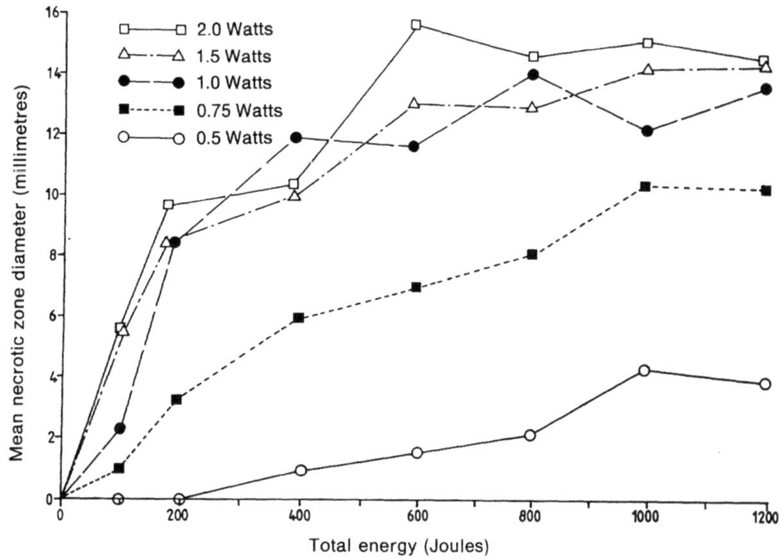

Fig. 9.1. Mean necrotic zone diameter versus total energy delivered for five different power settings, 3–4 days after ILH. Reproduced by permission of the Editor and Publishers of Gastroenterology (From MATTHEWSON et al. 1987)

1.5–4 W produced lesions of thermal necrosis of similar size to those described by MATTHEWSON et al. In all these cases resolution occurred by about 60 days, with a minute central char left. Comparison has been made with the injection of alcohol and this has been found to produce smaller and less predictable lesions of necrosis (VAN EYKEN et al. 1991). The use of a single fibre for ILH is simple, takes a reasonable time, 600 s in this type of work, and can be done percutaneously. The use of one fibre alone may be a drawback as the size of the resulting lesion of thermal necrosis is probably too small to be of clinical use. Multiple-fibre systems have been developed to overcome this.

For a multiple-fibre system to be of use there has to be as near an equal light output as possible from each fibre end so that an equal biological response can be predicted. If this were not the case then erratic tumour heating would occur. (It is conceivable that in the future fibre tip outputs will be deliberately calculated to be different to encompass tumour and anatomical variations, but I think that this is some way off). There are various technologies available that can provide multiple-fibre systems. The simplest (and most expensive) are multiple lasers or lasers built with a number of outputs and the beam divided. Optical beam splitters can be used but are expensive ($6000) and as there are several beam splits and fibre couplings to account for the equipment may need quite a lot of calibration each time it is used. An alternative (Wilson, personal communication) is the use of multiple fibres mounted on a moving mechanical rig so that each fibre is exposed in turn to the output beam of a laser. Another, perhaps simpler, method involves the combination of fibreoptics into star couplers. The technology for combining fibreoptics has developed in the telecommunications industry and been extended to, for example, local area computer networks. These techniques work well with small fibres (20–125 μm diameter) rather than the larger fibres used in medical laser work. With the fused biconic technique it is possible to join a number of fibres to a main one in such a way that by the removal of the cladding and the approximation of a fibre at a precalculated angle, a set amount of light exits from the main fibre to travel down the daughter fibres. This process is done under laser light transmission control so that the amount of light going into each fibre is controlled to achieve the desired splitting ratio of the input light. The fibres are then heat fused together and set in epoxy resin. The size of fibres used for medical laser work limits the number of fibres that can be coupled by this technique. The other limitation is that at each fibreoptic joint light is lost which at the wavelengths under discussion is converted into heat which could in theory damage the coupler. Cooling has not been used but could easily be; it has not been necessary to date. The great advantage of fibreoptic couplers is that the splitting ratio and thus the output ratio of the multiple fibres is preset and unalterable (STEGER et al. 1989). To use them they only have to be connected to the laser port and the outputs checked; there is no need for any further alteration or calibration. Figure 9.2 shows the static ratio of outputs for a four-fibre coupler made by Canstar of Canada and used extensively at

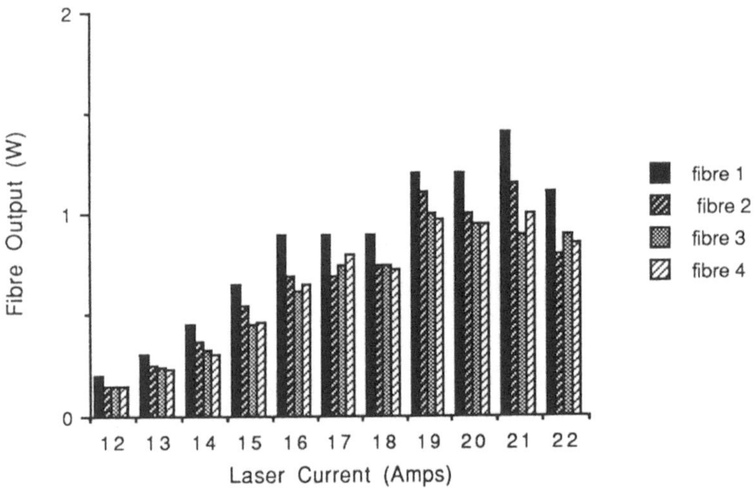

Fig. 9.2. The power outputs of the four output fibres of a 200-μm Canstar coupler at increasing laser operating currents transmitting 1064 nm laser light

the National Medical Laser Centre, University College in London (cost $440). To develop systems with more fibres other techniques may be needed, and an example of a stable seven-fibre system is shown in Fig. 9.3.

The exciting potential of multiple-fibre systems of the types discussed above is that in combination with further couplers and taking advantage of the fact that light can travel two ways in a fibreoptic, such systems could be used for both light delivery and sensation to allow monitoring of the tissue changes occurring during hyperthermia either by simple fluorescence or with biological tip modification.

With a four-fibre system, ILH was performed in canine liver to establish the parameters with which large areas of thermal necrosis could be produced (Steger et al. 1992a). Using 1.5 W for 670 s (4020 J in total) and a fibre spacing of 1.5 cm, lesions with dimensions of 3.6 × 3.1 × 2.8 cm were achieved in 75% of cases. There was no mortality and low morbidity. Healing occurred by 1 year. A dramatic rise in liver enzymes was seen with resolution to normal by a month. Figure 9.4 shows such a lesion at 7 days. It is on the basis of this type of experimental work that clinical studies have started.

In the canine pancreas single-fibre studies with laser parameters of 1–1.5 W for up to 1000 s resulted in lesions up to 18 mm in diameter whether the fibre was placed in the gland or in the major duct. With the multiple-fibre system used in the liver, the initial dimensions of the area affected were 6 × 3 × 1.7 cm, which had reduced to 4 × 3.5 × 2 cm at 1 week (Steger et al. 1987). All thermal damage was resolved by 9 months. The pathological changes were inflammatory in nature and care should be taken in interpreting these results as some of the response was probably inflammatory

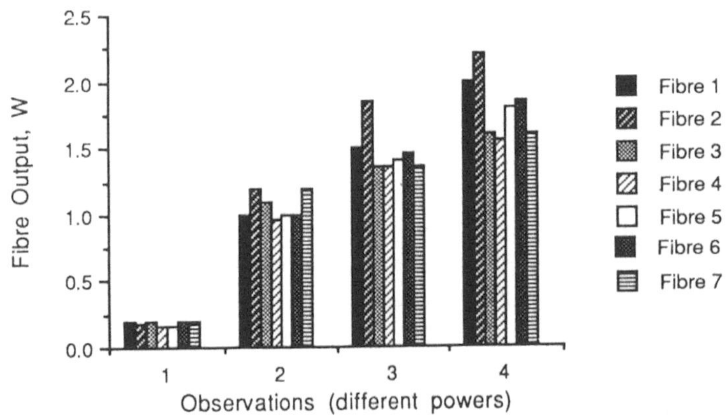

Fig. 9.3. Fibre outputs for increasing laser operating currents for a 1 × 7 fibre coupler (1064 nm laser light)

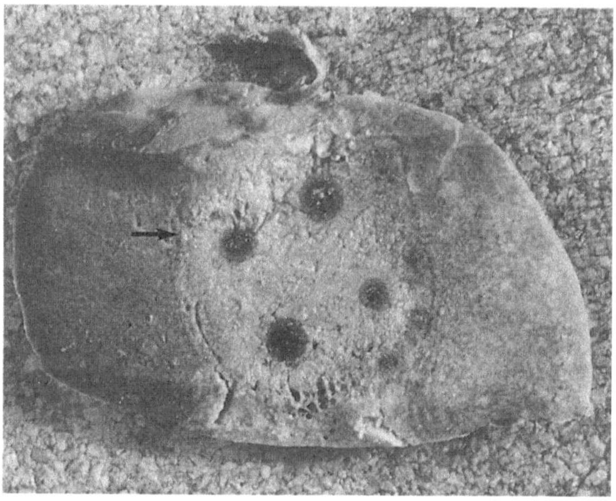

Fig. 9.4. A lesion of thermal necrosis produced using a four-fibre coupler, at 7 days. The four black spots are charring at the fibre sites. There is a clearly defined margin between the dead and surrounding normal liver →. Reproduced by permission of the Editor and Publishers of the British Journal of Surgery, Butterworth-Heinemann Ldt. (From STEGER et al. 1992a)

pancreatitis rather than purely thermal damage. However, there was a low morbidity and such studies indicate that it may not be unsafe to expose the normal pancreas to ILH.

Similar results have been found in the canine prostate, with thermal lesions of median size 1.5 cm for a single fibre and 2.2 cm for two fibres (STEGER and MCNICHOLAS 1990).

9.4.2 *Diffuser Tip Application*

HASHIMOTO et al. (1985, 1988, 1989) have used the Nd-YAG laser at higher powers (5–15 W) at open surgery with a modified quartz diffuser tip on the laser fibre for the treatment of hepatomas. This was after the treatment of any available surface of the tumour with 40–60 W. Ultrasound was used to guide the positioning of the fibre into the tumours. This was followed by a reduction in serum α-fetoprotein concentration and reduction of tumour size on CT scan. The same workers (HASHIMOTO et al. 1988, 1989) have reported the use of 5 W through a similar probe with temperatures in the range reported below, but do not give the dimensions of thermal necrosis caused.

There is great interest in altering the tip of the fibre to increase the area over which light is emitted as in theory this would reduce the undoubted point heat source effect that a simple fibre has with the cladding removed from the terminal few millimetres. Any alteration to the tip, however, alters the intrinsic strength of the fibre and greatly increases the chance of a break occurring. NOLSOE et al. (1992) described a cone frosted end to the fibre (diffuser tip) with which, using 4 W, lesions of up to 44 mm could be made. It should be noted that at 1.5 W the lesion size was not markedly larger than with a simple fibre.

9.4.3 *Computer-Controlled Sapphire Application*

KANEMAKI et al. (1988) reported the use of an artificial sapphire probe as a means of transmitting light into tumour tissue with a thermocouple placed about 6 mm away from the probe tip and the laser output controlled by a computerised feedback system from the thermocouple. The aim was to maintain the temperature at the thermocouple at 44°C. This work uses laser energy to provide temperatures in the range seen in conventional hyperthermia (41.5°–45°C) rather than at either a constant power or a higher power. It is unlikely that a point measurement of temperature 6 mm from the laser fibre is an indication either of overall tissue temperature or of that at the probe.

A similar probe has been used to cause ILH in canine muscle (PANJEHPOUR et al. 1990). The aim of the work was to use powers of 3–5 W for 30 min with the temperature controlled to that of conventional hyperthermia, 44°C. From the results, thermal damage occurred, but in a patchy manner rather than with the production of specific areas of necrosis.

The disadvantages of sapphire probes are that the diameter exceeds 2 mm, which is probably too large for percutaneous application, and that there can be damage at the fibre sapphire tip junction PANJEHPOUR et al. 1990; STEGER 1990) with loss of energy and sticking to tissue if deeply inserted. For the same input powers there was no increase in size of the area of thermal damage caused if a simple fibre and artificial sapphire probe were compared (STEGER 1990).

9.4.4 *High Power Application*

GODLEWSKI et al. (1988a, b) developed a device to use high powers (up to 100 W). In these studies the laser fibre was fed into a rigid metal handpiece 2.5 mm in diameter, with a lens at the end through which the laser beam was fired. This lens was cooled with circulating saline to prevent fibre damage. With this system lesions were made that had a central area of vaporization measuring 16–20 mm in diameter with coagulation around this to take the total lesion size to 2–3 cm. This was with ten 1-s shots of 100 W each, and so with a much shorter time than that reported by MATTHEWSON et al. (1987), but the same total energy dose.

9.5 Monitoring of Interstitial Laser Hyperthermia

9.5.1 Temperature

MATTHEWSON et al. (1987) recorded temperatures ranging from 70° to 100°C near the fibre tip down to 43°C at 6–8 mm away (Fig. 9.5). This correlated well with the diameter of the lesions of thermal necrosis produced. There is, however, great difficulty in recording temperatures in the immediate vicinity of a laser fibre; artefacts may be caused by a direct thermal effect on the temperature probe and by tissue disruption, causing an alteration in local conditions so that it is an artificial parameter that is being considered. The presence of charred tissue indicates that temperatures in the region of 350°C have been reached. GODLEWSKI et al. (1988b) found a similar drop in temperature to 43°C away from the central area of vacuolation.

STEGER et al. (1992a), in the production of large areas of necrosis, found temperatures that were well able to casue cell death (Fig. 9.6).

There is debate as to the precise mechanism of cell death caused by ILH. It may be due to (a) light penetrating tissue with conversion of photon energy into thermal energy or (b) absorption of light and high local temperatures over a small distance (1 mm) around the point of the fibre, as evidenced by charring and bubbles seen on ultrasound, with thermal diffusion away from this point. The fibre tip and area of high temperature in its immediate vicinity almost certainly act as a point heat source (STEGER et al. 1992b).

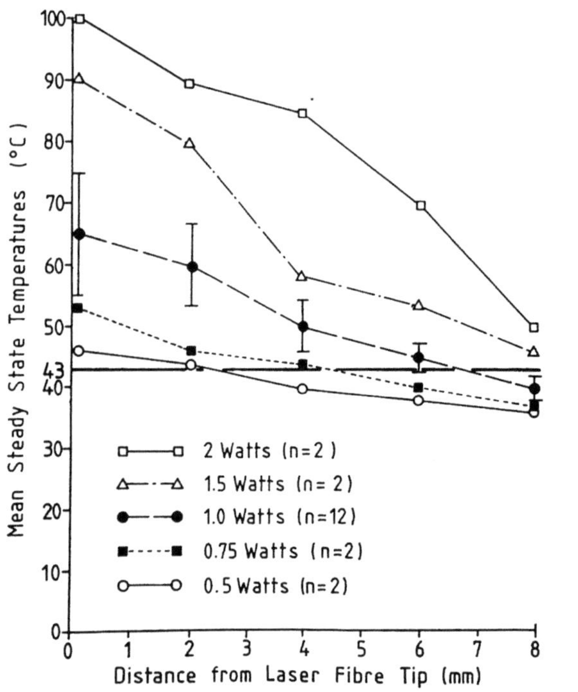

Fig. 9.5. Mean steady state temperatures versus distance from laser fibre tip for 0.5, 0.75, 1, 1.5 and 2 W. Standard deviations are given for 1 W. Reproduced by permission of the Editor and Publishers of Gastroenterology (From MATTHEWSON et al. 1987)

9.5.2 Ultrasound/Radiology

KANEMAKI et al. (1988) noted ultrasound changes after laser irradiation, the appearance of murine tumours seeming to change from hypoechoic to mixed hypo- and hyperechoic.

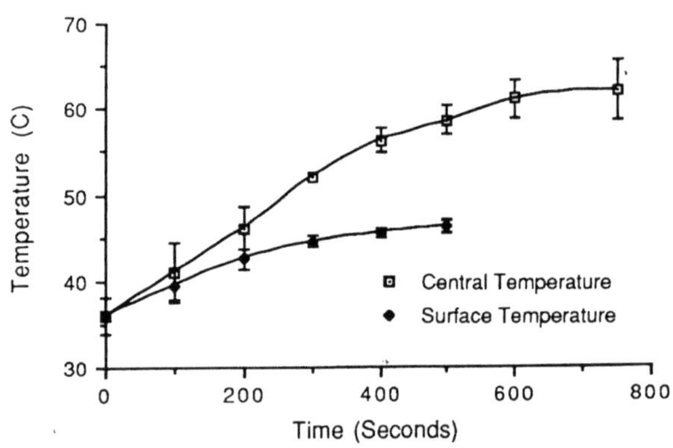

Fig. 9.6. Temperatures (± SD) recorded in the centre (10.5 mm from each fibre tip) and on the surface of the liver lobe (18.5 mm from each fibre tip) during creation of lesions of thermal necrosis with a four-fibre coupler (all with 1.5 W and a fibre spacing of 1.5 cm for 670 s). The surface recordings only ran to 500 s. Reproduced by permission of the Editor and Publishers of the British Journal of Surgery, Butterworth-Heinemann Ltd. (From STEGER 1992a)

Godlewski et al. (1988b) described ultrasound changes in the area irradiated. The effect of high power delivery was the development of an area of hyperechogenicity corresponding to the vaporised region with a surrounding hypoechoic ring. The delivery of such high powers (which do make use of the potential of laser energy) in a short time and the resulting vaporization make it impossible to study the appearances of the development of thermal change. Ultrasonic studies (U/S) of these lesions were carried out to the end of the study (120 days), and the point made that with central scarring and surrounding healing complete, resolution to normal was not seen on U/S.

With U/S the resolution of lesions of thermal necrosis caused by ILH can be described and followed (Bosman et al. 1991; Steger et al. 1992b; Dachman et al. 1990). When using 1–1.5 W it is possible to closely follow the development of thermal damage around the fibre (Steger et al. 1992b). With multiple-fibre ILH the development of overlap between fibres can be seen and the growth of such lesions followed (Steger et al. 1992b) to their resolution. Figure 9.7 shows the ultrasonic appearance of a lesion of thermal necrosis at 30 days. All of the aforementioned authors found that there was good correlation between ultrasonic appearances, temperature measurements and the development of thermal necrosis (compare Figs. 9.5–9.7 from the same set of experiments). The importance of this is that ultrasound allows real-time imaging of tissue changes during heating, which point temperature measurement does not, and is non-invasive.

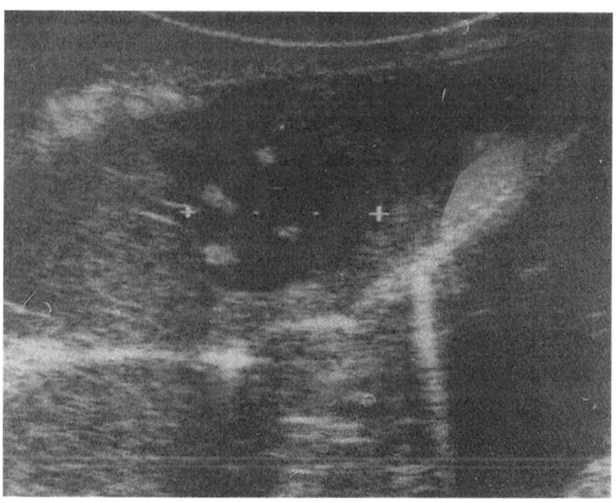

Fig. 9.7. U/S picture of a lesion at 30 days. The four areas of charring are clear, set in a hypoechoic surround, which has a clear margin with surrounding normal liver (+ to +). Reproduced by permission of the Editor and Publishers of the British Journal of Surgery, Butterworth-Heinemann Ltd. (From Steger et al. 1992a)

Magnetic resonance imaging (MRI) may well prove to be of great value in the imaging of ILH (Bleier and Jolesz 1991, personal communication). This could particularly relate to the edge of any area of thermal damage to study whether or not cell death has occurred. The technique may also be used as a method of measuring tissue temperature.

9.6 Clinical Experience

There is some limited clinical use of laser hyperthermia. Some of this is an extension of experimental work and in some cases laser energy has been used to destroy rather than to heat tumour in situ. Most of this work has been with cancers that were considered to be otherwise untreatable and therefore the results reflect this.

In the patients treated by Hashimoto et al. (1985), a modified fibre tip was used at laparotomy. Eight patients with hepatic colorectal metastases were treated, with subsequent reduction in serum carcinoembryonic antigen concentrations. No comment was made on the effect on patient survival. The artificial sapphire probe has also been used at laparotomy to vaporize secondary hepatic tumours. However, whilst computerized tomographic (CT) scanning showed evidence of necrosis, one patient died at operation from air embolism due to the paradoxical use of cooling gas to cool the sapphire probe (Schroder et al. 1989; Baggish and Daniell 1989). Both these approaches involve a laparotomy in patients with terminal disease, an approach some might question.

On the basis of the experimental work described above, low power multiple-fibre ILH with U/S monitoring was thought to be a feasible method by which to produce in situ necrosis in human hepatic and pancreatic tumours (Steger et al. 1989).

The experimental work on ILH showed that it was possible to cause discrete areas of thermal necrosis in normal canine liver of dimensions that were comparable to those of human tumours. This was achieved with one application of laser irradiation and the development of the area of thermal damage could be accurately monitored in real time with ultrasound. These two features represent an advance over other hyperthermic modalities that yield temperatures in a theoretically therapeutic range but with which the aim of treatment, the killing of tissue, has not been reported in the dimensions found possible with ILH (and possibly the other laser techniques discussed above).

Ten patients with 18 hepatic metastases and three with pancreatic cancers unsuitable for surgery have been treated. All applications were percutaneous with mild sedation and prophylactic antibiotic cover, with no complications and a hospital stay of 36–48 h. Those with liver tumours have been treated on one to four occasions (31 treatments in all), usually with four fibres simultaneously, depending on the size of the tumour, the response seen on serial follow-up with ultrasound and CT scans, and the development of new metastases. Response was seen in 44%, with more evidence of necrosis in tumours under 3 cm in diameter (MASTERS et al. 1992). In the pancreatic cancers there has been no effect on survival, but there has been post-mortem evidence of necrosis caused by treatment.

9.7 Conclusions and the Future

Interstitial laser hyperthermia applied percutaneously with ultrasound guidance is a method of causing precise amounts of tumour necrosis that can be accurately monitored in its formation. As a method of treating otherwise incurable disease it is relatively atraumatic and has had no morbidity to date. The temperatures are higher than in conventional hyperthermia. The use of laser energy allows this and means that the likelihood of causing necrosis is much greater with each treatment. The aim of treatment is to cause cell death and necrosis and to prevent continued tumour growth. Treatment times of 20–30 min and the ability to effectively reach deep-seated tumours are great advantages. Ultrasound monitoring permits precise localisation and dynamic real-time imaging of the changes that occur as a result of the higher temperatures.

This technique may have a role in the treatment of (liver and pancreatic) cancers as palliation to reduce tumour growth rate initially, in patients unable to receive curative surgery. Of other modalities that are used for the local treatment of liver tumours, cryotherapy requires a laparotomy and a 5- to 10-day hospital stay. Percutaneous alcohol injection is less precise than laser hyperthermia (VAN EYKEN et al. 1991) but is simple and cheap and can be done on a day case basis. However, the mere injection of alcohol is no guarantee that necrosis will develop. The three methods of causing local necrosis in liver tumours that are currently in use all have drawbacks. Alcohol injection is the cheapest and easiest but ILH on balance is more precise and has the great advantage that it can be monitored in its action more easily than the other two (MASTERS et al. 1991) and may be the better technique. Time will tell.

With laser techniques there are not the problems of patient and room isolation and risks to attendant medical personnel that have to be taken into account when using electromagnetic wave-induced hyperthermia. Hyperthermia caused by radiofrequency or microwave methods has been used as part of multimodality treatments, as a sensitiser for chemotherapy and radiotherapy, with little effect on the treated tumours (in the liver and pancreas). There are designs of microwave antennae for interstitial placement for which theoretical heating patterns are given. The use of any of these or other electromagnetic wave hyperthermia systems, including ferromagnetic seed implants and hot water circulating needles, which are two potential point heat source techniques, has not yet produced local hepatic necrosis of the dimensions seen with ILH.

Interstitial laser hyperthermia overcomes many of the problems seen with other hyperthermic applications, including those pertaining to tumour effect, side-effects and organ accessibility. It is too early to comment further on the therapeutic value of the technique. This method of laser hyperthermia is simple and does not need applicators or tip modifications or to be applied at operation. It can be easily repeated if need be, which is not the case with operative treatments, either laser hyperthermic or cryosurgical. ILH also offers great potential for the in situ treatment of a wide variety of tumours, including those of the adrenal, hyperparathyroid and prostate glands. As it is now possible to detect liver tumours (primary or secondary) much earlier than in the past, possibly even when they are asymptomatic, it becomes more pertinent than ever to be able to treat these tumours with a low complication rate. Low power ILH is a technique that meets this criterion.

With time the other techniques described here for causing local tissue necrosis, thermal and non-thermal, will develop further, as will laser hyperthermia. It should then be possible for comparative analyses to be carried out on both the techniques themselves and the long-term results of patient treatments. It is unlikely that any one treatment will be applicable in all circumstances. It is essential that the work carried out is well documented by means of phase II and III trials.

The impression that is beginning to appear from the laser literature is that with Nd-YAG laser powers in the region of 5 W it may be possible to produce larger dimensions of thermal necrosis (2–3 cm) around a single fibre than have so far been achieved, possibly with modification to the fibre tip but not with any probe addition to the fibre. The fibres would be part of a multiple-fibre system, thus allowing greater areas to be treated in one sitting. As more sophisticated multiple-fibre systems evolve, so treatment will be under interstitial fibre sensory feedback modification combined with real-time imaging and possibly control by ultrasound or MRI. These may be linked to a computer to form a feedback loop and modify a preset programme designed to treat a particular tumour of previously calculated dimensions. This type of in situ tumour debulking may be combined with other treatments such as chemotherapy.

It will be some time, I fear, before the development of an automated plug in treatment of short duration during which the patient and doctor chat over a cup of tea!

References

Baggish MS, Daniell JF (1989) Death caused by air embolus associated with Nd-YAG laser surgery and artificial sapphire tips. Am J Obstet Gynecol 161: 877–878

Bosman S, Phoa SSK Bosma A, van Gemert MJC (1991) Effects of percutaneous interstitial thermal laser on normal liver of pigs: sonographic and histopathological correlations. Br J Surg 78: 572–575

Bown SG (1983) Phototherapy of tumours. World J Surg 7: 700–709

Cummins L, Neuenberg M (1983) Thermal effects of laser radiation in biological tissue. Biophys J 42: 99–102

Dachman AH, McGee JA, Beam TE, Burris JA, Powell DA (1990) US guided percutaneous laser ablation of liver tissue in a chronic pig model. Radiology 25: 627–630

Davis M, Dowden J, Steger AC, Kapadia P, Whiting P (1989) A mathematical model for interstitial laser treatment of tumours using four fibres. Lasers Med Sci 4: 41–53

Dickinson MR, Charlton A, King TA, Freemont AJ, Bramley R (1991) Studies of er-YAG interactions with soft tissue. Lasers Med Sci 6: 125–132

Dowden JM, Davis M, Kapadia P, Matthewson K (1987) Heat flow in laser treatment by local hyperthermia. Lasers Med Sci 2: 211–221

Einstein A (1917) Zur Quantem Theorie der Strahlung. Physikalische Zeitschrift 18: 121–30. In: Elmsford A (ed) (1967) Old quantum theory. Pergamon, New York, pp 167–183

Godlewski G, Sambuc P, Eledjam JJ, Pignodel C, Ould-Said A, Bourgeois JM (1988a) A new device for inducing deep localised vapourisation in liver with the Nd-YAG laser. Lasers Med Sci 3: 111–117

Godlewski G, Rouy S, Pignodel C, Ould-Said A, Eledjam JJ, Bourgeois JM, Sambuc P (1988b) Deep localised Nd-YAG laser photocoagulation in liver using a new water cooled and echoguided handpiece. Lasers Surg Med 8: 501–509

Halldorsson T, Langerholc J (1978) Thermodynamic analysis of laser irradiation of biological tissue. Appl Optics 17: 3948–3958

Hashimoto D, Takami M, Idezuki Y (1985) In depth radiation therapy by YAG laser for malignant tumours in the liver under ultrasonic imaging (abstract). Gastroenterology 88: 1663

Hashimoto D, Yabe K, Uedera Y (1988) Ultrasonic guided laser therapy for liver cancers – experimental temperature measurements and clinical application. In: Waidelich W, Waidelich R (eds) Laser, optoelectronics in medicine. Proceedings of the 7th Congress International Society for Laser Surgery and Medicine 1987. Springer, Berlin Heidelberg New York, pp 168–171

Hashimoto D, Yabe K, Uedera Y (1989) Ultrasonographically guided lasers and spheric lasers. In: Riemann JF, Ell C (eds) Lasers in gastroenterology. International experiences and trends. Thieme, Stuttgart, pp 134–138

Hoye RC, Thomas LB, Riggle GC, Ketcham A (1968) Effects of Nd laser on normal liver and Vx2 carcinoma transplanted into the liver of experimental animals. J Natl Cancer Inst 41: 1071–1082

Kanemaki N, Tsunekawa H, Brunger C et al. (1988) Endoscopic Nd-YAG laserthermia: experimental study on carcinoma bearing BDF_1 mice. In: Waidelich W, Waidelich R (eds) Laser, optoelectronics in medicine. Proceedings of the 7th Congress International Society for Laser Surgery and Medicine 1987. Springer, Berlin Heidelberg New York, pp 200–203

Kubelka P (1948) New contributions to the optics of intensely light scattering materials J Opt Soc Am [A] 38: 448–457

Langerholc J (1979) Moving phase transitions in laser-irradiated biological tissue. Appl Optics 18: 2286–2293

Maiman TH (1960) Stimulated optical radiation in ruby. Nature 187: 4493–4494

Masters A, Steger AC, Bown SG (1991) Role of interstitial therapy in the treatment of liver cancer. Br J Surg 78: 518–523

Masters A, Steger AC, Lees WR, Walmsley KM, Bown SG (1992) Interstitial laser hyperthermia: a new approach for treating liver metastases. Br J Cancer 66: 518–522

Matthewson K, Coleridge-Smith P, Northfield TC, Bown SG (1986) Comparison of continuous wave and pulsed excitation for interstitial Nd-YAG induced hyperthermia. Lasers Med Sci 1: 197–201

Matthewson K, Coleridge-Smith P, O'Sullivan JP, Northfield TC, Bown SG (1987) Biological effects of intrahepatic Nd-YAG laser photocoagulation in rats. Gastroenterology 93: 550–557

Matthewson K, Barr H, Tralau C, Bown SG (1989) Low power interstitial Nd-YAG laser photocoagulation, studies in a transplantable fibrosarcoma. Br J Surg 76: 378–381

Matthewson K, Barton T, Lewin MR, O'Sullivan JP, Northfield TC, Bown SG (1988) Low power interstitial Nd-YAG laser photocoagulation in normal and neoplastic rat colon. Gut 29: 27–34

McKenzie AL (1990) Physics of thermal processes in laser-tissue interaction. Phys Med Biol 35: 1175–1209

Mordon SR, Brunetaud JM, Mosqet L, Charlier JR, Carpentier F, Bourez J, Migne J (1983) Pulsed Nd-YAG laser: study with an infrared camera, In: Joffe SN, Muckerheide MC, Goldman L (eds) ND-YAG laser in medicine and surgery. Elsevier Science, New York, pp 271–276
Mordon SR, Cornil AH, Brunetaud JM, Gosselin B, Moscetto Y (1987) Nd-YAG laser thermal effect: comparative study of coagulation in rat liver in vivo by continuous wave and high power pulsed lasers. Lasers Med Sci 2: 285–294
Mullins F, Hoye R, Ketcham AS, Kelly MG, O'Gara RW, McKnight WB, Jennings B (1967) Studies in laser destruction of chemically induced primate hepatomas. Am Surg 33: 298–303
Nakamura S, Nishiwaki Y, Suzuki S, Sakaguchi S, Yamashita Y, Ohta K (1990) Light attenuation of human liver and hepatic tumours after surgical resection. Lasers Surg Med 10: 12–15
Nishisaka T, Ozawa Y, Yonekawa M (1983) Analytical calculation of temperature distribution in biological tissue under laser irradiation In: Atsumi K (eds) New frontiers in laser medicine and surgery. Excerpta Medica, Amsterdam, pp 83–90
Nolsoe C, Torp-Pederson S, Olldag E, Holm HH (1992) Bare fibre low power Nd-YAG laser interstitial hyperthermia. Comparison between diffuser tip and non-modified tip. An in vitro study. Lasers Med Sci 7: 1–8
Panjehpour M, Overholt B, Milligan AJ, Swaggerty MW, Wilkinson JE, Klebanow ER (1990) ND-YAG laser induced interstitial hyperthermia using a long frosted contact probe. Lasers Surg Med 10: 16–24
Parrish JA, Deutsch TF (1984) Laser photomedicine. IEEE Quantum Electronics QE-20: 1386–1396
Patterson MS, Wilson BS, Wyman DR (1991a) The propagation of optical radiation in tissue. 1: Models of radiation transport and their application Lasers Med Sci 6: 155–168
Patterson MS, Wilson BS, Wyman DR (1991b) The propagation of optical radiation in tissue. II: Optical properties of tissues and resulting fluence distributions. Lasers Med Sci 6: 379–390
Schroder T, Puolakkainen PA, Hahl J, Ramo OJ (1989) Fatal air embolism as a complication of laser induced hyperthermia. Lasers Surg Med 9: 183–185
Steger AC (1990) Low power applications of the Nd-YAG laser in general surgery. MS Thesis, University of London
Steger AC, Bown SG (1989) Use of multiple fibre optic systems in the medical application of lasers. In: Katzir A (ed) The Proceedings of the SPIE-The International Society for Optical Engineering (SPIE Proceedings Series Volume 1067) Optical fibres in medicine IV, January 1989, pp 256–259
Steger AC, McNicholas T (1990) Interstitial hyperthermia of the prostate. In: McNicholas TA (ed) Lasers in urology. Springer, London
Steger AC, Barr H, Hawes R, Bown SG, Clark CG (1987) Experimental studies on low power laser interstitial hyperthermia for pancreatic cancer. Gut 28: A1382
Steger AC, Lees WR, Walmsley K, Bown SG (1989) Interstitial laser hyperthermia: a new approach to local destruction of tumours. Br Med J 299: 362–365
Steger AC, Lees WR, Shorvon P, Walmsley K, Bown SG (1992a) Multiple-fibre low-power interstitial laser hyperthermia: studies in the normal liver. Br J Surg 79: 139–145
Steger AC, Shorvon P, Walmsley K, Chisholm R, Bown SG, Lees WR (1992b) Ultrasound features of low power interstitial laser hyperthermia Clin Radiol: 46: 88–93
Svaasand L (1984) Thermal and optical dosimetry and photoradiation therapy of malignant tumours In: Cubeddu R, Andreoni A (eds) Porphorins in tumour phototherapy. Plenum, New York, pp 261–279
Svaasand LO, Boerslid T, Oeveraasen M (1985) Thermal and optical properties of living tissue: application to laser induced hyperthermia. Lasers Surg Med 5: 589–602
Townes CH, Schawlow A (1958) Infrared and optical lasers. Phys Rev, 2nd series, 112: 1940–1949
van Eyken P, Hiele M, Fevery J et al. (1991) Comparative study of low power Nd-YAG laser interstitial laser hyperthermia versus ethanol injection for controlled hepatic tissue destruction. Lasers Med Sci 6: 35–42
van Gemert MC, Henning JPH (1981) Model approach to laser coagulation of dermal vascular lesions. Arch Dermatol Res 270: 429–439
Waldow SM, Morrison PR, Grossweiner LI (1988) Nd-YAG laser-induced hyperthermia in a mouse tumour model. Lasers Surg Med 8: 510–514
Welch AJ (1984) The thermal response of laser irradiated tissue. IEEE J Quantum Electronics QE-20: 1471–1481
Wilson BC, Patterson MS (1986) The physics of photodynamic therapy. Phys Med Biol 31: 327–360
Yoon G, Welch AJ, Motammedi M, van Gemert CJ (1987) Development and application of three dimensional light distribution model for laser irradiated tissue. IEEE J Quantum Electronics QE-23: 1721–1732

10 Review of Intracavitary Hyperthermia Techniques

D. Roos

CONTENTS

10.1 Introduction

Intracavitary hyperthermia is one of three modalities which come under the heading of internal hyperthermia. The other two modalities are interstitial and perfusional hyperthermia. Internal hyperthermia in oncology and especially intracavitary hyperthermia is often combined with radiotherapy in the form of brachytherapy. As in brachytherapy, the aim with intracavitary hyperthermia is to limit the treatment to only the tumor volume and thereby to spare normal tissue surrounding the tumor.

It is clear that tumors located in body cavities can be treated by intracavitary hyperthermia techniques. One of the first groups (Mendecki et al. 1978) to discuss this treatment modality mentioned treatment sites such as the bladder, esophagus, and rectum. Since then numerous reports dealing with intracavitary hyperthermia have been published. Most of the reports describe applicator design together with measurements in phantoms and animals (Petrowicz et al. 1979; Sterzer et al. 1980; Mendecki et al. 1980; Scheiblich and Petrowicz 1982; Hand et al. 1982; Sugimachi et al. 1983a; Li et al. 1984; Roos et al. 1989; Astrahan et al. 1989; Diedrich and Hynynen 1989, 1990; Liru et al. 1990; Zhong et al. 1990). There are also some experimental clinical studies (Sugimachi et al. 1983b, 1988; Leybovich et al. 1987; Matsufuji et al. 1988; Wong et al. 1988; Valdagni et al. 1988; Schoracht et al. 1989; Sorbe et al. 1990), each with a few case reports. Additionally a few papers describe preliminary clinical work (Kochegarov et al. 1981; Li et al. 1982; Petrovich et al. 1985; Bichler et al. 1990; Sugimachi and Matsuda 1990; Berdov and Menteshasvili 1990).

A growing interest in the field of intracavitary hyperthermia, where hyperthermia is given alone without any form of radiotherapy, is use of the technique for the treatment of benign diseases like prostatic hyperplasia (Yerushalmi et al. 1985; Sapozink et al. 1990) and functional menorraghia (Phipps et al. 1990).

This paper is a review of the techniques used in intracavitary hyperthermia which have been discussed in the literature. Some aspects of thermometry in intracavitary hyperthermia are also presented.

10.2 Intracavitary Hyperthermia Techniques

Various techniques have been described to induce hyperthermia in tumors located in body cavities. The techniques involved use of radiofrequency electrodes, microwave antennas, ultrasound transducers, and hot source methods. Among these techniques, microwave antennas are the most commonly used, as can be seen in Fig. 10.1A, followed by radiofrequency electrodes, while ultrasound transducers and hot source techniques are not very frequently used. The esophagus is the most commonly reported treatment site, as can be seen in Fig. 10.1B, followed by pelvic sites like the rectum, uterine cervix, prostate, vagina, and bladder. Treatment sites like the trachea, bile duct, and nasopharynx are only mentioned on very rare occasions. It can be noted that microwave antennas

D. Roos, Ph.D., Department of Gynecologic Oncology, Örebro Medical Center Hospital, S-701 85 Örebro, Sweden

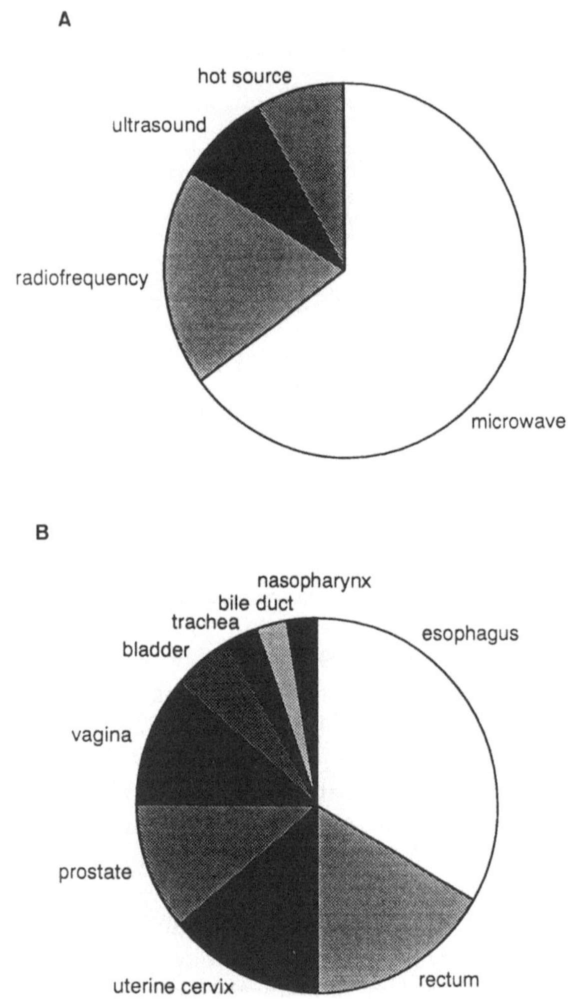

Fig. 10.1 A, B. Distribution of reported techniques (**A**) and treatment sites (**B**) in 30 papers

have been used in most treatment sites and that radiofrequency electrodes are mostly used in the esophagus. A survey of the reported intracavitary techniques is shown in Table 10.1.

10.2.1 Radiofrequency Electrodes

The heating by intracavitary radiofrequency electrodes is accomplished by a high frequency (typically 13.56 or 27 MHz) electrical field distributed between an internal and an external electrode. The electrodes are of different shape and size. The internal electrode is insulated and rod shaped. It is positioned at the treatment site and is small, with a diameter in the region of 10 mm. The external electrode, which often is a large plate or flexible belt, is positioned on the outside of the body. This arrangement concentrates the electrical field in the tissue close to the internal electrode. A good electrical contact is critical for the external electrode to avoid heating of the skin. The square of the electrical field is proportional to the SAR (specific absorption rate), which is the heat source. The SAR gradient is steep in the radial direction while a relatively even SAR distribution is obtained along the internal electrode. The technique has been used in the treatment of the esophagus (Sugimachi and Matsuda 1990) and bladder (Bichler et al. 1990). These applications of the technique are shown in Fig. 10.2.

10.2.2 Microwave Antennas

As can be seen in Fig. 10.1A, most work has been performed using microwave techniques i.e., insulated coaxial antennas. The frequencies commonly used have been 2450, 915, and 434 MHz. The basic principle for the action of these antennas is that a microwave current distributed on the antenna surface causes emission of an electromagnetic wave in the close vicinity of the antenna. The microwave power thus distributed in the surrounding tissue acts as a heat source. The antenna length must be carefully selected so that the applied microwave

Table 10.1. Survey of some characteristics of intracavitary hyperthermia techniques

	RF electrodes	Microwave antennas	Ultrasound transducers	Hot sources
Frequency (MHz)	13.56 27.12	434 915 2450	0.5–10	–
Mode of activity	em. power deposition	em. power deposition	acoustic power deposition	thermal conduction
Treatment sites	esophagus bladder cervix	esophagus rectum prostate vagina cervix	prostate rectum vagina	esophagus cervix

em. = electromagnetic

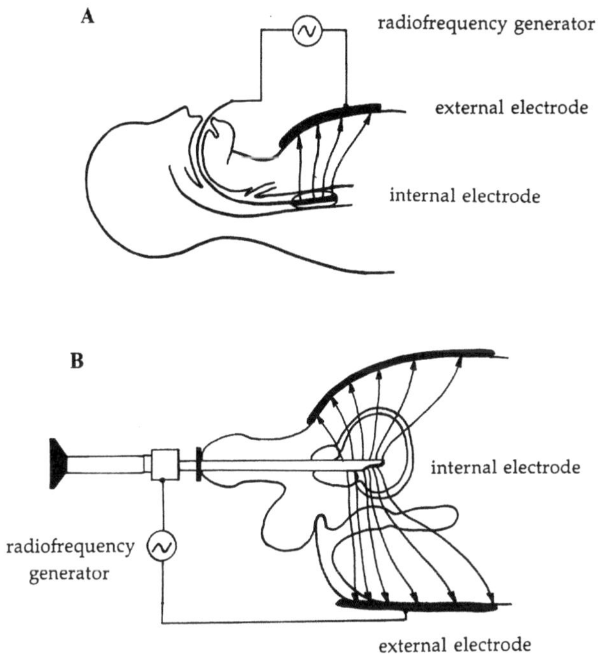

Fig. 10.2 A, B. Example of the use of radiofrequency electrodes for (**A**) treatment of the esophagus and (**B**) treatment of the bladder. The figures are redrawn from SUGIMACHI and MATSUDA (1990) and from BICHLER et al. (1990)

power is properly delivered into the surrounding tissue.

The shape of the microwave power distribution in the tissue, which is identical to the SAR distribution, is normally ellipsoidal and centered at the antenna feeding point. If no cooling system is present within the applicator the maximum temperature will always appear close to the applicator surface adjacent to the antenna feeding point. The length of a 50% SAR ellipsoidal contour is about 60 mm and the radial penetration at the feeding point is 10 mm (HAND et al. 1982) for an applicator operating at 915 MHz.

Theoretical calculations were performed for the SAR distribution as well as the resulting steady-state temperature distribution (BIFFI-GENTILI et al. 1991) produced by an applicator at 434 MHz. Internal water cooling was also included and it was demonstrated that a temperature peak appears at a radial distance of about 10 mm from the applicator surface. It was also shown that the tissue temperature close to the applicator surface could be altered by varying the temperature and flow rate of the cooling water.

Besides the coaxial antennas, helical structures terminating coaxial cables have been designed (ASTRAHAN et al. 1991). The action of these applicators is not yet completely understood and the design is therefore empirical. Clinical applications are, however, in the process of being developed.

The treatments of benign prostatic hyperplasia are normally performed using microwave antennas. In the case of transrectal heating (LINDNER et al. 1990) the applicator is positioned at the level of the prostate and temperatures are monitored in both the rectum and the prostatic urethra. Where a transurethral heating approach is used (BAERT et al. 1990) the applicator is positioned in the prostatic urethra together with temperature monitoring probes for both temperature control and temperature mapping along the urethra.

An example of the use of microwave antennas is shown in Fig. 10.3. SAR contour lines are shown for two vaginal applicators with no cooling applied.

10.2.3 Ultrasound Transducers

The heating produced by intracavitary ultrasonic applicators is based on the emission of a pressure wave in the ultrasound range (normally 0.5–10 MHz) from the applicator surface. The power distributed in the surrounding tissue is proportional to the square of the amplitude of the pressure. Intracavitary ultrasound applicators can be made with a suitable diameter and internal cooling by degassed water is normally included. A characteristic feature for the ultrasound technique is that multiple-element arrays can be designed (DIEDRICH and HYNYNEN 1989) to control the acoustic power distribution especially along the applicator. It has also been shown by simulation (DIEDRICH and HYNYNEN 1990) that the distant temperature peak position and the radial penetration in tissue can be varied by changing the frequency. For the frequency range 0.5–4 MHz the radial penetration was in the range 30–15 mm with constant cooling.

A schematic picture of a multielement ultrasound applicator is shown in Fig. 10.4.

10.2.4 Hot Source Techniques

One of the oldest reports on hyperthermia deals with intracavitary treatment of gynecologic tumors (WESTERMARK 1898). A hollow copper spiral was introduced vaginally and hot water was circulated

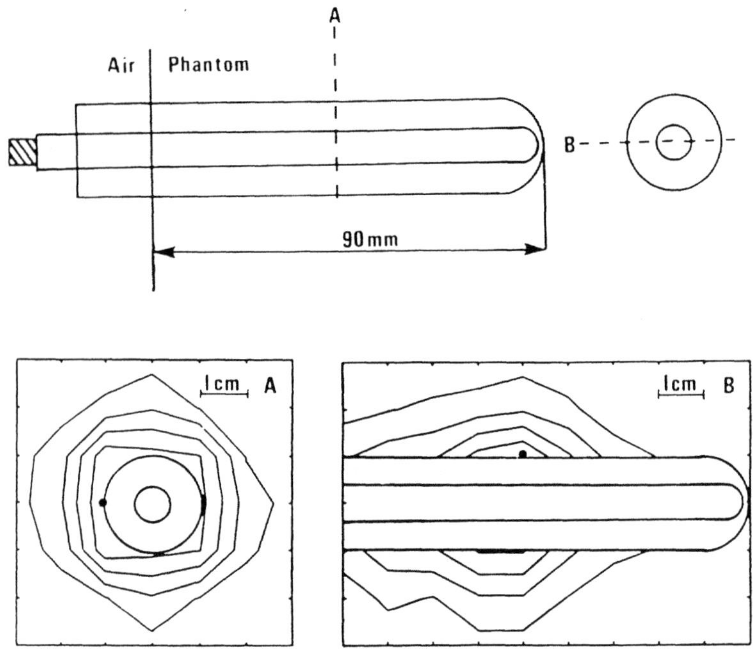

Fig. 10.3 A. SAR contour lines, for a 20 mm vaginal microwave applicator with symmetric heating pattern, measured at 915 MHz. The contour lines in both the transverse plane A and longitudinal plane B represents, going inwards, 20, 40, 60 and 80% of the maximum measured SAR value

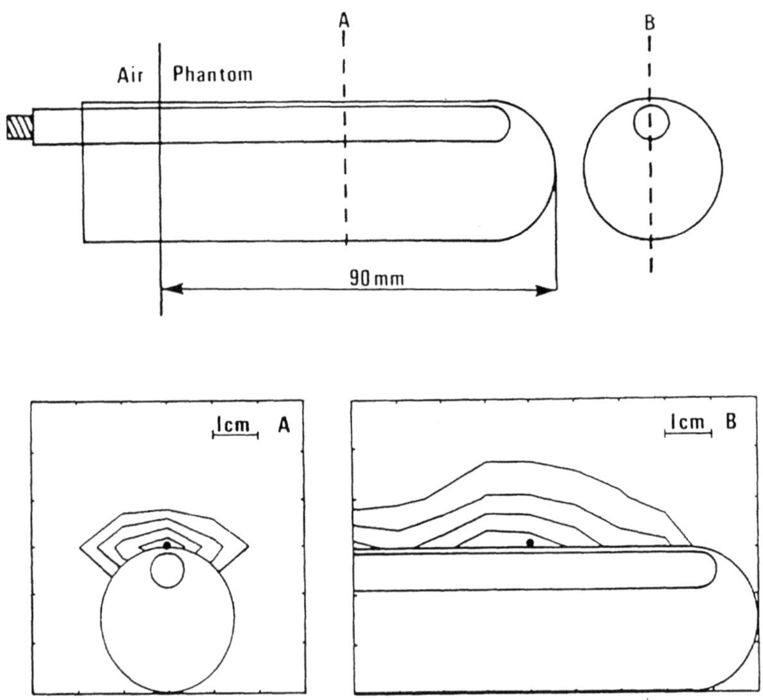

Fig. 10.3 B. SAR contour lines, for a 30 mm vaginal microwave applicator with asymmetric heating pattern, measured at 915 MHz. The contour lines in the transverse plane A represents, going inwards, 50, 60, 70 and 80% of the maximum measured SAR value. The contour lines in the longitudinal plane B represents, going inwards, 20, 40, 60 and 80% of the maximum measured SAR value

within the spiral. More recently, intracavitary hyperthermia by hot source techniques was presented by KOCHEGAROV et al. (1981) and SUGIMACHI et al. (1983). Both authors treated tumors of the esophagus by hot water perfusion of an esophageal tube or balloon. The radial penetration is poor but the method must be considered safe and relatively easy to perform. One advantage of the method is

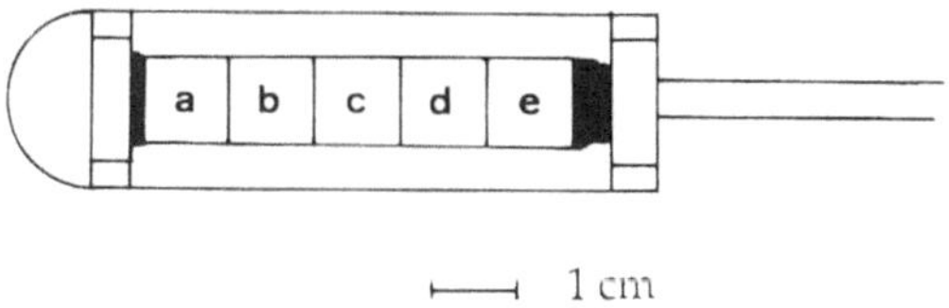

Fig. 10.4. Schematic picture of a linear array ultrasound applicator with five elements (*a–e*), redrawn from DIEDRICH and HYNYNEN (1989)

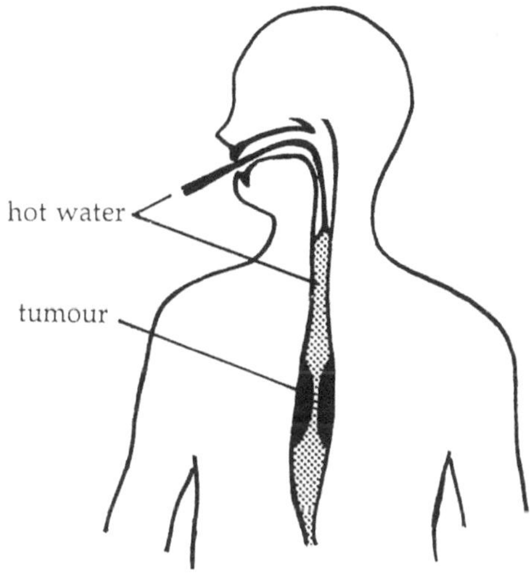

Fig. 10.5. Hot water perfusion for the treatment of carcinoma of the esophagus, redrawn from SUGIMACHI et al. (1983)

that the maximum temperature is always known. The application of an intracavitary hot source technique is illustrated in Fig. 10.5.

10.3 Thermometry in Intracavitary Hyperthermia

Invasive techniques such as thermistor, thermocouple, and fiberoptic probes are the most commonly used methods of thermometry in intracavitary applications. Measurements on the applicator surface are in general performed with probes either taped on the applicator or built-in.

Intratumoral temperatures are often difficult to register. In some treatment sites such as the vagina, probes can be interstitially inserted parallel to the applicator using a template. For the esophagus a similar procedure is probably not possible and therefore the intratumoral temperature data are not always given.

Noninvasive thermometry techniques based on radiometry, electrical impedance tomography, or ultrasound are therefore urgently needed in intracavitary hyperthermia. Noninvasive techniques will give better treatment control and ensure less trauma for the patient. The size and shape of the heated volume will be easier to estimate. Additionally, noninvasive thermometry will become a valuable complement to the ongoing work in thermal modelling of intracavitary hyperthermia applications.

10.4 Discussion

The described intracavitary hyperthermia techniques all show good examples of being able to adapt to a specific treatment site. A suitable diameter and shape for the applicator can be selected for the anatomic situation.

If we assume that the applicator is cylindrical, but not necessarily having a symmetric heat pattern around the axis, the radial penetration of the various techniques can be compared. The ultrasound technique has the greatest penetration, in the range of a few centimeters, followed by the microwave technique, while the radiofrequency technique has less penetration and the hot source technique has a penetration of only a few millimeters. It is, however, important to remember that the blood perfusion in the heated tissue greatly affects the heat pattern of any technique. It is therefore not wise to set up sharp boundaries, especially in terms of penetration, between techniques. It is more important that the selected techniques is flexible, comfortable, and easy to use so that there is no restriction in performing intracavitary hyperthermia. To reach this point the engineers, physicists, and physicians must continue to work in close collaboration, especially to improve the action of applicators and noninvasive thermometry.

References

Astrahan M, Sapozink M, Luxton G, Kampp T, Petrovich Z (1989) A technique for combining microwave hyperthermia with intraluminal brachytherapy of the oesophagus. Int J Hyperthermia 5: 37–51

Astrahan M, Imanaka K, Jozsef G et al. (1991) Heating characteristics of a helical microwave applicator for transurethral hyperthermia of benign prostatic hyperplasia. Int J Hyperthermia 7: 141–155

Baert L, Amaye F, Willemen P, Vandenhove J, Lauweryns J, Astrahan M, Petrovich Z (1990) Transurethral microwave hyperthermia for benign prostatic hyperplasia: preliminary clinical and pathological results. J Urol 144: 1383–1387

Berdov B, Menteshasvili G (1990) Thermoradiotherapy of

patients with locally advanced carcinoma of the rectum. Int J Hyperthermia 6: 881–890
Bichler K, Strohmaier W, Steimann W, Fluchter S (1990) Hyperthermia in urology. In: Gautherie M (ed) Interstitial, endocavitary and perfusional hyperthermia: methods and clinical trials. Springer, Berlin Heidelberg New York, p 43
Biffi-Gentili G, Gori F, Leoncini M (1991) Electromagnetic and thermal models of a water-cooled dipole radiating in a biological tissue. IEEE Trans Biomed Eng 38: 98–103
Diedrich C, Hynynen K (1989) Induction of hyperthermia using an intracavitary multielement ultrasonic applicator. IEEE Trans Biomed Eng 36: 432–438
Diedrich C, Hynynen K (1990) The development of intracavitary ultrasonic applicators for hyperthermia: a design and experimental study. Med Phys 17: 626–634
Hand J, Blake P, Hopewell J, Lambert H, Field S (1982) A coaxial applicator for intracavitary hyperthermia of carcinoma of the cervix. In: Gautherie M, Albert E (eds) Biomedical thermology. Liss, New York, p 635 (Progress in Clinical and Biological Research, vol 17)
Kochegarov A, Muratkhodzhaev N, Alimnazarov S (1981) Hyperthermia in the combined treatment of esophageal cancer patients. J Soviet Oncol 2: 17–22
Leybovich L, Emami B, Straube W, Schlessinger E, Nussbaum G, Devineni D, Sessions D (1987) Intracavitary hyperthermia: a newly designed applicator for tracheal tumours. Endocurietherapy/Hyperthermia Oncol 3: 23–29
Li D-J, Wang C-Q, Qui S-L, Shao L-F (1982) Intraluminal microwave hyperthermia in the combined treatment of esophageal cancer: a preliminary report of 103 patients. Natl Cancer Inst Monoge 61: 419–421
Li D-J, Luk K, Jiang H-B, Chou C-K, Hwang G-Z (1984) Design and thermometry of an intracavitary microwave applicator suitable for treatment of some vaginal and rectal cancers. Int J Radiat Oncol Biol Phys 10: 2155–2162
Lindner A, Siegel Y, Saranga R, Korzcak D, Matzkin H, Braf Z (1990) Complications in hyperthermia treatment of benign prostatic hyperplasia. J Urol 144: 1390–1392
Liru Z, Jianguo W, Zhongfa C, Guizhu W, Lingyi L, Weilian L (1990) 2450 MHz oesophagus applicator with multitemperature sensors and its temperature-control equipment. Int J Hyperthermia 6: 745–753
Matsufuji H, Kuwano H, Kai H, Matsuda H, Sugimachi H (1988) Preoperative Hyperthermia combined with radiotherapy and chemotherapy for patients with incompletely resected careinoma of the esophagus. Cancer 62: 889–894
Mendecki J, Friedenthal E, Botstein C, Sterzer F, Paglione R, Nowogrodski M, Beck E (1978) Microwave-induced hyperthermia in cancer treatment: apparatus and preliminary results. Int J Radiat Oncol Biol Phys 4: 1095–1103
Mendecki J, Friedenthal E, Botstein C, Paglione R, Sterzer F (1980) Microwave applications for localized hyperthermia treatment of cancer of the prostate. Int J Radiat Oncol Biol Phys 6: 1583–1588
Petrovich Z, Astrahan M, Lam K, Tilden T, Luxton G, Jepson J (1985) Intraluminal thermoradiotherapy with teletherapy for carcinoma of the esophagus. Endocurietherapy/Hyperthermia Oncol 4: 155–161
Petrowicz O, Heinkelman W, Erhart W, Wriedt-Lubbe I, Hepp W, Blumel G (1979) Experimental studies on the use of microwaves for localized heat treatment of the prostate. J Micorwave Power 14: 167–171
Phipps J, Lewis B, Roberts T, Prior M, Hand J, Elder M, Field S (1990) Treatment of functional menorraghia by radiofrequency-induced thermal endometrial ablation. Lancet 335: 374–376
Roos D, Hamnerius Y, Alpsten M, Borghede G, Friberg L (1989) Two microwave applicators for intracavitary hyperthermia treatment of cancer colli uteri. Phys Med Biol 34: 1917–1921
Sapozink M, Boyd S, Asrahan M, Jozsef G, Petrovich Z (1990) Transurethral hyperthermia for benign prostatic hyperplasia: preliminary clinical results. J Urol 143: 944–950
Scheiblich J, Petrowicz O (1982) Radiofrequency-induced hyperthermia in the prostate. J Microwave Power 17: 203–209
Schorcht J, Zimmerman M, Redmann M, Eberhart H (1989) Erste Erfahrungen mit kombinerten hochdosierten Afterloading-Kurzeitherapie und Hyperthermie beim nicht operierten Zervixkarcinom. Radiobiol Radiother (Berl) 30: 386–390
Sorbe B, Roos D, Karlsson L (1990) The use of microwave-induced hyperthermia in conjuction with afterloading irradiation of vaginal carcinoma. Acta Oncol 29: 1029–1033
Sterzer F, Paglione R, Nowodgrodzki M, Mendecki J, Friedenthal E, Botstein C (1980) Microwave apparatus for the treatment of cancer. Microwave J 25: 39–44
Sugimachi K, Inokuchi K, Kai H, Sogawa A, Kawai Y (1983a) Endotract antenna for application of hyperthermia to malignant lesions. Gann 74: 622–624
Sugimachi K, Inokuchi K, Kai H, Kuwano H, Matsuzaki K, Natsuda Y (1983b) Hyperthermo-chemo-radiotherapy for carcinoma of the esophagus. Jpn J Surg 13: 101–105
Sugimachi K, Matsuda H, Ohno S, Fukuda A, Matsuoka H, Mori M, Kuwano H (1988) Long term effects of hyperthermia combined with chemotherapy and irradiation for the treatment of patients with carcinoma of the esophagus. Surg Gyn & Obste 167: 319–323
Sugimachi K, Matsuda H (1990) Experimental and clinical studies of hyperthermia for carcinoma of the esophagus. In: Gautherie M (ed) Interstitial, endocavitary and perfusional hyperthermia: methods and clinical trials. Springer, Berlin Heidelberg New York, p 59
Valdagni R, Amichetti M, Christoforetti L (1988) Intracavitary hyperthermia: construction of individualized vaginal prototype applicators. Int J Hyperthermia 4: 457–466
Westermark F (1898) Über die behandlung des ulcerirenden cervikcarcinoms mittels konstanter wärme. Centralb Gynäkologie 22: 1335–1339
Wong J, Vora N, Chou C-K et al. (1988) Intracatheter hyperthermia and iridium-192 radiotherapy in the treatment of bile duct carcinoma. Int J Radiat Oncol Biol Phys 14: 359
Yerushalmi A, Fishelovitz Y, Singer D et al. (1985) Localized deep microwave hyperthermia in the treatment of poor operative risk patients with benign with prostatic hyperplasia. J Urol 133: 873–876
Zhong Q, Chou C-K, McDougall J, Chan K, Luk K (1990) Intracavitary hyperthermia applicators for treating nasopharyngeal and cervical cancers. Int J Hyperthermia 6: 997–1004

Part II
Treatment Control and Treatment Planning

11 Invasive Thermometry Practice for Interstitial Hyperthermia

J.W. HAND

CONTENTS

11.1 Introduction

The importance of thermometry (a) to monitor and control hyperthermia treatments and (b) to provide the quantitative information needed to develop prognostic parameters to aid planning and dosimetry cannot be overstated. Currently we must resort to the use of invasive probes to obtain the necessary temperature data. Several invasive thermometry techniques and practices have been developed for use in clinical hyperthermia but each is subject to one or more sources of artefact, and care is needed to ensure good practice and a high quality of thermometry (CETAS 1990; SAMULSKI and FESSENDEN 1990).

The purpose of this brief overview is to summarise guidelines and recommendations for good practice for thermometry in interstitial hyperthermia treatments. Other reviews of thermometry in interstitial hyperthermia are to be found in STAUFFER (1990) and the report of an ESHO task group (ESHO 1992).

11.2 Temperature Sensors

Thermocouples, thermistors, fibre-optic probes and devices which interact with and perturb electromagnetic fields minimally (e.g., miniature thermistors with high resistance leads) have been used as thermometers in interstitial hyperthermia treatments. Suggested minimum performance requirements of invasive thermometers used in clinical hyperthermia are summarised in Table 11.1.

Thermocouple thermometry offers adequate accuracy and stability and a relatively large number of channels at relatively low cost. Artefacts associated with interactions between thermocouples (and thermistors) and the quasi-stationary electric fields encountered in radiofrequency localised current field (RF-LCF) heating techniques may be readily reduced to acceptable levels (CHAKRABORTY and BREZOVICH 1982; CETAS 1990). The relative advantages and disadvantages of thermocouples and thermistors (e.g., magnitude of signal, stability, calibration requirements) are described by CETAS (1990) and SAMULSKI and FESSENDEN (1990). In practice, thermocouples have been used more frequently than thermistors for hyperthermia applications; an important advantage is the relative ease with which multisensor thermocouple probes may be constructed.

The use of thermocouples is an attractive cost-effective thermometric technique for RF-LCF-induced interstitial hyperthermia. Thermocouples

Table 11.1. Suggested minimum performance requirements for invasive thermometers used in interstitial hyperthermia treatments

Parameter	Suggested minimum performance
Resolution	0.1°C (for monitoring and control)[a]
Accuracy	±0.2°C (over range 30°–50°C)
Response time	≤ 3 s (for monitoring and control)[a]
Data rate	≤ 1 s to interrogate all sensors
	≤ 10 s between successive sets of readings
Drift	≤ 0.1°C per hour[b]
Artefact	≤ 0.2°C[c]

[a] Better resolution and faster response may be advantageous when determining specific absorption rate (CETAS 1990)
[b] Accuracy must be maintained from calibration to end of treatment
[c] Residual artefact after corrections have been made

J.W. HAND, Ph.D., Hyperthermia Clinic, MRC Cyclotron Unit, Hammersmith Hospital, Du Cane Road, London W12 OHS, UK also offer the most cost-effective solution to thermometry for hot source interstitial techniques (e.g., hot water tubes, ferromagnetic seeds) although the usual precautions to minimise electromagnetic-related artefacts must be taken in the case of induction heating of ferromagnetic seeds. An additional problem in this case is that commonly used thermocouples contain ferromagnetic material (e.g., constantan) (CETAS 1982).

At the higher frequencies used with microwave interstitial hyperthermia techniques, electromagnetically non-perturbing fibre-optic probes provide the most reliable and artefact-free thermometry. In addition to the elimination of electromagnetic-related artefacts, thermal smearing in the presence of large temperature gradients (see below) can be small due to the low thermal conductivity of the fibres. The use of minimally perturbing probes such as miniature thermistors with high resistance leads provided with some commercial hyperthermia systems is also recommended. However, most fibre-optic thermometers are expensive, offer relatively few channels, may present problems in terms of stability and can be subject to other forms of artefact, for example, if the fibres are bent sharply. A cheaper alternative is to use thermocouple probes which can provide adequate performance if artefacts are carefully characterised and the heating fields are turned off 2–3 s before temperatures are measured. Table 11.2 summarises the preference of thermometric technique according to the interstitial method of inducing hyperthermia employed.

11.3 Calibration

To guarantee the level of accuracy suggested in Table 11.1, thermometers should be calibrated against a local standard accurate to 0.01°–0.02°C and traceable to a national standard. The local standard often consists of precision mercury-in-glass thermometers or standard thermistors used in a well-stirred and regulated water bath. Since no thermometer is guaranteed to be drift-free, the local standard must include three thermometers so that drift in one of them can be detected. Alternatively, thermometric fixed points such as those listed in Table 11.3 may be used as the local standard.

A new International Temperature Scale (ITS-90) has replaced the International Practical Temperature Scale (IPTS-68); the values given in Table 11.3 are in terms of ITS-90. The differences between the scales may be expressed to within 0.001°C above 0°C by

$$t_{90} - t_{68} = \sum_{i=1}^{8} a_i \left(\frac{t_{68}}{630}\right)^i$$

where $a_1 = -0.148759$, $a_2 = -0.267408$, $a_3 = 1.080760$, $a_4 = 1.269056$, $a_5 = -4.089591$, $a_6 = -1.871251$, $a_7 = 7.438081$ and $a_8 =$

Table 11.2. Preferred method of thermometry according to interstitial hyperthermia technique

Preference	RF-LCF	Hot source	Microwave
1st	Thermocouples	Thermocouples	Fibre-optic probes
2nd	Thermistors	Thermistors	Minimally perturbing probes
3rd	Fibre-optic probes [a]	Fibre-optic probes [a]	Thermocouples [b]
4th	Minimally perturbing probes [a]	Minimally perturbing probes [a]	Thermistors [b]

[a] Not cost-effective for use with these heating techniques
[b] With suitable precautions and 2- to 3-s delay between power off and temperature measurement

Table 11.3. Fixed points for calibration of thermometers[a]

Substance	Fixed point		
H_2O	Triple point	0.01°C	± 0.0002°C
Diphenyl ether	Triple point	26.862°C	± 0.002°C
Gallium	Melting point	29.76476°C	± 0.002°C
$Na_2SO_4 \cdot 10H_2O$	Salt hydration point	32.367°C	± 0.002°C
Ethyl carbonate	Triple point	36.316°C	± 0.002°C
$Na_2HPO_4 \cdot 7H_2O$	Salt hydration point	48.209°C	± 0.007°C

[a] The triple point of water and the melting point of gallium are fixed points in the International Temperature Scale ITS-90. The uncertainties are those associated with maintaining the fixed points. Further details are to be found in CETAS (1990) and HAND (1990)

– 3.536296. These differences are ≈ 0.01°C in the region of 43°C.

SHRIVASTAVA et al. (1988) reported the findings of a survey of 166 thermometers in use in several hyperthermia clinics in the United States. Their results suggested that stringent quality control measures were needed to achieve 0.2°C accuracy. Common reasons for inaccuracy were faulty or infrequent calibration procedures, drifts in thermometer characteristics and artefacts.

The frequency at which calibrations should be performed varies from one type of thermometer to another. However, it is good practice to carry out pretreatment checks at one or two temperatures within or near the therapeutic temperature range on all thermometers.

11.4 Thermal Conduction Artefact

A particular problem in interstitial hyperthermia is the likely presence of large temperature gradients (on the order of 10°C cm^{-1}). Artefacts may arise due to thermal conduction along a probe placed in a large temperature gradient; their magnitudes are dependent upon the thermal conductivities and physical dimensions of the probe and catheter.

The problem is usually investigated by measuring the response of the probe to a step change in temperature (CARNOCHAN et al. 1986; DICKINSON 1985; SAMULSKI et al. 1985) although a cell in which a well-defined temperature gradient is maintained is being developed for direct measurement of errors due to conduction (BINI M. and OLMI R., personal communication, 1991). Errors for thermocouple probes are typically 0.05°–0.1°C per °C cm^{-1}; the error may also be expressed as an error length (typically 0.5–1 mm for thermocouples) equivalent to a misplacement of the sensor in the temperature gradient. The error lengths associated with manganin–constantan thermocouples are significantly smaller than those for copper–constantan thermocouples (DICKINSON 1985) (Fig. 11.1). Thermal smearing associated with a fibre-optic probe is low. SAMULSKI et al. (1985) point out that the error length is reduced by using probe–catheter combinations that have a thermal conductivity similar to that of the surrounding tissue and by ensuring there is good thermal contact between the probe, catheter and tissue. A close-fitting or liquid-filled sheath is recommended. An acceptable error length is ≤ 1.5 mm.

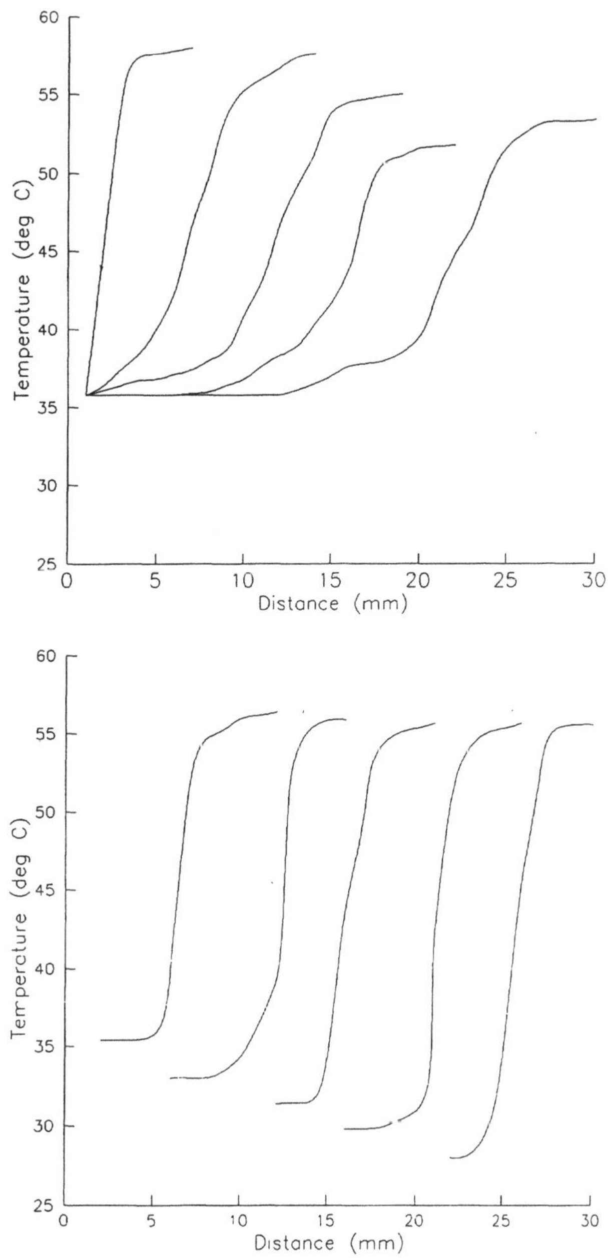

Fig. 11.1. Step response functions (SRFs) for copper-constantan (upper) and manganin constantan (lower) thermocouple arrays (after data of Dickinson (1985)). The thermocouples consisted of a common 50 μm diameter constantan wire and five wires of enamelled copper (60 μm) or manganin (50 μm). Junctions were soldered at 5 mm intervals and the complete arrays were placed within nylon sheaths (inner diameter 0.5 mm, outer diameter 0.63 mm). The thermocouples were moved through a small hole in a membrane from a hot region to a cold one. The junctions closest to the tips of each array are shown on the left in the figures above; these junctions exhibit the narrowest SRFs since heat can be conducted along the wires in only one direction at these points. These data illustrate (i) that the SRF is narrower for manganin-constantan than for copper-constantan and (ii) a widening of the SRF as we move away from tip (i.e., as the number of wires close to a junction increases)

11.5 Guidelines for Treatment Monitoring

The aim of thermometry when monitoring hyperthermia treatments is to provide detailed information concerning the temperature distribution; knowledge of this is a prerequisite for minimising the risk of damage to normal tissue, for determining thermal dose and for optimising treatment by determining the prognostic value of various thermal parameters. Guidelines which cover general requirements for thermometry in clinical hyperthermia (e.g., thermometer performance and calibration guidelines, preferred locations for temperature sensors in tumour and normal tissues and documentation required for hyperthermia treatments) include those proposed by HAND et al. (1989), SHRIVASTAVA et al. (1989) and DEWHIRST et al. (1990). Specific requirements for interstitial treatments are discussed by EMAMI et al. (1991).

Temperatures should be measured at locations representative of maximum and minimum tumour temperatures. In addition to monitoring within or close to electrodes or antennas (locations also required for control, see below), preferred locations are midway between two heat sources, centrally between four (or other subgroup of) heat sources, at the periphery of the tumour (deepest and lateral extremes), at tissue interfaces and in regions susceptible to overheating.

Table 11.4 lists recommendations by EMAMI et al. (1991) regarding the minimum number of thermometry catheters compatible with good practice. Each catheter may be loaded with a multisensor probe or a single sensor probe which is scanned to provide "thermal mapping" (GIBBS 1983; ENGLER et al. 1987). The suggested spatial interval between sensors or mapping points is 5 mm for catheter tracks < 5 cm and a maximum of 10 mm for longer tracks. It is recommended that the maximum interval between thermal mapping scans is 10 min; more frequent measurements should be made when possible.

Table 11.4. Minimum number of thermometry catheters (from EMAMI et al. 1991)

Number of heat sources	Centre of implant	Centre of 4 heat sources	Periphery of implant
3–8	1	0	1
9–16	1	1	1
17–32	1	2	1
More than 32	1	3	2

Whilst the recommendations for the minimum number of catheters are particularly suited to treatments involving microwave antennas, they become impractical for large implanted arrays often used with the RF-LCF technique (DEWHIRST et al. 1990). In these cases multisensor probes should be used and at least two non-heated catheters should be employed for thermal mapping along the tumour axis and in the peripheral region of the tumour. When possible, a perpendicular probe intersecting the central axis in the mid-plane at depth is also recommended.

In the case of ferromagnetic seeds, DEWHIRST et al. (1990) recommended that at least one seed temperature and the temperature profile along the central axis of each group of four seeds should be measured. This approach is also recommended when heating is achieved using hot water tubes. Invasive thermometry requirements for treatments involving thermally self-regulating seeds (i.e. those with a Curie point similar to the maximum temperature desired) can be relaxed only when experience shows that the thermoregulation of such systems under clinical conditions is adequate.

11.6 Guidelines for Treatment Control

Temperature sensors used for controlling interstitial hyperthermia systems should be located close to antennas if the feedback system is to have a fast response, a necessary requirement if good temporal regulation of temperature is to be achieved. Indeed, temperature sensors have been incorporated into electrodes (COSSET 1990; SAMULSKI and FESSENDEN 1990) and antennas and/or catheters (STROHBEHN and MECHLING 1986; TURNER 1986; SUN et al. 1989). However, care is needed when interpreting temperatures recorded in this way (ASTRAHAN et al. 1988) and temperatures close to electrodes or antennas are unlikely to be representative of the temperature in more distant regions of the implant. Thus it is also necessary with all systems to monitor within the implant and to correlate temperatures in those regions with temperatures close to the sources. Suggested locations for this sampling are midway between a pair, or centrally within a group, of electrodes or antennas. For safety reasons, temperatures from regions susceptible to overheating must also be sampled and used to limit power should they exceed predetermined levels.

The requirements for controlling interstitial hyperthermia treatments are system specific and thermometry must match the degrees of freedom available. For example, for RF-LCF systems, a control sensor is needed for each set (ideally each pair) of electrodes which can be powered independently. If a temperature sensor is provided in each electrode, full benefit of the high degree of flexibility offered with modern multiplexed RF-LCF systems can be achieved.

In the case of microwave antennas, a non-perturbing or minimally perturbing sensor placed closed to the junction of each antenna provides information for balancing power to antennas and for minimal temporal variation in temperature.

For hot water tube systems, the temperatures at the entrances and exits of each implant should be monitored. Ideally, there should be independent control of the temperature and flow of water through each implant. Curie-point ferromagnetic seeds are thermally self-regulating; however, a cautious approach requires that the temperature achieved by seeds should be verified by measurement or modelling.

References

Astrahan MA, Luxton G, Sapozink MD, Petrovich Z (1988) The accuracy of temperature measurements from within an interstitial microwave antenna. Int J Hyperthermia 4: 593–607

Carnochan P, Dickinson RJ, Joiner MC (1986) The practical use of thermocouples for temperature measurement in clinical hyperthermia. Int J Hyperthermia 2: 1–19

Cetas TC (1982) Invasive thermometry. In: Nussbaum GH (ed) Physical aspects of hyperthermia. American Institute of Physics, New York, p 231

Cetas TC (1990) Thermometry. In: Field SB, Hand JW (eds) An introduction to the practical aspects of clinical hyperthermia. Taylor & Francis, London, p 423

Chakraborty DP, Brezovich IA (1982) Error sources affecting thermocouple thermometry in RF electromagnetic fields. J Microwave Power 17: 17–28

Cosset JM (1990) Interstitial hyperthermia. In: Gautherie M (ed) Interstitial, endocavitary and perfusional hyperthermia. Springer, Berlin Heidelberg New York, p 1

Dewhirst MW, Philips TL, Samulski TV et al. (1990) RTOG quality assurance guidelines for clinical trials using hyperthermia. Int J Radiat Oncol Biol Phys 18: 1249–1259

Dickinson RJ (1985) Thermal conduction errors of manganin-constantan thermocouple arrays. Phys Med Biol 30: 445–453

Emami B, Stauffer P, Dewhirst MW et al. (1991) RTOG quality assurance guidelines for interstitial hyperthermia. Int J Radiat Oncol Biol Phys 20: 1117–1124

Engler MS, Dewhirst MW, Winget JW, Oleson JR (1987) Automated temperature scanning for hyperthermia treatment planning. Int J Radiat Oncol Biol Phys 13: 1377–1382

ESHO (1992) Interstitial and intracavitary hyperthermia: A task group report of the European Society for Hyperthermic Oncology. Tor Vergata Medical Physics Monograph Series, University of Rome Tor Vergata, Rome (in press).

Gibbs FA (1983) Thermal mapping in experimental cancer treatment with hyperthermia: description and use of a semiautomatic system. Int J Radiat Oncol Biol Phys 9: 1057–1063

Hand JW (1990) Technical aspects of quality assurance in clinical hyperthermia. Physica Medica 6: 7–15

Hand JW, Lagendijk JJW, Bach Andersen J, Bolomey JC (1989) Quality assurance guidelines for ESHO protocols. Int J Hyperthermia 5: 421–428

Samulski TV, Fessenden P (1990) Thermometry in therapeutic hyperthermia. In: Gautherie M (ed) Methods of hyperthermia control. Springer, Berlin Heidelberg New York, p 1

Samulski TV, Lyons BE, Britt RH (1985) Temperature measurements in high thermal gradients: II. Analysis of conduction effects. Int J Radiat Oncol Biol Phys 11: 963–971

Shrivastava PN, Saylor TK, Matloubieh AY, Paliwal BR (1988) Hyperthermia thermometry evaluation: criteria and guidelines. Int J Radiat Oncol Biol Phys 14: 327–335

Shrivastava P, Luk K, Oleson JR et al. (1989) Hyperthermia quality assurance guidelines. Int J Radiat Oncol Biol Phys 16: 571–587

Stauffer PR (1990) Techniques for interstitial hyperthermia. In: Field SB, Hand JW (eds) An introduction to the practical aspects of clinical hyperthermia. Taylor & Francis, London, p 344

Strohbehn JW, Mechling JA (1986) Interstitial techniques for clinical hyperthermia. In: Hand JW, James JR (eds) Physical techniques in clinical hyperthermia. Research Studies Press, Letchworth, p 210

Sun M, McCulloch M, Ikeda M (1989) Catheter-borne fiberoptic sensors and supporting instrumentation for effective temperature measurement and control during RF and microwave interstitial hyperthermia. In: Sugahara T, Saito M (eds) Hyperthermic oncology 1988, vol 1. Taylor & Francis, London, p 649

Turner PF (1986) Interstitial EM applicator/temperature probes. In: Robinson CJ, Kondraske GV (eds) Proceedings 8th Annual Conference of IEEE Engineering in Medicine and Biology Society, vol 3. IEEE, New York, p 1454

12 Noninvasive Thermometry Practice for Interstitial Hyperthermia

B. PREVOST, J.J. FABRE, J.C. CAMART, and M. CHIVE

CONTENTS

12.1 Introduction

In his summary lecture on the clinical studies presented at the International Hyperthermia meeting at AARHUS (Denmark) in 1984, N. BLECHEM wrote: "Interstitial thermoradiotherapy does currently seem to be the only technique for providing reasonably uniform heating in a smaller volume which is not actually very close to the surface . . . , but the precondition for successful clinical results is that hyperthermia treatments are carefully controlled". Reliable knowledge of the thermal dose requires that the temperature be accurately measured within a sufficient volume and with an adequate spatial resolution (STAUFFER et al. 1989).

Usually, temperature controls are invasively performed by using thermocouples or optical fibers. As a result, the temperature can be considered to be known with a good accuracy but only within a finite number of points. Outside these points of measurement, an approximation of the amplitude of the temperature gradients can be calculated.

In order to quantify clinical treatments, several techniques have been proposed for noninvasive temperature measurements (BOLOMEY and HAWLEY 1990). The major difficulty in comparing these techniques is that they are all at different stages of development: – X-ray computed tomography (CT), magnetic resonance imaging (MRI) and ultrasonic CT are well developed imaging techniques, only recently considered for application in temperature monitoring. – In contrast, electrical impedance tomography, active microwave imaging and other ultrasound methods are relatively recent modalities at an early stage of development (CETAS 1984). – Last but not least, microwave radiometry has been used for many years in human body temperature measurement (CHIVE et al. 1984; PLANCOT et al. 1987; BROWN and BARDATI 1991).

All of the considered modalities are influenced to a greater or lesser extent by other factors such as inhomogeneities of the tissue and physiological changes (for example, an increase in local blood flow). The major question relates to the stability of the thermometric parameter with respect to other influences. Moreover, the clinical context imposes other constraints such as innocuity which mainly depends on the ionizing properties of the concerned radiation (X-ray CT), duration of the image formation or time required to obtain the thermal information, compatibility with heating equipment, and cost.

The question of compatibility between various active imaging apparatuses (such as X-ray CT, MRI and ultrasonic CT) and metallic antennas used for interstitial or intracavitary hyperthermia has not yet been resolved, so that the risks of interference and interactions remain. Because of these practical considerations in clinical situations, only two techniques seem at present to be promising for a routine noninvasive temperature control system during interstitial or intracavitary hyperthermia: electrical impedance tomography and multiband microwave radiometry.

12.2 Electrical Impedance Tomography

The dielectric characterization of living tissues has been considered for a long time. Various points need to be borne in mind. First, the complex permittivity depends on the nature of the tissue or on

B. PREVOST, M.D.; Centre de lutte contre le Cancer, Oscar Lambret, 1 rue Frédéric Combemale, BP 307, F-59020 Lille Cedex, France
J.J. FABRE, Ph.D.; J.C. CAMART, M.S.; M. CHIVE, Ph.D.; I.E.M.N. CHS UMR 9929 CNRS, Université des Sciences et Technologies de Lille, Bât. P4, 59655 VILLENEUVE D'ASCQ, France

its constitution. It is convenient to distinguish between tissues with high water content, such as muscle, and tissues with low water content, such as fat. Second, for a given time, the complex permittivity strongly depends on the frequency. Third, for a given tissue at a given frequency many other factors are able to influence the complex permittivity. Among these factors, water content is probably one of the most important, but temperature variations and tissue modifications due to thermoregulatory mechanisms are also significant.

Such a situation explains the difficulties in effectively realizing absolute thermometry. But even if absolute measurement remains impossible, the variation of the images with temperature changes could yield interesting information on the heating process.

Impedance tomography operates at frequencies of a few tens to a few hundreds of kilohertz. At such low frequencies, the wavelength is much longer than the dimensions of the human body so that the quasistatic condition operates. Current and voltage on the surface of a given volume are measured to determine the distribution of resistivity within that volume. The imaging systems employed in all the experiments are very similar: a 16-electrode system with current drive of 5 mA at 50 kHz. Data acquisition times are rapid (8 to 10 s at present) and it is not necessary to switch off the heating in order to collect data (Griffiths et al. 1987). In clinical practice, measurements are performed by placing electrodes in contact with the skin in a ring around the part of the body to be measured (Persson et al. 1991). The spatial resolution is approximately 10% of the circular array diameter. In one measurement configuration, constant current drive is injected between two adjacent electrodes and the potential difference between all remaining pairs of electrodes is measured. The temperature resolution is around 1°C in vivo.

With a relatively low cost, simplicity of use and good compatibility with hyperthermia equipment, "electrical impedance tomography" can emerge as one of the most promising noninvasive hyperthermia control systems (Bolomey and Hawley 1990).

12.3 Electromagnetic Radiometry

Electromagnetic radiometry measures the natural electromagnetic emissions from the body due to its temperature. Since infrared measurements only give temperature information in a surface layer of tissue up to 0.1 mm thick, microwave radiometry was developed. Its application to medicine was first proposed in the early 1970s. More recently, since 1980, this technique has been investigated for monitoring of hyperthermia treatments (Chive 1990). A temperature resolution of 0.1°C is achievable for most present systems with a time constant of 2 s.

The radiometry technique measures the electromagnetic (EM) power spontaneously emitted by tissues and directly related to temperature. This measured EM power is the integral summation of the elementary EM power emitted by each subvolume situated in a volume coupled to the used antenna-sensor. The EM power value gives a temperature information by means of a calibration. The temperature pattern is then computed; thus the spatial resolution and the temperature resolution depend on the used radiometer, antenna sensor and on the dielectric characteristics of the volume under investigation. It is absolutely necessary to measure how the tissue volume contributes to the collected electromagnetic power. In accordance with the reciprocity principle, the coupled volume is determined by means of the radiative diagram of the used antenna in the frequency bandwidth of the radiometer (Fabre et al. 1990).

In the case of radiofrequency or perfusional interstitial hyperthermia, for the purpose of noninvasive thermometry the temperature is measured through an external applicator; thus the depth of view depends on the penetration depth and on the temperature resolution of the radiometer. Penetration depth is usually defined as the depth to which a signal can travel in tissue before it is attenuated by a factor 1/e. The majority of radiometer receivers operate with a center frequency in the range 1–5 GHz, where the spatial resolution is acceptable for most medical applications. Plane wave penetration depth is from about 1 to 4 cm in muscle; consequently it is possible to employ noninvasive thermometry from the body surface for tumors situated within this range (Chive 1990).

In the case of microwave interstitial hyperthermia, the problem is less pronounced because the same antenna is used both for heating and for temperature measurement employing an alternating method. As the spacing of implanted antennas is in the range of 1 to 1.5 cm, the technique is inherently suited to microwave radiometry.

The antenna is constituted from coaxial cable, the outer conductor of which is removed in order to achieve the radiating part (Fig. 12.1) (Fabre et al.

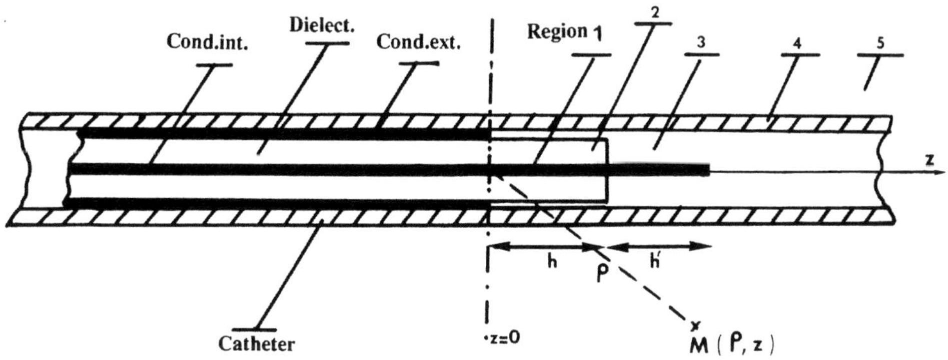

Fig. 12.1. Diagram of a radiating antenna made up from a coaxial cable inserted in an implanted plastic catheter. Numbers indicate the various regions taken into account in the theoretical calculation of the radiating pattern at the heating frequency and in the frequency bandwidth of the radiometers

1991). The aim of current attempts at optimization is to develop radiating antennas that will, during use, permit transfer of at least 90% of the microwave energy to the volume to be heated, thereby achieving matching in the electronic sense of the word. The matching must be obtained not only at the heating frequency but also in wide bandwidths around the central frequency of the radiometers used for temperature measurement and monitoring. The quality of the matching is tested by studying the evolution of the power reflection coefficient (S11 parameter) in the antenna input plane as a function of the frequency (Fig. 12.2).

From the electric field calculations at any point of the irradiated medium we can deduce the isopower lines around the antenna; we have then determined the SAR when the antenna is fed by a 3 GHz continuous wave (Fig. 12.3). This permits determination of the volume which contributes to the EM signal, directly related to the temperature, and measured through the antenna by a radiometer: we call it the coupled volume. In the first approximation this volume is limited by a cylinder of 6 cm height with a radius of 6 mm around the active length of the antenna (Fabre et al. 1989;

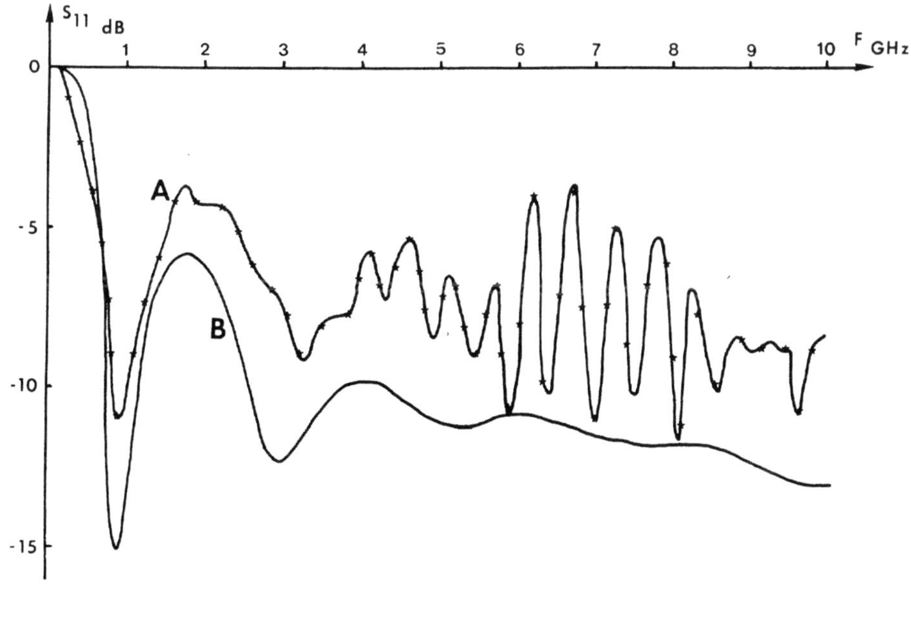

Fig. 12.2. Reflection coefficient in the input plane of the coaxial antenna as a function of frequency for h = 43 mm and h′ = 0. The coefficient is calculated from and measured on a polyacrylamide gel of the same dielectric characteristics as living tissues. *A*: experimental; *B*: theoretical

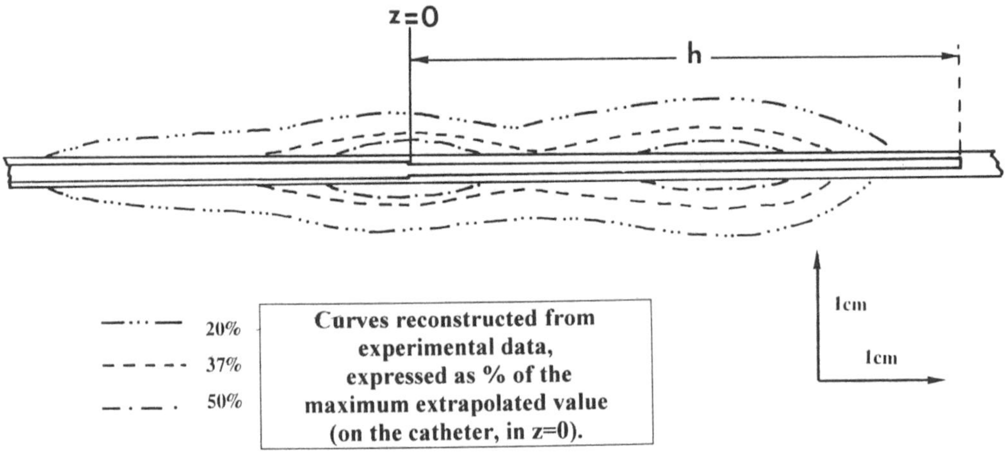

▲

Fig. 12.3. Radiative diagram of the coaxial antenna for h = 43 mm, h′ = 0 at 3 GHz around a catheter dipped in 6 g/l salted water: experimental lines are deduced from detected voltage obtained on a field mapping system

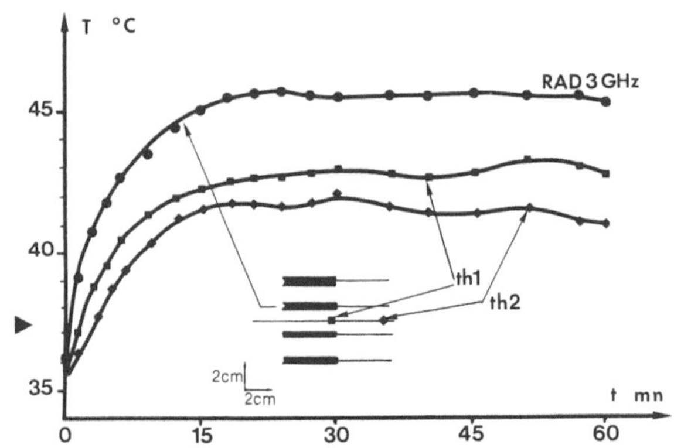

Fig. 12.4. Temperature during hyperthermia treatment of a breast tumor. Four parallel antennas were fed in phase making a plane (P = 16 W). One radiometric (RAD 3 GHz) and two thermocouple (th1, th2) measurements are shown ▶

Fig. 12.5. Reconstructed heating pattern in the cross-section plane of temperature maximum from measurements memorized during the session illustrated by Fig. 12.4

▼

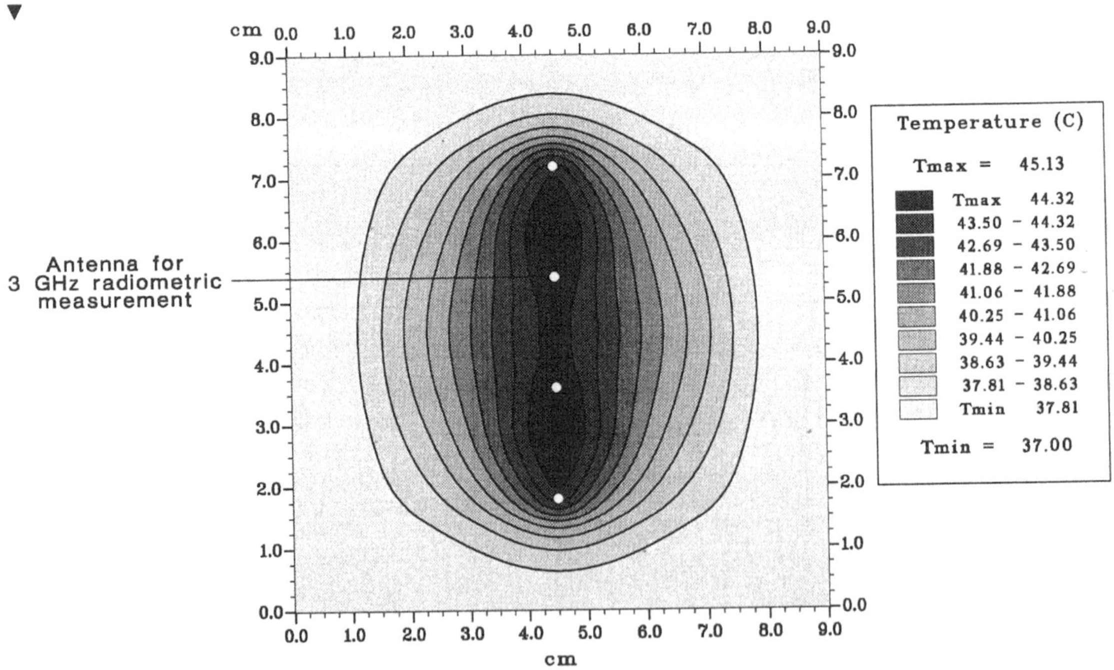

CHIVE 1990). When measuring the noise power collected by the antenna and a radiometer centered on 3 GHz (with 1 GHz bandwidth), this noise power is the integral summation of the elementary noise power emitted by each subvolume in the coupled volume and multiplied by a weighting coefficient depending on its distance from the antenna and on the 3 GHz radiative diagram of the antenna (DUBOIS et al. 1991).

When the antenna is fed by a 9 GHz wave, the coupled cylinder presents the same height but its radius is now about 3 mm. That is to say, a radiometer centered on 9 GHz gives temperature information in a smaller volume than does one centered on 3 GHz, which permits precise measurement of the temperature in the vicinity of the antenna. This measurement is used to control the temperature in the heated region during the hyperthermia session (Fig. 12.4) and also to drive the microwave power through the comparison with a temperature order (FABRE et al. to be published).

Memorized measurements allow a posteriori heating pattern reconstruction applying electromagnetism transfer radiation theory and the bioheat transfer equation (Fig. 12.5).

This technique has been integrated into a commercially available endocavitary hyperthermia system (PROSTCARE: prostate treatment by microwave hyperthermia. Bruker Co.) and into an experimental interstitial hyperthermia system (HIMCAR) usually used for clinical applications at the Cancer Center of Lille (PREVOST et al. 1989, 1990, 1991a, 1991b).

Dielectric characteristics of living tissues and several parameters used in the bioheat transfer equation are not constant with temperature: this fact has influence on the spatial resolution and the temperature accuracy of reconstructed heating patterns. Clinical experience has also shown that the device is very sensitive to environmental electromagnetic radiation. It is often necessary to operate the radiometer inside a shielded room.

12.4 Conclusion

The two noninvasive thermal control apparatuses discussed in this chapter have been applied with success to interstitial and endocavitary hyperthermia treatments. More importantly, it has been shown that noninvasive dosimetric devices can and must be integrated with specific heating approaches to realize the full potential of hyperthermia as a treatment for malignant disease.

References

Bolomey JC, Hawley MS (1990) Methods of hyperthermia control. Clinical thermology. Springer, Berlin Heidelberg New York

Brown VJ, Bardati F (1991) Noninvasive temperature measurement by multifrequency microwave radiometry. Simulated retrievals of Gaussian temperature pulses to access accuracy and resolution. Strahlenther Onkol 167: 328

Cetas TC (1984) Will thermometric tomography become practical for hyperthermia treatment? Cancer Res [suppl] 44: 4805s–4808s

Chive M, Plancot M, Giaux G, Prevost B (1984) Microwave hyperthermia controlled by microwave radiometry. Technical aspects and first clinical results. J Microwave Power 19: 233–241

Chive M (1990) Use of microwave radiometry for hyperthermia monitoring and as a basis for thermal dosimetry. Methods of hyperthermia control. Springer, Berlin Heidelberg New York, vol III, pp 113–128

Dubois L, Fabre JJ, Ledee R, Chive M, Moschetto Y (1991) Bidimensional reconstruction of temperature patterns from noninvasive microwave multifrequency radiometric measurements during microwave hyperthermia session: applications to thermal dosimetry. Innov Techn Biol Med 12: 126–146

Fabre JJ, Chive M, Dubois L et al. (to be published) 915 MHz microwave interstitial hyperthermia. Part I. Theoretical and experimental aspects with temperature control by multifrequency radiometry. Int J Hyperthermia

Fabre JJ, Playez E, Chive M et al. (1989) Microwave interstitial hyperthermia controlled by microwave radiometry: technical aspects, animal experiments and first clinical results. Proc IEEE EMBS, 11th Int Conf Seattle, USA, p 1150

Fabre JJ, Chive M, Dubois L et al. (1990) Microwave interstitial hyperthermia controlled by multifrequency microwave radiometry: phase I trials. Innov Techn Biol Med 11: 236–248

Fabre JJ, Camart JC, Dubois L et al. (1991) Microwave interstitial hyperthermia system monitored by microwave radiometry (HIMCAR) and dosimetry by heating pattern remote sensing. Proc Eur Microwave Conf, Stuttgart, pp 1409–1414

Griffiths H, Ahmed A (1987) Applied potential tomography for noninvasive temperature mapping in hyperthermia. Clin Phys Physiol 8 [suppl A]: 147–153

Persson BRR, Blad B et al. (1991) Noninvasive temperature distributions in hyperthermic oncology investigated by electrical impedance. Strahlenther Onkol 167: 327

Plancot M, Prevost B, Chive M, Fabre JJ, Ledee R, Giaux G (1987) A new method for thermal dosimetry in microwave hyperthermia using microwave radiometry for temperature control. Int J Hyperthermia 3: 9–19

Prevost B, Chive M, Fabre JJ,Vanseymortier L, Demaille A (1989) Hyperthermie interstitielle microonde avec contrôle de la température par radiométrie microonde. Bull Cancer (Paris) 76: 564

Prevost B, Chive M, Fabre JJ, Vanseymortier L, Dubois L

(1990) Technique d'hyperthermie interstitielle microonde contrôlée par radiométrie microonde à deux fréquences. Bull Cancer (Paris) 77: 608
Prevost B, Mirabel X, Coche B, Chive M, Fabre JJ, Sozanski JP (1991a) Hyperthermie interstitielle microonde combinée à la Curiethérapie dans le traitement des cancers de la langue. Bull Cancer (Paris) 78: 49
Prevost B, Mirabel X, Chive M, Fabre JJ, Dubois L, Sozanski JP (1991b) Clinical evaluation of a microwave interstitial hyperthermia system with microwave radiometry. Strahlenther Onkol 167: 344
Prevost B, De Cordoue-Rohart, Camart JC, Fabre JJ, Chive M, Sozanski JP (to be published) 915 MHz microwave interstitial hyperthermia. Part III. Phase II clinical results. Int J Hyperthermia
Stauffer PR, Sneed PK, Suen SA et al. (1989) Comparative thermal dosimetry of interstitial microwave and RF-LCF hyperthermia. Int J Hyperthermia 5: 307–318

13 Methods of Thermal Modeling and Their Impact on Interstitial Hyperthermia Treatment Planning

T.P. Ryan

CONTENTS

13.1 Introduction

What is the purpose of writing another chapter, or book for that matter, on hyperthermia principles involving temperature models and treatment planning? The answer is that the field is constantly changing as new technologies appear and refinements of current technologies occur. Additional mathematical models for thermal modeling have been developed since prior books or chapters have been published, with many of these now encompassing three-dimensional (3-D) calculations. Also, practical 3-D noninvasive thermal imaging systems are being developed which will be a boon to temperature control during hyperthermia treatments.

In clinical treatments, interstitial methods are applied both superficially and for deep-seated tumors. A distinct advantage of interstitial applicators is that there is no tissue coupling problem when compared with external applicators and if care is taken, no preferential superficial heating. Additionally, reflection from tissue–bone or tissue air interfaces that are encountered with external techniques is also avoided. Three main techniques for interstitial heating are (a) microwaves (MW) – power is deposited as a result of interaction between rapidly attenuated electromagnetic waves propagating from an array of antennas into tissue; (b) radiofrequency-local current field (RF-LCF) – an RF voltage is applied between pairs of electrodes, and currents that flow between the electrodes produce resistive heating within the tissues; and (c) conductive sources such as ferromagnetic seeds, hot water sources, or resistive heaters.

With interstitial implants, heating must be restricted to neoplastic tissue only, and normal tissue spared to avoid complications, including pain and skin ulceration at the catheter insertion points. In spite of the invasiveness of interstitial techniques, the ability to selectively heat tissue from the inside out is advantageous, especially in light of the compatibility with interstitial brachytherapy. The potential for sparing normal tissue is high, providing that the volumetric heating pattern remains within the intended treatment volume. For conformability of heating patterns to the intended treatment volume, interstitial techniques offer the advantage of arrays which will apply heat maximally in the tumor, and minimally in the normal tissue. No complex assembly of external applicators is necessary to factor a geometric gain to deposit power at depth. Indeed, some of our earlier patients at Dartmouth came into our clinic with 16–20 catheters

T.P. Ryan, M.S., Section of Radiation Oncology, Dartmouth-Hitchcock Medical Center, Lebanon, NH 03756, USA and Thayer School of Engineering, Dartmouth College, Hanover, NH 03755, USA exiting surgical puncture wounds. The tips of these long catheters resided directly in the tumor, and served as conduits to deposit power deep within the body, but precisely localized. External devices that measure temperatures are still under development and invasive procedures will be needed to afford internal temperature monitoring. Thus, the invasiveness of interstitial implants seems less problematic.

An advantage of interstitial systems in correlation with CT or MRI images, made after surgical implant, is that localization of tumor margins in relation to the catheter locations is defined spatially, which is crucial for treatment planning. A decision must be made in regard to the extent of the target treatment volume in 3-D, including both the imagable tumor and any additional margin that will be heated. Often from 1.0 to 2.0 cm is added at each boundary; thus a $3 \times 3 \times 3$ cm tumor may become a $5 \times 5 \times 5$ cm or $7 \times 7 \times 7$ cm target volume. It may be true though that treatment planning is of less importance if heat delivery systems are fixed, stationary ones that provide little flexibility in the redistribution of heat other than adjustment of a power knob.

During pretreatment planning power deposition is calculated, if applicable, for RF and MW arrays. Then temperature distributions are calculated and the implant can be iteratively changed to optimize temperature distributions. Following this pretreatment planning, the implant is typically done in the operating room and the implant and tumor are imaged again. The power deposition (if applicable) can be recalculated based on the actual implant and the predicted temperature distributions are calculated. Thermal models used in planning have evolved to be device-specific. For example, ferromagnetic seeds are regulated by either a set temperature or resistive sources which are controlled by a temperature feedback loop. For thermal predictions a conductive source model is necessary with heat sources placed in a grid and temperatures specified along the sources. An optimization is then done to spare normal tissue and achieve heating at therapeutic levels of the entire tumor volume within the confines of the fixed implant. This optimization scheme employs enhancements that depend on the modality of the heating:

1. MW – phase shifting, rotating phase, air or water cooled applicators, antenna type and frequency.
2. RF – active length of needle segments and water cooling.
3. Conductive sources – distribution of source temperatures throughout the implant. Ferromagnetic seeds require a choice of Curie point temperature seeds, hot water sources require decisions regarding water temperatures, and resistive heaters require similar decision making.

As hyperthermia systems become more refined and offer more flexibility, treatment planning systems must adapt and provide the umbrella encompassing all new enhancement techniques. Versatility is needed to provide optimization of the treatment variables, such as antenna design choice and frequency, air or water cooling, phase focusing, and individually adjustable power or temperature at each source. These enhancements, combined with noninvasive temperature monitoring in 3-D, will bring available hyperthermia techniques closer towards the ideal treatment system. Already the capability of treatment systems to control the distribution of temperatures far surpasses the ability to monitor this temperature distribution throughout the treatment volume in 3-D.

The requirements for a good hyperthermia treatment can be divided into clinical and engineering aspects. From the clinical aspect, the hyperthermia treatment must produce temperature elevations in a carefully delineated volume that encompasses the malignancy. From the engineering aspect, the temperature distribution should be controllable. In the presence of nonuniform blood flow, each source may require a different power level or source temperature setting to maintain constant local temperatures. Furthermore, the thermal dose should be steerable spatially so as to optimally distribute temperature throughout the treatment volume by temperature feedback techniques in real time during the treatment, to overcome factors such as varying blood flow, thermal conduction, and differing electrical properties.

Several enhancements to assist in thermal modeling and interstitial hyperthermia (IH) treatment planning are either available or under development:

1. Impedance imaging provides the distribution of the conductivity and permittivity of tumor and surrounding normal tissue which could be placed into a model to more accurately predict power deposition patterns, when applicable. This can also be done during the treatment at hyperthermic temperatures.

2. Blood flow regions in the treatment volume are divided up into three to seven distinct regions including core, rapidly proliferating margin, and surrounding normal tissue.

3. Imagable blood vessels found radiographically by digital subtraction techniques can be added to the patient specific thermal model in the imaging plane under study.

4. An important part of the temperature feedback system that controls clinical IH treatments is the placement of thermometry probes in the predicted locations of maximum or minimum heating to provide monitoring for extreme temperatures.

5. If a treatment #0 (brief test treatment) is performed, for subsequent treatments:

a) Certain catheters which may not have contained heating sources may have sources placed, and vice versa.

b) With microwave antennas the choice of a different antenna design may overcome overheating or underheating problems.

c) With ferromagnetic seeds, optimization of seed segment selection is possible to control distribution of temperatures along each catheter.

d) If pain is a limitation, sources can be cooled (applicable to microwave and RF only) or temperatures can be lowered in the case of ferromagnetic seeds or hot water or resistive sources, or phasing can be utilized with microwaves to eliminate hot spots.

6. There is a growing potential for viable thermal imaging systems to be incorporated into the treatment system, and feedback control to steer power and overcome changes in blood flow that are inhomogeneously distributed throughout the treatment region and vary during the treatment.

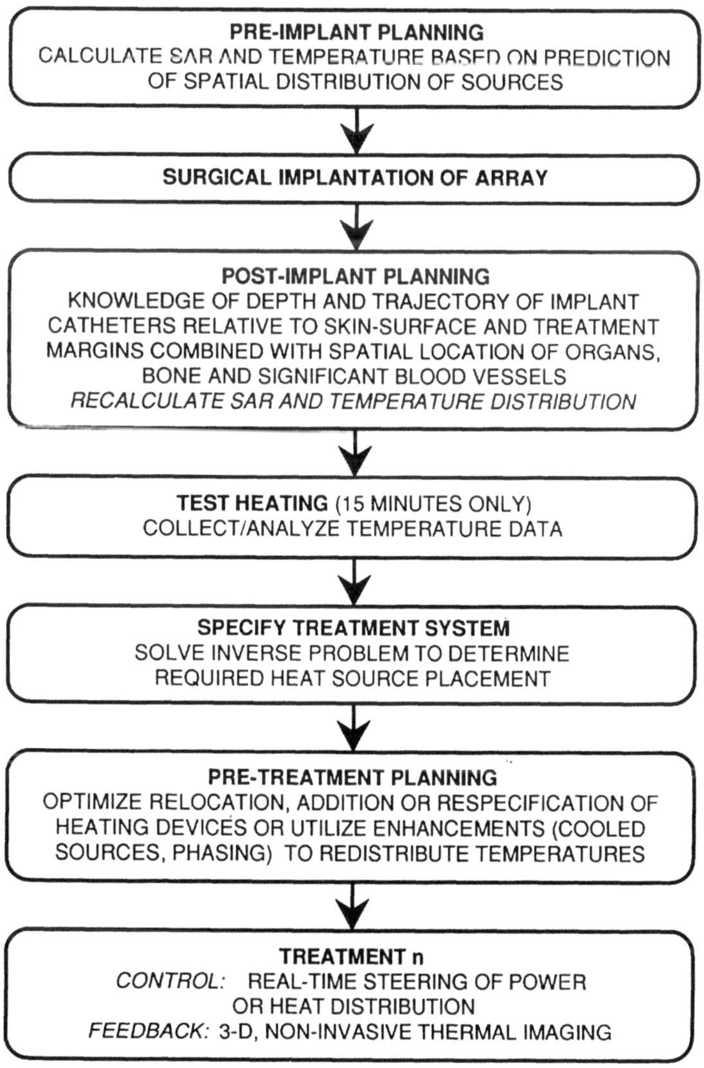

Fig. 13.1. Generalized flowchart of treatment planning implementation

13.2 Treatment Planning

Treatment planning will be divided into pre- and postimplant sections (see Fig. 13.1). In the preimplant work, the intended array geometry is planned after CT or MRI scans are obtained for the tumor, and decisions are made as to the extent of the treatment volume encompassing the imagable tumor. Postimplant treatment planning is done with the actual catheter geometry. All possible enhancements are manipulated in the thermal model to achieve evenly distributed heating. A discussion of generic devices follows, outlining the ideal treatment system. Following this, device-specific models are briefly introduced, including those that deposit power and hot sources that rely on thermal conduction to fill in between sources. Thermal models are discussed incorporating embedded tumors with different electrical and blood flow properties than normal tissue. The effects of heat on blood flow are discussed, and microcirculation models shown.

Noninvasive temperature monitoring is discussed, with several modalities showing initial promising results. The combination of (a) pretreat-

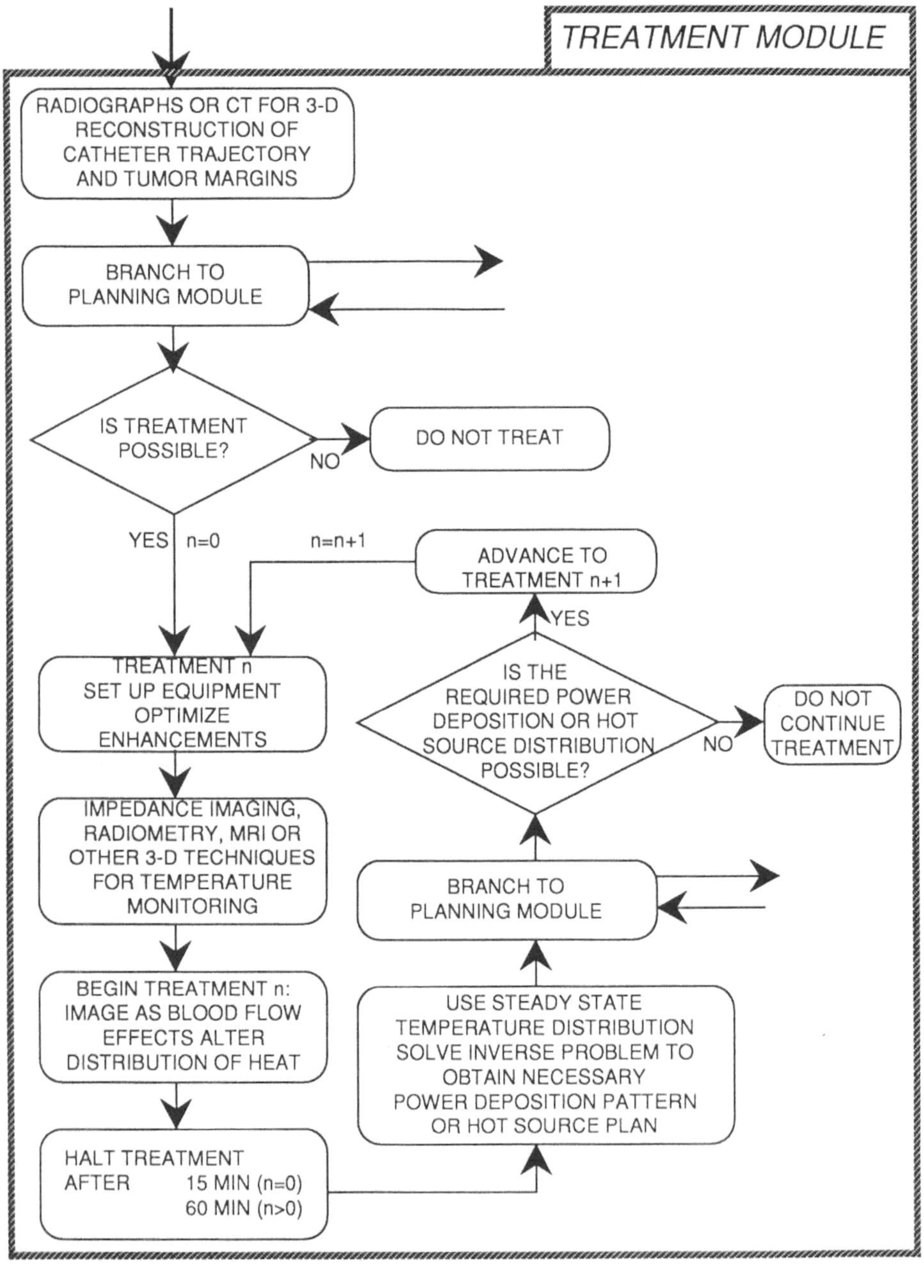

a

Fig. 13.2. Flowchart outlining treatment planning scheme

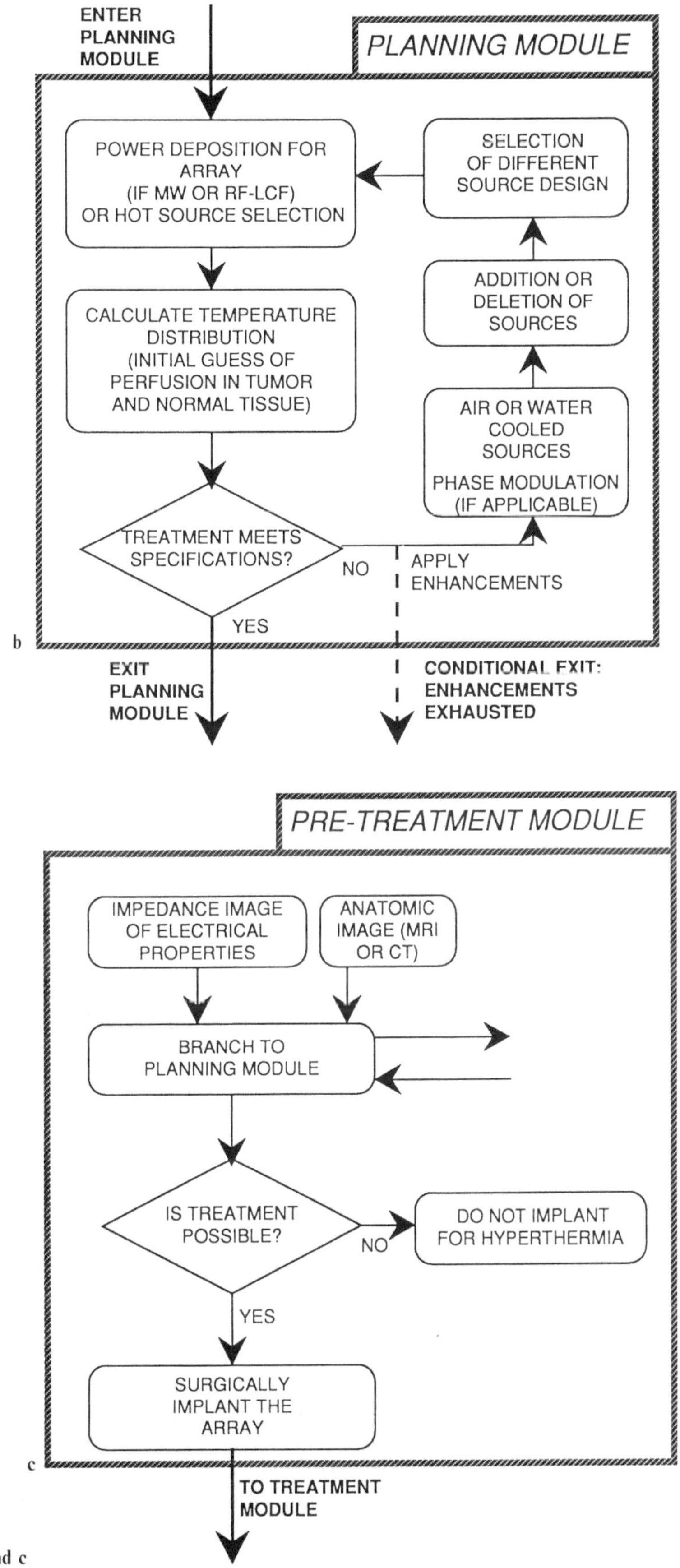

Fig. 13.2. b and c

ment planning, (b) a test heating of the patient, (c) noninvasive thermometry operating in real time, and (d) the ability to steer the heating pattern around the treatment volume will most likely result in better heat treatments. This improvement will stem in part from the extensive treatment planning process and in part from the noninvasive thermometry that will provide continuous evaluation of the treatment volume and surrounding normal tissue.

A significant part of the treatment planning process targets a treatment volume and uses inverse methods to calculate the required power deposition pattern or hot source distribution to obtain the desired temperature distribution. Whether or not it is possible to treat the patient should be evaluated at this step in the treatment planning.

13.2.1 Pretreatment Planning Module

The *pretreatment planning module* in Fig. 13.2 incorporates anatomic images assembled in 3-D with additional information on the distribution of conductivity and permittivity if MW or RF techniques are used. A branch to the planning module in Fig. 13.2 gives the opportunity to fine-tune the device- and modality-specific enhancements to optimize thermal distributions. If a successful treatment is possible then a surgical implant is done based on geometric recommendations of the pretreatment planning.

The planning module first calculates specific absorption rate (SAR) if MW or RF techniques are used. If conductive sources are used, the distribution of source temperatures is done at this time. An initial "guesstimate" is made for the various regions in the tumor model and temperatures are calculated. Enhancements are made such as water–air cooling, source modification or relocation, or phase modulation (if applicable) to approach treatment specifications. If no amount of enhancements can ensure an effective treatment, the patient is not treated.

Since more and more flexibility is being built into modern treatment systems, there is a need for a clear treatment goal and temperature distribution (Roemer 1991). An ideal treatment system would deposit power or place heat sources outside of the treatment region to preheat incoming blood and overcome thermal conduction effects. Also, the conformability of the power deposition field would allow power to be deposited on the edge of the treatment region to accomplish this. Ideal temperature distributions would provide a uniform therapeutic level inside the treatment volume and a rapid fall off outside of the treatment region. Factors such as tumor morphology, microscopic infiltrating boundary, and location of thermally significant blood vessels in the treatment volume should be considered. Some of the difficulty in computer simulations for treatment planning is the lack of adequate data, due in part to the fact that blood flow varies in both time and space. Thus, better methods for predicting perfusion before the treatment are needed, as also are methods for estimating the change in perfusion during the treatment (Strohbehn and Roemer 1984).

Hyperthermia treatment planning requires knowledge of both anatomic and physiologic characteristics of the patient. The energy deposition as well as energy removal patterns must be known because these result in the final temperature distribution. Concurrent thermal dosimetry is defined as calculating the complete temperature fields during the treatment and adjusting power deposition parameters to optimize the actual treatment. Conformability is the fundamental limitation of all hyperthermia treatments. What hyperthermia does not have in its favor is that there is not a significant difference in response to heat by tumor and normal tissue. Energy entering locally by power deposition sources must compensate for local losses due to blood perfusion; power or heating must be zero outside the treatment volume; and outer margins of the volume require additional power due to the conductive losses into normal tissue. These must all be incorporated into the model. Increasing the normal tissue blood flow causes normal tissue temperature to decay more rapidly, thus requiring more heat at the tumor edge, but will not affect the internal tumor temperatures once additional heat is added to the boundary. What complicates the process is that large vessels do not obey the bioheat equation and need to be analyzed separately. For the case of uniformly heated tumor, venous blood leaving the tumor is at the treatment temperature. To idealize the treatment though, arterial blood entering the tumor must also equal the treatment temperature. Thus, the vessels entering the tumor must be preheated (Strohbehn and Roemer 1984).

The power absorption ratio between tumor and normal tissue may range from 1 to 5, depending on frequency and tumor type (Joines et al. 1989). This is predicted from the dependence of conductivity and permittivity values on tissue types. Also, excess sodium and fluid in malignant tissue would yield greater values of conductivity and permittivity. NMR techniques indicate that water content of rat tumor was 36% greater than normal tissue which would also influence conductivity and permittivity values (SCHEPPS and FOSTER 1980). Additionally, density and specific heat of malignant tissue should be higher, so preferential heating may be higher than predicted (JOINES et al. 1989). Also, thermal conductivity of tissue is largely determined by water content which indicates there will be a difference here also. Lastly, permittivity and conductivity change with temperature. Experiments on excised tissue showed initial temperature rise to be greater in tumor than in normal tissue for the same power due to the greater electromagnetic absorption (JOINES et al. 1989). These factors argue strongly for an impedance imaging system that can map permittivity and conductivity, even at hyperthermic temperatures.

13.2.2 Treatment Planning Module

Treatment planning includes locating the tumor in the surrounding anatomy through CT imaging, MRI imaging, or related modalities. Thermal properties of each anatomic type are assigned in this stage. Power deposition is calculated (if applicable) and the actual blood flow values and distribution that would be present during treatment would ideally be known. Some tumors are difficult to image because of the problem of imaging vessels and perhaps this would be a place for digitial subtraction techniques to emphasize vessel structures, geometry, and trajectories.

The following problems confound the model in treatment planning. The effects of large blood vessels are not predicted in most of the current work, including the bioheat equation. In the analysis of tumor energy removal, the necrotic core in the center uses purely conductive methods and locations near large vessels or the highly perfused periphery are purely convective. At any point in a heated volume, the energy removal process can be dominated by either conduction or convection (blood flow), and the magnitude of the effects is not known. Treatment planning typically neglects physiology and anatomy of tumor that the actual treatment does not ignore. In mathematical simulations, often treatment limitations are that maximum allowable tumor or normal tissue temperature is exceeded. An ideal simulation program would incorporate 3-D efforts, realistic inhomogeneous tissues, realistic power deposition, the best and worst case of blood perfusion patterns, the effects of large blood vessels, variable arterial blood temperature, and the directional effects of blood flow. On the other hand, the limitations of 2-D analysis are that only the plane in the center of the power deposition field is commonly analyzed and the heat transfer in the axial direction is neglected, resulting in the neglect of lower power deposition. It was found that the difference between 2-D and 3-D simulations can be as much as 8°C, depending on perfusion values in tumor dimensions (CHEN et al. 1990) due to axial conduction. This becomes less important as perfusion values increase.

New images are created to specify the tumor and implanted array geometry in 3-D postimplant. After optimizing enhancements, if treatment is possible, the patient advances to treatment #0. This follows from a previous recommendation that a test heating be done with each patient after potential enrollment in the protocol to see whether the patient will be eligible for the study (STROHBEHN 1991). Following equipment setup (as specified in the planning module), the patient undergoes treatment #0, a test treatment. This test treatment validates the IH treatment planning optimizations and provides valuable data when used in conjunction with noninvasive thermometry. After 15 min, the treatment is halted and using the work of OCHELTREE and FRIZZELL (1987) and the steady-state temperature distribution, the required power deposition pattern is calculated and the model then branches to the planning module. If the power or heat distribution is possible to meet the criterion of percent of treatment volume ≥ 43°C, the patient advances to treatment #1 (60 min) and then subsequent treatments. A flexible heating system that allows control over the distribution of heat is necessary to be able to meet treatment specifications of volume heated $\geq 75\%$.

13.3 Generic Device Modeling

For devices that deposit power in tissue, the power deposition patterns need to be known or calculated prior to entering a thermal solver that provides temperature distribution. The transient bioheat transfer equation is written as follows (see appendix):

$$\rho_t c_t \frac{\partial T}{\partial t} = \nabla \cdot (k_t \nabla T) - c_b \rho_b m \rho_t (T - T_b) + Q_p + Q_m \quad (1)$$

13.3.1 General Requirements

OCHELTREE and FRIZZELL (1987) used a prospective thermal dosimetry approach. The steady-state bioheat transfer equation (PENNES 1948) was used along with the target temperature distribution, then calculations were made to find the required 3-D steady-state power deposition pattern. The strategy for clinical work was to choose the desired temperature patterns, calculate the needed power deposition patterns, then take available applicators and try to achieve these projected power patterns. The steady-state bioheat transfer equation was used, taking Eq. 1 and setting the time variant part to zero.

A given power distribution produces a single temperature distribution using the steady-state bioheat transfer equation. Conversely, a desired temperature distribution is associated with a single power distribution. Setting $Q_p = 0$ outside of the tumor, power deposition would be positive everywhere and uniform in the interior of the tumor. The result is constant power across the tumor with a delta function at the normal tissue–tumor boundary. This requires that significantly more heating must occur in the plane of the heating source tips which are at the tumor margin (TREMBLY and RYAN 1992). To achieve a more realistic model, a perfusion distribution is placed across the tumor and normal tissue, by assuming zero perfusion at the tumor center, 24 ml/100 g/min at the interface between tumor and normal tissue, and 9 ml/100 g/min in normal tissue, and then calculating the 3-D temperature distributions (OCHELTREE and FRIZZELL 1987).

In the study of the transient heat-up phase that precedes steady-state hyperthermia, the power deposition required to maintain steady-state temperatures was found to be insufficient to raise the temperatures to therapeutic levels in the first 10% of the heating session (OCHELTREE and FRIZZELL 1988). By using a time-dependent solution of the bioheat equation, Q_p was solved as a function of time. The study concluded that *different* power deposition patterns are required for initial heat-up [$Q_{p(t)}$] and for the steady-state portions of the treatment (OCHELTREE and FRIZZELL 1988).

13.3.2 Microwave Heating Devices

Power of the distribution of heat sources needs to be continuously adjustable for each heating source independently. More power will be required at the tumor periphery, where blood flow may be higher because of the vasculature structures as well as thermal conduction removing heat outwardly into normal tissue.

13.3.2.1 Power Deposition Models

Prior to utilization of various heating devices in a treatment planning program, those that deposit power must first be modeled. Models for the dipole antenna were presented by KING et al. (1983) and TREMBLY (1985), for multisection antennas by ISKANDER and TUMEH (1989), and for multinode antennas by TUMEH and ISKANDER (1989). The electric (**E**) field of each individual antenna is calculated and the complex **E** fields of all antennas are summed for arrays. The resulting magnitude is squared for power deposition. The model should also be able to handle nonparallel antennas.

For proper modeling, in situ measurements of dielectric properties of tissue are advantageous and more accurate since excised tissues rapidly change dielectrical properties due to the loss of membrane function and breakdown of cellular structure (OSTERHOUT 1922). There is also a loss of blood and moisture in the excised tissue. Impedance imaging has potential for providing this in situ information. The **E** field distribution $\vec{E}(\vec{r}, t)$ is described by:

$$\vec{E}(\vec{r}, t) = \sum_{i=1}^{N} \vec{E}_i(\vec{r}, t),$$

where $\vec{E}_i(\vec{r}, t)$ is the complex **E** field from the ith antenna, with phase and amplitude information (STROHBEHN et al. 1982). Thus, in the $z = 0$ plane (of the antenna junction) for homogeneous tissue

$$\begin{aligned}\vec{E}(\vec{r}) &= E(\rho, z)\\ &= j\omega\mu I_z(0)e^{j\theta}\left[\frac{z-h}{r_1}e^{-\gamma r_1} + \frac{z+h}{r_2}e^{-\gamma r_2} - j\frac{2z}{r_0}\sinh(\gamma_r h)e^{-\gamma r_0}\right]\vec{U}_\rho\\ &\quad - \frac{j\omega\mu I_z(0)e^{j\varnothing}}{4\pi|\gamma|}\left[\frac{e^{-\gamma r_1}}{r_1} + \frac{e^{-\gamma r_2}}{r_2} - j\frac{2}{r_0}\sinh(\gamma_r h)e^{-\gamma r_0}\right]\vec{U}_z,\end{aligned}$$

where

$\gamma^2 = -\varepsilon\mu\omega^2 + j\sigma\mu\omega$;

$\vec{r}(\rho, \theta, \phi) =$ location of **E** field;

$r =$ magnitude of $\vec{r}$;

$\varnothing = \tan^{-1}(\gamma_R/\gamma_I)$;

$r_0 = [\rho^2 + z^2]^{0.5}$;

$r_1 = [\rho^2 + (z-h)^2]^{0.5}$;

$$r_2 = [\rho^2 + (z+h)^2]^{0.5} . \quad (2)$$

The SAR is calculated as:

$$\mathrm{SAR} = \frac{\sigma}{2\rho}[|\vec{E}_z|^2 + |\vec{E}_r|^2] \text{ [W/kg]} . \quad (3)$$

Microwave antenna designs are diverse enough to have a dramatic effect on the distribution of power (RYAN 1991b). Single antennas, though, do not predict array performance and thus simulation and phantom measurements are necessary in several planes to adequately characterize array behavior. Catheter materials and wall thickness will also affect performance since thick-walled catheters cause the antenna's radially directed **E** field to fall off less rapidly (JONES et al. 1989; MECHLING et al. 1991a). Dramatic changes in heat distribution are obtained simply by substituting antenna designs during IH treatments. The difference between dipole and helical antennas in the brain have been shown, as well as dipole versus choke dipole antennas (RYAN 1991a). A requirement of new designs should be the ability to deposit power at the tips of the antennas, especially along the central array.

13.3.2.2 Phase Modulation

The intrinsic behavior of a four-antenna array at 915 MHz driven in-phase results in an SAR that is characteristically nonuniform, since the array dimensions are comparable to the wavelength in tissue with strong phase coherence effects. By placing a pair of antennas out-of-phase with the other pair, the central array phase shifts, and by rotating around the array, the fixed phase shift moves around within the interior of the array smoothing out the central hot spot (TREMBLY et al. 1986). The typical 100% central SAR section is reduced to a broad 30% area, theoretically, and 25%, experimentally, exhibiting no central peak. Thus, 90% of the array interior falls within 40%–50% SAR. Changing the driving phase will have the same effect at all points along the antennas. Asymmetry of temperature distribution due to either individual antenna performance or perfusion levels could be eliminated through the dwell time or power modualtion based on temperature feedback of sensors inside the array (TREMBLY et al. 1988). ISKANDER et al. (1990) modeled phase steering in a tumor with a 2 × 2 antenna array. They assigned tumor electrical properties to have a dielectric constant ($\varepsilon = 55$) and conductivity ($\sigma = 1.45$ S/m). Normal tissue was given the electrical properties of $\varepsilon = 42$ and $\sigma = 0.88$ S/m. Significant differences were found in the results with and without the tumor embedded in normal tissue, when a 25% difference in electrical properties was assigned to the tumor (FURSE and ISKANDER 1989).

13.3.2.3 Water or Air Cooling of Sources

Surface cooling of MW sources provides deeper penetration in tissue without overheating tissue in contact with the sources. GENTILE et al. (1991) modeled a water-cooled dipole antenna, neglecting the external casing since it is much smaller than a wavelength in tissue, and the wave number of the irradiating system was determined by the cooling liquid. Total heat transfer coefficient (U) is calculated as:

$$U = \left[\left(\frac{r_2}{h^* \cdot r_1}\right) + \left(\frac{r_2}{k_{is}}\right)\ln\left(\frac{r_2}{r_1}\right)\right]^{-1} \quad (4)$$

with dependency on the catheter wall thickness and thermal conductivity. Combining U and power deposition, the steady-state bioheat equation was solved by the alternating direction implicit method. Calculations were made with a range of values for coolant temperature, flow rates, and tissue perfusion levels. High perfusion levels caused a flattened radial distribution. Comparing the volume of tissue heated when the allowable maximum was 42.2°C, the case with cooling showed a 70% increase in the volume of tissue heated in the range of 40°–42.2°C. The temperature of the coolant was 10°C.

Development of a water-cooled microwave applicator for transurethral heating demonstrated that cooling greatly extends the radial heating pattern (RYAN et al. 1992) as shown in Fig. 13.3. The dotted line shows the predicted position of maximum temperature without cooling. The coolant temperature or flow rate are adjusted to flatten the curve. The peak temperature is moved away from the applicator 10–20 mm in both directions. By adjusting the coolant temperature and flow rate as well as microwave power, the temperatures would

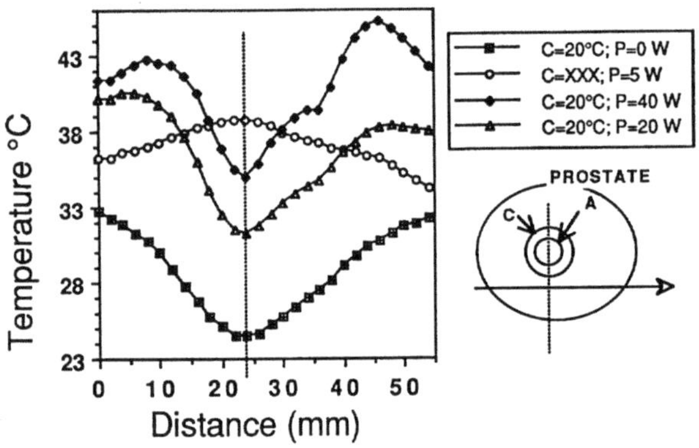

Fig. 13.3. Plot showing temperature pullbacks in a canine prostate with cooling either on (20°C, 100 ml/min flow) or off (XXX), and power equal to 0, 5, 20, or 40 W. The *vertical dashed line* indicates the center of the prostate in the plot and sketch. *A*, antenna; *C*, catheter in urethra

plateau with only 1°C variation over 30 mm (Ryan et al. 1992).

Eppert et al. (1991) used 2-D calculations in the junction plane of single antennas or arrays with air cooling of microwave antennas. Because the analysis was done in the junction plane at the center of the two dipole element segments, the results would vary only a few percent from the 3-D case. The model included heat flux from the tumor into the catheter as follows:

$$q_{tis} = \pi d_2 \int h_{oa}(T_t(x) - T(x))dx\,[\mathrm{W}]\,, \qquad (5)$$

where T = temperature of flowing air [K]; x = distance along catheter [m] (Eppert et al. 1991). Effective cooling occurred in the vicinity of individual antennas and tapered off as the array center was approached. The cooling had an effect radially over 6 mm. For single antenna work in vivo with air flow of 7.5 l/min at room temperature, it was found that the area heated to the target temperature increased by a factor of 4 when the temperature was measured at the antenna surface [A101]. The model showed that if water was substituted for air as the coolant, the antenna appears bare instead of insulated, reducing radial deposition of energy (Trembly et al. 1991).

13.3.2.4 Antenna–Tumor Size Ratio

Seegenschmidt et al. (1990) performed an interstitial clinical trial with 915 MHz microwave interstitial treatments. It was found that one of the most important prognostic factors was tumor volume. For larger volumes, typical implants may be insufficient to adequately provide a therapeutic thermal dose. They calculated the ratio of tumor volume to the antennas in the implant. Complete response was achieved in 20% of the patients with tumor volume greater than 10 cm^3/antenna, whereas complete response of 85% was achieved when the ratio was less than 10 cm^3/antenna (Seegenschmidt et al. 1990). The recommended spacing between non-cooled MW sources is 12–20 mm (Emami et al. 1991).

13.3.3 RF-LCF Devices

13.3.3.1 Power Deposition Model

By applying a voltage between implanted needles, an RF current is induced in tissue, resulting in joule heating. If RF needles are perfectly parallel, power deposition and temperatures in the longitudinal direction along the needles will tend to be uniform, at least when away from the plane of the implant tips. If needles converge, the currents will be greater, resulting in higher power deposition and higher temperatures. The convergence of the needles can be used to the clinician's advantage (Strohbehn 1987) since RF techniques are known to be sensitive to any deviations from parallelism between electrodes. Mechling and Strohbehn (1986) showed that SAR for an array of parallel RF electrodes is:

$$\mathrm{SAR}(r) = \frac{(\sigma/\rho)}{8\pi^2\omega^2|\varepsilon^*|^2}\left[\left(\sum_{i=1}^{m}\frac{I_i(x-x_i)^2}{r_i^2} + \sum_{i=1}^{m}\frac{I_i(y-y_i)^2}{r_i^2}\right)^2\right]. \qquad (6)$$

Calculations were done for a 2-D solution with the assumptions of homogeneity in electrical and thermal properties and infinitely long needles (Strohbehn 1983). The transient response was also investigated using the two time constants of the bioheat transfer equation: thermal conduction: $\tau_c = \rho_t c_t d_0^2/k$ and blood flow: $\tau_b = c_t/(m\rho_b c_b)$. Work at the University of Utah has shown that the problem of excessive heating around RF needles can be solved by circulating water at 13 ml/min through the hollow 18 gauge needles (Zhu and Gandhi 1988). For RF needles, recommended spacing between sources in tissue is 10–15 mm (Emami et al. 1991).

13.3.3.2 Cooled RF-LCF Source Model

PRIOR (1991) used the finite difference method and obtained a 2-D solution to the bioheat equation to model water-cooled RF sources. The model was composed of 1.0-mm-diameter needles, 1.0 cm grid spacing and BF of resting muscle ×1, ×5, and ×10. The maximum tolerable tissue temperature was 49°C. With the goal of encompassing the array at steady state in the 42°C isotherm, RF heating alone required the sources to be 49°C at the needle. Hot water alone required all the tubes to be at 49°C, with the array encompassed only by the 41°C isotherm. When RF and cold sources were combined and the sources were kept at 46°C, the array was encompassed by 43°C isotherm (1.0 cm spacing, 10 times normal BF). At 1.4 cm spacing, RF needles were 49°C, or if cooled were only 46°C (PRIOR 1991).

13.3.3.3 Power Optimization

ZHU and GANDHI (1988) used the impedance method and considered the treatment volume to be modeled by a 3-D network of equivalent impedances. Each impedance represents a subvolume of the target heat volume with constant permittivity and conductivity. A theoretical model for brain tumors used a target tumor in the brain with a skull, skin, and air interface. The goal was to achieve a minimum standard deviation in SAR distribution throughout the treatment volume. As part of the modeling process, they experimented with different tumor properties having higher or lower values of conductivity (0.1 or 0.4 S/m) than normal tissue (0.2 S/m). An initial guess for the placement of the RF needles was used and SAR was calculated. The standard deviation was then calculated and the needles moved around each cell which had 0.4 cm diameter and recalculated for minimization of the variance of the SAR in the tumor volume (ZHU and GANDHI 1988).

13.3.4 Conductive Heating

Heat sources that do not deposit power have also been modeled. Heating patterns for treatment planning derived from a conductive model are based on the finite difference solution to the bioheat transfer equation (SCHREIER et al. 1990) or a finite element model in 2-D (MECHLING and STROHBEHN 1986) in which $Q_p = 0$.

13.3.4.1 Hot Water Source Model

One form of conductive heating utilizes hot water tubes. SCHREIER et al. (1990) showed that temperature $T_m(x)$ is calculated at a given cross-section of the tube:

$$T_m(x) = \frac{8}{u_m d^2} \int_0^{\frac{d}{2}} u(r, x) T(r, x) r \, dr \, . \tag{7}$$

The rate of heat transfer radially through the wall of the tube is expressed as follows:

$$Q = N_u k \pi L (T_m - T_s) \, , \tag{8}$$

where L = length of tube at cross-section analyzed; k = thermal conductivity of water; T_m = mean water temperature at a cross-section of tube. The tubes are metal or plastic with a diameter of 1.6 mm, and 0.1 mm wall thickness. The tubes are spaced at 10 or 14 mm in a square grid, and the flow rate is 1.5 to 2.5 ml/s. In the model $T_w = 45.5$°C at 1.0 cm grid spacing, and the entire array is at 42°C (BF = 2.5 ml/100 g/min). If BF is increased by a factor of 10, T_w must be raised to 54°C. If a model of 1.4 cm spacing is used at a flow rate of 2.55 ml/s with resting muscle BF, then the required $T_w = 48$°C. The temperature at the wall of the heating tube is 1°C less than the water temperature. Blind-ended catheter techniques with the same flow and thermal properties have yet to be studied (SCHREIER et al. 1990)

13.3.4.2 Resistive Source Model

Another form of conductive heating utilizes resistive heaters (BABBS et al. 1990). DEFORD et al. (1991) reported on 22 patients with 31 hyperthermia treatments. They compared the measured versus the estimated temperatures predicted in their model and the resulting difference was 0.0° ± 0.4°C for temperature sensors within 1.0 mm of the minimum temperature locations. Other points 4–5 mm away (closer to a source) were off by as much as 5°C. The control algorithm incorporated a polynomial expression for droop (minimum temperature between sources) to bring these values to therapeutic levels. Droop = $T_{\text{target}} - T_{\min}/T_{\text{target}} - T_a$ and was found to be equal to $-827.5\sigma^2 + 72.9\sigma - 0.0006$ (DEFORD et al. 1991), where σ = heating catheter power/heating catheter temperature rise. The entire implant was done under CT guidance. Serial coronal scans were made to accurately locate thermometer sensors. Sagittal reconstruction was used to record the cross-sectional geometry, and measure distances between probes and heating elements (DEFORD et al. 1991).

13.3.4.3 Ferromagnetic Seed Model

The final conductive heat source discussed is ferromagnetic seeds, which operate by absorbing energy from an externally applied RF magnetic field (STAUFFER et al. 1984). The power absorbed by the implants of ferromagnetic material is

$$P_I = \pi a(\omega\mu/2\sigma)^{1/2} H_0 \cdot 10^{-2} \text{ [W/cm}^3\text{]} \qquad (9)$$

for a 1.0-cm-long cylindrical implant, normalized to 1.0 cm³ of tissue. It was found that lower frequencies should be used (less than 2 MHz) to take advantage of the values greater than 10 of P_I/P_T (power absorbed by the needles/power absorbed directly by tissue). STAUFFER et al. (1984) found the total energy absorbed by the implant in volume V of phantom material. For a semicylindrical volume of tissue heated by needles length L,

$$Q_{I/L} = c\rho \int_0^R \int_0^\pi \Delta T_0 \left(1 - \frac{r}{R}\right) r\,dr\,d\theta = \frac{\pi c \rho \Delta T_0 R^2}{6} \qquad (10)$$

In brain heating studies, extreme temperatures of 65°C were necessary to overcome the high blood flow and bring the tumor tissue greater than or equal to 43°C (STAUFFER et al. 1984). Extensive work has been done for conductive heating both in theoretical treatment planning and in clinical treatments (BREZOVICH et al. 1984).

The 2-D model used for treatment planning of ferromagnetic seed heating was found to be applicable to the 3-D case within 1 cm of the ends in the implants (CHIN and STAUFFER 1991). The model also compared axial spacing between seeds since radioactive brachytherapy sources may be alternately interspersed with ferromagnetic seeds for simultaneous treatment. The catheter wall thickness makes a significant difference in the heating of the seeds. The time to reach steady state was longer for single- (0.1 mm) or double-walled (0.25 mm) catheters than for bare seeds (TOMPKINS et al. 1992). In in vivo experiments, temperatures between seeds were lowered from 48.8°C to 47.7°C (single wall) and 45.3°C (double wall). Also, field misalignment may lower temperatures 2.5°C (75° misalignment) to 11.5°C (90° misalignment) (TOMPKINS et al. 1992).

Future models should incorporate different Curie point seed segments along each catheter to allow additional heat on the tumor periphery where the vasculature is hyperdeveloped, and to achieve a more evenly distributed therapeutic dose of heat (PRIOR 1991). There is a definitive need to heat more in the plane of the antenna tips of the implant. One way to do this is to load the ferromagnetic seeds as segments, thus inserting higher Curie seeds at the tip. Sometimes, unpredictable physiologic and anatomic constraints limit the array spacing, although recommended spacing between conductive sources is 10–13 mm (EMAMI et al. 1991).

13.4 Thermal Models

Several models have been worked on by different groups. These include arrays of sources in a tissue volume that has an embedded tumor. Additional work assigns layers of perfusion to the tumor and normal tissue interface, as well as a range of electrical properties (where applicable) in the tumor and thermal conductivity that may differ from normal tissue. Furthermore, studies have incorporated blood vessel models into the bioheat transfer equation by adding additional terms to incorporate vessel branching, blood flow directionality, thermally significant vessels, and countercurrent vessel pairs. The ultimate, but perhaps unattainable model, would incorporate all of the above using data from a target treatment that is patient specific. Unfortunately, tumor vasculature responds to heat in a non-linear fashion and quite unlike normal tissue. Thus, it may not be possible to model unless a test heating is done with the patient.

13.4.1 Microwave-Induced Thermal Model with Embedded Tumor

To provide an optimum and realistic treatment using hyperthermia, the tumor model requires accurate shape, electrical characteristics, and blood flow properties. MECHLING et al. (1991b; MECHLING and STROHBEHN 1992) developed a theoretical model which placed an array of four dipole antennas driven at 915 MHz into muscle tissue at various depths, and experimental verification was also shown (RYAN et al. 1990). The 3-D SAR patterns were calculated using the theory of KING et al. (1983) and TREMBLY (1985). The bioheat transfer equation was solved for the 3-D steady-state temperature distributions in cylindrical and ellipsoidal tumor models using a finite element method. In the cylindrical and elliptical models, tumors of 4 and 6 cm length were studied and the antenna junction plane was positioned in the center of the tumor. The tumor and the normal tissue were assumed to have the same thermal properties and dielectric properties ($\sigma = 1.28\ \Omega/m$ and $\varepsilon_r = 51.0$). The tumor diameter extended 1 cm beyond the diagonal dimension of the array. The boundary conditions were such that a constant temperature boundary was placed at the outermost boundaries in normal tissue, and a no flux boundary at the plane of insertion of the antennas. The results showed that there were some insertion depths that resulted in virtually no therapeutic heating in the tumor because of the effects of insertion depth on the shape of the 3-D SAR pattern, which caused most of the heating to occur in the normal tissue and not in the tumor (MECHLING et al. 1991a).

If the model has enough flexibility without changing the implant, the SAR pattern can be adjusted with the accompanying thermal dosimetry adjustment, simply by changing frequency for dipoles or helical antennas or by changing antenna design. If there is no solution available to the theory of some antenna types (i.e., helical, modified dipole) then the measured SAR pattern in the diagonal plane is used as input to the bioheat equation for thermal modeling (RYAN 1991b). In those cases where the maximum tumor temperature is a limiting factor in the analysis of MECHLING et al. (1991a, b; MECHLING and STROHBEHN 1992), phase rotation would lower the centrally overheated tumor and allow greater therapeutic penetration.

MECHLING et al. (1991a) also varied frequency (433, 915, or 2450 MHz) for cylindrical tumor models from 2 to 16 cm in length in 2-D. The 2450 MHz array had only 20% power at the center and maximum SAR was in the proximity of the antennas. These could be candidates for air or water cooling to avoid any pain limitation in the treatment. MECHLING and STROHBEHN (1986) also investigated antenna spacing for microwave antenna arrays spaced 1, 2, or 3 cm apart. The range of tumor–normal blood flow ratios in the model ranged from 0 to 40. This study was interested in investigating array spacing since minimizing the number of sources will lower the amount of trauma and complication rate (MECHLING and STROHBEHN 1986).

Three blood flow cases were examined: (a) homogeneous model: tumor blood flow was the same as normal blood flow with values of 0, 2.5, 5, 10, 20, 50, and 100 ml/100 g/min; (b) nonhomogeneous model: tumor and normal tissue had uniform blood flow but different values, normal tissue ranging from 2.5 to 100 and tumor ranging from 0 to 100 ml/100 g/min; and (c) concentric annulus tumor perfusion (CATP) model with a necrotic core of 0 perfusion in the tumor center, an intermediate region with half the perfusion of the normal tissue, and a peripheral zone containing a tumor margin with greater perfusion. The maximum allowable temperature in the model was 60°C in tumor and 44°C in normal tissue. Tumors were classified as small or large and assigned different ratios among necrotic core, intermediate perfusion zone, and highly perfused region.

13.4.2 RF-Induced Thermal Model

For the RF needle arrays, the maximum power density is at the electrodes and falls off radially as $1/R^2$ when 2-D models are explored. Also, RF needles decrease in temperature at the ends due to the divergence of the field lines and heat conduction draws heat away. Thus, it is recommended that RF needles be placed 1 cm beyond the tumor margin. At lower perfusion rates, thermal conduction dominates and smooth temperature distributions prevail. At higher perfusion rates (>20 ml/100 g/min), convection dominated thermal conduction and the temperature distribution resembled the SAR pattern of microwave antennas. If the blood flow equals 100 in normal tissue and 2.5 in the tumor, conduction dominates in the tumor and convection dominates in the surrounding normal tissue (MECHLING and STROHBEHN 1986). Cooling the array elements will help to evenly distribute temperature (PRIOR 1991). If the electrodes are spaced close together ($=1$ cm), in cases of higher perfusion (>20 ml/100 g/min), the temperature distribution becomes more evenly distributed (STROHBEHN 1983).

13.4.3 Thermal Significance of Blood Vessels

The bioheat equation does not account for the presence of large thermally significant blood vessels that may be either heat sinks or sources. It also does not account for the directionality of blood flow. To determine whether a vessel is thermally significant, the thermal equilibrium length of a vessel is calculated (MOOIBROEK and LAGENDIJK 1991):

$$\chi_{eq} = \left[\frac{\rho_{bl} c_{pbl}}{8k_{bl}}\right] \langle V \rangle D_v^2 \left[\frac{3}{4} + \frac{k_{bl}}{k_{tis}} \ln\left(\frac{D_c}{D_v}\right)\right]. \quad (11)$$

If vessel lengths are smaller than the thermal equilibrium length, these are considered thermally significant and need to be considered individually in the model. For individual blood vessels, capillaries are in thermal equilibrium with the surrounding tissue, small arteries and veins experience significant heat transfer, and larger vessels experience little heat transfer. The large number, architecture, and dimensional variety of the blood vessels in the treatment regions make it impractical to account for the contributions of individual vessels, except for larger arteries and veins. The individual arteries and veins are small relative to the macroscopic volume of interest; thus only the collective behavior is statistically considered. These considerations include thermal conductivity, specific heat, and blood perfusion. Vessel radii range in size from capillaries (4 μm), arterioles (10 μm), and venules (15 μm) to large arteries (1500 μm), large veins (3000 μm), and the aorta (5000 μm). The velocity in each vessel is roughly proportional to radius. Values for χ_{eq} are 2×10^{-7} m for capillaries, 2×10^{-6} m for venules, 5×10^{-6} m for arterioles, 5 m for large veins, and 4 m for large arteries. Thus, capillaries, arterioles, and venules equilibrate with tissue. To place the contributions of various vessels into perspective, let us consider the percent of vascular volume each occupies: capillaries (6.6%), venules (12%), arterioles (3%), large arteries (7%), large veins (24%), and aorta (3%) (CHEN and HOLMES 1980). Most of the heat exchange does not take place in the capillary beds, but rather after the blood leaves the terminal arterial branches, before entering the arterioles, with vessel sizes between 10 and 50 μm radii. CHEN and HOLMES (1980) provided additions to the bioheat transfer equation including heat transfer contributions of local perfusion velocity and effective thermal conductivity:

$$\rho c \frac{\partial T}{\partial t} = \nabla \cdot k \nabla T_k + W_j^*(T_a^* - T) - \rho_b c_b \vec{u}_p \cdot \nabla T + \nabla \cdot k_p \nabla T + q_m \quad (12)$$

To assess how quickly or along what lengths a thermally significant vessel will equilibrate with surrounding tissue, certain assumptions are made:

1. Tissue surrounding the vessel is at the treatment temperature.
2. Power is deposited directly into the vessel (i.e., into the blood).
3. The overall heat transfer coefficient equals the convective heat transfer coefficient.
4. Countercurrent vessel is at the treatment temperature.

The model showed that it is difficult or impossible to preheat vessels ≥ 1.0 mm with only local heating. With the vast number of small vessels that exist in any treatment volume, it would be an impossible task to include every vessel as well as capillaries for computation of temperature distributions. Even if the geometry of the microvasculature was known, the computation time would be very lengthy. The basic assumption of the bioheat transfer equation is that blood enters the treatment volume at arterial temperature and then exits at local tissue temperature. Tissue flow is not unidirectional since vessels are often combined in countercurrent pairs and vessel orientation is frequently isotropic. The k_{eff} model instead of the heat sink model is more suitable to the interaction between tissue-volume elements (CREZEE and LAGENDIJK 1990).

13.4.4 *Patient-Specific Microcirculation Models*

The model proposed by MOOIBROEK and LAGENDIJK (1991) handles vessels with irregular shapes or tapered geometry, and various vessel diameters. Typically, problems confronting thermal models involve heat conduction and convection in highly inhomogeneous tissue as well as heat-related physiological responses. This study concluded that convective heat transfer by blood flow is the dominant factor in the final temperature distribution. The bioheat transfer equation Eq. 1 is based on the idea that the influence of blood flow is described in terms of volumetrically distributed scalar heat sinks or sources. Thus, heat is added or withdrawn from tissue without an explicit convective heat transfer term. Large vessels are distributed throughout the tissue volumes involved in treatment planning. These vessels typically follow irregular pathways, branch continuously into smaller or larger vessels, and thus require some consideration, although countercurrent vessels formed from an arterial–venous pair reduce the need for individual description of medium-sized vessels. In the model, branching of a vessel is represented by three vessel segments with a common branching point. Vessel tapering is handled by segmenting a vessel with different diameters and flow values per segment and the model divides the tissue volume into cubic subdivisions including the blood vessels and its transient component. The transient thermal model provided a dynamic updating of all vessel segment data during the treatment run time.

A model by WEINBAUM and JIJI (1985) included thermally significant countercurrent vessels that have an arbitrary direction relative to tissue temperature gradients. The flowing blood in the countercurrent vessels retains a different memory of the neighboring tissue temperature due to the opposite directionality. The advantage in this bioheat model is that blood–tissue heat transfer can be directly related to the geometry of local vasculature and flow. In the traditional bioheat equation, it was found that the convective term due to blood flow was treated as a volumetric isotropic heat source and under normal physiologic conditions is negligible. This study showed that the primary mechanism by which flow in the microvasculature alters heat transfer in tissue is incomplete countercurrent exchange in the thermally significant vessels $\geq 40\ \mu m$ (WEINBAUM and JIJI 1985).

$$\overline{\rho c}\frac{\partial \theta}{\partial t} - \frac{\partial}{\partial x_i}\left[(k_{ij})_{eff}\frac{\partial \theta}{\partial x_j}\right] = \frac{\pi^2 n a^2 k_b^2}{4\sigma k}\mathrm{Pe}^2 l_j \frac{\partial l_i}{\partial x_i}\frac{\partial \theta}{\partial x_j} + q_m$$

where

$$k_{eff} = k\left(1 + \frac{\pi^2}{4\sigma k^2} n a^2 k_b^2 n a^2 k_b^2 \mathrm{Pe}^2\right) \tag{13}$$

where θ = mean tissue temperature and σ = shape factor.

The term *incomplete countercurrent exchange* is used since the energy transferred by conduction from an arterial surface to adjacent tissue is not equal to the energy transferred by conduction from the tissue to the venous surface. Since each countercurrent vessel travels from a region of different temperature, there is a net energy transfer when the vessels exist in a tissue temperature gradient which will have a component in the direction of flow (WEINBAUM and JIJI 1985).

These models are more accurate perhaps than the "bare" bioheat transfer equation, but several factors must be weighted. The time to construct the models for individual patient treatments must be considered. The computation time also becomes a factor. More importantly, the amount of information required is difficult to obtain from current imaging devices, especially in three dimensions, short of doing careful dissection and histologic analysis of the treatment volume, which is impractical. This implies that there are different levels of treatment planning and the limitations are not the models but the information required to allow the models to run.

13.4.5 Two-Dimensional Versus Three-Dimensional Thermal Models

When considering 2-D versus 3-D solutions to power deposition or heat transfer in thermal models, several factors must be weighted. The amount of computation power measured by computer size and execution time (minutes, hours, days) is a factor if individual patient treatments will be modeled. The second problem lies in the grid construction. If a realistic finite element model is used, for example, organ placement and other features that are obtained by manually outlining CT or MRI scans in a number of planes for final 3-D reconstruction could take more than 1–2 person-days. Lastly, the visualization of results in 3-D is more complex when attempting to display 3-D data on 2-D devices.

CHEN et al. (1990) placed actual patient CT data into a 3-D simulation, distributed power uniformly, and compared 2-D to 3-D temperature simulations using an inhomogeneous tissue model. It was found that 2-D models are valid when working in the center of a tumor if blood flow is greater than 6 ml/100 g/min. This is due to the higher blood flow values, and the fact that blood perfusion heat transfer overwhelms the effects of conduction in the z-direction. The predictions become inaccurate when near the tumor boundary, and thus 3-D simulations will be necessary for treatment planning. It was noted that the correct thermal conductivity values must be used for each tissue type: 0.4–0.6 W/m/°C for soft tissue, 1.16 W/m/°C for bone, and 0.2 W/m/°C for fat. The steady-state bioheat transfer equation does not account for the effects of major blood vessels which either sink or source heat, nor does it deal with the directionality of convective losses. In the model, each organ as a whole is assumed to have uniform thermal properties. The 2-D model assumes no energy transfer in the third dimension, an insulated boundary in the z-direction. If perfusion is homogeneous then the

2-D model is valid, though at higher perfusion rates blood perfusion heat transfer dominates conduction in the z-direction. Also, the 2-D model does not predict the lower temperatures at the tumor boundary where conduction in the z-direction is significant. When comparing the 2-D to the 3-D models, a maximum error of 10°–30°C was found in the center of the tumor in the 2-D case. If the tumor is less than 5 cm in axial length and blood perfusion is less than 3.0 ml/100 g/min, the error in the central plane is also very large and the results will be misleading in the 2-D case (CHEN et al. 1990).

13.4.6 Temperature Field Estimation

DIVRIK et al. (1984) estimated the complete temperature field from a few measured points. Difficulty in the correct estimation is compounded in volumes with tumor present because of the inhomogeneity of blood perfusion. The assumptions are that there exist a priori knowledge of thermal conductivity, density, specific heat of blood, tissue metabolism, power deposition patterns, arterial blood temperature, and the anatomy of the tumor and surrounding structures. The unknown parameters are the blood perfusion distribution and the temperature field. The study demonstrates the errors in temperature predictions when the following errors are induced into the model: power ($\pm 20\%$), thermal conductivity ($\pm 20\%$), boundary temperatures ($\pm 2°C$), arterial temperatures ($\pm 2°C$), and measured temperatures ($\pm 1°C$). The problem of inhomogeneity of tumor blood perfusion distribution and the lack of imaging systems to divide the tumor into zones of perfusion still remain. Validation of the model was done with animal experiments and showed convergence to better than 0.05°C.

Other work on temperature field estimation used initial guesses at the blood perfusion, and then the bioheat equation was used to predict the temperature field (CLEGG et al. 1985). If the error was large between the calculated points and measured values at the same points, the blood perfusion guess was changed by an optimization algorithm and the technique restarted. The optimization algorithm stopped when errors $\leq 0.01°C$. It was assumed that there are seven blood perfusion regions which have ratios to one known region. Clinical situations will be more complex since the perfusion is unknown and the geometry is 3-D. In addition, perfusion rates are time dependent; thus the transient method performed better than steady-state methods (CLEGG et al. 1985).

13.4.7 Hyperthermic Effects on Blood Flow: Empirical Studies

A blood vessel with isothermal flow will always act as an additional heat sink unless the blood temperature exceeds ambient tissue temperature. Tortuous and dilated vasculature would predispose a tumor to a decrease in blood flow as a direct effect of heat. Blood flow under hyperthermia conditions has been found by SEKINS et al. (1982) to increase in the thigh from 2.6 to 36 ml/100 g/min, in the forearm from 3.2 to 50 ml/100 g/min, and in the forearm skin from 8.4 to 280 ml/100 g/min.

Studies on tumor microcirculation found that there was an initial increase and then a decrease in tumor blood flow (REINHOLD and ENDRICH 1986). Stasis may also be observed although this may occur a few hours after the treatment. Also, vascular stasis depends on tumor type, rate of heating, and assay method. A systematic determination of vascular stasis and collapse due to heat dose still remains to be done. This argues for steered power controlled by way of a temperature feedback system.

It was found that the effective thermal conductivity is 50%–100% greater in mammary tumors due to blood supply. The vasculature of growing tumors is composed of two components: newly formed networks and preexisting networks of host tissue. The blood supply declined in about half of the tumors in the in vivo model with hyperthermia (SONG et al. 1980). The vascular volume in small tumors increases as a result of hyperthermia and the vascular volume in large tumors decreases as a result of hyperthermia. There was no appreciable change in blood flow in rats at 43°C for 1 h, as far as the differential effects on the tumor in vivo were concerned, but there was a vasodilatation effect that caused an increase in blood flow in skin in the normal tissue.

Another proposed perfusion model included five zones for the distribution of perfusion in the tumor volume (CRAVALHO et al. 1980): necrotic area with no vascularization, seminecrotic area with long capillaries without branching, stabilized tumor microcirculation inside the edge of the tumor (two to three arterioles, three to five venules), advancing tumor front with highest perfusion of all zones, and normal tissue. If power is only deposited in the fourth and fifth zones at a rate of 6.26 W/cm^3, the maximum temperature equals 42.7°C (CRAVALHO et al. 1980).

A study by MANTYLA et al. (1982) utilized xenon washout techniques and showed an increase in blood flow in superficial metastatic tumors from 20.1 to 31.3 ml/100 g/min prior to and 1 week following the first week of radiation therapy. WONG et al. (1988) utilized a tumor model with concentric regions composed of a 1.0-cm-diameter core, 1.2-cm intermediate annulus, and 0.3-cm outer shell surrounded by normal tissue. The study assumed the same density, permittivity, permeability, and electrical and thermal conductivity in all regions. The study did allow, though, for different blood flow parameters in each of the four regions.

Blood perfusion can increase by increasing the number of vessels, blood pressure, or vessel diameter or by decreasing blood viscosity or vessel length. Local response in normal tissue is to actively dilate heated vessels by relaxing vascular smooth muscles to increase flow. Neoplastic tissues lack this local control since vessels are devoid of smooth muscle. Normal tissue heated to 46°C and neoplastic tissue heated to 41°C both show a return to normal blood flow after 45 min (DUDAR and JAIN 1984). At higher temperatures, vascular stasis is often permanent in neoplastic vessels beyond 42°C. Their findings support the concept of temporal and functional blood flow inhomogeneity in the microcirculation of spreading tumors (ENDRICH et al. 1979). Blood flow in the well-vascularized peripheral tumor area is greater than the inner area of tumors (SONG et al. 1984). Rat muscle blood flow increased ninefold when heated to 45°C, and there was a sixfold increase at 44°C. Certain types of tumors have increased blood flow at low temperatures (i.e., 41°–42°C), but decreased blood flow over time or with further temperature increase. In tumor vasculature, vulnerability to heat is such that vascular stasis, occlusion, and hemorrhage are likely at 42°–43°C (SONG et al. 1984).

Another study measured RBC velocity and vessel lumen diameter in normal versus tumor tissue in rabbits (DUDAR and JAIN 1984). It was found that during hyperthermia, blood flow in normal tissue increased until a temperature of 45.7°C was reached, and at higher temperatures blood flow shuts down. Blood flow in the tumor increased until a temperature of 43°C was reached, and then began to decrease. Additionally, normal tissue vessels were able to increase the amount of blood flow by a factor of 6.8 (45.7°C) and tumor by only 2.1 (43.8°C). Vessel diameter in normal tissue may increase up to 50% but decrease slightly at temperatures exceeding 47°C. In the neoplastic tissue, no increase was seen (DUDAR and JAIN 1984).

These studies point out the difficulties in modeling a nonlinear system where the steady-state bioheat transfer equation, which assumes linear blood flow, will no longer suffice as a model.

13.5 Noninvasive Temperature Monitoring

Knowing the complete temperature field will assist in the evaluation of heat treatments since inhomogeneities exist in power or heat distribution, blood flow, and tissue electrical properties. Invasive methods for temperature measurements can only provide temperatures at a limited number of points. Implantation of many additional measurement catheters to get the true temperature distribution is overly traumatic to the patient and raises the risk of infection. Microwave radiometry has limitations due to the high frequencies used (GHz range) and the amount of attenuation in tissue (HALL et al. 1990). Some studies have used MRI sensitivity of T1 relaxation time to temperature (HALL et al. 1990) or molecular diffusion magnetic imaging (ZHANG et al. 1992). Problems arise in committing bulky and expensive apparatuses to temperature measurements; thus, use of CT or MRI systems may be ruled out at most institutions. Electrical impedance tomography (EIT) systems are truly portable and attach to the patients by small electrodes on the order of 4–8 mm in diameter. The entire EIT system equals the cost of a handful of CT or MRI patient scans.

13.5.1 Electrical Impedance Tomography for Noninvasive Imaging of Temperature

The EIT method utilizes electrodes driven by signals from 10 to 50 kHz with 5 mA currents (GRIFFITHS and AHMED 1987). Recent thermal imaging efforts map electrical conductivity changes with temperature, which are typically 2%/°C. Impedance mapping has the following advantages. EIT operates well in a strong electromagnetic or acoustic field, and its operation does not perturb hyperthermia applicators and there is efficient spatial temporal and thermal resolution. Temperature resolution of greater than 1°C has been reported

(CONWAY 1987). Electrodes are placed superficially around the treated region and internally within the heated region, current fields are configured, and the voltages measured. The electrical conductivity changes in tissues are then reconstructed and subtracted from a baseline with uniform temperature, prior to hyperthermia-induced gradients. Current is cosine distributed around the outer boundary of the phantom simulation. A linear array with eight contacts is also used for internal measurements and this doubles as a microthermocouple tract which justifies its existence as an implant catheter. Thus, this model combined invasive and noninvasive measurements (RYAN et al. 1991). An impedance imaging system was fabricated for the purpose of noninvasive temperature imaging (RYAN et al. 1991). Computer simulations show that significantly improved images can be made when internal electrodes are used in conjunction with implanted thermometry probes or catheters (PAULSEN et al. 1991). Impedance imaging is a new modality to examine the electrical properties of tissue prior to heating in order to do the appropriate treatment planning.

Figure 13.4a shows an actual CT-based image with exact electrical properties (conductivity and permittivity) distributed throughout the image. The large mass below the image center is tumor. Fat and bone are also visualized. The simulation in Fig. 13.4b is reconstructed by using surface and

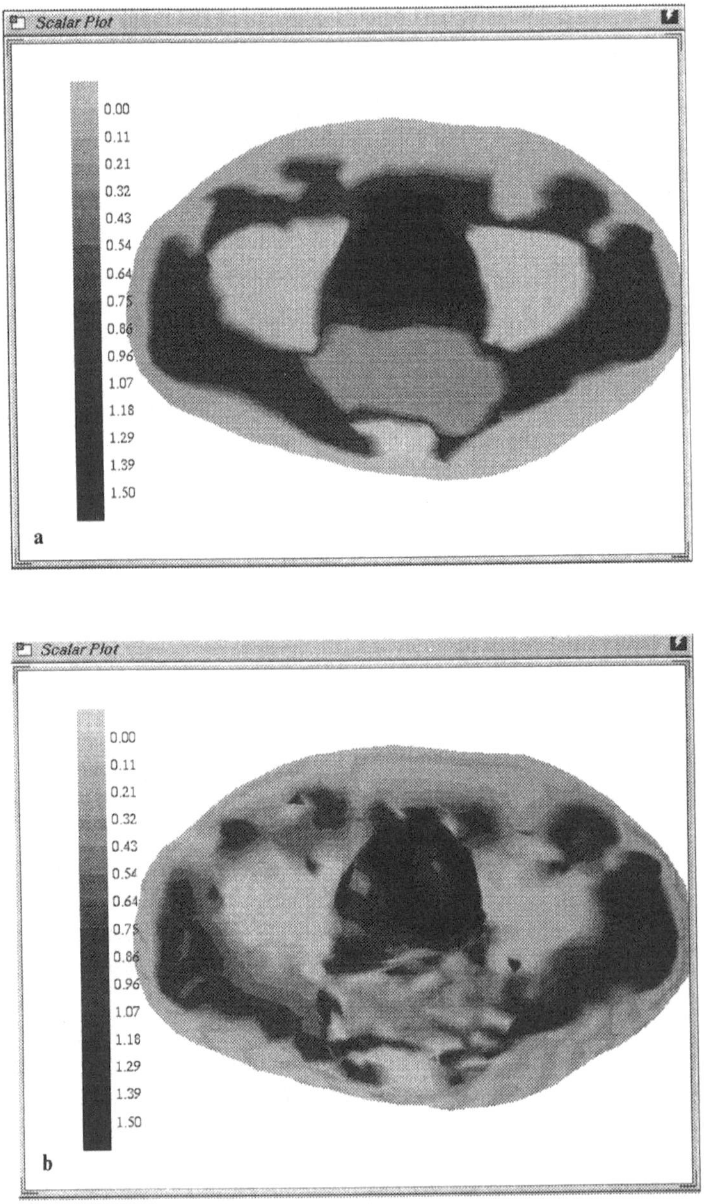

Fig. 13.4. **a** Exact electrical property distribution based on actual patient CT image. **b** Reconstructed distribution combining surface and internal electrodes

internal electrodes. Sixty-four superficial electrodes were placed around the periphery in addition to internal electrodes placed in the tumor and solved with a finite element model. The addition of the surface electrodes reduces reconstruction errors by an order of magnitude.

13.5.2 Microwave Radiometry and Ultrasound Tomography

Microwave radiometry has been developed as an atraumatic thermal dosimetry system based on radiometric temperature measurements and the superficial temperature at the applicator–tissue interface during heating (PLANCOT et al. 1987). Microwave thermography is possible because human tissue emits thermal radiation which, at microwave frequencies of centimeter or millimeter wavelengths, is proportional to temperature. In addition, microwave radiation can penetrate human tissue to several centimeters' depth. Radiometric temperature of a planar homogeneous or layered lossy medium can be calculated by integrating the thermal noise contribution of different normal path sections of the stratified lossy medium of interest (BARRETT and MYERS 1985). This follows from the equation

$$I(\nu) = \frac{2h\nu^3}{c^2}\,[e^{h\nu/kT} - 1]^{-1} \tag{14}$$

where ν = frequency of emitted radiation; h = Planck's constant; c = velocity of propagation; $I(\nu)$ = intensity of radiation; k = Boltzmann's constant (BARRETT and MYERS 1985). Thus, in the microwave range of frequencies, the intensity is proportional to the temperature of the emitter. This may penetrate several centimeters in depth if lower frequencies are used. Although waveguides are commonly coupled directly to the skin's surface, alternate techniques may incorporate parabolic reflectors or lenses that can scan the body from a distance.

A smart algorithm to estimate temperature profiles along the axis perpendicular to the skin surface has not yet been forthcoming. The difficulty lies in the inverse problem of estimating temperature profiles from measured radiometric data. The simulations using the sweep radiometer showed a sensitivity of greater than 0.1°C if used in a body model with homogeneous dielectric properties (CAMART et al. 1991). In France, more than 1300 heating sessions have been performed using radiometric temperature control performed noninvasively (PLANCOT et al. 1987).

Simulations were done with ultrasonic CT techniques which indicated that 1°C resolution is achievable (TOMIKAWA et al. 1988). For a 5°C temperature difference, a 10 m/s velocity difference is found. One drawback is the long measurement time due to the moving applicator and the applicator size of 1.5 cm diameter.

13.5.3 MRI Thermal Imaging

HALL et al. (1990) showed that the basis for MRI imaging of temperature lies in the relation

$$T1^T = T1^\infty \exp(-e\alpha/kT)\,. \tag{15}$$

It was found that the temperature coefficient of $T1$ was 1.5%/°C and the diffusion coefficient, 2.5%/°C (HALL et al. 1990). No temperature-dependent change in $T2$ was found (ZHANG et al. 1992). Molecular diffusion is more sensitive to temperature change and measurements within 0.2°C in regions of 0.3 cm^3 have been observed in phantom experiments when compared to fiberoptic thermometry (ZHANG et al. 1992).

13.6 Conclusions

Several factors in thermal modeling make treatment planning a difficult task. Although power deposition patterns of microwave antennas or RF needles can be predicted, a correct evaluation of the electrical properties of the normal and malignant tissue is needed for the model to accurately predict power deposition. This can be done by electrical impedance tomography. The other confounding problem may be that the small necrotic core might be found in treatment #1 but a larger necrotic core may be present in treatment #2 because of the first hyperthermia treatment. A new conductivity and permittivity image would be required. The next step of creating a thermal model using some adaptation of the bioheat transfer equation is confounded by the lack of blood perfusion distribution information in 3-D, and locations of thermally significant vessels and countercurrent vessel pairs. In addition, even if the distribution of perfusion is known, changes in perfusion values occur as a response to heat, varying significantly in tumor as opposed to normal tissue. A potential solution to these complex gaps in knowledge for the modeler is to attempt to model with as much information as possible, attempt a test heating utilizing all of the enhancements to optimize the selected heating modality, and to incorporate a noninvasive thermometry system to drive the heating system with dynamic control over the distribution of heat. The planning process may eventually become more abbreviated if thermal imaging such as EIT or MRI techniques give temperature feedback in real time, and the power distribution system can be adjusted accordingly.

Acknowledgments. The author is grateful to Joyce Mechling, Keith Paulsen, and Susan Scown for editorial review.

Appendix

w_b = blood perfusion rate ($kg/m^3/s = 6 \times ml/100\ g/min$)
I = antenna current
ε = dielectric constant of tissue
h = length of one dipole element
μ = magnetic permeability
$\vec{U}_\rho$ = unit vector in r direction
$\vec{U}_z$ = unit vector in z direction
$\vec{E}_r$ = radial component of **E** field (V/m)
σ = electrical conductivity (S/m)
ρ = density (kg/m^3)
$\vec{E}_z$ = longitudinal component of **E** field (V/m)
U = total heat transfer coefficient ($W/m^2/°C$)
h^* = convection coefficient of water
k_{is} = thermal conductivity of external casing = 0.15 (W/m/°C)
r_2 = radius of external casing
r_1 = radius of coolant column
d_2 = inner diameter of catheter (m)
T_t = outer catheter wall tissue temperature (K)
h_{oa} = overall conductive and convective heat transfer coefficient between tissue and air [$W/(m^2 \cdot K)$]
ε^* = complex dielectric constant (farad/m)
T_m = maximum temperature goal
T = local tissue temperature
t = time
$u(r, x)$ = local velocity of water
$T(r, x)$ = local temperature of water
u_m = mean velocity of water
T_w = water temperature
T_s = temperature at surface of tube
N_u = Nusselt number for dimensionless heat flux
a = radius
R = radius of needle
ΔT_0 = temperature change from baseline
ρ_t = density of tissue (kg/m^3)
ρ_b = density of blood (kg/m^3)
c_t = specific heat of tissue (W-s/kg-°C)
c_b = specific heat of blood (W-s/kg-°C)
k_t = thermal conductivity of tissue (W/m°C)
m = volumetric flow rate of blood per unit mass tissue (m^3/kg-s)
T_b = temperature of entering arterial blood (°C)
Q_p = q_p = power absorbed per unit volume of tissue (W/m^3) = $r_t \times$ SAR
Q_m = power generated by unit volume of tissue by metabolic processes (W/m^3)
χ_{eq} = thermal equilibrium length
r_{bl} = density of blood vessel
c_{pbl} = specific heat of blood vessel
k_{bl} = thermal conductivity of blood vessel
D_c = mean tissue diameter
D_v = mean vessel diameter
$\langle V \rangle$ = mean vessel flow velocity
W_j^* = total perfusion rate/unit volume tissue
T_a^* = temperature reached by T_b
$\vec{u}_p$ = mean perfusion velocity
k_p = perfusion conductivity
$\overline{\rho c}$ = average blood-tissue capacity
c = specific heat
n = density of vessel pairs crossing surface of control volume/unit area
k_b = thermal conductivity of blood
Pe = Peclet number
l = spacing between neighboring vessels (center to center)
$T1^T$ = $T1$ at the temperature T
α = activation energy of the relaxation process
d = tube diameter.

References

Babbs CF, Fearnot NE, Marchosky JA, Moran EJ, Jones JT, Plantenga TD (1990) Theoretical basis for controlling minimal tumor temperature during interstitial conductive heat therapy. IEEE Trans Biomed Eng 37: 662–672

Barrett AH, Myers PC (1985) Basic principles and applications of microwave thermography. In: Larson LE, Jacobi JH (eds) Medical applications of microwave imaging. IEEE, New York, pp 41–46

Brezovich IA, Atkinson WJ, Chakraborty DP (1984) Temperature distributions in tumor models heated by self-regulating nickel-copper alloy thermoseeds. Med Phys 11: 145–152

Camart JC, Morganti F, Fabre JJ, Chive M (1991) Microwave interstitial hyperthermia controlled by microwave radiometry: modeling of the temperature increasing versus time. In: Nagel JH, Smith WM (eds) Proceedings of the International Conference of IEEE Engineering in Medicine and Biology Society. IEEE, New York, pp. 991–992

Chen MM, Holmes KR (1980) Microvascular contributions in tissue heat transfer. Ann NY Acad Sci 335: 137–150

Chen ZP, Miller WH, Roemer RB, Cetas TC (1990) Errors between 2- and 3-dimensional thermal model predictions of hyperthermia treatments. Int J Hyperthermia 6: 175–191

Chin RB, Stauffer PR (1991) Treatment planning for ferromagnetic seed heating. Int J Radiat Oncol Biol Phys 21: 431–439

Clegg ST, Roemer RB, Cetas TC (1985) Estimation of complete temperature fields from measured transient temperatures. Int J Hyperthermia 1: 265–286

Conway J (1987) Electrical impedance tomography for thermal modeling of hyperthermic treatment: an assessment using in-vitro and in-vivo measurements. Clin Phys Physiol Meas [Suppl A] 8: 141–146

Cravalho EG, Fox LR, Kan JC (1980) The application of the bioheat equation to the design of thermal protocols for local hyperthermia. Ann NY Acad Sci 335: 86–97

Crezee J, Lagendijk JJW (1990) Experimental verification of bioheat transfer theories: measurement of temperature profiles around large artificial vessels in perfused tissue. Phys Med Biol 35: 905–923

Deford JP, Babbs CF, Patel UH, Bleyer MW, Marchosky JA, Moran CJ (1991) Effective estimation and computer control of minimum tumor temperature during conductive interstitital hyperthermia. Int J Hyperthermia 7: 441–453

Divrik AM, Roemer RB, Cetas TC (1984) Inference of complete tissue temperature fields from a few measured temperatures: an unconstrained optmization method. IEEE Trans Biomed Eng 31: 150–160

Dudar TE, Jain RK (1984) Differential response of normal and tumor microcirculation to hyperthermia. Cancer Res 44: 605–612

Emami B, Stauffer P, Dewhirst MW et al. (1991) RTOG quality assurance guidelines for interstitial hyperthermia. Int J Radiat Biol Oncol Phys 20: 1117–1124

Endrich B, Reinhol HS, Gross JF, Intaglietta M (1979) Tissue perfusion inhomogeneity during early tumor growth in rats. J Natl Cancer Inst 62: 387–396

Eppert V, Trembly BS, Richter HJ (1991) Air cooling for an interstitial microwave hyperthermia antenna: theory and experiment. IEEE Trans Biomed Eng 38: 450–460

Furse CM, Iskander MF (1989) Three dimensional electromagnetic power deposition in tumors with interstitial antenna arrays. IEEE Trans Biomed Eng 36: 977–986

Gentile DB, Gori F, Leoncini M (1991) Electromagnetic and thermal models of a water-cooled dipole radiating in a biological tissue. IEEE Trans Biomed Eng 38: 98–103

Griffiths H, Ahmed A (1987) Applied potential tomography for non-invasive temperature mapping and hyperthermia. Clin Phys Physiol Meas [Suppl A] 8: 147–153

Hall AS, Prior MV, Hand JW, Young IR, Dickinson RJ (1990) Observation by MR imaging of in-vivo temperature changes induced by radiofrequency hyperthermia. J Comput Assist Tomogr 14: 430–436

Iskander MF, Tumeh AM (1989) Design optimization for interstitial antennas. IEEE Trans Biomed Eng 36: 236–247

Iskander MF, Tumeh AM, Furse CM (1990) Evaluation and optimization of the electromagnetic performance of interstitial antennas for hyperthermia. Int J Radiat Oncol Biol Phys 18: 895–902

Joines WT, Shrivastava S, Jirtle R (1989) A comparison using tissue electric properties and temperature rise to determine relative absorption of microwave power in malignant tissue. Med Phys 16: 840–844

Jones KM, Mechling JA, Strohbehn JW, Trembly BS (1989) Theoretical and experimental SAR distributions for interstitial dipole antenna arrays used in hyperthermia. IEEE Trans Microwave Theory Tech 37: 1200–1209

King RWP, Trembly BS, Strohbehn JW (1983) The electromagnetic field of an insulated antenna in a conducting or dielectric medium. IEEE Trans Microwave Theory Tech 31: 574–583

Mantyla MJ, Toivanen JT, Pitkanen MA, Rekonen AH (1982) Radiation-induced changes in regional blood flow in human tumors. Int J Radiat Oncol Biol Phys 8: 1711–1717

Mechling JA, Strohbehn JW (1986) A theoretical comparison of the temperature distributions produced by three interstitial hyperthermia systems. Int J Radiat Oncol Biol Phys 12: 2137–2149

Mechling JA, Strohbehn JW (1992) Three dimensional theoretical SAR and temperature distributions created in brain tissue by 915 and 2450 MHz dipole antenna arrays with varying insertion depths. Int J Hyperthermia (in press)

Mechling JA, Strohbehn JW, France LJ (1991a) A theoretical evaluation of the performance of the Dartmouth IMAAH system to heat cylindrical and ellipsoidal tumor models. Int J Hyperthermia 7: 465–483

Mechling JA, Strohbehn JW, Ryan TP (1991b) Three-dimensional theoretical temperature distributions produced by 915 MHz dipole antenna arrays with varying insertion depths in muscle tissue. Int J Radiat Oncol Biol Phys 22: 131–138

Mooibroek J, Lagendijk JJW (1991) A fast and simple algorithm for the calculation of convective heat transfer by large vessels in 3-dimensional inhomogeneous tissue. IEEE Trans Biomed Eng 38: 490–501

Ocheltree KP, Frizzell LA (1987) Determination of power deposition patterns for localized hyperthermia: a steady-state analysis. Int J Hyperthermia 3: 269–279

Ocheltree KP, Frizzell LA (1988) Determination of power deposition patterns for localized hyperthermia: a transient analysis. Int J Hyperthermia 4: 281–296

Osterhout WJV (1922) Injury, recovery and death in relation to conductivity and permeability. Lippincott, Philadelphia

Patel UH, Deford UA, Babbs CF (1991) Computer-aided design and evaluation of novel catheters for conductive interstitial hyperthermia. Med Biol Eng Comput 29: 25–33

Paulsen KD, Moskowitz MJ, Ryan TP (1991) A combined invasive-non invasive conductivity profile reconstruction approach for thermal imaging in hyperthermia. In: Nagel JH, Smith WM (eds) Proceedings of the International Conference of IEEE Engineering in Medicine and Biology Society. IEEE, New York, pp 323–324

Pennes HH (1948) Analysis of tissue and arterial blood temperatures in the resting human forearm. J Appl Phys 1: 93–122

Plancot M, Prevost B, Chive M, Fabre JJ, Ladee R, Giaux G (1987) A new method for thermal dosimetry in microwave hyperthermia using microwave radiometry for temperature control. Int J Hyperthermia 3: 9–19
Prior MV (1991) Comparative study of RF-LCF and hotsources interstitial hyperthermia techniques. Int J Hyperthermia 7: 131–140
Reinhold HS, Endrich B (1986) Tumor microcirculation as a target for hyperthermia. Int J Hyperthermia 2: 111–137
Roemer RB (1990) Thermal dosimetry. In: Gautherie M (ed) Clinical thermology, thermal dosimetry and treatment planning. Springer, Berlin Heidelberg New York, pp 119–214
Roemer RB (1991) Optimal power deposition in hyperthermia. I. The treatment goal: the ideal temperature distribution: the role of large blood vessels. Int J Hyperthermia 7: 317–341
Ryan TP (1991a) Techniques for heating brain tumors with implantable microwave antennas. In: Heiter GL (ed) Proceedings of IEEE MTT-S International Microwave Symposium, vol 2. IEEE, New York, pp. 791–794
Ryan TP (1991b) Comparison of six microwave antennas for hyperthermia treatment of cancer: SAR results for single antennas and arrays. Int J Radiat Oncol Biol Phys 21: 403–413
Ryan TP, Mechling JA, Strohbehn JW (1990) Absorbed power deposition for various insertion depths for 915 MHz interstitial dipole antenna arrays: experiment versus theory. Int J Radiat Oncol Biol Phys 19: 377–387
Ryan TP, Moskowitz MJ, Paulsen KD (1991) The Dartmouth electrical impedance tomography system for thermal imaging. In: Nagel JH, Smith WM (eds) Proceedings of the International Conference of IEEE Engineering in Medicine and Biology Society. IEEE, New York, pp 321–322
Ryan TP, Hoopes PJ, Jonsson E, Heaney J (1992) Use of a water-cooled microwave applicator for transurethral prostate heating: techniques for in-vivo temperature analysis. In: Gerner EW (ed) Hyperthermic oncology, vol 1. ICHO, Tucson, p 267
Schepps JL, Foster KR (1980) The UHF and microwave dielectric properties of normal and tumor tissues: variation in dielectric properties with tissue water content. Phys Med Biol 25: 1149–1159
Schreier K, Budihna M, Lesnicar H et al. (1990) Preliminary studies of interstitial hyperthermia using hot water. Int J Hyperthermia 6: 431–444
Seegenschmidt MH, Sauer R, Fietkau R, Karlsson UL, Brady LW (1990) Primary advanced and local recurrent head and neck tumors, effective management with interstitial thermal radiation therapy. Radiology 176: 267–274
Sekins KM, Emery AF, Lehmann JF, MacDougall JA (1982) Determination of perfusion field during local hyperthermia with the aid of finite element thermal models. J Biomech Eng 104: 272–279
Song CW, Kang MS, Rhee JG, Levitt SL (1980) Effective hyperthermia on vasculature function in normal and neoplastic tissues. Ann NY Acad Sci 335: 35–47
Song CW, Lokshina A, Rhee JG, Patten M, Levitt SH (1984) Implication of blood flow in hyperthermic treatment of tumors. IEEE Trans Biomed Engin 31: 9–16
Stauffer PR, Cetas TC, Fletcher AM, Deyoung DW, Dewhirst MW, Oleson JR, Roemer RB (1984) Observations on the use of ferromagnetic implants for inducing hyperthermia. IEEE Trans Biomed Engin 31: 76–90
Strohbehn JW (1983) Temperature distributions for RF electrode hyperthermia systems: theoretical predictions. Int J Radiat Oncol Biol Phys 9: 1655–1667
Strohbehn JW (1987) Interstitial techniques for hyperthermia. In: Field SB, Franconi C (eds) Physics and technology of hyperthermia. Martinus Nijhoff, Boston, pp 211–239
Strohbehn JW (1991) An engineer looks at hyperthermia. In: Dewey WC, Edington M, Fry RJM, Hall EJ, Whitmore GF (eds) Proceedings of the Ninth International Radiation Research Meeting, vol 2. Academic, San Diego, pp 14–25
Strohbehn JW, Roemer RB (1984) A survey of computer simulation of hyperthermia techniques. IEEE Trans Biomed Eng 31: 136–149
Strohbehn JW, Trembly BS, Douple EB (1982) Blood flow effects on the temperature distributions from an invasive microwave antenna array used in cancer therapy. IEEE Trans Biomed Engin 29: 649–661
Tomikawa W, Numata M, Yamada H, Nakamura H (1988) Measurement of internal temperature distribution using ultrasonic CT – in case of eccentric heat source existence. Acoust Soc Jpn 2: 777–778
Tompkins DT, Partington BP, Steeves RA, Bartholow SD, Paliwal BR (1992) Effect of implant variables on temperatures achieved during ferromagnetic hyperthermia. Int J Hyperthermia 8: 241–251
Trembly BS (1985) The effects of driving frequency and antenna length on power deposition within a microwave antenna array used for hyperthermia. IEEE Trans Biomed Eng 32: 152–157
Trembly BS, Ryan TP (1992) Review of interstitial microwave hyperthermia techniques. In: Gerner EW (ed) Hyperthermia oncology, vol 2. ICHO, Tucson (in press)
Trembly BS, Wilson AH, Sullivan MJ, Stein AD, Wong TZ, Strohbehn JW (1986) Control of the SAR pattern within an interstitial microwave array through a variation of antenna driving phase. IEEE Trans Microwave Theory Tech 34: 568–571
Trembly BS, Wilson AH, Havard JM, Sabatakakis K, Strohbehn JW (1988) Comparison of power deposition by inphase 433 MHz and phase-modulated 915 MHz interstitial antenna array hyperthermia systems. IEEE Trans Microwave Theory Tech 36: 908–916
Trembly BS, Douple EB, Hoopes PJ (1991) The effect of air cooling on the radial temperature distribution of a single microwave hyperthermia antenna in-vivo. Int J Hyperthermia 7: 343–354
Tumeh AM, Iskander MF (1989) Performance comparison of available interstitial antennas for microwave hyperthermia. IEEE Trans Microwave Theory Tech 37: 1126–1133
Weinbaum S, Jiji LM (1985) A new simplified bioheat equation for the effect of blood flow on local average tissue temperature. J Biomech Eng 107: 131–139
Wong TZ, Mechling JA, Jones EL, Strohbehn JW (1988) Transient finite element analysis of thermal models used to estimate SAR and blood flow in the homogeneously and non-homogeneously perfused tumor models. Int J Hyperthermia 4: 571–592
Zhang Y, Samulski TV, Joines WT, Mattiello J, Levin RL, LeBihan D (1992) On the accuracy of non-invasive thermometry using molecular diffusion magnetic imaging. Int J Hyperthermia 8: 263–274
Zhu XL, Gandhi OP (1988) Design of RF needle applicators for optimum SAR distributions in irregularly shaped tumors. IEEE Trans Biomed Eng 35: 382–388

14 Thermal Modeling for Interstitial Hyperthermia: General Comparison Between Radiofrequency, Microwave, and Ferromagnetic Techniques

K.S. Nikita and N.K. Uzunoglu

CONTENTS

14.1 Introduction

In this chapter current modeling methods in respect of interstitial hyperthermia techniques are examined. Computational techniques for electromagnetic fields and thermal distributions are described briefly. Proposals are put forward for more accurate modeling techniques, and different hyperthermia techniques are compared.

In any hyperthermia modeling procedure, two distinct but closely related topics must be addressed: electromagnetic (or ultrasound) field computation and the prediction of temperature distribution inside the tissues to be heated. The results of the electromagnetic (ultrasound) modeling procedure are needed to compute the temperature distribution.

The formulation of the electromagnetic field problem associated with the energy deposition inside the tissues calls for special numerical/analytical techniques depending on the type of hyperthermia technique being used. Low frequency current fields are analyzed using electrostatic techniques based on the Laplace equation. The microwave linear radiators need to be analyzed using dynamic field theory, taking into account the propagation of waves inside a lossy medium generated from a current distribution placed inside a tissue medium and isolated with a thin dielectric tube. Finally, in the case of ferromagnetic seed hyperthermia techniques, low frequency electromagnetic field modeling techniques can be employed to take into account the coupling between implants and loop radiators operating at low frequencies.

Until now, in modeling temperature distribution inside tissues heated by interstitial hyperthermia sources, the bioheat equation has usually been employed under the assumption of a homogeneous tissue medium. The complications arising from highly inhomogeneous and vascularized tissues have not been considered seriously.

14.2 Electromagnetic Field Modeling Techniques

In the following the three different hyperthermia modality modeling techniques are examined.

14.2.1 Radiofrequency Electrodes

Two types of radiofrequency (RF) electrode interstitial hyperthermia systems are employed: (a) low frequency current probes and (b) capacitive electrode systems. In the former case frequencies as low as 0.5 MHz are employed to heat tissues by using the Joule phenomenon. Capacitive electrode systems are based on similar physical principles, but in this case capacitive coupling is employed.

In modeling RF electrode hyperthermia energy deposition, the Laplace equation is applied to determine the quasistatic field distribution inside the tissue medium (Strohbehn 1983; Uzunoglu and Nikita 1988). To this end, assuming an arbitrary tissue medium, the electric field at a given point r inside the tissue medium is computed to be:

$$E(r) = \sum_i I_i F_i(r) , \qquad (1)$$

K.S. Nikita, Ph.D.; N.K. Uzunoglu, Ph.D.; Department of Electrical and Computer Engineering, National Technical University of Athens, 42 Patison St., GR-10682 Athens, Greece where I_i is the ith probe current and $F_i(r)$ is a response function. Then the power delivered per unit volume is computed from $W = \sigma E^2/2$, where σ is the tissue conductivity.

14.2.2 Microwave Radiators

Interstitial antennas are basically uniformly insulated or multisection insulated radiators immersed in the conductive medium of tissue. These antennas are end-fed by coaxial transmission lines and hence may be approximately treated as monopole antennas. The calculation of the radiation characteristics of these antennas involves two major steps. The first is related to modeling and calculating the current and the charge distributions along the antennas, whereas the other is related to the calculation of the radiation fields in the conductive medium. In computing the current and charge distribution along insulated antennas, a theory based on a lossy transmission model developed by KING et al. (1983) can be employed. In this model the interstitial applicator is simulated as a symmetrical dipole. An asymmetrical dipole model has also been proposed by ZHANG et al. (1988) for the interstitial applicator. These two models are currently used to simulate interstitial applicators. The radiation field can be computed by using fundamental relations of electromagnetic radiation theory.

Although some single antenna designs have been modeled theoretically (JAMES et al. 1989; JONES et al. 1989; RYAN et al. 1990; TREMBLY 1985; TREMBLY et al. 1986; ZHANG et al. 1988), only dipole antennas have been modeled in arrays (JAMES et al. 1989; JONES et al. 1989; RYAN et al. 1990; TREMBLY 1985; TREMBLY et al. 1986; ZHANG et al. 1990).Theoretical modeling of helical antennas used in hyperthermia has not yet appeared in the literature.

14.2.3 Ferromagnetic Seeds

The coupling between a loop antenna and a ferromagnetic seed can be computed by using electromagnetic field analysis technique (COTTIS et al. 1990). However, when Curie temperature-regulated ferromagnetic seeds are employed, provided that sufficient power is delivered to ferromagnetic seeds, there is no need to model the coupling of magnetic energy into ferromagnetic medium. Only thermal modeling is needed in this case.

The review of the present status of electromagnetic modeling of interstitial hyperthermia shows that:

1. Mostly homogeneous tissue medium approximation is employed to compute deposited power.
2. The coupling between low frequency current probes or between microwave antennas is assumed to be negligible. This approximation should be verified experimentally.
3. Only recently have three-dimensional techniques been presented. Further work is needed to reduce the computation time and cost.

14.3 Thermal Modeling

Until now in almost all published reports the conventional bioheat transfer equation has been used to formulate the heat transfer problem. This equation was introduced by PENNES (1948) and is given by:

$$\rho c \frac{dT}{dt} = \nabla \cdot (k \nabla T(r)) + P - B \qquad (2)$$

where ρ (kg m^{-3}) and c (J kg^{-1} °C^{-1}) are the density and specific heat of the tissue, respectively, k (W m^{-1} °C^{-1}) is the thermal conductivity coefficient, P (W m^{-3}) is the absorbed power density, and $B = w_b c_b (T - T_b)$ is the heat sink term, with w_b (kg m^{-3} s^{-1}) the volume perfusion rate, c_b the specific heat of the blood, and T_b the temperature of the arterial blood entering the heated volume.

The conventional bioheat transfer equation has been solved by employing analytical (STROHBEHN 1983; UZUNOGLU and NIKITA 1988) or numerical (CHIN and STAUFFER 1991; WONG et al. 1988; MECHLING et al. 1991) techniques in order to estimate temperature distributions provided by interstitial hyperthermia systems. In the case of RF electrodes (STROHBEHN 1983; UZUNOGLU and NIKITA 1988) and microwave antennas (MECHLING et al. 1991), the bioheat equation is solved with an external source term. In the case of Curie temperature-regulated ferromagnetic seeds (CHIN and STAUFFER 1991), a constant temperature boundary condition is employed on the source–tissue interface.

The conventional bioheat transfer theory neglects all heat transfer related to distributed circulation. A comprehensive discussion of the strengths and limitations of Eq. 2 can be found in a work published by LAGENDIJK (1990). Several researchers have developed alternative formulations to the conventional bioheat transfer equation which attempt to take into account the effects of the vascular architecture of tissues. An equivalent heat conductivity model with a reduced blood flow heat removal has been suggested for use with present applications (LAGENDIJK 1990), and is given by the following equation:

$$\rho c \frac{dT}{dt} = \nabla \cdot (k_{\text{eff}} \nabla T(r)) + P - fB , \quad (3)$$

with k_{eff} the effective thermal conductivity describing both the intrinsic thermal conductivity and the heat transfer by the medium-sized vessels. The factor f ranges from 0 to 1, depending on the unknown heat escape in the venous vessels. Large vessel heat transfer must be taken into account separately. Estimation of capillary lengths inside tumors is an important topic that needs to be examined. In estimating the thermal properties of tissues, dynamic thermal response techniques could be extremely useful.

Finite difference techniques are suitable tools in computing temperature distributions inside tissues because of the capability of computing transient phenomena and modeling of discrete vessels. A three-dimensional numerical thermal model has been developed by MOOIBROEK and LAGENDIJK (1991) in which large vessels are taken into account.

It seems that fundamental work is needed to evaluate further the basic theory governing the thermal behavior of tissues and more attention must be paid to the following issues: (a) tissue inhomogeneity and (b) nonlinear properties associated with thermal conductivity and blood flow rate.

14.4 Comparison Between Interstitial Radiofrequency, Microwave, and Ferromagnetic Hyperthermia Techniques

In the following, an inventory of current interstitial hyperthermia techniques will be presented, including the advantages and disadvantages of each technique (EMAMI et al. 1991).

The temperature distributions provided by RF electrode hyperthermia systems are affected by operational factors (amplitude and phase of current excitation), physical characteristics, and spacing of the electrodes, as well as the electrical and thermal properties of tissues (STROHBEHN 1983; UZUNOGLU and NIKITA 1988). A critical issue with these systems is the necessity of positioning the implant electrodes parallel to each other. Failure to do so will lead to excessive heating of regions where the electrodes are close together and poor heating where they are farther apart. Multiple-element (segmented) electrodes have been developed to provide some control over the longitudinal SAR distribution (PRIONAS et al. 1988). Spacing of electrodes is extremely critical in order to avoid cold spots.

Microwave antennas have the capability of depositing power at some distance away. Therefore relatively few sources are needed to heat the target volume.

There are certain constraints in the proper use of dipole antennas, such as the dependence of heating length upon frequency (JAMES et al. 1989; TREMBLY 1985) and the dependence of shape and location of the heated volume upon insertion depth (DENMAN et al. 1988; JAMES et al. 1989; RYAN et al. 1990). Another clinical restraint relates to the poor heating of the region located close to the tip of the antenna (LEE et al. 1986), which means that the antenna must be inserted beyond the deep margin of the tumor. Recent design improvements, including enlarged tips, choke sections, modified dipoles, and helical coil configurations, alleviate the above problems (LEE et al. 1986; LIN and WANG 1987; WU et al. 1987). A further potentially useful feature of microwave antennas is the capability of using phase control in order to provide desired temperature distributions (TREMBLY et al. 1986; ZHANG et al. 1990). Helical antennas are not insertion depth sensitive, provide enhanced tip heating, and can produce controlled heating patterns of various lengths (WU et al. 1987), but they cannot yet be driven in phase to yield predictable peak regions of deposited power.

Use of ferromagnetic seeds provides good temperature control. Because of the mechanism of tissue heating from thermal conduction hot sources, this modality is especially sensitive to thermal conductivity and blood flow variation within the tumor. Seed spacing may be critical, especially in high blood flow situations (CHIN and STAUFFER 1991). The choice of Curie point temperature is also a critical issue.

Temperature distributions computed by solving the steady state conventional bioheat transfer equation are presented in Figs. 14.1–3 for the three types of interstitial hyperthermia systems.

In Fig. 14.1 the effect of blood flow variation is shown for a two-electrode RF hyperthermia system. It is observed that the decrease in blood flow tends to spread the temperature to larger volumes.

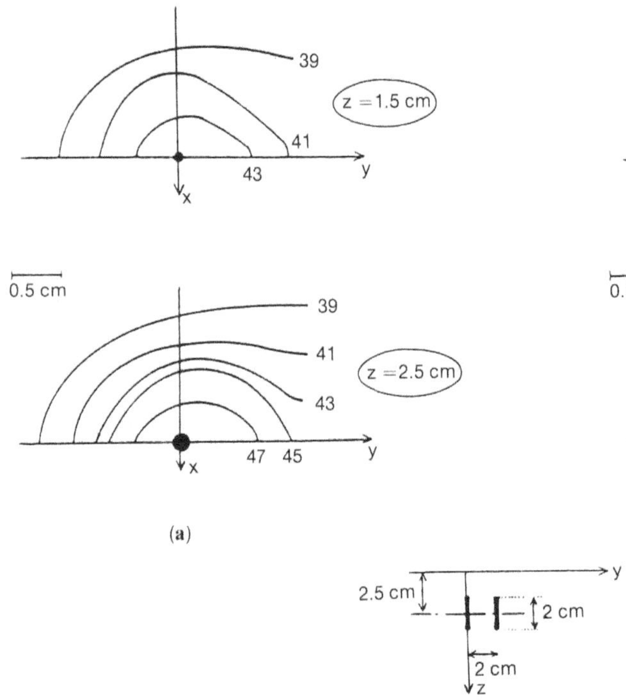

▲
Fig. 14.1 a, b. Temperature distributions at two $z =$ constant planes of a two-electrode radiofrequency hyperthermia system. The blood mass flow rate is **a** $10\,kg/m^3/s$ and **b** $5\,kg/m^3/s$. Because of the symmetry, the isothermal curves are shown only on a single quadrant on two $z =$ constant horizontal planes. (From UZUNOGLU and NIKITA 1988)

Fig. 14.2 a, b. Temperature distributions produced by four 915-MHz antennas in a 2 × 2 cm array. **a** The blood flow is 2.7 ml/100 g/min in the tumor and in the normal tissue. **b** The blood flow is 80 ml/100 g/min in the normal tissue and 20 ml/100 g/min in the tumor. The increment in isotherms is 1°C and the *shaded region* has therapeutic temperatures > 43°C. (From MECHLING et al. 1991)
▼

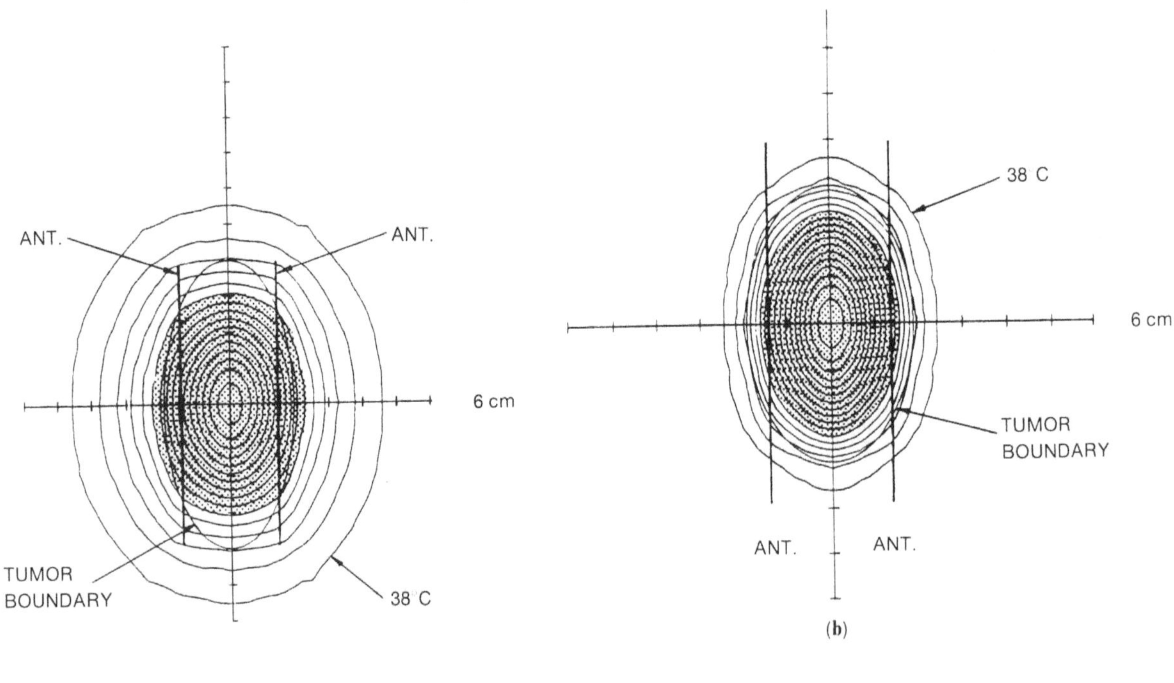

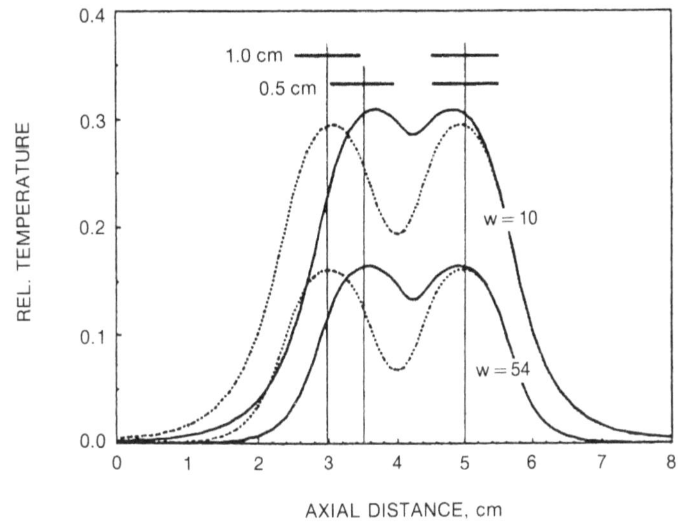

Fig. 14.3. The longitudinal temperature profile at 0.5 cm from the ferromagnetic seed axis of two seeds as a function of axial separation and perfusion rate. Temperature profiles are normalized to the seed surface temperature. The perfusion rates stimulated are 10 and 54 ml/100 g/min. The *solid lines* represent seed separations of 0.5 cm whereas the *dotted lines* represent 1-cm separations. (From CHIN et al. 1991)

The performance of a 2 × 2 cm array consisting of four 915-MHz antennas to heat ellipsoidal tumor models is shown in Fig. 14.2. The effect of different blood flow values between tumor and normal tissue is examined. The maximum temperature in the normal tissue is the limiting factor when the tumor blood flow rate is considered to be equal to that of normal tissue, while the maximum allowable temperature in the tumor is limiting when the ratio of the normal tissue blood flow and the tumor blood flow is large.

In Fig. 14.3 the longitudinal temperature profiles for two ferromagnetic seeds are shown for different blood perfusion rates. The results shown indicate that the uniformity of temperature diminishes with increasing blood perfusion and implant spacing.

14.5 Conclusions

It is definitely too early to designate a single technique of choice for interstitial hyperthermia. The present status of modeling for interstitial hyperthermia seems to have several open areas such as:

1. Development of three-dimensional and efficient computational algorithms to determine the deposited energy from interstitial hyperthermia radiators. The same requirement exists for the computation of temperature distribution by taking into account tissue inhomogeneities, blood flow, and the details of the blood vessels.
2. Development of a general and realistic treatment planning system to optimize the placement of interstitial radiators in hyperthermia treatments.

References

Chin RB, Stauffer PR (1991) Treatment planning for ferromagnetic seed heating. Int J Radiat Oncol Biol Phys 21: 431–439

Cottis PG, Melas AI, Uzunoglu NK (1990) Analysis of energy coupling into spheroidal ferrite implants for hyperthermia applicators. IEEE Trans Microwave Theory Tech 38: 1259–1267

Denman DL, Foster AF, Leuis GC et al. (1988) The distribution of power and heat produced by interstitial microwave antenna arrays: II. The role of antenna spacing and insertion depth. Int J Radiat Oncol Biol Phys 14: 537–545

Emami B, Stauffer P, Dewhirst MW et al. (1991) RTOG quality assurance guidelines for interstitial hyperthermia. Int J Radiat Oncol Biol Phys 20: 1117–1124

Iskander MF, Tumeh AM, Furse MS (1990) Evaluation and optimization of the electromagnetic performance of interstitial antennas for hyperthermia. Int J Radiat Oncol Biol Phys 18: 895–902

James B, Strohbehn JW, Mechling JA, Trembly BS (1989) The effect of insertion depth on the theoretical SAR patterns of 915 MHz dipole antenna arrays for hyperthermia. Int J Hyperthermia 5: 733–747

Jones KM, Mechling JA, Trembly BS, Strohbehn JW (1988) SAR distributions for 915 MHz interstitial microwave antennas used in hyperthermia for cancer therapy. IEEE Trans Biomed Eng 35: 851–857

Jones KM, Mechling JA, Strohbehn JW, Trembly BS (1989) Theoretical and experimental SAR distribution for interstitial dipole antenna arrays for hyperthermia. IEEE Trans Microwave Theory Tech 37: 1200–1209

King RWP, Trembly BS, Strohbehn JW (1983) The electromagnetic field of an insulated antenna in a conducting or dielectric medium. IEEE Trans Microwave Theory Tech 31: 574–583

Lagendijk JJW (1990) Thermal models: principles and implementation. In: Field SB, Hand JW (eds) An introduction to the practical aspects of clinical hyperthermia. Taylor and Francis, London, pp 478–512

Lee DJ, O'Neill MJ, Lam K, Rostock R, Lam W (1986) A new design of microwave interstitial applicator for

hyperthermia with improved treatment volume. Int J Radiat Oncol Biol Phys 12: 2003–2008
Lin JC, Wang YJ (1987) Interstitial microwave antennas for thermal therapy. Int J Hyperthermia 3: 37–47
Mechling JA, Strohbehn JW, France LJ (1991) A theoretical evaluation of the performance of the Dartmouth IMAAH system to heat cylindrical and ellipsoidal tumour models. Int J Hyperthermia 7: 465–483
Mooibroek J, Lagendijk JJW (1991) A fast and simple algorithm for the calculation of convective heat transfer by large vessels in three dimensional inhomogeneous tissues. IEEE Trans Biomed Eng 38: 490–501
Pennes HH (1948) Analysis of tissue and arterial blood temperature in resting forearm. Appl Physiol: 93–122
Prionas SD, Fessenden P, Kapp DS, Goffinet DR, Hahn GM (1988) Interstitial electrodes allowing longitudinal control of SAR distributions. In: Sugahara T, Saito M (eds) Proceeding of the 5th international symposium on hyperthermic oncology. Taylor and Francis, London, p 707
Ryan TP, Mechling JA, Strohbehn JW (1990) Absorbed power deposition for various insertion depths for 915 MHz interstitial dipole antenna arrays: experiment versus theory. Int J Radiat Oncol Biol Phys 19: 377–387
Strohbehn JW (1983) Temperature distributions from interstitial RF electrode hyperthermia systems: Theoretical predictions. Int J Radiat Oncol Biol Phys 9: 1655–1667
Trembly BS (1985) The effects of driving frequency and antenna length on power deposition within a microwave antenna array used for hyperthermia. IEEE Trans Biomed Eng 32: 152–157
Trembly BS, Wilson AH, Sullivan MJ, Stein AD, Wong TZ, Strohbehn JW (1986) Control of the SAR pattern within an interstitial microwave array through variation of antenna driving phase. IEEE Trans Microwave Theory Tech 34: 568–571
Uzunoglu NK, Nikita KS (1988) Estimation of temperature distribution inside tissues heated by interstitial RF electrode hyperthermia systems. IEEE Trans Biomed Eng 35: 250–256
Wong TZ, Mechling JA, Jones EL, Strohbehn JW (1988) Transient finite element analysis of thermal methods used to estimate SAR and blood flow in homogeneously and nonhomogeneously perfused tumour models. Int J Hyperthermia 4: 571–592
Wu A, Watson M, Sternick ES, Bielawa RJ, Carr KC (1987) Performance characteristics of a helical microwave interstitial antenna for local hyperthermia. Med Phys 14: 235–237
Zhang Y, Dubal NV, Takamoto-Hampleton R, Joines WT (1988) The determination of the electromagnetic field and SAR pattern of an interstitial applicator in a dissipative dielectric medium. IEEE Trans Microwave Theory Tech 36: 1438–1444
Zhang Y, Joines WT, Oleson JR (1990) The calculated and measured temperature distribution of a phased interstitial antenna array. IEEE Trans Microwave Theory Tech 38: 69–77

15 Thermal Modeling for Intracavitary Heating

M. Chive, J.C. Camart, and F. Morganti

CONTENTS

15.1 Introduction

The past decade has witnessed increased interest in the application of electromagnetic techniques for intracavitary hyperthermia treatment of cancer of the prostate (Mendecki et al. 1980; Fabre and Chive 1988; Roos 1988), esophagus (Zhang et al. 1990; Liu et al. 1991), and vagina (Li et al. 1991; Valdagni et al. 1988; Zhong et al. 1990), as well as of other benign prostatic diseases (Astrahan et al. 1989, 1991; Sapozink et al. 1990). The applicators designed for these treatments have generally been based on the use of coaxial antennas in association with a water cooling system in order to avoid overheating and burns at the applicator–tissue interface. The computed and measured SAR distributions (in phantom equivalent to muscle tissue) permit determination of the tissue volume which will be heated at the therapeutic temperature level (42°–43°C). The computed SAR patterns can be determined from the theory of King et al. (1975) in conjunction with the numerical procedure of Casey and Bansal (1986) which calculates the electric field produced by a dipole antenna coupled with a multilayered medium (cooling water, catheter, and tissue). Then, using the bioheat transfer equation, it is possible to model the thermal gradient which occurs in the steady state (plateau phase) during microwave hyperthermia induced by these applicators. In this paper we present the electromagnetic and thermal models of two specific microwave intracavitary applicators used for transurethral and rectal hyperthermia of the prostate. However, these models can be adapted and generalized for all types of microwave intracavitary coaxial applicator.

M. Chive, Ph.D., Professor; J.C. Camart, Ph.D.; F. Morganti, Ph.D.; IEMN, UMR CNRS 9929 Département Hyperfréquences et Semiconducteurs, Bât. P4, Université des Sciences et Technologies de Lille, F-59655 Villeneuve d'Ascq Cédex, France

15.2 The Microwave Intracavitary Applicators and Their Electromagnetic Model

15.2.1 The Urethral Applicator

The urethral applicator comprises a microwave dipole antenna associated with a Foley-type urological catheter as shown in Fig. 15.1. The microwave antenna is made of a flexible coaxial cable ($\Phi \approx 2.2$ mm) at the end of which the outer conductor has been removed at a length h to yield a radiative antenna of active length $l = 2h$. The plane $z = 0$ where the external conductor ends is called the junction plane or node plane. This flexible antenna is inserted in a balloon-type urological catheter of which the external diameter is about 6 mm (18 French); this catheter is filled with cooling liquid (water) which enters by a small catheter and flows in the annular region between the antenna and the catheter, as shown in Fig. 15.1. A thermocouple glued to the surface of the catheter and located in the junction plane of the antenna ($z = 0$) allows control of the temperature at the applicator–tissue (urethra) interface during hyperthermia.

The radiative part h of the antenna has been optimized to operate at the heating frequency (915 MHz) in order to obtain a good matching for the applicator (antenna + catheter filled with the cooling water) when it is coupled with an acrylamide phantom. This applicator can also be used as

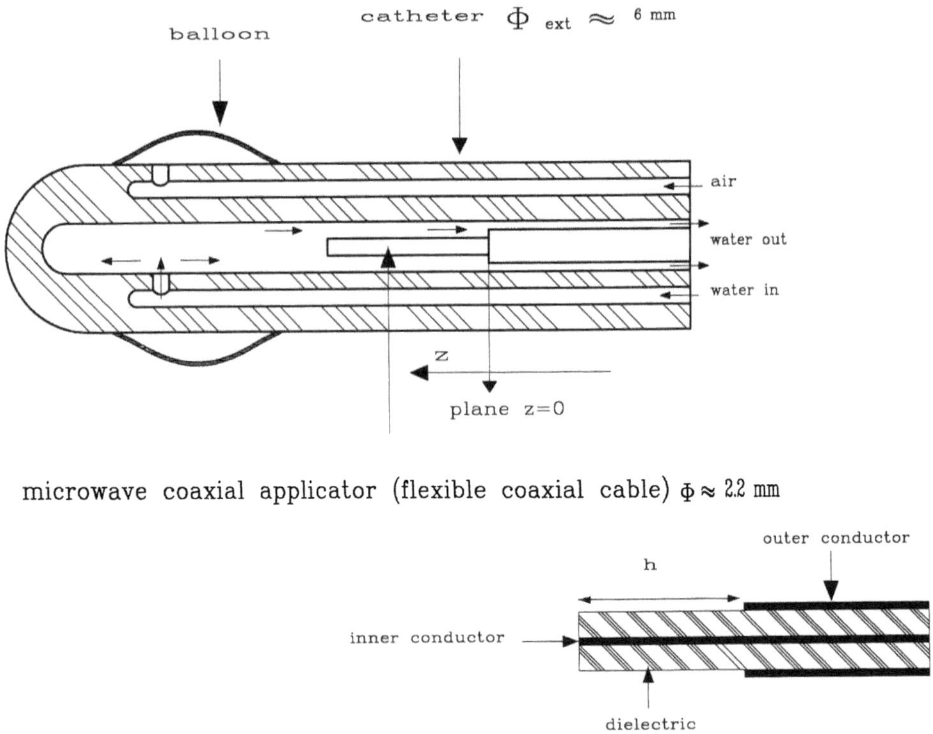

Fig. 15.1. Schematic diagram of the urethral applicator comprising a microwave coaxial antenna and a catheter with an air balloon and flowing water for cooling

a receiving antenna for radiometry at 3 GHz to measure temperature (FABRE and CHIVE 1988).

As intimated above, to determine the absorbed power (and then the SAR patterns) in the biological tissue, the theory of KING et al. (1975) can be used in conjunction with the numerical procedure of CASEY and BANSAL (1986). This formalism calculates the electromagnetic field produced by a dipole antenna surrounded by a multilayered medium comprising the cooling water flowing in the catheter, the catheter, and the tissues. This electromagnetic model is well known and has been used by various authors (e.g., GENTILI et al. 1991) to determine the electric field value E_m in each point of the medium and then to obtain the absorbed power in the tissue $P_m = \frac{1}{2}\sigma_m |E_m|^2$ (with σ_m the conductivity of the tissue – here the prostatic tissue).

Figure 15.2 shows the SAR distribution (longitudinal and transverse) obtained with the present numerical method in prostatic tissue for the applicator under consideration. Dielectric characteristics of the prostatic tissue have been measured from an excised prostatic gland at room temperature over a large frequency range (0.1–4 GHz) (CHAPOTON and LEGRAND, unpublished work, 1991). For this model the dielectric constants of the different media at the heating frequency of 915 MHz are summarized in Table 15.1.

15.2.2 The Rectal Applicator

The rectal applicator consists of one or two coaxial dipole antennas and a metallic reflector which focuses the radiated microwave energy into the prostate. The antennas, made of a semirigid coaxial cable (UT 85), are of the same type as the urethral antenna. The antennas and the metallic reflector are inserted in a Teflon tube which includes a cooling system (i.e., flowing water; cf. Fig. 15.3).

To calculate the electric field created in the tissue by the single antenna or by the two antennas fed in phase, in association with the metallic reflector,

Table 1. Dielectric parameters at 915 MHz

	ε_r'	$\varepsilon_r'' = \dfrac{\sigma}{\omega\varepsilon_0}$
Muscle	49	21.2
Prostate	41	8.8

Thermal parameters of the muscle tissue:
$c_t \cdot \rho_t = 4.18\ 10^6\ \mathrm{J\,m^{-3}\,°C^{-1}}$
$k_t = 0.45\ \mathrm{W\,m^{-1}\,°C^{-1}}$
c_t = specific heat; ρ_t = tissue density; k_t = thermal conductivity

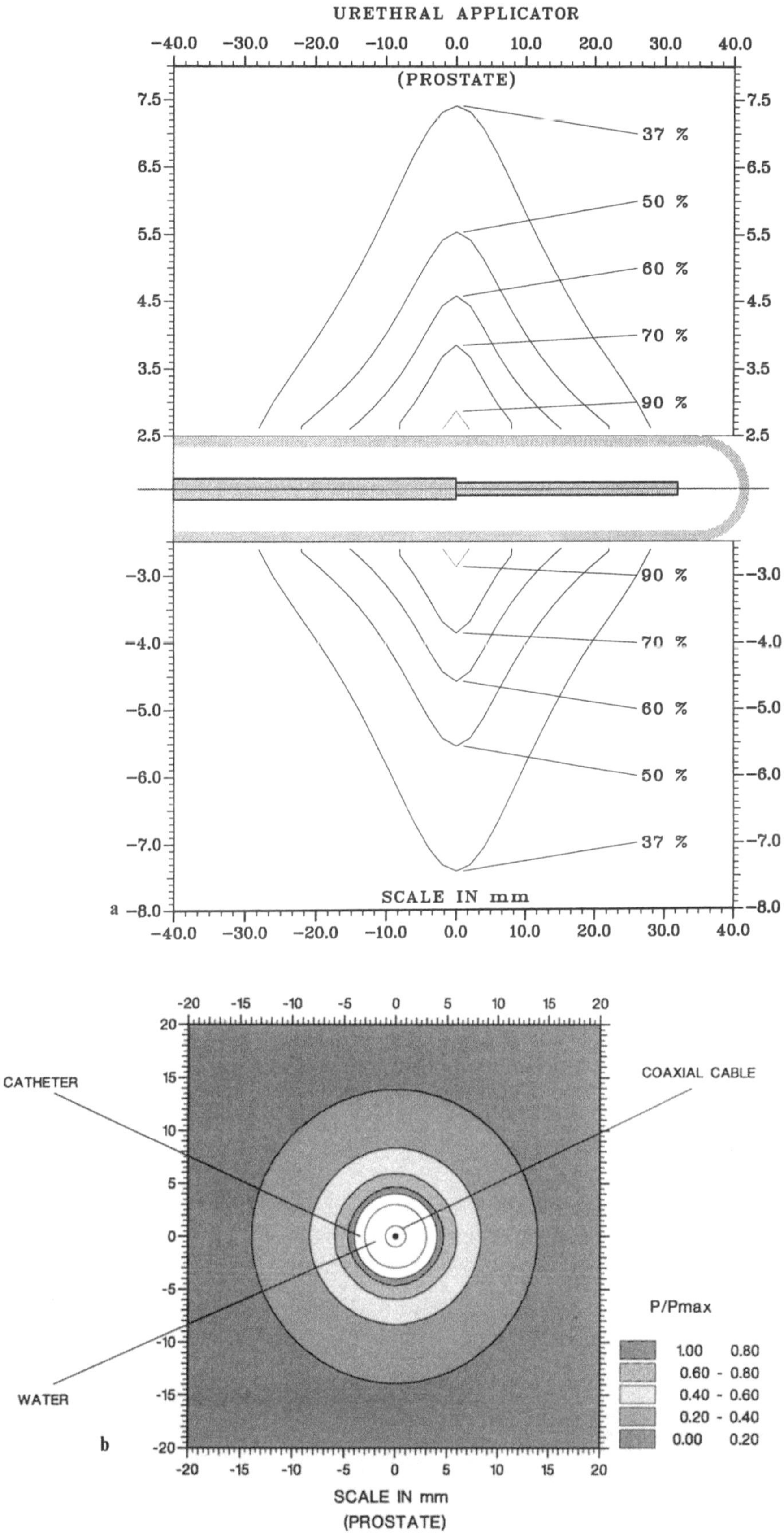

Fig. 15.2 a, b. Longitudinal and transverse SAR patterns for the prostatic tissue at 915 MHz.
a Londitudinal SAR in the prostatic tissue.
b Transverse SAR (in the plane $z = 0$)

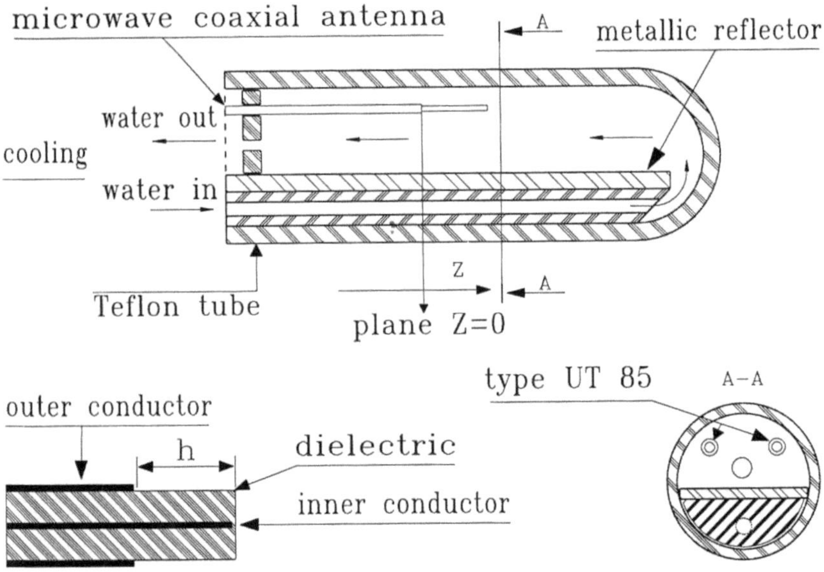

Fig. 15.3. Schematic diagram of the rectal applicator (two antennas) with metallic reflector and flowing water for cooling

a numerical procedure based on the finite differences method has been used to solve the Maxwell equation (RINE et al. 1990). The total electric field E_{tot} in the tissue is decomposed into an incident field E_{in} and a scattered field E_{scat}. The incident field exists in the free space (constituted of the cooling water) in the absence of a metallic reflector, the Teflon tube, and the prostatic tissue (scattering bodies). The scattered field results from the reirradiation of the EM energy due to the current induced on the metallic reflector when it is exposed to the incident field. The expression of the total electric field E_{tot} can be written as:

$$E_{tot} = E_{in} + E_{scat} \,. \tag{1}$$

This relation combined with the Maxwell curl equations allows deduction of the inhomogeneous wave vector equation:

$$\nabla\nabla E_{scat} - \omega^2 \mu \varepsilon_i^* E_{scat} = \omega^2 \mu (\varepsilon_i^* - \varepsilon_j^*) E_{in} \,, \tag{2}$$

where ω is the angular frequency, μ is the magnetic permeability, and ε_i^* and ε_j^* are the complex permittivities of two consecutively considered media: water $\varepsilon_i^* = \varepsilon_1^*$ – Teflon $\varepsilon_j^* = \varepsilon_2^*$; Teflon $\varepsilon_i^* = \varepsilon_2^*$ – prostatic tissue $\varepsilon_j^* = \varepsilon_3^*$.

Assuming, as in KING et al.'s theory, that in the plane $z = 0$ the components E_x and E_y can be neglected as compared with the component E_z for each field E_{in} and E_{scat}, Eq. 2 can be simplified and written as:

$$\nabla\nabla E_{zscat} + k^2 \varepsilon_{ri}^* E_{zscat} = k^2 (\varepsilon_{ri}^* - \varepsilon_{rj}^*) E_{zin} \,, \tag{3}$$

where k is the wave number $\omega^2 \mu_0 \varepsilon_0$ and $\varepsilon_{ri}^* = \dfrac{\varepsilon_i^*}{\varepsilon_0}$, $\varepsilon_{rj}^* = \dfrac{\varepsilon_j^*}{\varepsilon_0}$.

The solution of Eq. 3 allows determination of the total field E_{tot} at each point of the tissue and subsequent calculation of the corresponding absorbed power:

$$P_m = \frac{1}{2} \sigma_m |E_{ztot}|^2 .$$

The SAR distribution in the plane $z = 0$ can then be determined and referred to the maximum computed value obtained on the Teflon tube.

Figure 15.4 shows the SAR patterns in muscle tissue for the single- and double-antenna rectal applicators. It is seen that the latter gives a larger heated volume.

15.3 The Thermal Model

When the absorbed microwave power in the tissue is calculated, the temperature distribution can be obtained by the numerical solution of the bioheat transfer equation (PENNES 1948; DUBOIS et al. 1991):

$$\rho_t c_t \frac{dT}{dt} = k_t \nabla^2 T + Q_a + v_s (T_a - T) + Q_m \,,$$

where ρ_t is the tissue density ($\mathrm{kg\,m^{-3}}$), c_t is the

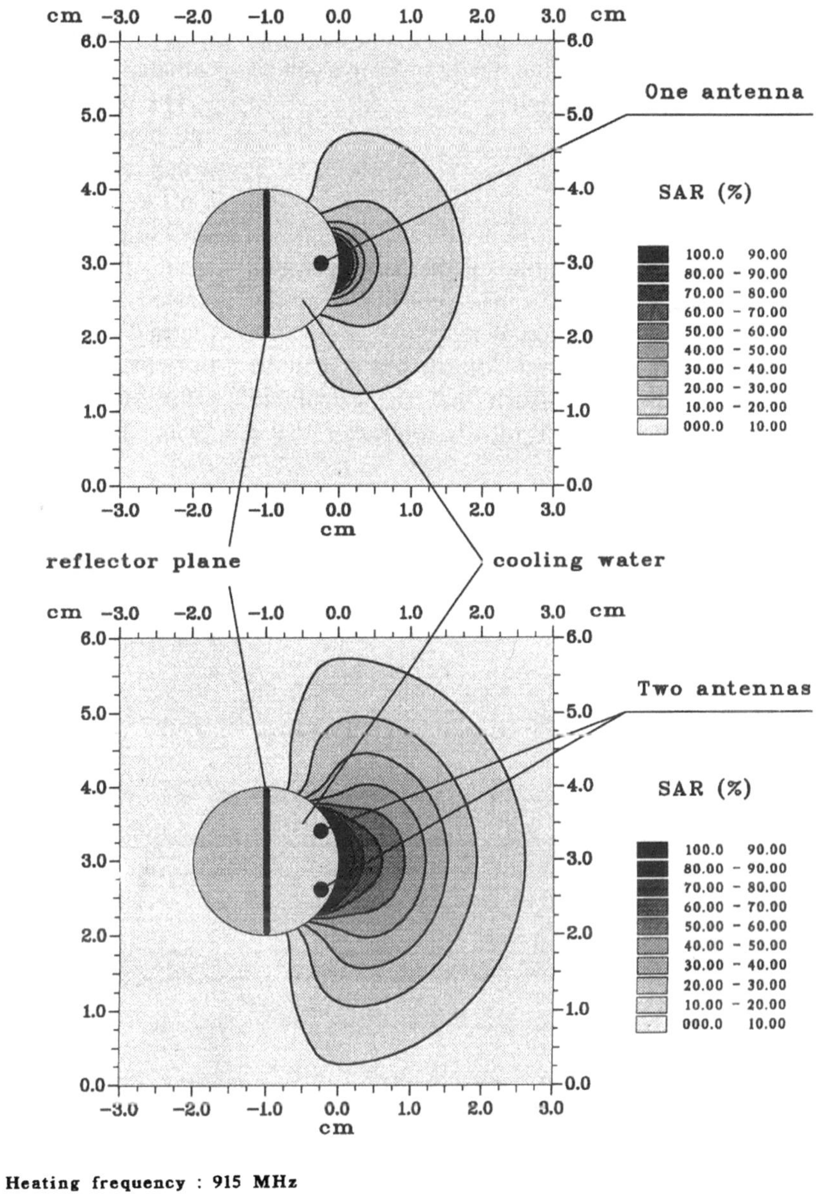

Fig. 15.4. SAR patterns in muscle tissue for the single- and double-antenna rectal applicators, computed in the plane $z = 0$ at 915 MHz

specific heat of the tissue ($\mathrm{J\,kg^{-1}\,°C^{-1}}$), Q_a is the heat generated by the absorbed microwave power P_m [$Q_a = P_m$ ($\mathrm{W\,m^{-3}}$)], v_s is the heat exchange parameter between the blood and the tissue ($\mathrm{W\,m^{-3}\,°C^{-1}}$), T_a is the temperature of blood entering the tissue, T is the temperature of the tissue, and Q_m is the heat due to the metabolism ($\mathrm{W\,m^{-3}}$). The aforementioned term v_s is expressed by the relation $v_s = [c_b - W_b]$ where c_b is the specific heat of blood ($\mathrm{J\,kg^{-1}\,°C^{-1}}$) and W_b is the rate of blood perfusion ($\mathrm{kg\,m^{-3}\,s^{-1}}$). The term Q_m can be neglected as it is insignificant compared to Q_a (DUBOIS et al. 1991).

In the steady state (during the plateau phase of the hyperthermia session) the temperature distribution $T(x, y, z)$ is independent of the time, so the bioheat equation is then written as:

$$k_t \nabla^2 T + Q_a + v_s(T_a - T) = 0 .$$

This equation is solved by a numerical procedure based on the finite differences method, taking into account the following boundary conditions:

- The temperature in depth is equal to the arterial blood temperature $T_a = 37°\mathrm{C}$.

– Due to the cooling water in the catheter a thermal equilibrium is obtained at the applicator–tissue interface in the steady state; this can be expressed by the relation

$$k_t \frac{\partial T}{\partial r} = H[T(r) - T_e],$$

where T_e is the temperature of the cooling water and H is the total heat transfer coefficient at the applicator–tissue interface (W m^{-1} °C^{-1}).

The term H is not well known but it can be adjusted in the model such that the calculated superficial temperature T_s (at the applicator–tissue interface) is equal to the temperature obtained with the thermocouple glued to the surface of the catheter in the plane $z = 0$.

The term v_s is also undetermined in the model and depends on the vascularization of the tissue, which changes during hyperthermia: it is fixed a priori to begin the computation. If radiometry is used to control and monitor the temperature in the tissue during hyperthermia, it has been demonstrated that the term v_s can be adjusted in the thermal model in order to obtain a good correlation between the measured radiometric temperature and the computed one (GIAUX and CHIVE 1986; CHIVE 1990; DUBOIS et al. 1991).

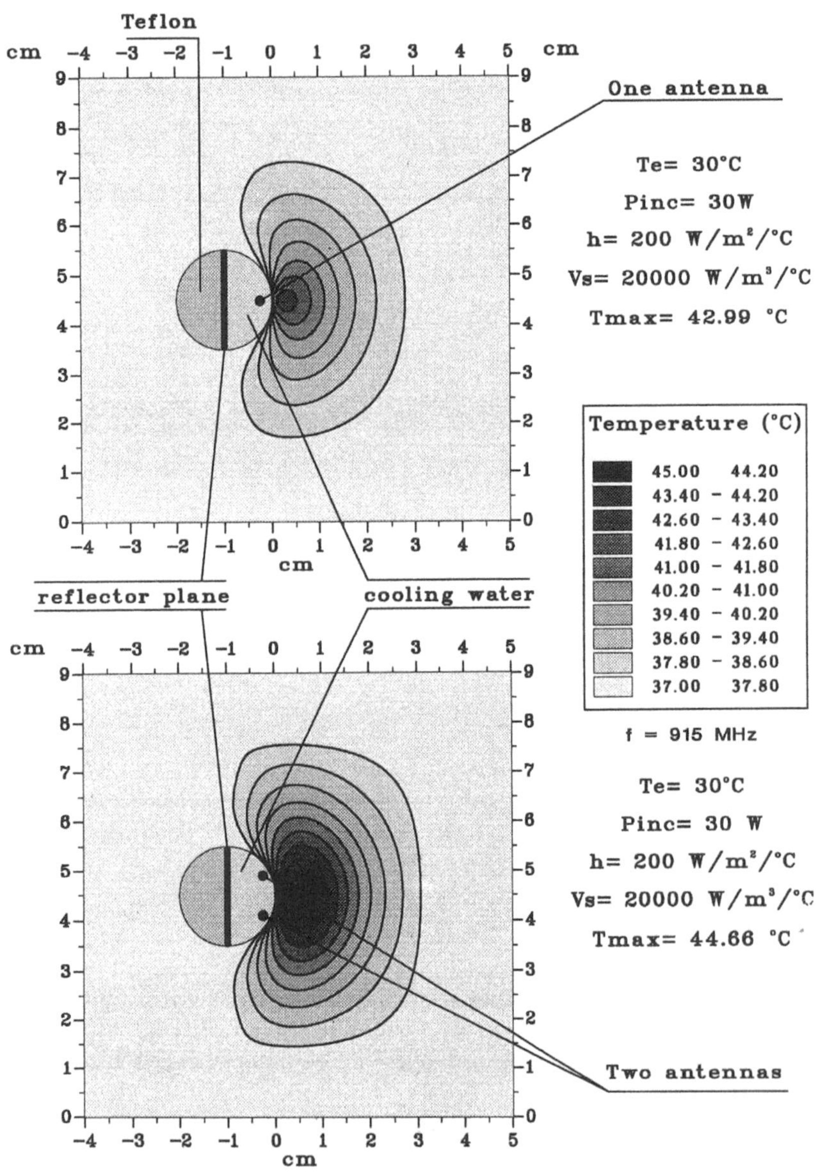

Fig. 15.5. Steady-state isothermal profiles in the plane $z = 0$ for the two rectal applicators (computation has been done for muscle tissue heated at 915 MHz with an incident power of 30 W

15.4 Examples and Discussion

In order to illustrate the model achieved, Fig. 15.5 shows the steady-state isothermal profiles obtained during a hyperthermia session with the two different rectal probes. The computation of the isotherms has been performed in the junction plane $z = 0$ of the coaxial antennas, with the cooling water thermostated at 30°C. The thermal parameter H has been chosen to obtain a temperature at the probe–prostatic tissue interface not higher than 42°C.

Each applicator was fed with an incident microwave power of 30 W, with v_s fixed at a value of 20 000 W m^{-3} °C^{-1}. This corresponds to a classical value in this type of model and yields a heated zone with a temperature of 43°C to 45°C.

Comparison of the results obtained with the single coaxial probe applicator and double-antenna applicator (15 W per antenna; antennas fed in phase) shows the advantage of the latter applicator. The heated zone at the therapeutic temperature level (41°–42°C) is larger and deeper with the double-antenna probe than with the single-antenna applicator under the same conditions. If the isothermal pattern is compared with the SAR pattern shown in Fig. 15.4, it can be noted that the isopower zone of 30%–40% in each case corresponds approximately to the therapeutically heated zone.

It may be concluded that the discussed type of intracavitary focusing applicator, made with coaxial antennas operating at 915 MHz, allows heating of a small volume of tissue (2–2.5 cm thick and 3–4 cm in length).

The thermal simulation that can be achieved for the urethral applicator shows that the radial thickness of the heated zone at the therapeutic temperature level (42°C) is about 1–1.5 cm, which also corresponds to the SAR isopower zone of 30% (Fig. 15.2).

15.5 Conclusion

The main problems of thermal modeling can be summarized as follows:

1. It is necessary to know the dielectric and thermal characteristics of the tissue to be heated.
2. The power deposition due to each type of applicator must be calculated exactly in three dimensions in order to ascertain the tissue volume which will probably be heated at the therapeutic level. To increase this volume, a new type of applicator such as a strip-slot applicator needs to be designed, since the performance of coaxial antenna applicators is limited.
3. Thermal modeling based on the bioheat equation can give interesting information but two parameters are unknown: the heat exchange term H at the applicator–tissue interface and the blood flow term v_s. These terms can be adjusted in the thermal model using, as imposed data, the temperature measurements (by thermocouples and radiometry for example) achieved during hyperthermia.

If the above conditions are satisfied, use of the thermal model described in this chapter allows identification of the most probable thermal pattern in the tissue under consideration during hyperthermia (in the steady state).

References

Astrahan M, Sapozink MD, Cohen D, Luxtron G, Kampp TD, Boyd S, Petrovitch Z (1989) Microwave applicator for transurethral hyperthermia of benign prostatic hyperplasia. Int J Hyperthermia 5: 286–296

Astrahan M, Imanaka K, Jozsef G, Ameye F, Baerts L, Sapozink MD, Boyd S, Petrovitch Z (1991) Heating characteristics of a helical microwave applicator for transurethral hyperthermia of benign prostatic hyperplasia. Int J Hyperthermia 7: 141–155

Casey JP, Bansal R (1986) The near field of an insulated dipole in a dissipative medium. IEEE Trans Microwave Theory Tech 34: 459–463

Chive M (1990) Use of microwave radiometry for hyperthermia monitoring and as a basis for thermal dosimetry. In: Gautherie M (ed) Clinical technology method of hyperthermia. Springer, Berlin Heidelberg New York, pp 113–128

Dubois L, Fabre JJ, Ledee R, Chive M, Moschetto Y (1991) Bidimensional reconstruction of temperature patterns from noninvasive microwave multifrequency radiometric measurements during microwave hyperthermia session: applications to thermal dosimetry. Innov Tech Biol Med 12: 126–146

Fabre JJ, Chive M (1988) Intracavitary multiapplicator for microwave hyperthermia and radiometry. Innov Tech Biol Med 9 (special no. 2): 116–120

Giaux G, Chive M (1986) Microwave oncologic hyperthermia combined with radiotherapy and controlled by microwave radiometry. Recent Results Cancer Res 101: 75–87

Gentili GB, Gori F, Leoncini M (1991) Electromagnetic and thermal models of a water coded dipole radiating in a biological tissue. IEEE Trans Biomed Eng 38: 98–103

King RWP, Trembly RS, Strohbehn JW (1975) The electromagnetic field of an insulated antenna in a conducting or dielectric medium. IEEE Trans Antennas Propagation 2

Li DJ, Chou CK, Luk KM, Wang JH, Xie CF, Macdougall JAN, Huang GZ (1991) Design of intracavitary microwave applicators for the treatment of uterine cervix carcinoma. Int J Hyperthermia 7: 693–701

Liu RL, Zhang EY, Gross EJ, Cetas T (1991) Heating pattern of helical microwave intracavitary oesophageal applicator. Int J Hyperthermia 7: 577–586

Mendecki J, Friedenthal E, Botstein C, Paglione R, Sterzer F (1980) Microwave applicators for localized hyperthermia of cancer of the prostate. Int J Radiat Oncol Biol Phys 6: 1583–1588

Pennes HH (1948) Analysis of tissue and arterial blood temperatures in the resting human forearm. J Appl Physiol 1: 93–122

Rine GP, Samulski TV, Grant W, Wallen CA (1990) Comparison of two dimensional numerical approximation and measurement of S.A.R. in a muscle equivalent phantom exposed to a 915 MHz slab-loaded waveguide. Int J Hyperthermia 6: 213–225

Roos DJF (1988) Interstitial and intracavitary microwave applicators for hyperthermia treatment of cancer. Technical report no. 183. Chalmers University of Technology, Göteborg (Sweden)

Sapozink MD, Boyd S, Astrahan M, Jozef G, Petrovich Z (1990) Transurethral hyperthermia for benign prostatic hyperplasia: preliminary clinical results. J Urol 143: 944–950

Valdagni R, Amichetti M, Cristoforetti L (1988) Intracavitary hyperthermia: construction and heat pattern of individualized vaginal prototype applicators. Int J Hyperthermia 4: 457–466

Zhang Liru, Wei Jianguo, Cheng Zhong FA, Wang Guizhu, Liu Lingy, Li Weilian (1990) 2450 MHz oesophagus applicator with multi temperature sensors and its temperature control equipment. Int J Hyperthermia 6: 745–753

Zhong QR, Chou CH, Macdougall JA, Chan KW, Luk KH (1990) Intracavitary hyperthermia applicators for heating nasopharyngeal and cervical cancer. Int J Hyperthermia 6: 997–1004

16 Thermal Modeling of Vascular Patterns and Their Impact on Interstitial Heating Technology and Temperature Monitoring

J. MOOIBROEK, J. CREZEE, and J.J.W. LAGENDIJK

CONTENTS

16.1 Introduction

In interstitial hyperthermia we rely for temperature measurements on thermocouples placed either inside the catheter lumen and/or a limited distance from the catheters. It would be very helpful if this limited spatial temperature information could be extended through use of reliable thermal models to obtain and control the three-dimensional (3-D) temporal temperature distribution. Needless to say, these models could also be used for pretreatment planning purposes. A prerequisite of a thermal model for biological tissues is that it describes conductive and convective heat transport adequately, with emphasis on the latter as it has long been established that this is the predominant heat transfer mode. In nearly all papers on interstitial hyperthermia, the contribution of convective heat transport has been taken into account according to the proposal of PENNES (1948), i.e., the conventional bioheat transfer equation. However, consensus has been achieved (VALDAGNI et al. 1990) on the necessity of including at least a large vessel description as such vessels are important structures causing underdosage. Based on an extensive study on the thermal equilibration length of individual vessels, we have adopted a tripartition of the vascular system with respect to heat transfer: (a) large vessels, (b) intermediately sized vessels and (c) microcirculation. Each category is characterized by a specific description: category (a) must be treated on an individual basis (MOOIBROEK and LAGENDIJK 1991) and category (c) by a continuum parameter termed k_{eff} (CHEN and HOLMES 1980; LAGENDIJK 1984; WEINBAUM and JIJI 1985). The intermediately sized vessels still pose some difficulties but we are investigating a mathematical method which connects the two aforementioned formulations in terms of tensorial heat transfer coefficients. The present contribution will focus on a physical description of individual vessels, which, depending on the available vascular information, can easily be extended to complex vascular patterns. In the first part we will concentrate on the effect of the number and density of catheters and the catheter diameter, the influence of k_{eff} on the temperature distribution, and the type of boundary conditions selected when no discrete vessels are present. Subsequently countercurrent vessel pairs with different diameter and flow running at different orientations with respect to the catheters will be considered. An example of how to manipulate the temperature distribution in the immediate vicinity of a countercurrent vessel pair will be presented, and finally the results of a hypothetical vessel structure will be given. For reasons of simplicity, water tube heating was selected as the heat source mode.

J. MOOIBROEK, Ph.D.; J. CREZEE, Ph.D.; J.J.W. LAGENDIJK, Ph.D.; Department of Radiotherapy, University Hospital Utrecht, Heidelberglaan 100, NL-3584 CX Utrecht, The Netherlands

16.2 Materials and Methods

16.2.1 Basics of Discrete Vessel Model

Due to the limited space available, the basics of our thermal model will be outlined on a pictorial basis. For more details the reader is referred to MOOIBROEK and LAGENDIJK (1991). Figure 16.1a presents the physical problem together with its mathematical formulation. The 3-D object space is decomposed into an inhomogeneous tissue space in which heat transfer is conductive and a vessel space

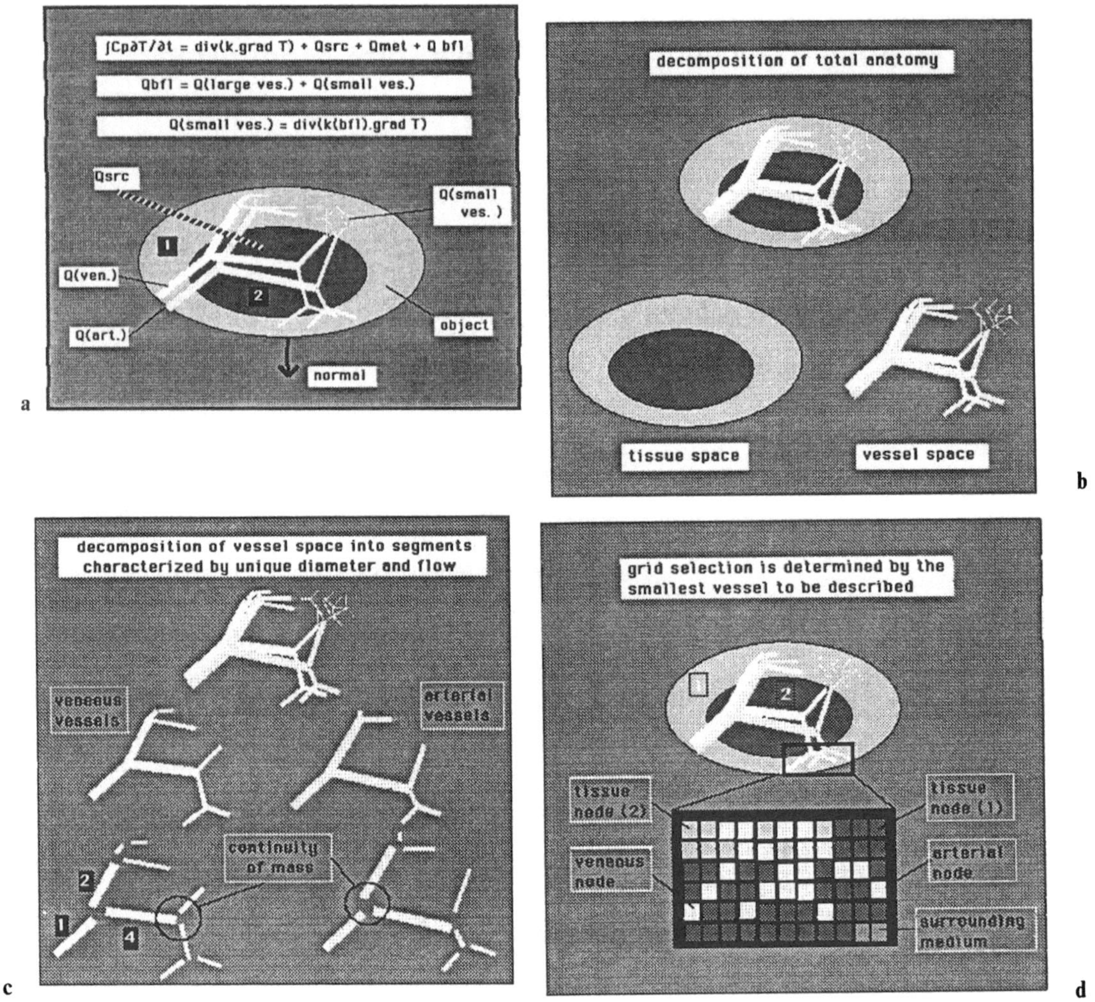

Fig. 16.1 a–d. Mathematical formulation of the physical problem (**a**) and subsequent decomposition into tissue and vessel space (**b, c**), followed by definition of applied grid (**d**)

for the description of convective heat transport (Fig. 16.1b). The latter is in turn separated into an arterial and a venous branching structure. Our model is based on a segmental description of vessel portions each of which has a unique diameter and flow; therefore to each a unique number is assigned corresponding to a vessel table entry for temporal updating of thermal and flow parameters (Fig. 16.1c).

Finally, the total space is covered by a cubical grid (Fig. 16.1d) which enables the conversion of the partial difference equation into one using finite differences. We selected a multitime level explicit finite difference method which generates the 3-D transient temperature distribution very rapidly.

16.2.2 Calculations

The model situation studied was a homogeneous muscle-like tissue covered by $64 \times 64 \times 40$ cubical nodes of 1 mm each side. Volumetric catheter density was varied by raising the numbers from 2×2 to 5×5 in a centrally located subvolume of $30 \times 30 \times 40\ \mathrm{mm}^3$. This coincides with catheter spacings of 30 to 8 mm. Catheter diameter was 1 or 2 mm, while water flow was kept constantat 10 cm/s. To mimic the influence of the microcirculation, the effective thermal conductivity k_{eff} was taken to be two and five times the intrinsic value of resting muscle. The thermal parameters which were kept constant in each calculation were: the density $\rho = 1030\ \mathrm{kg\,m^{-3}}$, the specific heat capacity $C_p = 3960\ \mathrm{J\,kg^{-1}\,°C^{-1}}$, and $k_{\mathrm{intr}} = 0.6\ \mathrm{W\,°C^{-1}\,m^{-1}}$. In the first part of this study isothermic ($T = 37°\mathrm{C}$) boundary conditions were imposed on the four planes parallel with the catheters while the other two were assumed to be adiabatic. These conditions were changed afterwards using heat transfer coefficients which virtually extend the object dimensions.

16.3 Results

In the following section the theoretical results will be presented in a qualitative way to grant the reader better insight into the impact of different parameters on the stationary temperature distribution. Figure 16.2a shows the model configuration on the basis of which the results displayed in panels b, c, and d of Fig. 16.2 were derived. One panel consists of 12 different calculations, each of which represents the two-dimensional temperature distribution in the midplane ($z = 20$) of the model, which is normal to the tube orientation. Results in the planes parallel to the selected one are identical due to: (a) model symmetry, (b) the equivalence of entrance and exit temperatures enforced by high tube water flow (10 cm/s), and (c) the adiabatic boundary conditions imposed on planes $z = 1$ and $z = 40$. For all three panels in Fig. 16.2 the layout is the same, i.e., starting at the upper left corner and proceeding along a row indicates increasing volumetric heat source density, while the columns correspond to different k_{eff} values ranging from one to five times the value of k_{intr} of resting muscle. The effect of using different tube diameters is illustrated by comparing the temperature distributions in panel 2b ($d_{tube} = 1$ mm) and panel 2c ($d_{tube} = 2$ mm). If the temperature distribution in the

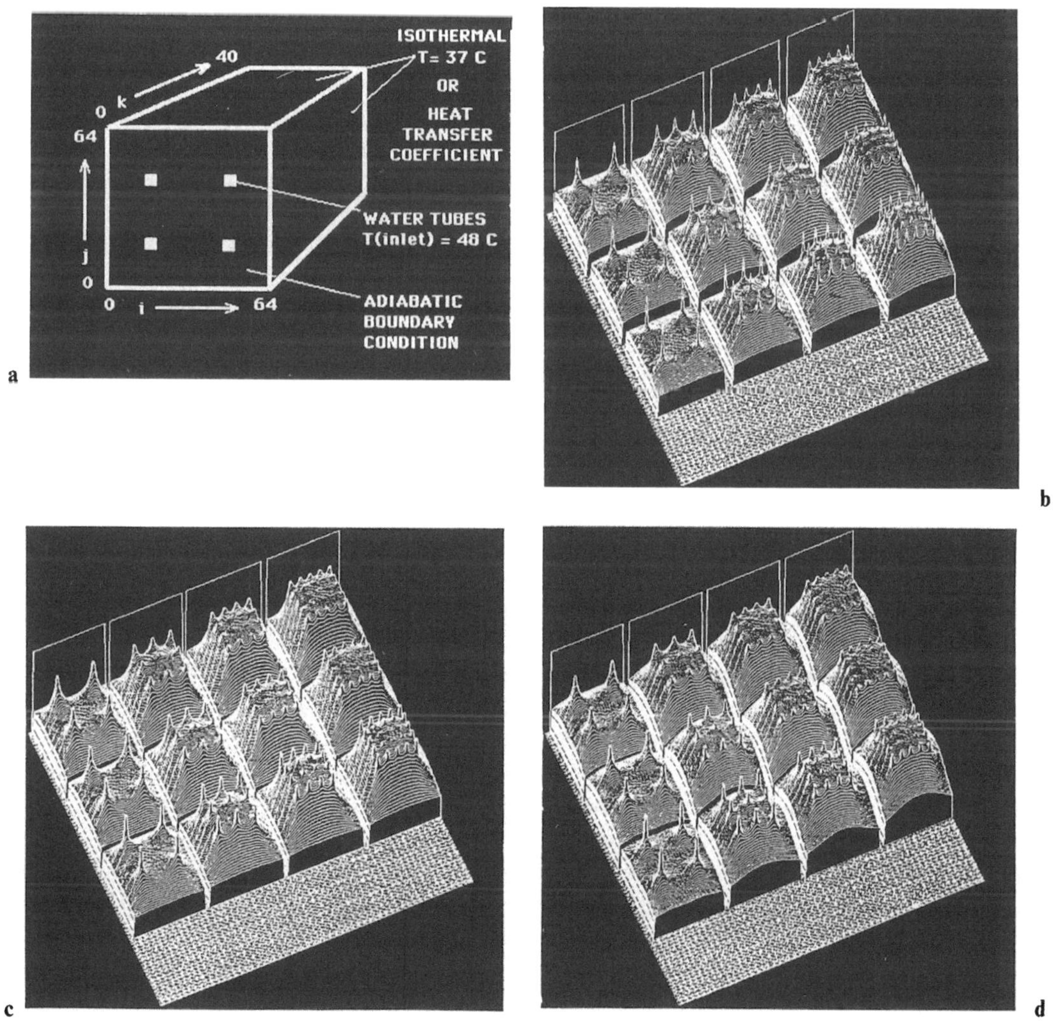

Fig. 16.2. a Overview of the model configuration. **b–d** Stationary temperature distributions in the midplane of the model for 1-mm catheters (**b**), 2-mm catheters (**c**), and changed boundary conditions (**d**). See text for detailed explanation
▼

inner region spanned by the tubes is taken as a qualitative measure, then the distribution improves considerably after raising the source density and it is obvious that higher k_{eff} values are accompanied by lower absolute values of the temperatures but cause no change in their distribution. This drop in temperature can be easily compensated for by increasing the strength of the heating sources. In the former two cases isothermic boundary conditions, i.e., $T_{bound} = 37.0°C$, were imposed on the four planes parallel to the tubes. This may have led to some underestimation of the stationary temperature distribution with respect to an actual clinical situation where the 37.0°C isotherm is determined by the physical problem and its location is not known beforehand. Therefore we performed a series of computations changing the heat transfer coefficient h (W °C^{-1} m^{-2}) at the bounding surfaces. Results for $h = 20$ and $h = 40$ corresponding to virtual extensions of the object dimensions of 15 and 7.5 cm, respectively, did not differ significantly; therefore the case of $h = 20$ was selected to show that temperature distribution has improved in the whole region, especially for the higher k_{eff} values.

So far the effect of blood flow has only been accounted for by changing the k_{eff} values. The impact of discrete countercurrent vessel pairs oriented parallel or normal to tube tracks ($n = 16$) is investigated in Fig. 16.3. In order to compare the impact of counter vessel flow, the undisturbed temperature distribution in plane $j = 32$ has been displayed in the leftmost column. The column in the middle shows the results in the same plane for a vessel pair ($d = 2$ mm) with a flow velocity of 10 cm/s and running in parallel (upper block) or orthogonally (middle block). The lowest block in each row is a different representation of the same result of the middle block, thus improving visualization. The rightmost column displays the effect of smaller vessels ($d = 1$ mm) with lower flow, i.e., 1 cm/s. From Fig. 16.3 it is clear that in the high flow case no equilibration of the vessel blood temperature with surrounding tissue has occurred, while in the low flow case the blood temperature rises from 37°C at the entrance towards 45.6°C at the exit of a vessel.

The aforementioned high flow case has been used to examine how the stationary temperature distribution can be improved. Panel a of Fig. 16.4 shows the results of plane $z = 20$ for the undisturbed situation. In this and subsequent panels the image data have been manipulated by window leveling such that temperature values above 44°C are displayed white. From panel b it is clear that a centrally located vessel pair results in a colder area with a minimal tissue temperature of 39.8°C located between the vessels while the maximum tissue temperature amounts to 46.2°C. Shifting the vessel pair out of the center and into the immediate neighborhood (panel c) of a water tube changes the shape of the colder area while the temperature minimum for this case reads 40.1°C. A substantial improvement was obtained when the water temperatures of the four nearest tubes were increased, i.e., the closest to 52°C and the others to 50°C (panel d). For this particular case the highest tissue temperature amounted to 47.6°C while the lowest was 40.9°C, which again was located between the vessel pair.

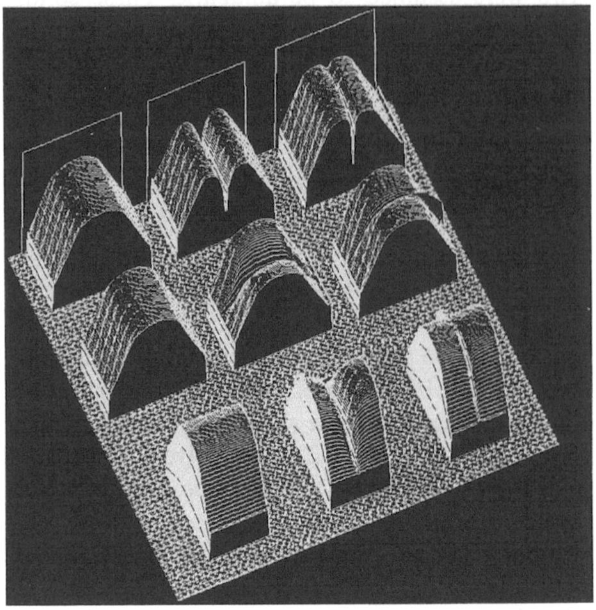

Fig. 16.3. Temperature distribution in a plane perpendicular to the water tubes for vessel pairs with high and low blood flow oriented parallel or orthogonal to the tubes

The spatial disturbance induced by a hypothetical countercurrent vessel network is depicted in Fig. 16.5, which is a selection of those planes ($n = 16$) containing a vessel segment. Panel a gives an overview of these 16 transverse planes of the model configuration, of which some ($13 < z < 21$) clearly exhibit the location of the vessel structure. The network consists of a short countercurrent vessel pair ($d = 3$ mm) branching into two pairs ($d = 2$ mm), each of which ends in two smaller vessel pairs ($d = 1$ mm). The arterial part of the network is imaged black while the venous part is dotted. Applying the same window leveling for the 44°C isotherm as was used in Fig. 16.4, a good qualitative

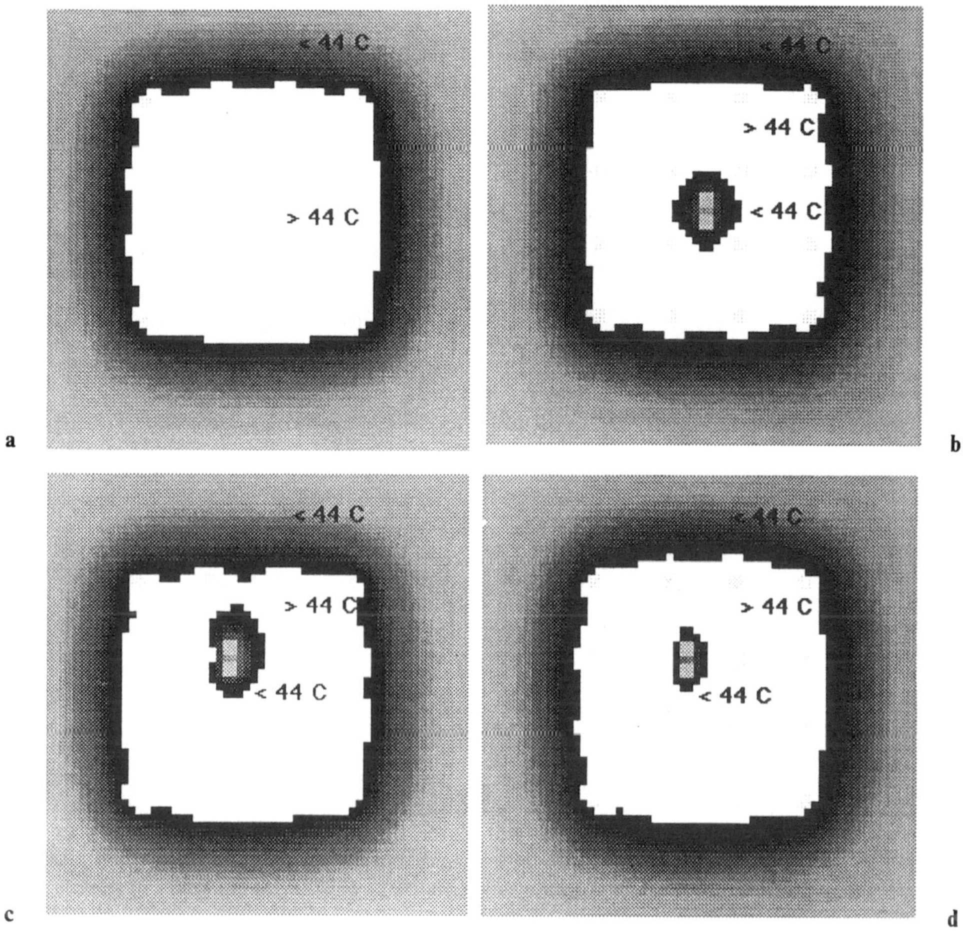

Fig. 16.4 a–d. Example to show the improvement in temperature distribution in the same plane as Fig. 16.3 following displacement of the vessel pair and increase in the water temperature of the tubes nearest to the vessel pair

impression is obtained of the temperature distortion, which is clearly associated with the vessel structure. It can also be inferred from this figure that the arterial part remains at low temperatures and that the venous outlet temperature has increased significantly. When the water temperature of the four tubes in the lower left corner was raised to 52°C we obtained the results illustrated in panel 5c, showing a significant improvement. However, in this case the maximum temperature was 49.1°C, located near the four tubes and extending over their total lengths. It is obvious from such observations that interstitial techniques require radial as well as longitudinal control of the power deposition. Figure 16.6 is a magnification of the 8-th block in panels 5b and 5c which shows the local temperature distortion in more detail.

16.4 Discussion

Some of the conclusions which may be derived from the presented results are trivial and well-known to experienced interstitial hyperthermia physicists, e.g., the effect of catheter diameter and density on thermal distribution. The results obtained with different k_{eff} values show that the temperature distributions remained nearly the same but that the absolute values decreased with increasing k_{eff}. In the case of a homogeneous tissue this fall in temperature can be easily compensated for by raising the water temperature. Another aspect of relevance to the temperature distribution is the fact that in highly perfused tissues the vessel wall temperatures, which reflect the minimum tissue temperature, may increase. This feature has been studied analytically by CREZEE and LAGENDIJK (1992). If the tissue volume to be heated is perfused heterogeneously and/or is characterized by an inhomogeneous distribution of the thermal conductivity, the maximal allowable tube temperature is a

b

c

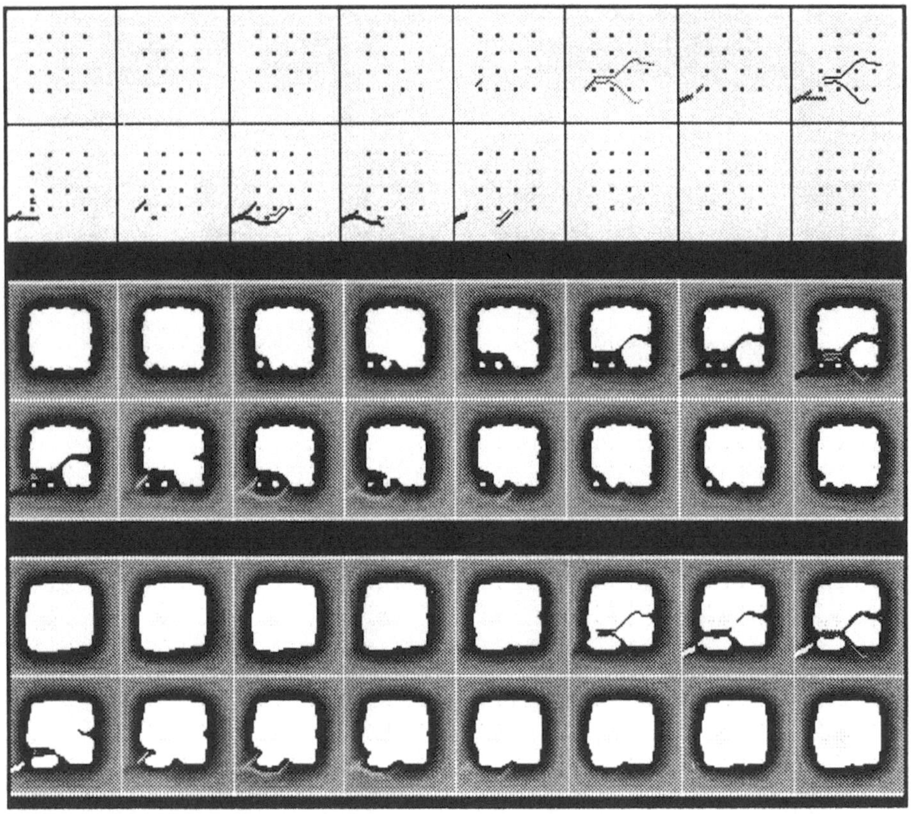

Fig. 16.5 a–c. Theoretical temperature distribution in a muscle-like phantom (*gray*) containing a countercurrent vessel network (panel **a**) heated by a matrix of 16 water tubes (*black dots*). Out of a total of 40 planes, 16 have been selected to display the location and architecture of the countercurrent vessel structure. Panel **b** is the stationary temperature distribution in these 16 transverse planes when all tubes have the same entrance temperature (48°C). Panel **c**: same as for panel **b** but now the water temperature of the four tubes in the *lower left corner* has been raised to 52°C

a

b

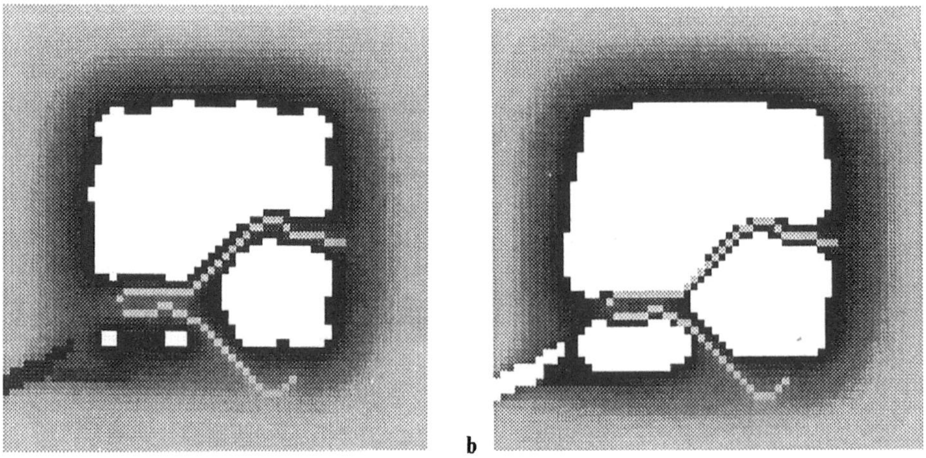

Fig. 16.6 a, b. Enlarged view of the 8th block in the *upper rows of panels 5b and 5c*. **a** The two courses dotted *light gray* correspond to the 1-mm arteries while the *dark gray area* in the *lower left corner* is associated with venous outlet temperature. **b** Raising the water temperature of some tubes improves the spatial distribution and results in higher venous outlet temperature

determined by the location where the maximum temperature occurs. In general this implies that besides radial control, the heating sources must also have axial control of the temperature distribution.

From the presented results it is concluded that in general catheter spacings of 10–15 mm should be sufficient to raise the temperature of the volume between the catheters to the desired level. However, in the presence of large vessels this conclusion no longer holds and temperature control must be achieved by adapting the source strengths which are closest to the vessels and/or by raising the local catheter density. This calls for pretreatment planning (see this volume, Chap. 20) based on anatomical and physiological data in respect of the vessels. During this process, attention should also be given to a proper definition of the imposed boundary conditions. Although no general conclusions can be derived from the few examples presented, we are of the opinion that more uniform tumor temperatures may be derived when the catheters are placed in close proximity to the largest vessels and, insofar as is possible, in parallel with them. The final conclusion of this theoretical work is obvious: In vivo tests (see this volume, Chap. 19) and acquisition of clinical data for the verification of the underlying theories are indispensable and are therefore to be strongly encouraged.

Acknowledgment. This work was supported by a grant from the Dutch Cancer Society.

References

Chen MM, Holmes KR (1980) Microvascular contributions in heat transfer. Ann NY Acad Sci 335: 137–151

Crezee J, Lagendijk JJW (1992) Temperature uniformity during hyperthermia: the impact of large vessels. Phys Med Biol 37(6): 1321–1337

Lagendijk JJW (1984) A new theory to calculate temperature distributions in tissues, or why the "bioheat transfer" equation does not work. In: Overgaard J (ed) Hyperthermic oncology 1984. Taylor & Francis, London, pp 507–510

Mooibroek J, Lagendijk JJW (1991) A fast and simple algorithm for the calculation of convective heat transfer by large vessels in three dimensional inhomogeneous tissues. IEEE Trans Biomed Eng 38: 490–501

Pennes HH (1948) Analysis of tissue and arterial blood temperatures in the resting human forearm. J Appl Physiol 1: 93–122

Valdagni R, Amichetti M, Antolini R et al (1990) International consensus meeting on hyperthermia. Final Report. Int J Hyperthermia 6: 839–877

Weinbaum S, Jiji LM (1985) A new simplified bioheat equation for the effect of blood flow on local average tissue temperature. ASME J Biomech Eng 107: 131–139

17 Thermal Modeling of Heterogeneous Tumours with Irregular Microwave Antenna Arrays

A. McCowen and K.L. Clibbon

CONTENTS

17.1 Introduction

A major challenge for hyperthermia engineers and physicists is the prediction of temperature distribution both inside the tumour and in the external tissue in which the radiating microwave antenna array is embedded. There are two distinct aspects to solving this problem. There is firstly the task of determining the complex interaction of the microwave electromagnetic energy within the antenna array in order to calculate the SAR; it is this aspect of the problem that will be discussed in this chapter. Secondly there is the question of how the supplied heating is distributed by the local tissue and this aspect is discussed elsewhere.

There have been a number of recent papers – notably by Trembly (1985), Wong et al. (1986) and Zhang et al. (1988) – concerning the prediction of SAR distributions in interstitial microwave dipole antenna arrays. Mathematical expressions have been developed to compute the theoretical SAR distributions within "ideal" arrays of parallel dipole antennas embedded in homogeneous medium. These predictions have been shown to give reasonably good agreement with measurements made in homogeneous phantoms. However, the work to extend both the modeling capability and phantom measurements to heterogeneous media is thwarted. Firstly, construction of and subsequent measurements within a more realistic heterogeneous phantom are impractical and thus theoretical predictions will form the only practical means of assessing the performance of a particular array configuration in a given situation. Secondly, the mathematical expressions used to compute the radiated electric fields, as used by Trembley (1985) etc., on their own will be inadequate for the heterogeneous case since they have been developed by assuming a superposition of the radiated fields from the different dipole antennas in a uniform medium. When the problem is heterogeneous with tumour tissue, muscle, fat and/or bone all local to the antenna region, then a complex microwave electromagnetic scattering problem will need to be solved to determine the resulting SAR distribution.

Such complex scattering problems can only be solved by reverting to the fundamental electromagnetic equations of Maxwell, which in turn need to be solved using numerical techniques such as finite element, finite difference and method of moments. In this chapter we summarise the recent work of the Computational Electromagnetic Group at Swansea in which we had two specific aims. Firstly, to model a "non-ideal" microwave interstitial dipole array which would be more realistic than the "ideal" arrays previously reported in the literature. To this end we have allowed each antenna to be positioned and skewed independently so as to form a completely arbitrary array. Secondly, to solve the heterogeneous electromagnetic scattering problem within the antenna array. The next two sections of this chapter summarise how these aims were achieved and some of our initial findings are discussed.

17.2 Antenna Array

The configuration of a single embedded and insulated dipole of the type under consideration in this work is shown in Fig. 17.1. The radiated electric field from such a dipole can be determined from expressions derived by King et al. (1983). These expressions are valid only for symmetric dipoles, i.e., $h_1 = h_2$, and have been further developed by

A. McCowen, B.Sc., M.Sc., Ph.D.; K.L. Clibbon; Department of Electrical and Electronic Engineering, University College of Swansea, Singleton Park, Swansea SA2 8PP, UK

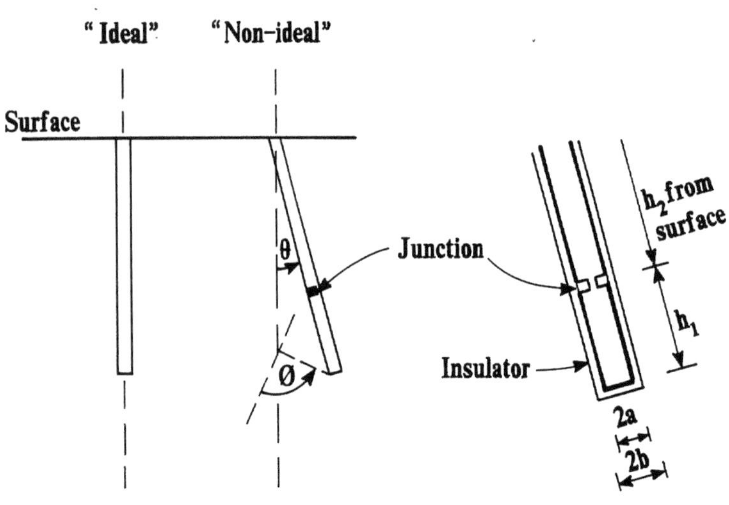

Fig. 17.1. "Ideal" and "non-ideal" configuration of an insulated microwave dipole antenna

ZHANG et al. (1988) to be applicable to non-symmetric dipoles, i.e., $h_1 \neq h_2$. Since the total field within an array is computed by the super position of the radiated fields from each antenna then the total computational effort required to determine an SAR distribution is directly proportional to the number of dipoles in the array. Using ZHANG'S expressions, the calculation of the electric field distribution within an array is computationally very expensive and further modifications to the expressions have recently been made by MCCOWEN and CLIBBON (unpublished work) to significantly reduce the computational effort. The expressions for the radiated electric field include all the variables shown in Fig. 17.1 and in addition depend on the permittivity of the background, lossy dielectric medium and also the frequency of operation. To allow for an arbitrary array we have included the facility to specify the location of the junction of each dipole as well as its skew (θ, ϕ) relative to an "ideal" configuration.

For two or more dipoles forming the array, the total radiated electric field is determined by the superposition of the individual fields from each of the dipoles. In an "ideal" array in which each of its antennas are fed in-phase, the constructive interference of the radiated electric fields results in a dome-shaped SAR distribution which peaks at the phase centre coinciding with the physical centre of the array. The steepness of the dome-shaped SAR distribution within the array is dependent on the frequency of operation and the lengths of the dipoles and such results have been well documented by TREMBLY (1985).

The placement of the individual microwave dipoles is very often determined by radiology considerations and an "ideal" array configuration is unrealistic. To demonstrate the degradation in SAR distribution due to a "non-ideal" array, we have used the antenna and tissue parameters listed in Table 17.1. Figure 17.2 shows the SAR distribution within an "ideal" arrangement of four symmetric dipoles arranged in a 3-cm square array. The SAR distribution is shown over a 1.2-cm square centred in the middle of the plane intersecting the dipole junctions. Assuming the dipole junctions are implanted 5 cm from the surface, if one of these dipoles is now skewed at the surface by just 5° in the θ-plane along the diagonal, then the shifting of the phase centres is sufficient to reduce the peak heating by 20%. What is more significant here is that even this slight skewing has resulted in a one-sided SAR distribution which may lead to a region that is inadequately heated.

17.3 Modeling Inhomogeneities

To solve the electromagnetic scattering associated with the heterogeneous problem of an embedded tumour in a background medium, we have used fast-Fourier transform (FFT)-based algorithms to solve the electric field integral equation (EFIE)

Table 1. Antenna and tissue parameters

Parameter description	Symbol	Value
Complex permittivity of external medium	$\left(\varepsilon_{ext} - j\frac{\sigma_{ext}}{\omega\varepsilon_0}\right)$	42-j17
Frequency of operation		915 MHz
Diameter of inner conductor	2a	0.66 mm
Diameter of insulator	2b	2.0 mm
Permittivity of insulator	ε_i	2.0
Halflength of symmetric dipole	h_2	3.0 cm

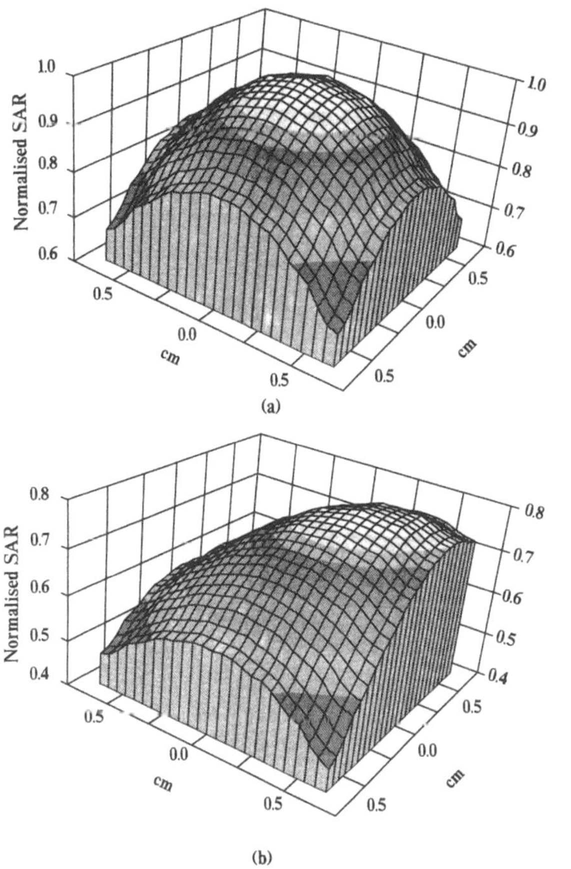

Fig. 17.2. **a** Normalised SAR distribution in the plane of the dipole junctions in an "ideal" 2 × 2 array. **b** "One-sided" SAR distribution within the same 2 × 2 array as in **a** with one of the dipoles skewed by 5°

which is basically discretised as in a method of moments scheme. This technique, of which there are several forms (see TRAN and MCCOWEN 1991), is at present probably the most efficient method of solving the computationally expensive problem associated with three-dimensional dielectric scatterers.

The tumour and any other region with different electrical characteristics, specified by $(\varepsilon_r - j\sigma_r/\omega\varepsilon_0)$ against the background medium permittivity of $(\varepsilon_{ext} - j\sigma_{ext}/\omega\varepsilon_0)$, is modeled by the following equivalent current sources:

$$J = [(\sigma_r - \sigma_{ext}) + j\omega\varepsilon_0(\varepsilon_r - \varepsilon_{rext})]E_T \,, \tag{1}$$

where E_T is the total electric field.

The EFIE for this heterogeneous model becomes

$$\frac{J}{(\sigma_r - \sigma_{ext}) + j\omega\varepsilon_0(\varepsilon_r - \varepsilon_{ext})} + \iiint\limits_{scatterer} GJ\,dv = E_i \tag{2}$$

where J is the unknown equivalent current distribution within the tissue and E_i is the known incident electric field radiated from the dipole array. As discussed in Sect. 17.2, an E_i can be determined for a "non-ideal" configuration of dipoles and hence Eq. 2 can be solved to determine the resultant current density distribution which in turn yields the SAR distribution. The method of moments has been used to discretise Eq. 2 to yield a set of linear equations which can be expressed in matrix form as follows

$$[G]\,[J] = [E_i] \,, \tag{3}$$

where $[G]$ is the known impedance matrix, $[E_i]$ is the known vector of incident electric field and $[J]$ is the vector of the unknown equivalent current densities. In this scheme scatterers are usually discretised using samples spaced at intervals of $\lambda/10$ throughout the volume, where λ is the electric wavelength in the dielectric medium. Scatterers with a feature size of the order of λ will generate an extremely large system of equations in (3) which cannot be solved using standard matrix inversion techniques, even with the most modern powerful workstations. For example, at 915 MHz the electric wavelength in muscle of relative permittivity 42-j17 is just under 5 cm so that any scatterer with a feature size of greater than just a few centimetres will generate a problem which is computationally expensive to solve.

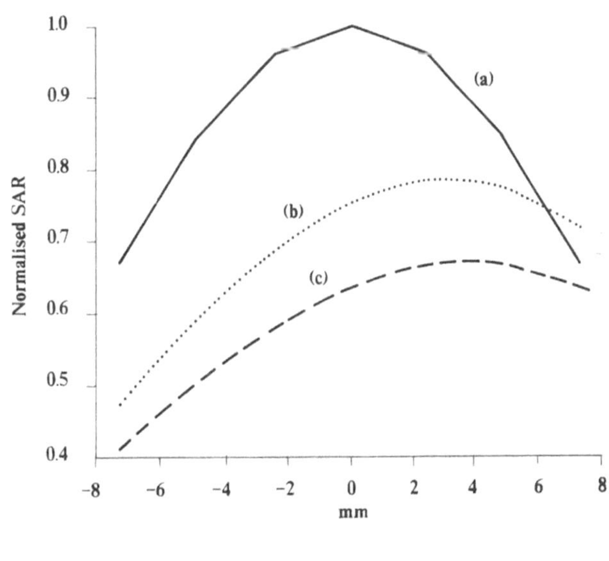

Fig. 17.3. Normalised SAR distributions along a diagonal transect of *(a)* an "ideal" 2 × 2 array in a uniform medium of permittivity 42-j17; *(b)* as for *(a)* with a 1.2-cm-diameter tumour of permittivity 55-j27 at the centre of the array

A detailed discussion of the FFT-based algorithms used to overcome the problem of solving Eq. 3 is inappropriate here and the reader is referred to Tran and McCowen (1991) and McCowen and Tran (1991) for the details.

To demonstrate the use of this facility we have modeled a 1.2-cm-diameter tumour of permittivity 55-j28 placed at the centre of the skewed array described in Sect. 17.2 and tabulated in Table 17.1. Figure 17.3 shows the SAR distribution across the tumour along the diagonal transect of the antenna array. The figure clearly shows a further degradation of the SAR distribution due to the inhomogeneity of the problem.

References

King WPK, Trembly BS, Strohbehn JW (1983) The electromagnetic field of an insulated antenna in a conducting or dielectric medium. IEEE Trans Microwave Theory Tech 31: 574–583

McCowen A, Tran TV (1991) Matrix interpretation of the spectral iteration technique for 3D dielectric scatterers in the resonance region. IEE Proc-H 138: 219–224

Tran TV, McCowen A (1991) A comparative study of a class of FFT-based methods for the computation of electromagnetics scattering from 2 and 3D objects. IEE Int Conf CEM'91: 238–240

Trembly BS (1985) The effects of driving frequency and antenna length on power deposition within a microwave antenna array used for hyperthermia. IEEE Trans Bio Med Eng 32: 152–157

Wong TZ, Strohbehn JW, Jones KM, Mechling JA, Trembly BS (1986) SAR patterns from an interstitial microwave antenna – array hyperthermia system. IEEE Trans Microwave Theory Tech 34: 560–567

Zhang Y, Nilesh VD, Randall T-H, William TJ (1988) The determination of the electromagnetic field and SAR pattern of an interstitial applicator in a dissipative dielectric medium. IEEE Trans Microwave Theory Tech 36: 1438–1443

18 Thermal Modeling for Brain Tumors

M. SEEBASS, W. SCHLEGEL, P. WUST, and J. NADOBNY

CONTENTS

18.1 Introduction

Interstitial stereotactic brain tumor therapy is the field of research in a cooperative project between the Department for Biophysics and Medical Radiation Physics at the German Cancer Research Center in Heidelberg and the Department of Stereotactic Neurosurgery at the University Hospital of Cologne. As a part of this project, the use of hyperthermia to enhance the effects of radiotherapy is being investigated. In brain tumor therapy the number of applicators has to be as small as possible; thus microwave antennas are the most suitable applicators, as has been shown by comparative calculations (STROHBEHN and MECHLING 1986).

A three-dimensional (3-D) computer simulation program has been developed to study the effects of treatment parameters (number and locations of antennas, amplitudes and phases of feeding voltages) and tissue properties (heat conductivity, specific heat, blood perfusion) on the temperature distribution.

M. SEEBASS, Ph.D., Konrad Zuse-Zentrum für Informationstechnik Berlin, Abteilung Numerische Software-Entwicklung, Heilbronner Straße 10, W-1000 Berlin 31, Germany
W. SCHLEGEL, Ph.D., Deutsches Krebsforschungszentrum, Abteilung Biophysik und Medizinische Strahlenphysik, Im Neuenheimer Feld 280, W-6900 Heidelberg, Germany
P. WUST, M.D.; J. NADOBNY, Ph.D.; Klinikum Rudolf Virchow, Freie Universität Berlin, Strahlenklinik und Poliklinik, Augustenburger Platz 1, W-1000 Berlin 65, Germany

18.2 Method

Four steps are required to perform a hyperthermia simulation. Initially, a 3-D finite elements (FE) grid is generated. Secondly, the electromagnetic field of the antennas is calculated, from which the power deposition pattern is derived. The bioheat transfer equation is applied to compute the temperatures achieved in tissue. Finally, the 3-D temperature distributions are visualized and quantitatively evaluated.

18.2.1 Grid Generation

Since the FE method is used for temperature calculation, a 3-D FE grid is needed. The grid is based on contours which are drawn into a set of the patient's computed tomographic (CT) scans. The CT scans cover a region at least 2 cm above and below the tumor margin. The slice distance should be 2 mm.

Grid generation starts with the creation of two-dimensional (2-D) grids (consisting of triangular elements) for some selected CT slices. Based on the 2-D grids a coarse 3-D grid is generated: The space between consecutive 2-D grids is filled with tetrahedron elements. Finally, the 3-D grid is refined, i.e., each element is divided into smaller elements. The element size determines the precision of the calculated temperature distribution.

18.2.2 Field Calculation

To apply an interstitial microwave hyperthermia treatment, plastic catheters are implanted into the tumor, in which the microwave antennas are inserted. The catheter walls provide electrical insulation between the antennas and the surrounding tissue. Thus, the theory of insulated dipoles in dissipative media (KING et al. 1983) can be applied to calculate the antenna fields, if the surrounding tissue is assumed to be an electrically homogeneous medium. According to this theory, the system of antenna, catheter, and surrounding tissue is modeled by a transmission line. For improvement of field calculation the transmission line model has been generalized from cylindrical antennas to more complicated antenna designs, e.g., antennas consisting of several cylindrical sections with different radii, conical antennas, or antennas with sleeve sections. If more than one antenna is used, a superposition of the antenna fields is performed. The simulation program allows arbitrary antenna positions in space. From the total electric field inside tissue the absorbed power per volume element is calculated.

18.2.3 Temperature Calculation

Temperature calculation is based on the bioheat transfer equation (BHTE), the standard model of heat transport in tissue (PENNES 1948). The BHTE is a balance equation for the heat which enters and leaves each tissue volume element. The heat transport by blood is described in a simplified manner. It is assumed that heat is exchanged between blood and surrounding tissue only in the capillary bed. In the simulation program a solution of the stationary BHTE is calculated.

The parameters of the BHTE, such as heat conductivity, specific heat, and blood perfusion, can be specified for each tissue compartment. In addition, boundary conditions on the body surface have to be stated.

The FE discretization of the BHTE results in a linear equation system that is iteratively solved by a preconditioned conjugate gradient algorithm.

18.2.4 Evaluation

Using the evaluation procedures, the temperature distribution can be visualized and a quantitative rating given. Thus evaluation provides a means of choosing the best among several antenna configurations. The following evaluative methods have been implemented:

1. The temperature distribution in transverse, frontal parallel, and sagittal parallel sections can be displayed in combination with corresponding CT data.

2. In a 3-D representation the target volume is shown as a closed surface and the isotherms as "ribbons." Thus, it can be recognized whether the isotherms totally enclose the target volume.

3. Temperature-volume histograms for target and healthy tissue can be generated. The volume heated to temperatures greater than T is shown as a function of temperature T. The histogram provides a quantitative assessment of the temperature distribution.

18.2.5 Optimization

Based on the results of evaluation, an algorithm for optimization of antenna parameters (locations, amplitudes, and phases) was developed. The part of the tumor heated to above 42°C is maximized under the constraint

$$V_{t,<42} = V_{h,>43} ,$$

where $V_{t,<42}$ is the volume of tumor tissue heated to less than 42°C and $V_{h,>43}$ is the volume of healthy tissue heated to above 43°C.

18.3 Results

Based on CT data of patients treated with interstitial radiotherapy, several hyperthermia simulation studies were performed. The target volume was 2–11 cm^3, the total volume included in the simulation 500–850 cm^3. The antenna type used was a cylindrical antenna with extended inner conductor (KING et al. 1983) at a frequency of 915 MHz. The influence of different antenna numbers (two to four) on the temperature distribution was investigated for tumor perfusions between 0 and 20 ml/kg/s (twice of normal brain perfusion). For each case the antenna parameters (locations, amplitudes, phases) were optimized. The results of hyperthermia simulations can be summarized as follows:

1. With increasing antenna number the temperature distribution improves. The physician has to find a compromise between improved treatment and higher risk to the patient due to increased number of implants. If tumor blood flow is less than or equal to 4.5 ml/kg/s, two or three antennas are sufficient to heat more than 90% of the target volume to therapeutic temperatures (i.e., > 42°C)

while the thermal load to healthy tissue (temperatures > 43°C) is kept at an acceptable level.

2. With increasing tumor blood flow (relative to normal tissue perfusion) the temperature distribution worsens, and the part of the target volume heated to therapeutic temperatures decreases.

The optimal antenna configuration mainly depends on the location and size of the target volume; it is only weakly influenced by tumor blood flow.

Figures 18.1–18.3 show as an example the results for a treatment using three antennas. Brain and tumor blood flow were assumed to be 9 and 4.5 ml/kg/s, respectively.

A complete hyperthermia simulation (excluding optimization) can be performed on a computer workstation like a DECstation 5000 within about 30 min. The hyperthermia simulation program was installed at the University Hospital of Cologne in March 1990, and hyperthermia treatments will commence there in the near future.

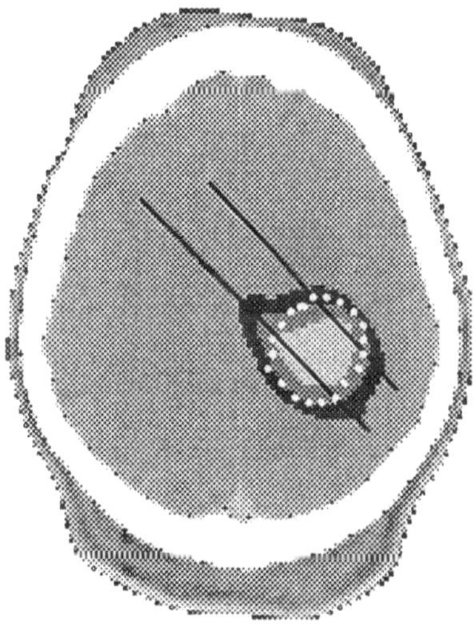

Fig. 18.1. Temperature distribution in a transverse section (colorwash representation). *Dark gray*, 40°–42°C; *gray*, 42°–45°C; *light gray*, > 45°C; *white dots*, contour of target volume; *black lines*, projections of antennas

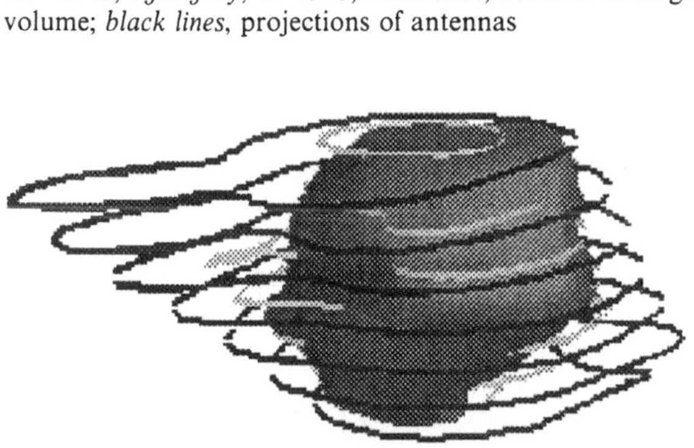

Fig. 18.2. Three-dimensional representation of temperature distribution. *Gray*, target volume; *dark gray*, 40°C isotherms; *light gray*, 42°C isotherms

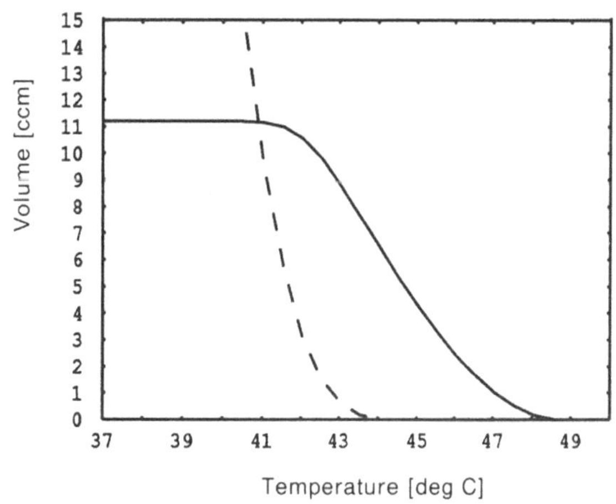

Fig. 18.3. Temperature–volume histogram. *Solid line*, target volume; *dashed line*, healthy tissue

18.4 Discussion

The hyperthermia modeling presented is based on theoretical models of electromagnetic field generation and heat transport in tissue. The validation of these models by experimental data has been investigated in the literature: The theory of insulated dipole antennas in dissipative media is the basis for field calculation. The group who first applied this theory to hyperthermia modeling (King et al. 1983) also performed phantom measurements of the power deposition patterns (Wong et al. 1986). Good agreement was found between the theory and experimental data.

The results of temperature calculation cannot be compared directly to phantom measurements because no realistic phantom for perfused tissue is available. Since the BHTE is based on a simplified model of heat transport by blood that does not specifically include the effects of large blood vessels, errors in temperature modeling primarily must be expected in the vicinity of large blood vessels (Lagendijk 1987).

The results of hyperthermia simulations suggest:

1. For most clinical applications two or three antennas are sufficient to heat 90%–95% of the target volume (2–11 cm^3) to therapeutic temperatures (> 42°C) while thermal load to healthy tissue is kept at an acceptable level. However, this conclusion might be too optimistic if inhomogeneous tumor blood flow cases are considered

(e.g., low blood flow in the center; high blood flow in the periphery).

2. Tumor blood flow has only a small influence on the optimal antenna configuration. Thus, treatment planning and optimization can be performed even if tumor blood flow is not exactly known. Again, it is emphasized that only homogeneous tumor blood flow cases were simulated.

For future developments of the hyperthermia simulation program the following topics need to be investigated:

1. Inclusion of tissue inhomogeneities in electromagnetic field calculations.
2. More efficient optimization routines.
3. Use of temperatures measured during hyperthermia treatments for retrospective analysis.
4. Solution of the time-dependent BHTE for modeling the warm-up and cool-down phases of hyperthermia treatments.
5. Implementation of an improved model of heat transport by blood. As a first step the large blood vessels should be included in the model separately. Three-dimensional imaging of blood vessels can be done by NMR angiography.

18.5 Conclusion

The 3-D hyperthermia simulation program presented is based on a finite elements solution of the bioheat transfer equation. The accuracy of the calculated temperature distributions is mainly restricted by the simplifications in modeling heat transport by blood. A complete simulation can be performed on a computer workstation within 30 min.

Acknowledgment. This work was supported by Deutsche Forschungsgemeinschaft (DFG), grant Schl 249/1-2.

References

King RWP, Trembly BS, Strohbehn JW (1983) The electromagnetic field of an insulated antenna in a conducting or dielectric medium. IEEE Trans Microwave Theory Tech 31: 574–583

Lagendijk JJW (1987) Heat transfer in tissues. In: Field SB, Franconi C (eds) Physics and technology of hyperthermia. Martinus Nijhoff, Dordrecht, pp 517–552 (NATO ASI Series E: Applied Sciences, No. 127)

Pennes HH (1948) Analysis of tissue and arterial blood temperatures in the resting human forearm. J Appl Physiol 1: 93–122

Strohbehn JW, Mechling JA (1986) Interstitial techniques for clinical hyperthermia. In: Hand JW, James JR (eds) Physical techniques in clinical hyperthermia. Research Studies Press, Letchworth, pp 210–287

Wong TZ, Strohbehn JW, Jones KM, Mechling JA, Trembly BS (1986) SAR patterns from an interstitial microwave antenna-array hyperthermia system. IEEE Trans Microwave Theory Tech 34: 560–567

19 Thermal Model Verification in Interstitial Hyperthermia

J. CREZEE, J. MOOIBROEK, and J.J.W. LAGENDIJK

CONTENTS

19.1 Introduction

In vivo tests are essential for the development and evaluation of interstitial hyperthermia systems, especially because determination of the three-dimensional temperature distribution during clinical treatment is impossible: Minimal temperatures are expected to occur somewhere between the needles, requiring an extensive set of thermocouple catheters in addition to the applicator catheters. Usually the number of catheters implanted is already a compromise between the need for a small catheter spacing to ensure uniform temperatures and the wish to prevent excessive trauma to the patient. Any extra catheters available one might prefer to use for extra interstitial needles to improve temperature homogeneity. One must therefore be able to rely on the accuracy and correctness of the computed small scale temperature distribution.

19.2 Thermal Models

Different bioheat transfer models have been proposed, three of which are discussed here: two continuum models and a discrete vessel model. The main difference between these is the way blood flow is incorporated:

1. The widely used bioheat equation of PENNES (1948) uses a heat sink term B to represent heat transport by convection. In each volume element:

$$\rho_t \cdot c_t \frac{dT}{dt} = \operatorname{div}(k_t \operatorname{grad}(T)) - B + P \ (\mathrm{W\,m^{-3}}) ,$$

where T is the temperature (°C), ρ_t the density (kg m^{-3}), c_t the specific heat (J kg^{-1} °C^{-1}), and k_t the thermal conductivity of tissue (W °C^{-1} m^{-1}). $B = w_b c_b [T - T_{art}]$, with w_b the volumetric perfusion rate (kg m^{-3} s^{-1}), c_b the specific heat of blood, and T_{art} the arterial blood temperature. P is the heat produced by the external heating system; metabolic heat production is neglected.

2. The k-effective model (CHEN and HOLMES 1980; LAGENDIJK 1984; WEINBAUM and JIJI 1985) includes small vessel blood flow (diameters $<$ ca. 0.5 mm) in a tensorial enhanced effective tissue conductivity k_{eff}.

$$\rho_t \cdot c_t \cdot \frac{dT}{dt} = \operatorname{div}(k_{eff} \operatorname{grad}(T)) + P \ (\mathrm{W\,m^{-3}}) .$$

3. The discrete large vessel model simulates the thermal behavior by large, thermally unequilibrated vessels with diameters larger than 0.5 mm by modeling these vessels discretely (MOOIBROEK and LAGENDIJK 1991; this volume, Chap. 16).

19.3 Model Predictions

The above three models yield very different predictions for the steady-state temperature distribution during interstitial heating, especially at high blood flow rates. According to the conventional bioheat equation (1), conduction becomes negligible in comparison to the convective heat sink term B; therefore $B \approx P$, and the temperature elevation $(T - T_{art}) \sim P/w_b$. At high but uniform perfusion $(T - T_{art})$ takes the shape of the power absorption

J. CREZEE, Ph.D.; J. MOOIBROEK, Ph.D.; J.J.W. LAGENDIJK, Ph.D.; Department of Radiotherapy, University Hospital Utrecht, Heidelberglaan 100, NL-3584 CX Utrecht, The Netherlands distribution; the desired uniform temperature rise consequently requires a uniform power deposition. In most interstitial heating systems, power deposition is restricted to the neighborhood of the applicators, resulting in high temperatures near the needles but a cool spot in between (BABBS et al. 1990; BREZOVICH and ATKINSON 1984; HAND et al. 1992; MECHLING and STROHBEHN 1986; SCHREIER et al. 1990; STAUFFER et al. 1989; STROHBEHN et al. 1982; STROHBEHN 1983; UZUNOGLU and NIKITA 1988). According to the k_{eff} model (2), high blood flow results in high tissue conductivity, but the shape of the temperature distribution does not change as long as the energy deposition is increased to compensate for the higher heat removal. For interstitial heating this means reasonably uniform temperatures, without cool spots (CREZEE and LAGENDIJK 1990; CREZEE et al. 1991). According to the discrete large vessel model (3), a large vessel entering the heated volume may produce a cold tract along its course (LAGENDIJK 1982). This effect resembles temperature predictions by the heat sink model (1), but with far more uncertainty regarding presence, location, and magnitude of cool spots, which depend strongly on vessel size and flow velocity. The considerable difference between these predictions emphasizes the need for verification of simulated temperature distributions.

19.4 Parameters to be Tested

Model predictions are tested by determining and verifying a number of thermal parameters – not just the temperature distribution itself, but also the perfusion rate w_b, the effective tissue conductivity k_{eff}, and the thermal equilibration length X_e for single and countercurrent large vessels. X_e is a measure of the distance it takes before the blood in a vessel reaches thermal equilibrium with the surrounding tissue and gives an indication of how large the preheated margin of normal tissue around the tumor must be in order to prevent a cold tract caused by a large vessel entering the heated volume. The determination of these parameters should take place in different types of tissue, with varying vessel flow, diameter, and density, and can be achieved in the following way:

1. The temperature distribution requires detailed temperature data. True model verification is difficult using just a single temperature point near the expected location of the temperature minimum.

2. w_b is obtained from the transient temperature after a stepwise increase or decrease in the applied power. If the conduction term is assumed to be negligible, the temperature will adapt exponentially according to Eq. 1: $T(t) = T(\infty) + \{T(0) - T(\infty)\}$ $\exp(-t/\tau)$, with time constant τ and $w_b = \rho_t c_t / c_b \tau$ (MILLIGAN et al. 1983).

3. k_{eff} is also determined using the transient temperature after a stepwise change of power. The best method is from the heat diffusion rate $\alpha = k_{eff}/\rho_t c_t$. With interstitial hyperthermia α can be found using the time delay τ_w before the temperature starts to rise at a certain distance from the needles after the heating has been switched on, provided power deposition is concentrated near the needles: $k_{eff} \sim \tau_w^{-1}$ (Fig. 19.1). A second possibility is using the time constant τ of the subsequent temperature curve, $k_{eff} \sim \tau^{-1}$ (CREZEE and LAGENDIJK 1990; CREZEE et al. 1991).

4. X_e requires temperature measurements in or along large vessels.

19.5 Phantoms

Designing a phantom suitable for thermal model tests is not simple. The behavior of large, thermally significant vessels, with diameters >ca. 0.5 mm, can be tested using conventional phantoms with individual vessels drilled into them. The smallest vessels, with diameters <0.1 mm (e.g., capillaries), contribute little to heat transport and can be simulated with a slightly enhanced effective tissue con-

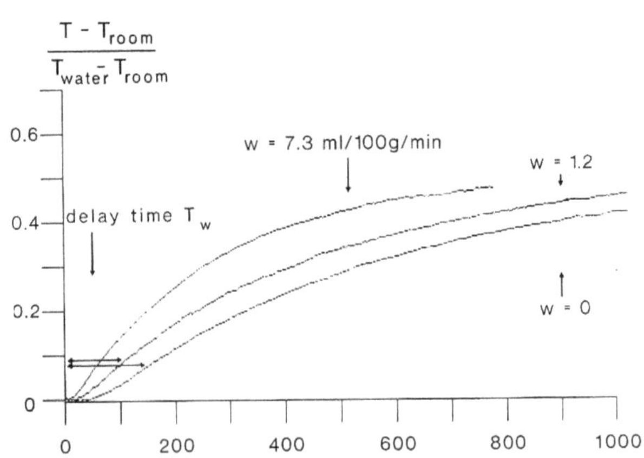

Fig. 19.1. Example of the delayed temperature response in isolated perfused bovine tongue at 6 mm from a hot water tube which is raised in temperature at $t = 0$. Perfusion rates vary between 0 and 7.3 ml/100 g/min

ductivity because the capillary flow is directed randomly. The remaining intermediate size vessels, with diameters of between 0.1 and 0.5 mm, are still thermally significant, but also are too small and numerous to be simulated in a conventional phantom: perfused human or animal tissues are more suitable, either in vivo or in vitro. Perfusion control is desirable, facilitating separation of convective and the intrinsic tissue heat transfer. Vessels should be of human size or larger. The contribution to bioheat transfer by the largest category of vessels will be much smaller in a small animal than in humans; as large vessels are thermally very significant, small animals cannot be a good model to simulate the human situation. Finally the (vascular) geometry must be known – the location and flow velocity of individual large vessels, the mean flow in the smaller ones, and whether the flow is isotropic or there is a mean flow direction. This can be achieved using computed tomography, magnetic resonance imaging/magnetic resonance angiography, casts and angiography.

19.6 Examples of Model Tests

We can distinguish two types of experiments: in vitro, using isolated perfused organs, or in vivo with or without the ability to control perfusion. Each category has its advantages.

19.6.1 In Vitro Tests

The use of isolated perfused organs ensures full control over blood flow, but it can be difficult to keep the vasculature intact once the organ is separated from the normal circulation. This requires the organ to be flushed with special perfusates: the kidney, liver, and spleen, for example, can be kept patent indefinitely using an alcohol fixation method (HOLMES et al. 1984). BOS et al. (1991) perfused isolated muscle tissue with a saline solution.

CREZEE et al. (1991) used a 2 × 2 interstitial hot water tube system (T_{water} = 39°C, tube outer diameter 2.0 mm, spacing 16 mm) to heat isolated perfused bovine tongues (n = 7). This method will

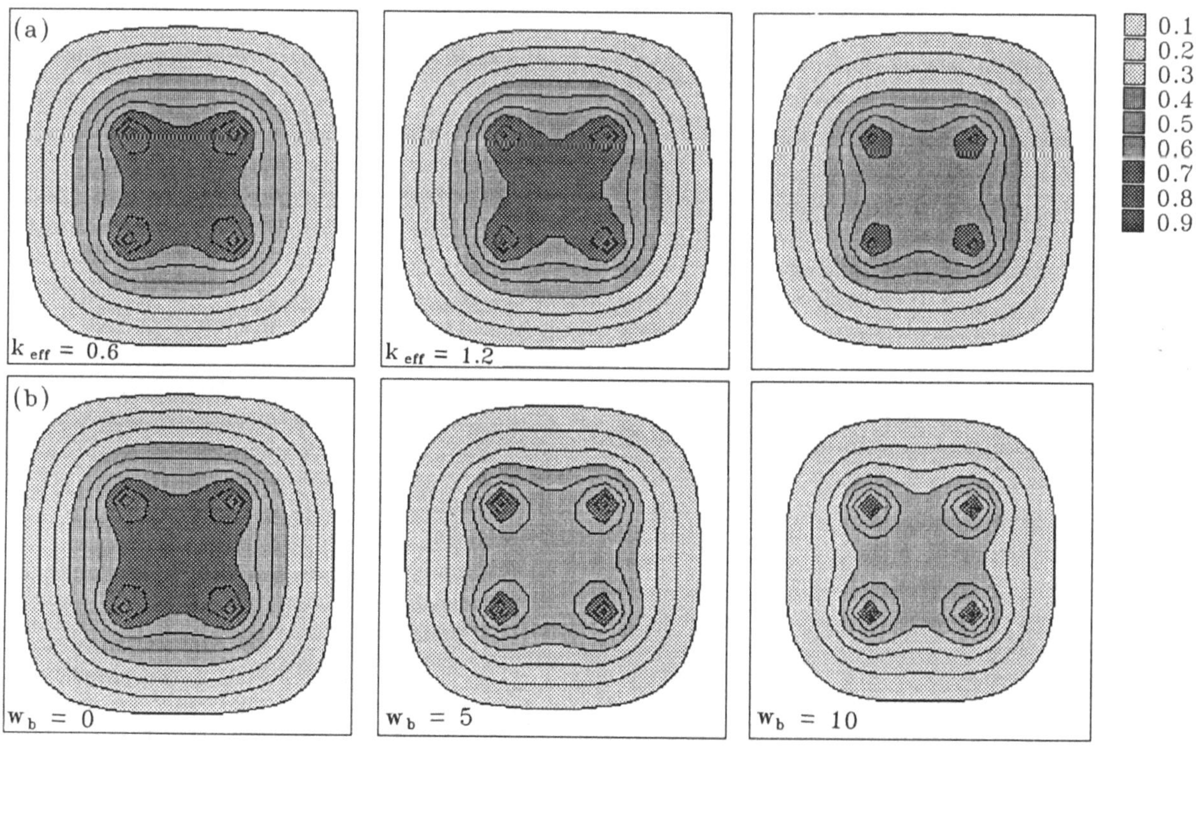

Fig. 19.2. a Simulated steady-state temperature distribution in an area of 5.5 × 5.5 cm heated by 2 × 2 hot water tubes. *Light* and *dark shading* indicates areas where the normalized temperature exceeds 0.3 and 0.7, respectively. $k_t = k_b = 0.6$ W K^{-1} m^{-1}, $\rho_t = 10^3$ kg m^{-3} and $c_t = c_b = 4 \cdot 10^3$ J kg^{-1}K^{-1}. Heat sink model prediction (1) with w_b = 0, 5, and 10 ml/100 g/min. **b** k_{eff} model (2) with k_{eff} = 0.6, 1.2, and 3.0 W K^{-1} m^{-1}. (Reprinted with permission of the Institute of Physics)
▼

not distort equipment, temperature control is simple, and there is no need to model any electromagnetic absorption. The tongue was flushed at room temperature with a saline solution (Bos et al. 1991), with flow ranging between 0 and 17 ml/100 g/min. The stationary temperature distribution in a plane perpendicular to the needle array was mapped with five to eight single thermocouples (diameter 50 µm) with a spacing of 4 or 8 mm. Three-dimensional transient and steady-state temperature distributions were also simulated, using both the conventional bioheat transfer equation (1) and the k_{eff} model (2); the resulting temperature distributions are given in normalized temperatures $(T - T_{room})/(T_{water} - T_{room})$ in Fig. 19.2. For zero blood flow the predictions are identical. As blood flow increases, the temperature at the center of the array starts to behave quite differently, decreasing according to the heat sink theory (1), but remaining constant according to the k_{eff} model (2).

Two examples of experimental temperature distributions are shown in Fig. 19.3, both measured at a blood flow rate w_b of 0 and at ca. 7.5 ml/100 g tissue/min (w_b was determined from the ratio between total blood flow and tongue weight). The effective conductivity k_{eff} at $w_b = 7.5$ ml/100 g/min was estimated using the transient temperature response and was about 2.0 times the intrinsic conductivity for the first example and 1.6 for the second.

Four out of seven temperature distributions resembled Fig. 19.3a, which agrees quite well with the k_{eff} prediction. Two others were somewhat distorted and lower; Fig. 19.3b shows the only case with low central temperatures. This was attributed to the presence of a large vessel in the heated volume. Analysis of the transient temperature data suggested that k_{eff} was on average twice the intrinsic tissue conductivity k_t for a tissue blood flow of 10 ml/100 g/min.

Conclusion. A 16-mm spacing proved sufficient for adequate heating between the needles at normal blood flow rates, in the absence of large vessels. Accurate temperature predictions require that large vessels are modeled discretely.

19.6.2 In Vivo Tests

In general, in vivo tests have the disadvantage of lacking perfusion control, complicating attempts to separate convection and conduction. Not only is the absolute blood flow level difficult to determine, but perfusion will probably display time- and temperature-dependent behavior. For other modes of hyperthermia in vivo tests have been reported where some form of perfusion control was maintained (e.g., De Young et al. 1986 for kidney), but to our knowledge these methods have not been used for testing interstitial techniques.

Schreier et al. (1990) heated pig and rabbit thigh in vivo with a 4 × 4 hot water tube array (Handl-Zeller et al. 1986). The spacing between the needles was 10 (rabbit/pig) or 14 mm (pig), and the water temperature T_{water} 45.5° or 48°C. The stationary temperature was measured at three points within the array and compared with predictions by a numerical model based on the conventional bioheat transfer equation (1). No analysis of transient temperatures was performed. Cool spots with temperatures of 41.1°C occurred within the array for $T_{water} = 45.5$°C and a spacing of 14 mm. In general, temperatures agreed reasonably with the predicted values if perfusion was assumed not to exceed 0.45 $kg\,m^{-1}s^{-1}$, a value expected for resting muscle, which seems quite low for tissue at hyperthermic temperatures. An exception was the case with a spacing of 10 mm: for $T_{water} = 48$°C the average tissue temperature was nearly 2°C higher than predicted, e.g., at the center $T = 47.2$°C versus a predicted value of 45.4°C! The temperature distribution was more uniform at $T_{water} = 48$°C than at 45°C, suggesting that the contribution of heat sink-like heat removal is relatively lower at 48°C. There are two possible explanations for this: (a) vasoconstriction at 48°C, and hence a smaller heat sink, or (b) vasodilatation, causing enhancement of effective tissue conductivity and thereby reducing the relative contribution of heat sink. We must note, however, that the latter experiment was only carried out in the rabbit, and the result may not apply to the human situation.

Conclusion. Hot water tubes are feasible in regions of moderate blood flow. For a needle spacing of

Fig. 19.3. a Example of an array implant in a tongue. The thermocouples were inserted approximately in the plane of the main artery and its branches. The figure is based on both angiography and dissection data. Steady-state temperature distribution was present in the area indicated; normalised temperatures. Blood flow 0 and 7.3 ml/100 g/min. **b** Another example. Note the presence of a large vessel within the array. Blood flow 0 and 7.4 ml/100 g/min. One thermocouple was not functioning at the higher perfusion rate. (Reprinted with permission of the Institute of Physics)

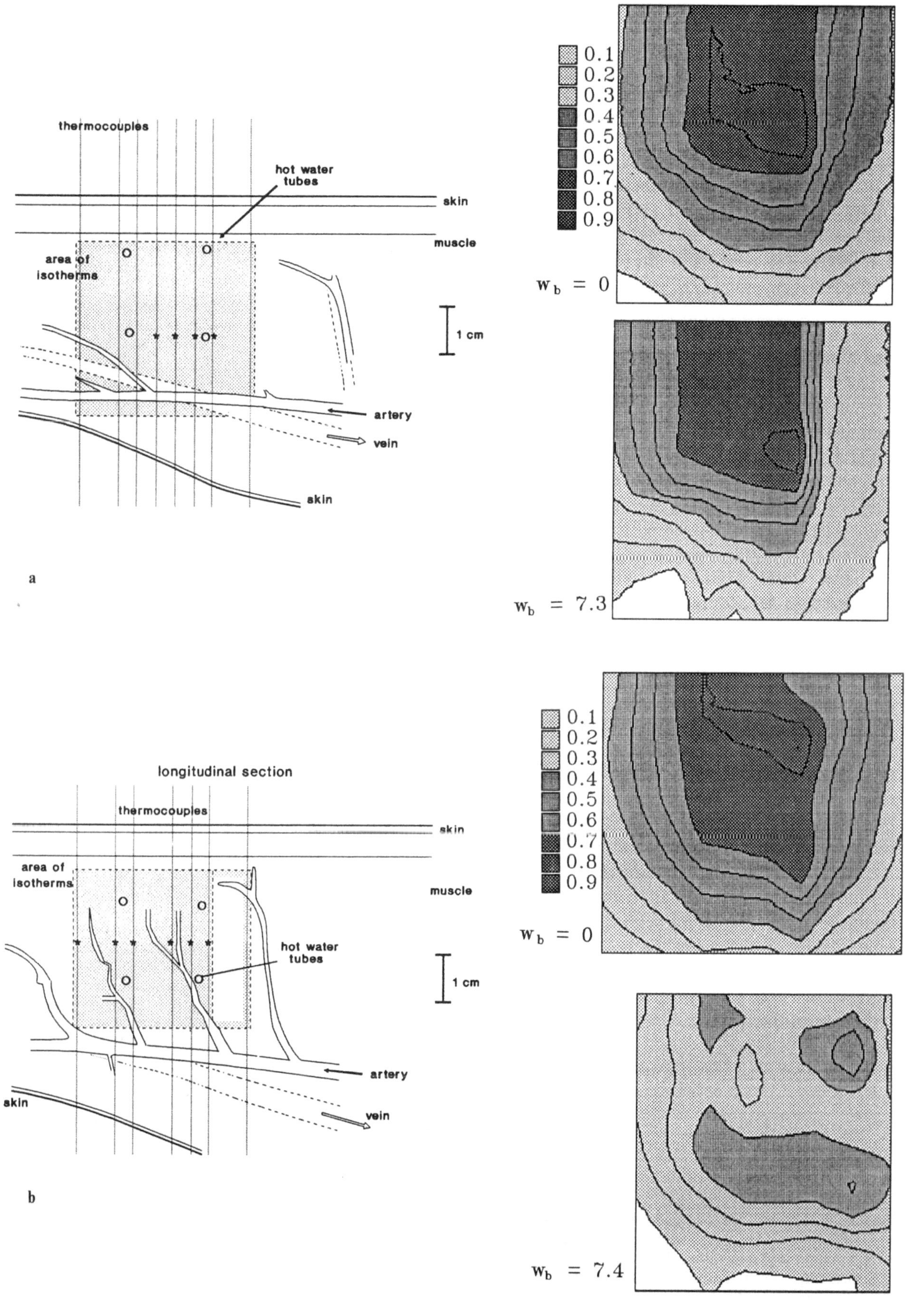
thermocouples
hot water tubes
skin
muscle
area of isotherms
1 cm
artery
vein
skin
a
0.1
0.2
0.3
0.4
0.5
0.6
0.7
0.8
0.9
$w_b = 0$
$w_b = 7.3$
longitudinal section
thermocouples
skin
area of isotherms
muscle
hot water tubes
1 cm
artery
skin
vein
b
0.1
0.2
0.3
0.4
0.5
0.6
0.7
0.8
0.9
$w_b = 0$
$w_b = 7.4$

10 mm a water temperature of 45°C suffices, but a spacing of 14 mm requires that T_{water} is raised to 48°C to achieve minimal tumor temperatures above 42.5°C.

Clinical treatments which include thermal data from both applicator and additional thermometry catheters can be useful for model tests. Some clinicians do use extra thermometry catheters, e.g., GOFFINET et al. (1990) and DEFORD et al. (1991), but usually because no reliable temperature data were available from the heating catheters themselves.

19.7 Conclusion

Although there is still much to be done on experimental verification of model predictions for interstitial hyperthermia, we may already conclude that the conventional bioheat transfer equation is incapable of correctly predicting the small scale temperature distribution in individual treatments. For an accurate quantitative prediction of the temperature the large vessels (diameter > 0.5 mm) should be modeled discretely, for instance using the numerical large vessel model of MOOIBROEK and LAGENDIJK (1991). The required detailed anatomical and vascular data, especially size, flow velocity, and direction of discrete large vessels, are expected to be available in the near future (this volume, Chap. 20). The representation of intermediate size vessels will probably consist of a tensorial enhanced effective tissue conductivity, possibly combined with a small heat sink, but this matter requires more tests. The relation between conductivity and vessel size, density, and blood flow also remains to be tested.

Underdosage caused by individual large vessels could be compensated by heating a larger tissue volume and/or increasing the power deposited in or close to that vessel (LAGENDIJK 1990; CREZEE and LAGENDIJK 1992), for hot water tubes this implies a reduction of the spacing.

Acknowledgment. This research was supported by a grant from the Dutch Cancer Society.

References

Babbs CF, Fearnot NE, Marchosky JA, Moran CJ, Jones JT, Plantenga TD (1990) Theoretical basis for controlling minimal tumor temperature during interstitial conductive heat therapy. IEEE Trans Biomed Eng 37: 662–672

Bos CK, Crezee J, Mooibroek J, Lagendijk JJW (1991) A perfusion technique for tongues to be used in bioheat transfer studies. Phys Med Biol 36: 843–846

Brezovich IA, Atkinson WJ (1984) Temperature distributions in tumor models heated by self-regulating nickel–copper alloy thermoseeds. Med Phys 11: 145–152

Chen MM, Holmes KR (1980) Microvascular contributions in tissue heat transfer. Ann NY Acad Sci 335: 137–151

Cosset JM, Bichler K-H, Strohmaier WL et al. (1990) Interstitial, endocavitary and perfusional hyperthermia. Methods and clinical trials. Springer, Berlin Heidelberg New York, pp 1–41

Crezee J, Lagendijk JJW (1990) Experimental verification of bioheat transfer theories: measurement of temperature profiles around large artificial vessels in perfused tissue. Phys Med Biol 35: 905–923

Crezee J, Lagendijk JJW (1992) Temperature uniformity during hyperthermia: the impact of large vessels. Phys Med Biol 37: 1321–1337

Crezee J, Mooibroek J, Bos CK, Lagendijk JJW (1991) Interstitial heating: experiments in artificially perfused bovine tongues. Phys Med Biol 36: 823–833

Deford JA, Babbs CF, Patel UH, Bleyer MW, Marchosky JA, Moran CJ (1991) Effective estimation and computer control of minimum tumour temperature during conductive interstitial hyperthermia. Int J Hyperthermia 7: 441–454

DeYoung DW, Kundrat MA, Cetas TC (1986) In vivo kidneys as preclinical thermal models for hyperthermia. Proceedings of the IEEE/9th Annual Conference of the Medical and Biological Society (Boston: IEEE No. 87CH2513-0): 994–996

Goffinet DR, Prionas SD, Kapp DS et al. (1990) Interstitial ^{192}Ir flexible catheter radiofrequency hyperthermia treatments of head and recurrent pelvic carcinomas. Int J Radiat Oncol Biol Phys 18: 199–210

Hand JW, Trembly BS, Prior MV (1992) Physics of interstitial hyperthermia. Radiofrequency and hot water tube techniques. In: Urano M, Douple E (eds) Hyperthermia and oncology, vol 3: Interstitial hyperthermia. European Book Service, de Meern, pp 99–134

Handl-Zeller L, Kärcher KH, Schreier K, Handl O (1986) Beitrag zur optimierung interstitieller hyperthermiesysteme. Strahlentherapie 163: 460–463

Holmes KR, Ryan W, Weinstein P, Chem MM (1984) A fixation technique for organs to be used as perfused tissue phantoms in bioheat transfer studies. Adv Bioeng ASME WAM: 9–10

Lagendijk JJW (1982) The influence of blood flow in large vessels on the temperature distribution in hyperthermia. Phys Med Biol 27: 17–23

Lagendijk JJW (1984) A new theory to calculate temperature distributions in tissues, or why the "bioheat transfer" equation does not work. In: Overgaard J (ed) Hyperthermic oncology 1984. Taylor & Francis, London, pp 507–510

Lagendijk JJW (1990) Thermal models: principles and implementation. In: Field SB, Hand JW (eds) An introduction to the practical aspects of clinical hyperthermia. Taylor & Francis, London, pp 478–512

Mechling JA, Strohbehn JW (1986) A theoretical comparison of the temperature distributions produced by three interstitial hyperthermia systems. Int J Radiat Oncol Biol Phys 12: 2137–2149

Milligan AJ, Conran PB, Ropar MA, McCulloch HA, Ahuja RK, Dobelbower RR (1983) Predictions of blood flow from thermal clearance during regional hyperthermia. Int J Radiat Oncol Biol Phys 9: 1335–1343

Mooibroek J, Lagendijk JJW (1991) A fast and simple algorithm for the calculation of convective heat transfer by large vessels in three dimensional inhomogeneous tissues. IEEE Trans Biomed Eng 38: 490–501

Pennes HH (1948) Analysis of tissue and arterial blood temperatures in the resting human forearm. J Appl Physiol 1: 93–122

Schreier K, Budihna M, Lesnicar H et al. (1990) Preliminary studies of interstitial 1 hyperthermia using hot water. Int J Hyperthermia 6: 431–444

Stauffer PR, Sneed PK, Suen SA, Satoh T, Matsumoto K, Fike JR, Philips TL (1989) Comparative thermal dosimetry of interstitial microwave and radiofrequency-LCF hyperthermia. Int J Hyperthermia 5: 307–318

Strohbehn JW (1983) Temperature distributions from interstitial rf electrode hyperthermia systems: theoretical predictions. Int J Radiat Oncol Biol Phys 9: 1655–1667

Strohbehn JW, Trembly BS, Douple EB (1982) Blood flow effects on the temperature distributions from an invasive microwave antenna array used in cancer therapy. IEEE Trans Biomed Eng 29: 649–661

Uzunoglu NK, Nikita KS (1988) Estimation of temperature distribution inside tissues heated by interstitial RF electrode hyperthermia systems. IEEE Trans Biomed Eng 35: 250–256

Weinbaum S, Jiji LM (1985) A new simplified bioheat equation for the effect of blood flow on local average tissue temperature. ASME J Biomech Eng 107: 131–139

20 Future Developments in Respect of Thermal Modeling, Treatment Planning, and Treatment Control for Interstitial Hyperthermia

J.J.W. LAGENDIJK, J. MOOIBROEK, and J. CREZEE

CONTENTS

20.1 Introduction

Progress in the clinical use of hyperthermia depends fundamentally on knowledge of the actual three-dimensional (3-D) temperature/thermal dose distributions in the heated tissues. Invasive thermometry alone cannot provide the high spatial resolution (< 0.5 cm) necessary to determine the steep thermal gradients in vascularized tissues, especially around the larger vessels (LAGENDIJK 1990; ROEMER 1990a). Recently great progress has been made in computing the 3-D temperature distribution (MOOIBROEK and LAGENDIJK 1991). However, the development of accurate 3-D hyperthermia treatment planning systems is still hindered by the complexity of tissue blood flow and the lack of information on normal and pathological vessel network properties of individual patients (LAGENDIJK 1990; ROEMER 1990a).

Interstitial hyperthermia (IHT) is the ideal test site for hyperthermia treatment planning owing to (a) the possibility of achieving detailed 3-D temperature mapping because of the number of catheters inserted and (b) the relatively small volumes to be heated, with potentially well-defined vascular networks. In IHT of brain, breast, and head and neck tumors in particular, the expectation is that hyperthermia treatment planning can be realized. High quality 3-D magnetic resonance imaging (MRI) and angiography (MRA) using head coils and surface coils are expected to supply both the anatomical and the vascular structures with such a resolution that the present discrete vessel thermal model will be able to calculate the temperature distribution (MOOIBROEK and LAGENDIJK 1991).

In the near future, IHT treatment planning will start with the catheter/electrode positions in 3-D. The SAR calculation, which will depend, of course, on the heating technique used, will be performed in a fully heterogeneous 3-D tissue space using segmented MRI and/or computed tomographic (CT) data. The resulting temperature distribution will be calculated on the basis of the SAR distribution, the 3-D anatomy, and the perfusion distribution and vascular network information down to at least the 0.5 mm vessel diameter level using MRA techniques. Computer techniques will allow 3-D multimodality display of anatomy (tissues, vessels, blood flow parameters), electrode positions, SAR, and the resulting temperature together with the interactive choice of electrode positions and spatial SAR control. In vivo pulse/transient techniques will supply tissue parameters such as the effective thermal conductivity. Future heating techniques must provide flexibility in SAR distribution and treatment control at a spatial scale of 1 cm (CREZEE and LAGENDIJK 1992). Treatment control will be achieved via corrected temperature measurements performed from inside the brachytherapy catheters backed up with on-line modeling information. The need for extra invasive probes for thermometry catheters, leading to increased trauma, will be absent.

In the remaining part of this chapter we will try to investigate this "heaven" and to define the present status and real developments to be expected in the near future.

J.J.W. LAGENDIJK, Ph.D.; J. MOOIBROEK, Ph.D.; J. CREZEE, Ph.D.; Department of Radiotherapy, University Hospital Utrecht, Heidelberglaan 100, NL-3584 CX Utrecht, The Netherlands

20.2 Three-Dimensional Brachytherapy Electrode/Catheter Definition

Three-dimensional reconstruction of catheter/source positions is already standard in brachytherapy planning. Data from CT or film or, in the near future, on-line directly from the image intensifier, can be used for the 3-D position reconstruction. Sophisticated image processing techniques can be used to visualize the 3-D geometry of the catheters in the anatomy. On-line reconstruction will become important for interactive catheter positioning and on-line treatment planning.

20.3 Determination of Anatomy for SAR Calculation

For both 3-D CT and 3-D MRI, the present small volume resolution is better than 2.5 mm and sufficient for the determination of the 3-D anatomy. Geometrical accuracy for CT is perfect; for MRI care must be taken in using external markers for catheter positioning due to geometrical distortion by susceptibility artifacts (Bhagwandien et al. 1992). All radiofrequency (RF) and microwave techniques require details of the dielectric structure for accurate computation of the SAR. Segmentation according to gray scales is possible with CT, but no data are available about the possible relation between Hounsfield units and the dielectric constants. However, the major difference in dielectric properties is between tissues of low water content and high water content (Guy 1971). This can be defined relatively easily and automatically by both CT and MRI. MRI can provide the water content of tissues and, in the near future, may provide the dielectric structure directly (Higer and Bielke 1990).

20.4 SAR Computation

The clinical application of SAR modeling of IHT is still in its infancy; progress in 3-D has only been made in local current field. (LCF) IHT. Most of the present experience is with two-dimensional models of homogeneous phantoms. The complex 3-D distributions around irregular LCF implants in inhomogeneous tissues are, from a theoretical point of view, not difficult to obtain. However, models to perform these extensive calculations have not been described in the literature. In homogeneous three-dimensional situations the Laplace equation $\mathrm{grad}(\mathrm{div}\,\mathbf{V}) = 0$ can be solved easily by numerical methods (Lagendijk 1990, 1991). The needles must be described as fixed potential lines (LCF voltage sources) or fixed current sources [LCF capacitive coupled systems (Visser et al. 1989; Deurloo et al. 1991)]. In heterogeneous structures, the voltage distribution is described by $\mathrm{div}[(\sigma + jw\varepsilon)\,\mathrm{grad}\,\mathbf{V}] = 0$, which can be solved using numerical techniques such as the impedance method (Sowinski and Van Den Berg 1990; Zhu and Gandhi 1988). However, because of the small diameter of the needles, small grid sizes must be applied to ensure accurate description of the high SAR peaks directly around the needles and especially around the needle tips. For low frequencies, the complex part may be omitted and the model is straightforward; for 27 MHz, however, the complex part must be considered too, which, unfortunately, will result in larger programs with longer computation time.

Interactive treatment planning is at least possible within the LCF environment. Fast source summation techniques allow interactive SAR calculation in homogeneous situations.

20.5 Thermal Modeling

Heat transport related to blood flow dominates bioheat transfer. The presence of large vessels and inhomogeneities in blood flow are the major causes of temperature nonuniformity which may result in underdosed areas in the tumor and unsuccessful treatment (Valdagni et al. 1990). This makes it of utmost importance that heat transfer by blood flow is described correctly in the thermal models (for reviews, see Chato 1990; Lagendijk 1990; Roemer 1990a).

In recent years great progress has been made (a) in the development and verification of heat transfer theories for vascularized tissues (Chen and Holmes 1980; Weinbaum and Jiji 1985; Crezee and Lagendijk 1990; Crezee et al. 1991; this volume, Chap. 19) and (b) in computing the 3-D temperature distribution in tissues containing discrete branching vessels (Mooibroek and Lagendijk 1991; this volume, Chap. 16). However, thermal modeling is still hindered by the complexity of tissue blood flow and the lack of information on normal and pathological vessel network properties of individual patients (Lagendijk 1990; Roemer 1990a). A quantitative prediction of the temperature requires that anatomical data, particularly discrete large vessels (diameter $> \approx 0.5$ mm), are incorporated into the numerical model. Smaller vessels may be described by the effective thermal conductivity continuum theory (CREZEE and LAGENDIJK 1990). Uncertainty exists about the type and level of errors which will occur at the transition from the discrete large vessel description towards the effective thermal conductivity continuum model. This area is presently attracting much attention. Ultimately the errors in the temperature distributions predicted will depend greatly on the quality of the angiography techniques used and the degree of resolution which can be achieved in the model.

Recent developments in digital subtraction angiography (DSA) and in particular MRA can be used to supply the vascular data. During the last 2 years, MRA has entered the clinical routine and evolved as a noninvasive technique which, at specific body sites, e.g., cerebral vessel anatomy, can compete with other standard angiographic methods (SCHMALBROCK et al. 1990; PAVONE et al. 1990; MASARYK et al. 1989; EDELMAN et al. 1989a). By optimizing the hardware and using special pulse sequences and/or contrast agents (Gd-DTPA), it is expected that this will also become the case for other body sites such as the abdomen, pelvis, and extremities (KIM et al. 1990; FRUCHT et al. 1989; EDELMAN et al. 1989b). A major advantage of MRA over other methods is its capability to image not only the 3-D arterial architecture but also the venous vessel anatomy (CHAKERES et al. 1990; KIM and CHO 1990; EDELMAN et al. 1989b).

The quantification of blood flow by MRA shows the same evolutionary trend as depicted above, but with some phase lag. Its state of art has been reviewed in the workshop on magnetic resonance of blood flow held in Philadelphia (USA) (SMRM Workshop 1990). Promising clinical results have been reported by HAACKE et al. (1990) and LAUB (1990) with emphasis on the cerebral blood flow.

One of the remaining problems with respect to thermal modeling is how to represent both the vessel architecture and the flow in such a way that they can be loaded into a hyperthermia treatment planning system. For DSA several techniques have been developed to reconstruct vessel architecture from 2-D or 3-D vessel imaging data (SUN 1989). The one which matches the segmental approach of vessels (MOOIBROEK and LAGENDIJK 1991) is the work presented by SMETS (1990) and VANDERMEULEN (1991), which also gives the state of art in this particular field of investigation.

In Utrecht we will, in collaboration with Nucletron International, incorporate our thermal model (MOOIBROEK and LAGENDIJK 1991) into an IHT Planning System in order to predict, control, and evaluate the temperature distribution in the tumor and in the healthy tissue. We plan to incorporate the complete 3-D anatomy with a spatial resolution of 1 mm. For regular implants, $10 \times 10 \times 10$ cm^3 volumes with $100 \times 100 \times 100$ nodes seem feasible. This will allow us to insert discrete vessels down to about the 0.5 mm diameter scale. Modern Unix workstations can easily handle this amount of data while special algorithms (MOOIBROEK and LAGENDIJK 1991) can speed up computation. General purpose parallel processing systems which can increase the speed of computation further are entering the Unix market (e.g., SUN 600 series). Present applications are limited by the 3-D angiography and not by computer power. Speed and degree of interaction will become important because predicted areas of underdosage may require direct insertion of extra catheters during implantation.

20.6 Three-Dimensional Thermometry

Thermometry can be performed at a large number of locations without increasing trauma because of the array of catheters and/or needles inserted for IHT. LCF electrodes can easily be made compatible with thermocouples' thermometry using common catheters. Disturbance of the thermometry due to RF/microwave interference, self-heating of the electrodes, and thermal conduction by the the electrode must be investigated carefully (RYAN et al. 1989) but can be solved in most cases by RF filtering and a good description of heat flow within and around the electrode/catheter. The incorporation of the catheters and electrodes/antennas in thermal models will permit accurate prediction of the complete temperature field provided that, as described above, blood flow is incorporated correctly in the model too. Maximum temperatures will often occur at the needles, particularly when a larger spacing is used. Thus, depending upon the accuracy of the model used, additional thermometry sensors may be required in extra catheters to verify the thermometry and thermal modeling.

Invasive thermometry can be used for SAR measurements and evaluation of the local blood flow (ROEMER et al. 1985; LAGENDIJK et al. 1988;

ROEMER 1990b), while the effective thermal conductivity, an important parameter, can be measured using the transient temperature effect between needles. This information is essential as input data for accurate thermal modeling (CREZEE et al. 1991).

20.7 Conclusions

As stated in the Introduction, IHT is the ideal test site for hyperthermia treatment planning due to the unique situation of a relatively large number of available catheters and the relatively small volumes to be heated. However, progress in IHT treatment planning will depend greatly on the progress being made in imaging techniques, while progress in its clinical application will also depend on the flexibility and reliability of future IHT systems.

References

Bhagwandien R, van Ee R, Beersma R, Bakker CJG, Moerland MA, Lagendijk JJW (1992) Numerical analysis of the magnetic field for arbitrary permeability distributions in 2D. Magn Reson Imag 10: 299–313

Chakeres DW, Schmalbrock P, Brogan M, Yuan C, Cohen L (1990) Normal venous anatomy of the brain: demonstration with gadopentetate dimeglumine in enhanced 3-D MR angiography. ANJR 11: 1107–1118

Chato JC (1990) Fundamentals of bioheat transfer. In: Gautherie M (ed) Thermal dosimetry and treatment planning. Springer, Berlin Heidelberg New York, pp 1–56

Chen MM, Holmes KR (1980) Microvascular contributions in tissue heat transfer. Ann NY Acad Sci 335: 137–151

Crezee J, Lagendijk JJW (1990) Experimental verification of bioheat transfer theories: measurement of temperature profiles around large artificial vessels in perfused tissue. Phys Med Biol 35: 905–923

Crezee J, Lagendijk JJW (1992) Temperature uniformity during hyperthermia: the impact of large vessels. Phys Med Biol 37(6): 1321–1337

Crezee J, Mooibroek J, Bos CK, Lagendijk JJW (1991) Interstitial heating: experiments in artificially perfused bovine tongues. Phys Med Biol 6: 843–846

Deurloo IKK, Visser AG, Morawska M, van Geel CAJF, van Rhoon GC, Levendag PC (1991) Application of a capacitive-coupling interstitial hyperthermia system at 27 MHz: study of different applicator configurations. Phys Med Biol 36: 119–132

Edelman RR, Wentz K, Mattle HP et al. (1989a) Intracerebral arteriovenous malformations: evaluation with selective MR angiography and venography. Radiology 173: 831–837

Edelman RR, Wentz KU, Mattle H, Zhao B, Liu C, Kim D, Laub G (1989b) Projection arteriography and venography: initial clinical results with MR. Radiology 172: 351–357

Frucht H, Doppman JL, Norton JA et al. (1989) Gastrinomas: comparison of MR imaging with CT, angiography and US. Radiology 171: 713–717

Guy AW (1971) Analyses of electromagnetic fields induced in biological tissues by thermographic studies on equivalent phantom models. IEEE Trans Microwave Theory Tech 19: 205–214

Haacke EM, Masaryk TJ, Wielopolski PA (1990) Optimizing blood vessel contrast in fast three-dimensional MRI. Magn Reson Med 14: 202–221

Higer HP, Bielke G (eds) (1990) Tissue characterization in MR imaging; clinical and technical approaches. Springer, Berlin Heidelberg New York

Kim JH, Cho ZH (1990) 3-D MR angiography with scanning 2-D images – simultaneous data acquisition of arteries and veins (SAAV). Magn Reson Med 14: 554–561

Kim D, Edelman RR, Kent KC, Porter DH, Skillman JJ (1990) Abdominal aorta and renal artery stenosis: evaluation with MR angiography. Radiology 174: 727–731

Lagendijk JJW (1990) Thermal models: principles and implementation. In: Field SB, Hand JW (eds) An introduction to the practical aspects of clinical hyperthermia. Taylor & Francis, London, pp 478–512

Lagendijk JJW (1991) A 3-d SAR model for voltage and current source LCF interstitial hyperthermia systems. Strahlenther Onkol 167: 329

Lagendijk JJW, Hofman P, Schipper J (1988) Perfusion analyses in advanced breast carcinoma during hyperthermia. Int J Hyperthermia 4: 479–495

Laub G (1990) Displays for MR angiography. Magn Reson Med 14: 222–229

Masaryk TJ, Modic MR, Ross JS et al. (1989) Intracranial circulation: preliminary clinical results with three-dimensional (volume) MR angiography. Radiology 171: 793–799

Mooibroek J, Lagendijk JJW (1991) A fast and simple algorithm for the calculation of convective heat transfer by large vessels in three dimensional inhomogeneous tissues. IEEE Trans Biomed Eng 38: 490–501

Pavone P, Di Cesare E, Di Renzi P, Marsili L, Ventura M, Spartera C, Passariello R (1990) Abdominal aortic aneurysm evaluation: comparison of US, CT, MRI, and angiography. Magn Reson Imag 8: 199–204

Roemer RB (1990a) Thermal dosimetry. In: Gautherie M (ed) Thermal dosimetry and treatment planning. Springer, Berlin Heidelberg New York, pp 119–214

Roemer RB (1990b) The local tissue cooling coefficient: a unified approach to thermal washout and steady-state 'perfusion' calculations. Int. J Hyperthermia 6: 421–430

Roemer RB, Fletcher AM, Cetas TC (1985) Obtaining local SAR and blood perfusion data from temperature measurements: steady-state and transient techniques compared. Int J Radiat Oncol Biol Phys 11: 1539–1550

Ryan TP, Samulski TV, Lyons BE, Lee E, Holdren D, Fessenden P, Strohbehn JW (1989) Thermal conduction effects associated with temperature measurements in proximity to radiofrequency electrodes and microwave antennas. Int J Radiat Oncol Biol Phys 16: 1557–1564

Schmalbrock P, Yuan C, Chakeres DW, Kohli J, Pelc NJ (1990) Volume MR angiography: methods to achieve very short echo times. Radiology 175: 861–865

Smets C (1990) A knowledge-based system for the automatic interpretation of blood vessels on angiograms. Thesis. Katholieke Universiteit, Leuven

SMRM Workshop (1990) Magnetic resonance imaging of blood flow. Magn Reson Med 14: 171–315

Sowinski MJ, Van Den Berg PM (1990) A three-dimensional iterative scheme for an electromagnetic capacitive applicator. IEEE Trans Biomed Eng 37: 975–986

Sun Y (1989) Automated identification of vessel contours in coronary arteriograms by an adaptive tracking algorithm. IEEE Trans Med Imag 8: 78–88

Valdagni R et al. (1990) International consensus meeting on hyperthermia, final report. Int J Hyperthermia 6: 837–878

Vandermeulen D (1991) Methods for registration, interpolation of three dimensional medical imaging data for use in 3-D display, 3-D modelling and therapy planning. Thesis. Katholieke Universiteit, Leuven

Visser AG, Deurlo IKK, Levendag PC, Ruifrok ACC, Cornet B, van Rhoon GC (1989) An interstitial hyperthermia system at 27 MHz. Int J Hyperthermia 5: 265–276

Weinbaum S, Jiji LM (1985) A new simplified bioheat equation for the effect of blood flow on local average tissue temperature. ASME J Biomech Eng 107: 131–139

Zhu Xi-Li, Gandhi Om P (1988) Design of RF needle applicators for optimum SAR distributions in irregular shaped tumors. IEEE Trans Biomed Eng 35: 382–388

Part III
Review of Clinical Experience

21 Rationale for Interstitial Thermoradiotherapy for Tumors in the Head and Neck Region

R. Fietkau, G.G. Grabenbauer, and M.H. Seegenschmiedt

CONTENTS

21.1 Introduction

The objective of both interstitial hyperthermia and interstitial radiotherapy is to increase local control. The main advantage of *brachytherapy* is that it delivers a high dose to a well-circumscribed area without excessive irradiation to the surrounding structures. For head and neck tumors, low dose rate radioactive sources are used in nearly all institutions; a dose of 20–30 Gy can be applied within 3–5 days at a rate of 30–70 cGy/h. According to Hall (1985), the radiobiology of low dose irradiation is characterized by increased repair of sublethal and lethal damage. This is responsible for the broad initial shoulder of the cell survival curve during acute low dose rate exposure. Consideration also has to be given to the "inverse dose rate effect," i.e., for a limited range of dose rates the survival curve steepens again as cells progress through the cell cycle and pile up at a G_2 block, which is a radiosensitive phase during which the cells cannot divide. A further lowering of the dose rate allows cells to escape the G_2 block and divide. Cell proliferation may then occur during protracted exposure. Whether pulsed high dose rate interstitial therapy can match all the effects of continuous low dose rate irradiation is the subject of ongoing investigations (Brenner and Hall 1991).

Hyperthermia is based on two main biological effects: First, hyperthermia has cytotoxic effects at temperatures above 42.5°–43°C. Second, hyperthermia offers radiosensitizing effects at temperatures above 41°C; this can be mainly attributed to decreased repair of sublethal and potentially lethal damage. This complementary interaction of hyperthermia and radiotherapy provides a strong biological rationale for their combined clinical application, especially since the two interstitial methods can be easily combined without major modifications of either technique.

In searching for a potential field of clinical application for interstitial thermoradiotherapy it is first necessary to review the local control rates for different treatment strategies, different tumor sites, and different tumor stages. Secondly an ethical question has to be raised: What rate of local or regional recurrence is acceptable? In this context one has to consider the extent to which a local recurrence influences the quality of life of these patients. The third step is a statistical consideration: What local control rate must be achieved to increase the survival rate of patients? Or, which palliative response suffices to justify the use of hyperthermia?

In this chapter we will not discuss the following questions: What is the cost-effectiveness of interstitial hyperthermia? What results of interstitial hyperthermia have been published and do these results indeed indicate a possible role of hyperthermia in oncology? Are there sufficient patients available for randomized or nonrandomized studies? Can adequate heating and temperature monitoring be achieved with currently available technology in specific tumor sites?

R. Fietkau, M.D.; G.G. Grabenbauer, M.D.; M.H. Seegenschmiedt, M.D.; Strahlentherapeutische Klinik, Universität Erlangen-Nürnberg, Universitätsstraße 27, W-8520 Erlangen, Germany

21.2 Implantation Techniques and Tumor Regions Accessible for Implantation

A variety of techniques are in clinical use for interstitial radiotherapy. The most important ones are the plastic tube technique (Syed and Feder 1977) and the use of rigid steel needle implants, i.e., guide gutters (Pierquin et al. 1991). The advantage of guide gutters or steel needle implants with the help of templates is that the implantation geometry is automatically predetermined by the inherent spacing between the branches or the hollows of the template. Thus parallelism between the needles can be easily achieved and maintained. On the other hand, rigid needle implants cause the patient significant discomfort during a treatment course of 3–5 days. Moreover, straight implants are not possible in all sites. Using plastic applicators, curved implants, such as loops and arches, are easily achieved. This is very helpful given the complex anatomy of the head and neck region. Especially tumors of the base of tongue, tonsillar region, oropharyngeal wall, uvula, and soft palate represent straightforward indications for the use of plastic applicators.

The interstitial heating technique is predetermined by the applied brachytherapy technique. Microwave techniques, hot water perfusion techniques, and ferromagnetic seeds can be applied using plastic applicators, whereas with rigid steel needle implants only radiofrequency techniques and hot water perfusion techniques can be used. Specific advantages and disadvantages of the various techniques and quality assurance have recently been reviewed by Emami et al. (1987) and Seegenschmiedt and Sauer (1992), and the interested reader is referred to these overviews.

Carcinomas of the floor of the mouth, mobile tongue, lip, buccal mucosa, and base of the tongue are easily accessible for implantation. We recommend that implantation is performed under general anesthesia in the operating room in order to obtain an exact overview of the tumor region and the extension of the tumor during the surgical procedure. Moreover, "optimal" implant geometry with parallelism of applicators and equidistant spacing is then easier to achieve.

Implantation of carcinomas of the tonsillar region, lateral or posterior wall of the oropharynx, or neck nodes is sometimes difficult due to the proximity of the carotid artery, which may be damaged by the needles. However, bleeding from the carotid artery can be stopped by careful compression and tamponade; surgical intervention is required only exceptionally. Nevertheless, before implantation one must be sure that the carotid artery is not infiltrated by the tumor; this can be demonstrated by computed tomographic scans. During the implantation procedure or removal of the catheters, or even later, hemorrhage can occur at the implantation site which cannot be easily controlled by any means.

To date, implantation of carcinomas of the hypopharynx, larynx, and nasopharynx is nearly impossible owing to anatomical restrictions. Implantation of the cartilage structures, i.e., thyroid cartilage or arytenoid cartilage, is not advisable because of the risk of cartilage necrosis which can lead to pharyngocutaneous fistulas. We have sometimes performed an implantation for supraglottic cancers if we found residual tumor in the base of the tongue following surgery.

At the time of applicator explantation, it must be ensured that appropriate facilities and sufficient staff are available so that immediate anesthesia and emergency surgery can be performed in response to any resulting hemorrhage, with prompt aspiration, should this prove necessary.

21.3 Results of Treatment of Primary Tumors

21.3.1 Early Tumor Stages

Early stage tumors are defined in this context as T1 or T2 tumors according to the UICC classification criteria (Table 21.1). One must be aware that the results of different authors are influenced by their specific staging method and the staging system used, the follow-up period, and the definition of local control and local recurrences, all of which vary quite considerably (Parsons et al. 1990). In general the results of most publications cannot be compared directly. With regard to this problem, we have tabulated the follow-up times and the relative and absolute numbers of recurrences. To summarize the local recurrence rates according to the life-table method was nearly impossible, because these values were not mentioned in many references. As we have focused our interest on local recurrence, the nodal status is not discussed in this chapter. Nevertheless, most tumors of the neck must be treated by neck dissection and/or radiotherapy.

Table 21.1. Comparison of the different classification systems of the American Joint Committee on Cancer (AJCC 1983/1988) and of the UICC (1985/1987). In their last edition UICC and AJCC made several major changes in the previous N classifications to have a world wide uniform TNM system. The staging system of the primary tumour did not change between 1982 and 1988

Oro-Pharynx		*Lip and Oral Cavity*	
Tx	Primary tumor cannot be assessed	Tx	Primary tumor cannot be assested
To	No evidence of primary tumor	To	No evidence of primary tumor
Tis	Carcinoma in situ	Tis	Carcinoma in situ
T1	Tumor 2 cm or less in greatest dimension	T1	Tumor 2 cm or less in greatest dimension
T2	Tumor more than 2 cm but not more than 4 cm in greatest dimension	T2	Tumor more than 2 cm but not more than 4 cm in greatest dimension
T3	Tumor more than 4 cm in greatest dimension	T3	Tumor more than 4 cm in greatest dimension
T4	Tumor invades adjacent structures, e.g. through cortical bone, soft tissues of the neck, deep (extrin-sic) muscle of tongue	T4	Tumor invades adjacent structures. Lip: e.g. through cortical bone, tongue, skin of neck. Oral cavity: through cortical bone, into deep (extrinsic) muscle of tongue, maxillary sinus, skin

N status	*UICC 1985*	*AJCC 1983*	*UICC 1987*	*AJCC 1988*
N/pNx	[------------ Regional lymph nodes cannot be assessed ------------]			
N/pNo	[------------ No regional lymph node metastasis ------------]			
N/pN1	Metastasis in movable ipsilateral lymph nodes	[-------- Metastasis in a single ipsilateral lymph node, 3 cm or less in greatest dimension --------]		
N/pN2	Metastasis in movable contralateral or bilateral lymph nodes	[----- *N2A* Metastasis in a single ipsilateral lymph node > 3 cm but not more than 6 cm -----] [----- *N2B* Metastasis in multiple ipsilateral lymph nodes, none more than 6 cm -----]		
			N2C Metastasis in bilateral or contralateral lymph nodes, none more than 6 cm	
N/pN3	Fixed regional lymph node(s)	*N3A* Massive homolateral node(s), at least one > 6 cm *N3B* Bilateral clinically positive nodes (each side should be staged separately) *N3C* Contralateral clnically positive node(s) only	[--- Metastasis in a lymph node > 6 cm ---]	

Distant Metastases	
Mx	Presence of distant metastasis cannot be assessed
Mo	No evidence of distant metastases
M1	Evidence of distant metastases

21.3.1.1 Tumors of the Oral Cavity

T1 and T2 tumors can be treated by surgery alone, or by interstitial or external beam radiotherapy alone. Moreover, different combinations of these strategies are used. Tables 21.2–21.5 show the results achieved with these modalities, as assessed by the rates of local recurrence. After surgery (Table 21.2), local recurrences occur in 0%–20% (T1) and 0%–28% (T2). Especially French groups have reported excellent local control rates after interstitial therapy alone (Table 21.3). Local recurrences were reported in 3%–18% for T1 and 10%–56% for T2 stages. Intraoral cone radiation

Table 21.2. Percentage of local recurrences after surgery alone for carcinomas of the oral cavity. Successful salvage therapies are not considered

Reference	Site	Surgical therapy	Local recurrences T1		T2		T3		Follow-up
AKINE et al. (1991)	Tongue	Partial glossectomy	–	–	–	(8%)	–		3 yr[b]
GRANDI et al. (1993)	Floor of the mouth	3 × intraoral excision; 29 × intraoral + suprahyoid resection; 7 × hemimandibulectomy	10/39 (T1 + T2)			(26%)	–		?
GUERRY et al. (1986)[a]	Oral cavity	Laser resection	5/33	(15%)	0/5		–		>3 yr
JOHNSON et al. (1980)	Tongue	?	3/28	(11%)	–		–		?
LEIPZIG et al. (1982)	Tongue	?	2/22	(9%)	1/16	(7%)	–		?
MARKS et al. (1983)	Floor of the mouth	Local excision	4/7	(57%)	–		–		?
NATHANSON et al. (1989)	Tongue	Partial glossectomy	10/58	(17%)	–		–		>2 yr
O'BRIEN et al. (1986)	Tongue	Partial glossectomy	3/67	(4.5%)	5/30	(17%)	–		Median 10 yr
SCHRAMM et al. (1980)	Floor of the mouth	Transoral surgical excision, mandibular resection	0/28	–	–	–	–		>2 yr
WHITEHURST and DROULIAS (1977)	Tongue	Local excision	15/82	(18%)	8/28	(28%)	2/14	(14%)	5 yr
YCO and CRUICKSHANK (1986)	Floor of the mouth	Partial glossectomy or hemiglossectomy	4/20	(20%)	–	–	–		>5 yr

[a] Some patients irradiated
[b] Actuarial local control

therapy has been used instead of interstitial implantation in selected patients with small superficial lesions (Table 21.5). Moreover, local control rates of 80%–90% have been obtained for T1 tumors (WANG 1989). KORB et al. (1991) have reported their experience with surgery and pre- or postoperative radiotherapy (Table 21.5). After 3 years they had obtained adjusted local control rates of 83% (T1) and 67% (T2). In our department we have used a combination of enoral surgery and interstitial and external beam radiotherapy (FIETKAU et al. 1991a). After a median follow-up of 17 months no local recurrences had occurred in patients with T1 tumors, and only one was seen in 20 patients with T2 tumors (rate: 5%). In comparison with the aforementioned results the local control rates achieved with external beam radiotherapy alone (Table 21.5) or in combination with interstitial implantation (Table 21.4) are worse. Local recurrences have been reported in 23%–38% of patients with T1 tumors and 20%–64% with T2 tumors.

21.3.1.2 Tumors of the Oropharynx

Brachytherapy is less frequently performed for oropharyngeal tumors than for oral cavity carcinomas. Moreover oropharyngeal tumors often involve the ipsilateral and contralateral neck nodes since some lymphatics cross the midline. In these cases interstitial radiotherapy is always used as a boost to the primary tumor site before or, as in most cases, after external beam irradiation. The comprehensive analysis (Table 21.6) for carcinomas of the base of tongue shows local recurrences in 0%–15% (T1) and 12%–41% (T2) of cases. The value of interstitial boost therapy is the subject of controversy in the literature. In a literature review, FOOTE et al. (1990) compared the results of combined interstitial and external beam therapy versus external beam irradiation alone and found no difference in terms of local control. After external beam irradiation alone, local recurrences are reported in 4%–22% (T1) and 10%–53% (T2) of cases (Table 21.7). FOOTE et al. (1990) concluded that interstitial implantation is not essential for successful radiotherapeutic management of base of tongue carcinomas. In contrast, HOUSSET et al. (1991) reported that local failures occurred twice as often in patients with base of tongue carcinomas (T1/T2) treated by external beam irradiation alone (43%) as in patients treated with implantation plus external beam

Table 21.3. Percentage of local recurrences after interstitial radiotherapy alone for squamous cell carcinomas of the oral cavity. Successful salvage treatments are not considered

<table>
<tr><th rowspan="2">Reference</th><th rowspan="2">No. of cases</th><th rowspan="2">Nuclides</th><th rowspan="2">Follow-up</th><th colspan="2">Local recurrences</th></tr>
<tr><th>T_1</th><th>T_2</th></tr>
<tr><td>AYGUN et al. (1984)[a]</td><td>14</td><td>^{226}Ra</td><td>> 2 yr</td><td>1/9 (11%)</td><td>0/5 –</td></tr>
<tr><td>BENK et al. (1990)[b]</td><td>85</td><td>^{192}Ir</td><td>?</td><td>–</td><td>10/85 (12%)</td></tr>
<tr><td>LEFEBVRE et al. (1990)[b]</td><td>263</td><td>^{192}Ir</td><td>?</td><td>2/89 (3%)</td><td>19/174 (11%)</td></tr>
<tr><td>MAZERON et al. (1990b)[b]</td><td>121</td><td>^{192}Ir</td><td>Median 10 yr</td><td>8/57 (18%)</td><td>10/64 (16%)</td></tr>
<tr><td>MAZERON et al. (1990a)[a]</td><td>116</td><td>^{192}Ir</td><td>> 11 mo</td><td>3/46 (7%)</td><td>20/70 (29%)</td></tr>
<tr><td>PERNOT et al. (1990a)[b]</td><td>70</td><td>^{192}Ir</td><td>5 yr Local control</td><td>–</td><td>– (10%)</td></tr>
<tr><td>WENDT et al. (1990a)[b]</td><td>17</td><td>^{192}Ir</td><td>> 2 yr</td><td>1/8 (12.5%)</td><td>5/9 (56%)</td></tr>
<tr><td>MAZERON et al. (1991)[a,b]</td><td>279</td><td>^{192}Ir</td><td>Mean 51 mo</td><td>14/134 (10%)</td><td>25/145 (17%)</td></tr>
<tr><td>KORB et al. (1991)[b]</td><td>11</td><td>^{192}Ir
^{226}Ra
^{198}Au</td><td>3 yr</td><td colspan="2">(29%)</td></tr>
</table>

[a] Floor of the mouth
[b] Mobile tongue

Table 21.4. Percentage of local recurrences after combined interstitial and external beam radiotherapy for squamous cell carcinomas of the oral cavity. Successful salvage therapies are not considered

<table>
<tr><th rowspan="2">Reference</th><th rowspan="2">No. of cases</th><th rowspan="2">Nuclides</th><th rowspan="2">Follow-up</th><th colspan="4">Local recurrences</th></tr>
<tr><th>T_1</th><th>T_2</th><th>T_3</th><th>T_4</th></tr>
<tr><td>AKINE et al. (1991)[a]</td><td>?</td><td>^{192}Ir/^{226}Ra</td><td>3 yr[c]</td><td>(12%)</td><td>(9%)</td><td>–</td><td>–</td></tr>
<tr><td>AYGUN et al. (1984)[b]</td><td>40</td><td>^{226}Ra</td><td>> 2 yr</td><td>3/9 (33%)</td><td>5/15 (33%)</td><td>6/9 (66%)</td><td>7/7 (100%)</td></tr>
<tr><td>BENK et al. (1990)[a]</td><td>25</td><td>^{192}Ir</td><td>?</td><td>–</td><td>16/25 (64%)</td><td>–</td><td>–</td></tr>
<tr><td>DEARNALEY et al. (1990)[a,b]</td><td>149</td><td>^{192}Ir/^{137}Cs</td><td>Mean 59 mo</td><td colspan="2">23%[d]</td><td colspan="2">75%</td></tr>
<tr><td>KORB et al. (1991)[a]</td><td>21</td><td>^{192}Ir/^{226}Ra/ ^{198}Au</td><td>3 yr</td><td colspan="4">(33%)</td></tr>
<tr><td>LEFEBVRE et al. (1990)[a]</td><td>78</td><td>^{192}Ir</td><td>?</td><td colspan="4">17/78 (22%)[e]</td></tr>
<tr><td>MARKS et al. (1983)[b]</td><td>44</td><td>?</td><td>?</td><td>5/14 (36%)</td><td>3/15 (20%)</td><td>4/15 (26%)</td><td>–</td></tr>
<tr><td>MENDENHALL et al. (1989)[a]</td><td>28</td><td>^{226}Ra</td><td>> 2 yr</td><td>–</td><td>13/31 (39%)</td><td>–</td><td>–</td></tr>
<tr><td>NOWAK et al. (1990)[a,b]</td><td>35</td><td>^{192}Ir</td><td>Median 41 mo</td><td colspan="2">16/35 (46%)</td><td></td><td></td></tr>
<tr><td>PERNOT et al. (1990)[a]</td><td>77</td><td>^{192}Ir</td><td>5 yr Local control</td><td>–</td><td>(51%)</td><td>–</td><td>–</td></tr>
<tr><td>PUTHAWALA et al. (1981)[a]</td><td>26</td><td>^{192}Ir</td><td>> 28 mo</td><td colspan="2">4/13 (31%)</td><td colspan="2">7/13 (54%)</td></tr>
<tr><td>WANG (1989)[a]</td><td>49</td><td>^{226}Ra/^{192}Ir</td><td>5 yr[c]</td><td>(23%)</td><td>(54%)</td><td>–</td><td>–</td></tr>
<tr><td>WENDT et al. (1990a)[a]</td><td>70</td><td>^{226}Ra</td><td>> 2 yr</td><td>2/8 (25%)</td><td>16/62 (25%)</td><td>–</td><td>–</td></tr>
</table>

iRT, interstitial radiotherapy; eRT, external beam radiotherapy
[a] Mobile tongue
[b] Floor of the mouth
[c] Actuarial local control
[d] iRT or iRT + eRT
[e] cT1-4 cN2-3 treated by eRT + iRT; cT3 N0 and cT1-3 N1 treated by iRT alone

irradiation (20.5%) GOFFINET et al. (1985a) compared interstitial plus external beam irradiation and surgery plus external beam irradiation. A higher rate of local recurrence was found in the surgically treated group (5/14) (cf. 2/14 in the implanted group).

Other regions of the oropharynx are in most instances treated with external beam radiotherapy alone or with combined surgery and radiotherapy. Results of implantation are only sporadically reported. PERNOT et al. (1990b) reported a locoregional control rate at 5 years of 76% in a series of 270 patients with carcinomas of the palatotonsillar area. In smaller series of tumors of the tonsillar region, MAZERON et al. (1987c) and PUTHAWALA et al. (1985) achieved local control in 80%–100% (T1 and T2). Local control rates of 80%–90% were reported by MAZERON et al. (1987) for cancer of the

Table 21.5. Percantage of local recurrences after use of different treatment modalities for squamous cell carcinomas of the oral cavity. Successful salvage treatments are not considered

Reference	No. of cases	Follow-up	Therapy	Local recurrences			
				T1	T2	T3	T4
AKINE et al. (1991)[a]	31	3 yr[c]	IOI	(23%)	(50%)	–	–
WANG (1989)[a]	73	5 yr[c]	IOI+eRT	(10%)	(15%)	–	–
AYGUN et al. (1984)[b]	55	>2 yr	eRT	–	–	18/26[d]	24/29[d]
ILDSTAD et al. (1983)[a]	58		eRT	3/11 (27%)	11/23 (48%)	5/10 (50%)	10/14 (71%)
KORB et al. (1991)[a]	25	3 yr[c]	eRT	33% (T1–T2)		–	–
LEIPZIG et al. (1982)[a]	53	?	eRT	3/8 (38%)	8/14 (57%)	22/31 (71%)[d]	
WENDT et al. (1990a)[a]	7	>2 yr	eRT	–	5/7 (71%)	–	–
WHITE and BYERS (1980)	63		eRT	0/8	9/38 (23%)	12/17 (70%) (T3–T4)	
GRANDI et al. (1983)[b]	36	?	Surg+eRT±CT		11/36 (31%) (T2–T3)		
KORB et al. (1991)[a]	37	3 yr[c]	Surg+eRT	(17%)	(33%)	0/4	
LEIPZIG et al. (1982)[a]	13	?	Surg+eRT	–	–	2/13 (15%)[d]	
MARKS et al. (1983)[b]	63	?	Surg+eRT	1/12 (8%)	4/30 (13%)	6/21 (29%)	
WAZER et al. (1989)[a,b]	12	?	Surg+eRT	–	–	1/6[d]	2/6[d]

IOI, intraoral cone irradiation; eRT, external beam radiotherapy; Surg, surgery; CT, chemotherapy
[a] Oral tongue
[b] Floor of the mouth
[c] Actuarial local control
[d] Stage III, IV

Table 21.6. Percentage of local recurrences after combined interstitial and external beam radiotherapy for squamous cell carcinomas of the base of the tongue. Results of salvage treatments are not considered

Reference	No. of cases	Nuclide	Follow-up	Local recurrences			
				T_1	T_2	T_3	T_4
CROOK et al. (1988)	48	^{192}Ir	5 yr	2/13 (15%)	10/35 (29%)	–	–
GARDNER et al. (1987)	34	^{226}Ra	>2 yr	0/13	5/8	2/8	1/5
GOFFINET et al. (1985a)	14	^{192}Ir	Mean 32 mo	2/14 (14%) (T1–T4)			
HARRISON et al. (1989)	16	^{192}Ir	8–29 mo	0/4	1/6	1/6	–
HOUSSET et al. (1987)	29	^{192}Ir	>4 yr	0/6	6/23 (26%)	–	–
LUSINCHI et al. (1989)	108	^{192}Ir	5 yr	2/18 (11%)	16/39 (41%)	16/51 (31%)	–
PUTHAWALA et al. (1987)	70	^{192}Ir	?	0/2	2/16 (12%)	10/40 (25%)	4/12 (33%)
VIKRAM et al. (1985)	10	^{192}Ir	1–5 yr	0/1	0/2	0/7	–
HOFFSTETTER et al. (1986)	108	^{192}Ir	3 yr	(22%) (T1–T2)		–	–

Table 21.7. Percentage of local recurrences after external beam radiotherapy alone for squamous cell carcinomas of the base of the tongue. Successful salvage treatments are not considered

Reference	No. of cases	Follow-up	Local recurrences			
			T1	T2	T3	T4
BLUMBERG et al. (1979)	32	>2 yr	0/5	2/10 (20%)	7/13 (54%)	3/4
FOOTE et al. (1990)	84	>2 yr	1/9 (11%)	3/30 (10%)	6/31 (19%)	9/14 (64%)
GARDNER et al. (1987)	90	>2 yr	2/9 (22%)	8/23 (35%)	7/29 (24%)	14/29 (48%)
HOUSSET et al. (1987)	54	>4 yr	4/19 (21%)	19/35 (54%)	–	–
JAULERRY et al. (1991)	131	5 yr	1/22 (4%)	20/45 (46%)	38/64 (63%)	–
SPANOS et al. (1976)	174	>2 yr	3/32 (9%)	14/49 (29%)	14/64 (22%)	14/29 (48%)

soft palate and uvula and by ESCHE et al. (1988) for carcinoma of the uvula.

21.3.2 Advanced Tumor Stages

In this context we define T3/T4 tumors (Table 21.1) as locally advanced tumors. No differentiation was made between various subregions of the head and neck, because there are no great differences in treatment strategies, biological behavior, or clinical results. Moreover a clear differentiation is sometimes impossible and is therefore omitted from many publications. Classical therapeutic options are external beam radiotherapy alone or in combination with surgery. However, surgical resection of these advanced tumors results in mutilating defects which have to be reconstructed – if this is at all possible – with complicated flap techniques. Despite all efforts results are still poor, even if postoperative irradiation is given. Conventional fractionated radiotherapy alone yields the same unsatisfactory results in terms of locoregional control and overall survival (Tables 21.4–21.6)

In the last decade two new radiotherapeutic modalities have been introduced: hyperfractionated, accelerated radiotherapy and concurrent radiotherapy and chemotherapy. Hyperfractionation, based on the better repair of small single fractions, permits a higher total tumor dose, with equivalent normal tissue tolerance over an unchanged overall treatment time. In a randomized trial of the EORTC (HORIOT et al. 1988), oropharyngeal carcinomas (stage T3N0 and T3N1) were treated by conventional fractionation (2 Gy/day up to 70 Gy) or by hyperfractionation (2 × 1.2 Gy/day up to 80 Gy). Locoregional control after 5 years was clearly superior in the hyperfractionation group (56% vs. 38%). A further change in fractionation was triggered by the clinical observation that overall treatment time is the most predictive factor for tumors of the same stage receiving adequate total doses exceeding 55 Gy. Prolongation of overall treatment time by 10 days resulted in an increase in locoregional recurrences of 20%–25%. This can be entirely explained by tumor proliferation over the treatment time, taking into consideration the short potential doubling times (median: 4.9 days) of squamous cell carcinomas of the head and neck (WILSON et al. 1988; BEGG et al. 1990). Naturally, the overall treatment time can be shortened by means of accelerated fractionation. SAUNDERS et al. (1989) employed radiation three times daily with single doses of 1.6 Gy. Within 3 weeks a total dose of 54 Gy had been given. After treatment of 45 patients with advanced T3/T4 tumors, the authors reported a complete remission rate of 80%. However, after 2 years the local control rate had fallen to 55%.

In more than 50% of cases, squamous cell carcinomas in the head and neck region respond to cisplatin-containing chemotherapy schedules with complete or partial remission. This led to the implementation of combined chemotherapy and radiotherapy. While sequential radio- and chemotherapy has been shown to be no better than classical strategies alone (STELL and RAWSON 1990), concurrent application of radio- and chemotherapy is promising. In a randomized study, ADELSTEIN et al. (1990) demonstrated that the rate of NED survival was significantly better after concurrent radio- and chemotherapy than after sequential treatment. The treatment of advanced tumors (stage III and IV) with different schedules resulted in complete remission rates of 70%–88% (Table 21.8). However, patients with complete remission suffer locoregional recurrences in ca. 20%–40% of cases, and the long-term locoregional control rate is no more than 60%.

Interstitial radiotherapy of advanced tumors is performed by only a few brachytherapy centers. Mostly implantation is used as a boost *after* external beam radiotherapy. This sequence has the

Table 21.8. Results of concurrent radio- and chemotherapy for advanced tumors in the head and neck region. Successful salvage treatments are not considered

Reference	No. of cases	Follow-up	Complete remission	Locoregional failures after complete remission	Overall locoregional failures
ADELSTEIN et al. (1990)	24	3 yr	21/24 (88%)	4/21 (20%)	7/24 (30%)
FIETKAU et al. (1991b)	47	>2 yr	34/47 (72%)	8/34 (34%)	17/47 (37%)
MARCIAL et al. (1990)	124	4 yr	88/124 (71%)	35/88 (40%)	71/124 (57%)
WENDT et al. (1990b)	58	>2 yr	48/58 (83%)	8/48 (17%)	16/58 (28%)

advantage that the response of the tumor to the external beam radiotherapy can be evaluated. Implantation can be avoided for patients who achieve complete remission, i.e., specifically patients with small residual tumors can be submitted to implantation. This selection may in part explain the high local recurrence rates of 25%–66% (T3) and 33%–100% (T4) after combined interstitial and external beam radiotherapy (Tables 21.4, 21.6). Nevertheless, interstitial therapy is effective, as shown by our own data. Nineteen patients with T3/4 carcinomas of the oral cavity were treated after external beam irradiation, combined in 11 cases with concurrent and in seven cases with sequential chemotherapy. Interstitial hyperthermia was employed in 12 of the 19 patients. Before implantation only three patients had achieved a complete remission, proving the negative selection. In contrast after implantation 11 (57%) showed complete regression of the tumor. Nevertheless, after a follow-up of 6–66 months (median 16 months) local failures were noted in 12 of the 19 (63%) patients.

Summarizing these trials, the long-term locoregional control rates of advanced tumors achieved by all treatment strategies are below 60%. Or, put another way, at least 40% of patients with advanced tumors will suffer from locoregional residual disease or recurrent tumors.

21.4 Treatment of the Neck

As far as the staging of regional lymph node metastases is concerned, the classifications of the AJCC (1983/1988) and of the UICC (1985/1987) differ in specific details (Table 21.1). Reviewing clinical results in the literature is therefore quite difficult. In the following section the specific classification system is mentioned for each reference.

The clinically negative neck can be equally controlled by surgery or external beam radiotherapy. The overall results are excellent; neck recurrences are reported in only 3%–14% of patients (Bataini et al. 1990; Cox 1985; Mendenhall and Million 1986).

Control rates for the clinically positive neck depend on the nodal size, the number of involved nodes, and the treatment. Single nodes smaller than 3 cm can be controlled by external beam radiotherapy alone in 79%–92% of cases (Bataini et al. 1990; Mendenhall et al. 1984). However, if node size exceeds 3 cm, the neck recurrence rate increases to 25%–100% after radiotherapy alone (Bataini et al. 1990; Mendenhall et al. 1984). Combining surgery, i.e., neck dissection, and radiotherapy yields neck control rates of 75%–92% (Jesse and Fletcher 1977; MD Anderson staging system). Mendenhall et al. (1986; AJCC staging system 1983), who treated the neck by surgery and radiotherapy, made a further differentiation of neck control according to metastatic node size. If the nodal size was below 4 cm, neck recurrences occurred in 9%–18%, but if the diameter was above 4 cm, the percentage of neck recurrences increased to 25%–50%.

Interstitial radiotherapy was performed by Goffinet et al. (1985c) using intraoperatively implanted iodine-125 seed Vicryl suture implants. Regional control was achieved in 10 of 13 (77%) previously untreated patients. Thirty patients were treated for a neck failure; regional control was achieved in 23 (77%).

21.5 Treatment of Recurrent Tumors

As shown in the previous sections, patients with head and neck cancer, and especially those with advanced lesions, have a high risk of locoregional recurrences. Secondary tumors have been reported in about 15%. Many of these patients had undergone multimodality treatment including primary surgical extirpation, external beam irradiation, and/or multiagent chemotherapy. Of course, the nature and sequelae of these previous therapies have a major impact on the decision of the radiation oncologist as to whether retreatment is possible. Housset et al. (1991) reported the same risk of soft tissue necrosis with second treatment (28% –33%) as with primary therapy consisting of surgery and radiotherapy or radiotherapy alone. However, the primary radiation doses were different: 45 Gy for surgery and radiotherapy versus 72 Gy after exclusive radiotherapy.

The major concern of reirradiation is the tolerance of normal tissues. For example, after a previous course of radiotherapy the spinal cord cannot be irradiated again because the tolerance dose has already been reached. The vascular flow is altered and reduced after irradiation due to fibrosis and rarefaction of blood vessels. Fibrosis of the skin, underlying tissues, and muscles leads to restriction of the neck flexibility. As a consequence of these side-effects the dose and volume of a second course of radiotherapy have to be significantly reduced;

Table 21.9. Results of external beam radiotherapy for recurrent or secondary head and neck carcinomas

Reference	No. of cases	Therapy	Follow-up	Site	Local control	Survival
LANGLOIS et al. (1985)	35	eRT		Head and neck	46%	19% (2 yr)
LEVENDAG et al. (1992)	55	eRT ± Surg ± CT	>3 y	Head and neck	29%	20% (5 yr)
MCNEESE and FLETCHER (1981)	30	eRT		Nasopharynx	(33%)	–
SKOLYSZEWSKI et al. (1980)	20	eRT		Head and neck	–	70% (3 yr)
YAM and GU (1982)	162	eRT		Nasopharynx	–	23% (5 yr)

eRT, external beam radiotherapy; Surg, surgery; CT, chemotherapy

the delivery of cytotoxic drugs must be even more seriously reduced. Thus chemotherapy may offer some temporary palliation, but the long-term control is quite disappointing. Surgical resection of small recurrent tumors is possible, but for advanced tumors in most cases impossible due to the local extent of the tumor. Salvage rates of only 15%–20% are reported.

According to a review by LANGLOIS et al. (1988), external beam reirradiation yielded a low local control rate of 20%–40% (Table 21.9). Better results have been achieved for recurrent nasopharyngeal carcinomas. Treatment of nodal relapses always yielded poor results. Furthermore, the fact that a high dose of reirradiation is needed limits the use of external beam irradiation. By contrast, when using interstitial radiotherapy it is again possible to deliver a sufficient radiation dose. Table 21.10 shows that complete remissions can be achieved in ca. 20%–60% of patients. In general, local control is inversely proportional to the size of the tumor while the incidence of necrosis increases in direct relation to it.

21.6 Reduction of Side-effects of Interstitial Therapy

Achieving tumor control is the main goal of every cancer therapy, followed by the objective of avoiding normal tissue complications. The main complications of interstitial therapy are soft tissue necrosis and osteoradionecrosis. Fistulas, carotid ruptures, or bleedings are rare and in most cases develop as a complication of soft tissue necrosis and osteoradionecrosis. These side-effects have to be distinguished from locally recurrent or progressing tumors showing the same symptoms. Nearly all complications after interstitial therapy need prolonged supportive care. Soft tissue necrosis can be resolved by conservative treatment, but most other side-effects require surgical treatment. The high incidences of soft tissue necrosis (14%–30%) and osteoradionecrosis (6%–13%) (Table 21.11 and 21.12) justify the search for prognostic parameters and appropriate treatment modifications to reduce these complications.

The incidence of necrosis after interstitial therapy is influenced by a variety of clinical factors. The most important seem to be tumor size and dose rate. MAZERON et al. (1991) found an increasing incidence from 25% (T1) to 39% (T2b) depending upon tumor stage. Moreover, necrosis was related to dose rate independently of dose. For recurrent tumors, HOUSSET et al. (1991) and MAZERON et al. (1987b) also found a correlation between incidence of necrosis and tumor volume.

Other factors mentioned in the literature are:

1. *Site of the primary tumor.* MAZERON et al. (1991) reported an incidence of 28% for mobile tongue tumors and 58% for floor of the mouth tumors.
2. *Neglect of oral hygiene and dental care.* This is equally as important for the development of complications as the dose–time factors of the implantation (OLCH et al. 1988). According to DEARNALEY et al. (1991), a multivariant analysis showed smoking to be most closely correlated with side-effects; 35% of smokers developed complications compared to 20% of nonsmokers.
3. *Technical aspects of implantation.* CROOK et al. (1989) observed an increase in necrosis when the spacing between the seed ribbons was too large. WENDT et al. (1990a) found that severe complications were more likely to occur after combined interstitial and external beam irradiation.
4. *The time interval between initial treatment and attempted salvage.* According to HOUSSET et al. (1991) this is an important factor for recurrent or secondary tumors. Mucosal necrosis developed in 43% undergoing salvage irradiation after less than 18 months compared to 23% receiving second

Table 21.10. Results of interstitial radiotherapy for recurrent or secondary head and neck carcinomas

Reference	No. of cases	Nuclide	Therapy	Follow-up	Site	Local control	Survival
Fietkau et al. (1991c)	25	^{192}Ir	iRT ± Surg ± eRT	Median 27 mo	Head and neck	14/25 (56%)	26% (2 yr)
Fontanesi et al. (1989)	23	^{192}Ir	iRT	4–34 mo	Head and neck	16/18 (89%)	–
Goffinet et al. (1985b)	34	^{125}I	Surg + iRT	1–30 mo	Head and neck	20/34 (59%)	Mean 11 months
Langlois et al. (1988)	123	^{192}Ir	iRT/iRT + eRT	5 yr	Oropharynx Mobile tongue	(59%)	24% (5 yr)
Levendag et al. (1992)	18	^{192}Ir	iRT ± eRT ± Surg ± HT	> 3 yr	Head and neck	(50%)	20% (5 yr)
Liberman et al. (1989)	39	^{125}I	Surg + iRT	Median 28 mo	Head and neck	–	29% (5 yr)[a]
Mazeron et al. (1987b)	70	^{192}Ir	iRT	?	Oropharynx	51/69 (74%)	14% (5 yr)
Puthawala et al. (1981)	31	^{192}Ir	iRT	> 2 yr	Mobile tongue Base of tongue	12/31 (39%)	–
Puthawala et al. (1990)	108	^{192}Ir	iRT + HT	Median 30 mo	Head and neck	81/108 (75%)	–
Son et al. (1989)	25	^{125}I	iRT/iRT + eRT	3 yr	Head and neck	(78%)	48% (3 yr)
Vikram et al. (1986)	15	^{125}I	iRT	2 yr	Nasopharynx	(55%)	–

Surg, surgery; iRT, interstitial radiotherapy; eRT, external beam radiotherapy; HT, hyperthermia
[a]Disease-free survival

treatment after more than 18 months. This was not confirmed by Mazeron et al. (1987b) or Langlois (1987).

Surprisingly, most authors found no direct correlation between dose and incidence of complications (Dearnaley et al. 1991). Mazeron et al. (1991) observed a correlation between dose and complication rate only for dose rates below 50 cGy/h. However, these reports typically refer to the implantation of small tumors of less than 3–5 cm in diameter, where implantation was the sole treatment modality. If T3 or T4 tumor volumes have to be implanted, we believe that reduced doses need to be used, otherwise complications may increase markedly. The same holds true for implantation of recurrent or secondary tumors after prior radiotherapy. Radiation dose is restricted because of the limited normal tissue tolerance. Table 21.12 shows that soft tissue necrosis occurs in 16%–66% of cases following salvage interstitial radiotherapy. Using the radiosensitizing potential of hyperthermia it may be possible to reduce the interstitial dose without reducing the effect of the interstitial therapy.

21.7 Goals of Increased Local Control

Increasing local control has two major objectives:

1. Improved survival of patients
2. Improved quality of life

The first point can be discussed with reference to objective facts and figures. However, nearly no objective data exist in respect of the second point. Nevertheless, we will try to show that an important gain for the patient is indeed achieved.

21.7.1 Influence of Local Control on Survival

If permanent local control is achieved, various factors influence the patient's survival time:

1. Regional control
2. Incidence of distant metastases
3. Death from intercurrent disease
4. Development of secondary malignancies

Suit (1982) tried to estimate the increase in survival if locoregional failure were to be completely eliminated. Suit's analysis was applied to the 1985 American Cancer Society statistics by Kapp (1986). It was

Table 21.11. Side-effects of interstitial radiotherapy for oral cavity carcinomas

Reference	Tumor site	Nuclides	Therapy	Soft tissue necrosis	Osteoradio-necrosis	Overall side-effects
AYGUN et al. (1984)	Floor of the mouth	^{226}Ra	iRT/iRT+RT	–	–	17%
BENK et al. (1990)	Tongue	^{192}Ir	iRT/iRT+RT	–	–	34% (29/84)
DECROIX and GHOSSEIN (1981)	Tongue	^{226}Ra	iRT	29%	9%	–
HAIE et al. (1983)	Tongue	^{192}Ir	iRT	14%	6%	–
LEFEBVRE et al. (1990)	Tongue	^{192}Ir	iRT	–	–	19% (49/263)
MAZERON et al. (1990b)	Tongue	^{192}Ir	iRT/iRT+RT	–	–	26% (32/121)
MAZERON et al. (1990a)	Floor of the mouth	^{192}Ir	iRT	17% (16/95)	11% (10/95)	–
MENDENHALL et al. (1989)	Tongue	^{226}Ra	iRT/iRT+RT	–	–	42% (13/31)
PERNOT et al. (1990a)	Tongue	^{192}Ir	iRT/iRT+RT	–	–	11% (16/147)
PUTHAWALA et al. (1981)	Tongue	^{192}Ir	iRT+RT	19% (5/26)	8% (2/26)	27% (7/26)
WANG (1989)	Tongue	^{226}Ra/^{192}Ir	iRT+RT	30% (3/10)	13% (3/23)	–
WENDT et al. (1990a)	Tongue	^{226}Ra	iRT/iRT+RT	–	–	41%–60%

iRT, interstitial radiotherapy; eRT, external beam radiotherapy

Table 21.12. Side-effects of interstitial radiotherapy for recurrent or secondary tumors

Reference	Tumor site	Therapy	Soft tissue necrosis	Osteoradio-necrosis
FIETKAU et al. (1991)	Head and neck	iRT/Surg+iRT pRT+iRT	20% (5/25)	8% (2/25)
FONTANESI et al. (1989)	Head and neck	iRT	(11/23)[a]	–
HAYE et al. (1983)	Base of tongue	iRT	66% (14/20)	–
HOUSSET et al. (1991)	Base of tongue	iRT single course	43% (9/21)	–
		Split course	16% (3/19)	–
LANGLOIS et al. (1988)	Oropharynx Mobile tongue	iRT	23% (28/123)	–
LEVENDAG et al. (1992)	Head and neck	iRT±eRT±Surg±HT	72% (13/18)	–
MAZERON et al. (1987b)	Oropharynx	iRT	27% (14/51)	–
SYED et al. (1977)	Oropharynx Oral cavity	iRT	20% (6/29)	–
SYED et al. (1978)	Head and neck	iRT	30% (19/64)	–

iRT, interstitial radiotherapy; Surg, surgery; eRT, external beam radiotherapy; HT, hyperthermia
[a] Including fistulas, carotid rupture

estimated that 41% ($n = 3900$) of those patients ($n = 9500$) dying from head and neck cancer had locoregional failure as a major cause of death. Taking into account the percentage of patients who present with untreatable disease (24%) and the percentage who would subsequently die from distant metastases (27%) or other causes (49% of patients with uncomplicated locoregional control), it was calculated that elimination of locoregional failure would yield approximately 2600 additional survivors or, put another way, would reduce annual deaths from head and neck cancer by about 28%.

21.7.2 Influence of Local Control on Quality of Life

The efficacy of a particular therapy cannot be measured only by reference to survival rates. Another endpoint of evaluation must be quality of life. Two different questions have to be clearly distinguished:

1. Can interstitial thermoradiotherapy offer good palliation by achieving a partial response in patients with locally advanced incurable tumors?
2. Is it worthwhile achieving local control although the life expectancy of the patients will not be prolonged?

Despite an increasing number of publications suggesting that thermo-radiotherapy provides effective palliation for patients with cancer, most studies have measured only tumor and normal tissue response. However, the fact that a higher number of partial responses can be achieved with the aid of thermo-radiotherapy cannot be extrapolated into the assumption that combined treatment offers better quality of life (NIELSEN et al. 1992). Only two studies (KAI et al. 1988; KAKEHI et al. 1990) have investigated this matter, and both found a better quality of life after hyperthermia. However, in both studies the method of assessment was validated and the evaluations were based solely upon the judgments of physicians (NIELSEN et al. 1992).

As no literature data exist on question 2 above, we have to discuss this point theoretically. The life expectancy of patients whose form of cancer has a high incidence of distant metastases is not prolonged by achieving local control of the tumor. However, the patient with local control has a better quality of life than does a patient with locoregional tumor growth. Owing to the special anatomy of the head and neck region, regrowth of local or regional tumors can create disastrous problems for patients. Mastication and swallowing are impaired by tumor infiltration, and obstruction of the digestive pathway will ensue, i.e., patients are only able to take in semisolid or liquid meals and eventually cease to eat at all. Pain is caused by infiltration of nerves and bony structures or by infections and ulceration of soft tissues or bone. Foul odor and destruction of the face by infections and tumor growth cause the patients to be treated as outcasts. In contrast, distant metastases of the lung or liver are asymptomatic over a long period. Pain caused by bone metastases can be successfully managed by radiation therapy. Of course, we are aware of the difficulties related to the concept of "quality of life." This term includes a large number of factors which vary in their importance to different patients and which also depend on the tumor status and the success of therapy. Patients who have achieved complete remission may accept more treatment side-effects. In summary, locoregional control is not only a prerequisite for long-term survival but is also necessary for good quality of life in otherwise dismal therapeutic situations.

21.8 Summary: Indications for Interstitial Thermoradiotherapy in the Head and Neck Region

Tumors in the head and neck region can be treated with different modalities – surgery, chemotherapy, or interstitial and external beam irradiation, or combinations of these classic regimens. The major task is how to integrate interstitial thermoradiotherapy within this framework of multimodal therapy. Three aspects have to be discussed concerning the necessity of introducing an additional therapy:

1. The *percentage of local or regional recurrences.* It is generally accepted that if recurrences occur in more than 20% of cases, further treatment modalities must be inaugurated.
2. The *distribution of the locoregional recurrences.* To give an example: BATAINI et al. (1990) analyzed the site of recurrences in 437 patients with oropharyngeal carcinomas treated by external beam radiotherapy. Of the recurrences, 28% occurred only at the site of the primary and 21% only in the neck. Combined locoregional recurrences were noted in 25%. Twenty-six percent of all patients suffered from distant metastases. Summarizing, 74% of the recurrences were locoregional. Single-site recurrences occurred in 49%, and such recurrences are, of course, an indication for additional therapy. However, locoregional recurrences at multiple sites have to be dealt with cautiously. If there is no chance of achieving a complete remission or at least a very effective palliative result, then there is no place for additional therapy, if the primary has been treated by interstitial thermoradiotherapy, the neck metastases must be controlled by other modalities (surgery, external radiotherapy). If this is impossible, there is no additional role for interstitial thermoradiotherapy.
3. The *incidence of treatment side-effects.* If standard therapy has side-effects in more than 20% –30% of cases, alteration of the treatment strategy has to be considered, with the goal of reducing toxicity.

According to these rules, *early tumor stages* – defined as T1 or T2 – can be successfully treated with various methods as shown in Sect. 21.3.1. The choice of therapy will differ among oncologists according to experience or preference. In these tumor stages there is no need for additional therapy.

Advanced primary tumors – defined as T3 or T4 – are characterized by local recurrences in more than 20% of cases. By means of interstitial radiotherapy it is possible to deliver a boost to the primary, complementary to the external beam irradiation. In principle there are two ways of involving interstitial radiotherapy within the framework of multimodal therapy – before or after the other modalities. As shown in Sect. 21.3.2, most brachytherapy centers have chosen the second way, given the advantage that only residual tumors have to be implanted.

A disadvantage of implanation *after* external beam irradiation is the break which is necessary because of acute mucosal reactions. Given the well-known fast proliferation rate of squamous cell carcinomas of 2–4 days (potential doubling time, BEGG et al. 1990), this break can cause 4–14 doublings of the tumor cells. Therefore brachytherapy must kill more cells than expected after external beam radiotherapy. This may also explain the high recurrence rates observed with this sequence. Since the dose of interstitial radiotherapy is limited because of the previous external beam irradiation, a radiosensitizing agent like hyperthermia is necessary and useful. Furthermore, hyperthermia may be helpful because of the negative selection of the tumors which have not responded very well to previous therapy.

To shorten the break between the two modalities and to avoiding tumor repopulation, we would promote implanation *before* external beam therapy. After application of a moderate dose of 20 Gy, external beam irradiation can be started within a week. The disadvantage of this sequence is that all patients with accesible tumor must be implanted. Hyperthermia is necessary to maximize the effect of the low interstitial dose. To our knowledge this theoretical sequence has not been investigated up to now on a routine clinical basis.

Neck nodes up to 4 cm in diameter can be controlled by combined surgery and radiation. Interstitial thermoradiotherapy can be used as a boost dose after external beam radiotherapy if surgical removal is not possible or if residual tumor remains after surgery.

Treatment of recurrences involves a lot of problems, as mentioned in Sects. 21.5 and 21.6. Because of limited radiation tolerance we see an indication for interstitial thermoradiotherapy in nearly all cases. An exception is the small tumor which has been completely (= R0) resected; in this instance interstitial radiotherapy alone is sufficient as an adjuvant therapy.

References

Adelstein DJ, Sharan VM, Earle AS et al. (1990) Simultaneous versus sequential combined technique therapy for squamous cell head and neck cancer. Cancer 65: 1685–1691

Akine Y, Tokita N, Ogino T et al. (1991) Stage I–II carcinoma of the anterior two thirds of the tongue treated with different modalities: a retrospective analysis of 244 patients. Radiother Oncol 21: 24–28

Aygun C, Salazar OM, Sewchand W, Amornmarn R, Prempree T (1984) Carcinoma of the floor of the mouth: A 20-year experience. Int J Radiat Oncol Biol Phys 10: 619–626

Bataini JP, Bernier J, Jaulerry C, Brunin F, Pontvert D (1990) Impact of cervical disease and its definitive radiotherapeutic management on survival: experience in 2013 patients with squamous cell carcinomas of the oropharynx and pharyngolarynx. Laryngoscope 100: 716–723

Begg AC, Hofland I, Bartelink H et al. (1990) The predictive value of cell kinetic measurements in a European trial of accelerated fractionation in advanced head and neck tumours: an interim report. Int J Radiat Oncol Biol Phys 19: 1449–1453

Benk V, Mazeron JJ, Grimard L et al. (1990) Comparison of curietherapy versus external irradiation combined with curietherapy in stage II squamous cell carcinomas of the mobile tongue. Radiother Oncol 18: 339–347

Blumberg AL, Fu KK, Philips TL (1979) Results of treatment of carcinoma of the base of the tongue. The UCSF experience 1957–1976. Int J Radiat Oncol Biol Phys 5: 1971–1976

Brenner DJ, Hall EJ (1991) Conditions for the equivalence of continuous to pulsed low dose rate brachytherapy. Int J Radiat Oncol Biol Phys 20: 181–190

Cox JD (1985) Management of clinically occult (N0) cervical lymph node metastases by radiation therapy. In: Chretein PB, Johns ME, Shedd DP, Strong EW, Ward PH (eds) Head and neck cancer, vol 1. Decker, Philadelphia, pp 151–155

Crook J, Mazeron JJ, Marinello G, Walop W, Pierquin B (1989) Prognostic factors of local outcome for T1, T2 carcinomas of oral tongue treated by iridium-192 implantation – the Creteil experience. Int J Radiat Oncol Biol Phys 17 [Suppl, 1]: 170

Crook J, Mazeron JJ, Marinello G et al. (1988) Combined external irradiation and interstitial implantation for T1 and T2 epidermoid carcinomas of base of tongue: the Creteil experience (1971–1981). Int J Radiat Oncol Biol Phys 15: 105–114

Dearnaley DP, Dardoufas C, A'Hearn RP, Henk JM (1991) Interstitial irradiation for carcinoma of the tongue and floor of the mouth: Royal Marsden Hospital Experience 1970–1986. Radiother Oncol 21: 183–192

Decroix Y, Ghossein N (1981) Experience of the Curie Institute in treatment of cancer of the mobile tongue. Cancer 47: 496–508

Emami B, Perez CA, Leybovich L, Straube W, von Gerichten D (1987) Interstitial thermoradiotherapy in the treatment of malignant tumours. Int J Hyperthermia 3: 107–118

Esche BA, Haie CM, Gerbaulet AP, Eschwege F, Richard JM, Chassagne D (1988) Interstitial and external radiotherapy in carcinoma of the soft palate and uvula. Int J Radiat Oncol Biol Phys 15: 619–625

Fietkau R, Grabenbauer GG, Iro H, Müller RG, Farmand M, Altendorf-Hofmann A, Sauer R (1991a) Interstitielle und perkutane Strahlentherapie nach begrenzten chirurgischen Eingriffen beim Mundhöhlenkarzinom. Strahlenther Onkol 167: 591–598

Fietkau R, Iro H, Grabenbauer GG, Altendorf-Hofmann A, Sauer R (1991b) Simultane Radio-Chemotherapie mit

Cisplatin und 5-Fluorouracil bei fortgeschrittenen KopfHals-Tumoren. Strahlenther Onkol 167: 693–700

Fietkau R, Weidenbecher M, Spitzer W, Sauer R (1991c) Temporary and permanent brachycurie therapy in advanced head and neck cancer – The Erlangen experience. In: Sauer R (ed) Interventional radiation therapy techniques – brachytherapy. Springer, Berlin Heidelberg New York

Fontanesi J, Hetzler D, Ross J (1989) Effect of dose rate on local control and complications in the reirradiation of head and neck tumors with interstitial iridium-192. Int J Radiat Oncol Biol Phys 17: 365–369

Foote RL, Parsons JT, Mendenhall WM, Million RR, Cassisi NJ, Stringer SP (1990) Is interstitial implantation essential for successful radiotherapeutic treatment of base of tongue carcinoma? Int J Radiat Oncol Biol Phys 18: 1293–1298

Gardner KE, Parsons JT, Mendenhall WM, Million RR, Cassisi NJ (1987) Time-dose relationships for local tumor control and complications following irradiation of squamous cell carcinoma of the base of tongue. Int J Radiat Oncol Biol Phys 13: 507–510

Goffinet DR, Fee WE, Jr, Wells J, Austin – Seymour M, Clarke D, Mariscial JM, Goode RL (1985a) 192-Iridium pharyngoepiglottic fold interstitial implants. The key to successful treatment of base tongue carcinoma by radiation treatment. Cancer 55: 941–948

Goffinet DR, Martinez A, Fee WE (1985b) 125-I Vicryl suture implants as a surgical adjuvant in cancer of the head and neck. Int J Radiat Oncol Biol Phys 11: 399–402

Goffinet DR, Paryani SB, Fee WE (1985c) Management of patients with N3 cervical adenopathy and/or carotid artery involvement. In: Chretein PB, Johns ME, Shedd DP, Strong EW, Ward PH (eds) Head and neck cancer, vol 1. Decker, Philadelphia, pp 159–162

Grandi C, Chiesa F, Cervia M, Sala L, Barbano PR, Molinari R (1983) Surgery versus combined therapies for cancer of the anterior floor of the mouth. Head Neck Surg 6: 653–659

Guerry TL, Silverman S, Dedo HH (1986) Carbon dioxide laser resection of superficial oral carcinoma: indications, technique, and results. Ann Otol Rhinol Laryngol 95: 547–555

Haie C, Gerbaulet A, Wibault P, Chassagne D, Marandas P (1983) Resultates de la curietherapie et de l'association radiotherapie transcutanee-curietherapie dans 155 cas de cancer de la langue mobile. Actualites de carcinologie cervico-faciale 9: 53–57

Hall EJ (1985) The biological basis of endocurietherapy. The Henschke Memorial Lecture 1984. Endocuriether Hyperther Oncol 1: 141–152

Haye C, Mazeron JJ, Chassagne D, Gerbaulet A, Marandas P (1983) Curietherapie de rattrapage des tumeurs de la base de langue. J Eur Radiother 4: 139–142

Harrison LB, Sessions RB, Strong EW, Fass DE, Nori D, Fuks Z (1989) Brachytherapy as part of definitive management of squamous cancer of the base of tongue. Int J Radiat Oncol Biol Phys 17: 1309–1312

Hoffstetter S, Malissard L, Forcard JJ, Pernot M (1986) A propos de 108 cas traites au Centre Alexis Vautrin. J Eur Radiother 7: 101–110

Horiot JC, Le Fur R, Nguyen TN, Schraub S, Chenal C, De Pauw M, Van Glabbeke M (1988) Two fractions per day versus single fraction per day in the radiotherapy of oropharynx carcinoma: results of an EORTC randomized trial. 7th Annual Meeting of the European Society for Therapeutic Radiology and Oncology, abstract Nr. 438

Housset M, Baillet F, Dessard-Diana B, Martin D, Miglianico L (1987) A retrospective study of three treatment techniques for T1–T2 base of tongue lesions: surgery plus postoperative radiation, external radiation plus interstitial implantation and external radiation alone. Int J Radiat Oncol Biol Phys 13: 511–516

Housset M, Baillet F, Delanian S et al. (1991) Split course interstitial brachytherapy with a source shift: the results of a new iridium implant technique versus single course implants for salvage irradiation of base of tongue cancers in 55 patients. Int J Radiat Oncol Biol Phys 20: 965–971

Ildstad ST, Bigelow ME, Remensnyder JP (1983) Squamous cell carcinoma of the mobile tongue. Clinical behavior and results of current therapeutic modalities. Am J Surg 145: 443–449

Jaulerry C, Rodriguez J, Brunin F, Mosseri V, Pontvert D, Brugere J, Bataini JP (1991) Results of radiation therapy in carcinoma of the base of the tongue. The Curie Institute experience with about 166 cases. Cancer 67: 1532–1538

Jesse RH, Fletcher GH (1977) Treatment of the neck in patients with squamous cell carcinoma of the head and neck. Cancer 39: 868–872

Johnson MJT, Leipzig B, Cummings CW (1980) Management of T1 carcinoma of the anterior aspect of the tongue. Arch Otolaryngol 106: 249–251

Kai H, Matsufuji H, Okudaira Y, Sugimachi K (1988) Heat, drugs and radiation given in combination is palliative for unresectable oesophageal cancer. Int J Radiat Oncol Biol Phys 14: 1147–1152

Kakehi M, Ueda K, Mukojima T, Hiraoka M, Seto O, Akanuma A, Nakatsugawa S (1990) Multiinstitutional clinical studies on hyperthermia combined with radiotherapy and chemotherapy in advanced cancer of deep-seated organs. Int J Hyperthermia 6: 719–740

Kapp DS (1986) Site and disease selection for hyperthermia clinical trials. Int J Hyperthermia 2: 139–156

Korb LJ, Spaulding CA, Constable WC (1991) The role of definitive radiation therapy in squamous cell carcinoma of the oral tongue. Cancer 67: 2733–2737

Langlois D, Eschwege F, Kramar A, Richard JM (1985) Reirradiation of head and neck cancer. Radiother Oncol 3: 27–33

Langlois D, Hoffstetter S, Malissard L, Pernot M, Taghian A (1988) Salvage irradiation of oropharynx and mobile tongue about 192-iridium brachytherapy in Centre Alexis Vautrin. Int J Radiat Oncol Biol Phys 14: 849–853

Lefebvre LJ, Coche-Dequeant B, Castelain B, Prevost B, Buisset E, Ton Van J (1990) Interstitial brachytherapy and early tongue squamous cell carcinoma management. Head Neck 12: 232–236

Leipzig B, Cummings CW, Chung CT, Johnson JT, Sagerman RH (1982) Carcinoma of the anterior tongue. Ann Otol Rhinol Laryngol 91: 94–97

Levendag PC, Meeuwis CA, Wijthoff SJM, Visser AG (1992) Reirradiation of recurrent head and neck cancers: external versus interstitial radiation therapy. Activity 6: 3–10

Liberman F, Park R, Lee D-J, Goldsmith M (1989) Resection plus iodine-125 seed implantation for recurrent head and neck carcinomas. Int J Radiat Oncol Biol Phys: 227

Lusinchi A, Eskandri J, Son Y et al. (1989) External irradiation plus curietherapy boost in 108 base of tongue carcinomas. Int J Radiat Oncol Biol Phys 17: 1191–1197

Marcial VA, Pajak TF, Mohiuddin M et al. (1990) Concomitant cisplatin chemotherapy and radiotherapy in advanced mucosal squamous cell carcinoma of the head and neck cancer. Long-term results of the Radiation Therapy Oncology Group Study 81–17. Cancer 66: 1861–1868

Marks JE, Lee F, Smith PG, Ogura JH (1983) Floor of the mouth cancer: patient selection and treatment results. Laryngoscope 93: 475–480

Mazeron JJ, Crook J, Mahot P et al. (1987a) Mise au point sur la radiotherapie exlusive des T1 et T2 de l árche velo-amygdalienne. Ann Otolaryngol Chir Cervicofac 104: 197–203

Mazeron JJ, Langlois D, Glaubiger D et al. (1987b) Salvage irradiation of oropharyngeal cancers using iridium 192 wire implants: 5-year results of 70 cases. Int J Radiat Oncol Biol Phys 13: 957–962

Mazeron JJ, Marinello G, Crook J et al. (1987c) Definitive radiation treatment for early stage carcinoma of the soft palate and uvula: the indications for iridium 192 implantation. Int J Radiat Oncol Biol Phys 13: 1829–1837

Mazeron JJ, Grimard L, Raynal M et al. (1990a) Iridium-192 curietherapy for T1 and T2 epidermoid carcinomas of the floor of the mouth. Int J Radiat Oncol Biol Phys 18: 1299–1306

Mazeron JJ, Crook JM, Marinello G, Walop W, Pierquin B (1990b) Prognostic factors of local outcome for T1, T2 carcinomas of oral tongue treated by iridium 192 implantation. Int J Radiat Oncol Biol 19: 281–285

Mazeron JJ, Simon JM, Le Pechoux C et al. (1991) Effect of dose rate on local control and complications in definitive irradiation of T1-2 squamous cell carcinomas of mobile tongue and floor of mouth with interstitial iridium-192. Radiother Oncol 21: 39–47

McNeese M, Fletcher GH (1981) Retreatment of recurrent nasopharyngeal carcinoma. Radiology 138: 191–193

Mendenhall WM, Million RR (1986) Elective neck irradiation for squamous cell carcinoma of the head and neck: analysis of time-dose factors and causes of failure. Int J Radiat Oncol Biol Phys 12: 741–746

Mendenhall WM, Million RR, Bova FJ (1984) Analysis of time-dose factors in clinically positive neck nodes treated with irradiation alone in squamous cell carcinoma of the head and neck. Int J Radiat Oncol Biol Phys 10: 639–643

Mendenhall WM, Million RR, Cassis NJ (1986) Squamous cell carcinoma of the head and neck treated with radiation therapy: the role of neck dissection for clinically positive neck nodes. Int J Radiat Oncol Biol Phys 12: 733–740

Mendenhall WM, Parsons JT, Stringer SP, Cassisi NJ, Million RR (1989) T2 oral tongue carcinoma treated with radiotherapy: analysis of local control and complications. Radiother Oncol 16: 275–281

Nathanson A, Agren K, Lind MG et al. (1989) Evaluation of some prognostic factors in small squamous cell carcinoma of the mobile tongue: a multicenter study in sweden. Head Neck 11: 387–392

Nielsen OS, Munro AJ, Warde PR (1992) Assessment of palliative response in hyperthermia. Int J Hyperthermia 8: 11–12

Nowak PJCM, Levendag PC, Visser AG (1990) Brachytherapy failure analysis of floor of mouth and oral tongue. Endocuriether Hyperther Oncol 6: 1–9

O'Brien CJ, Lahr CJ, Soong SJ, Gandour MJ, Jones JM, Urist MM, Maddox WA (1986) Surgical treatment of early – stage carcinoma of the oral tongue – would adjuvant treatment be beneficial? Head Neck Surg 8: 401–408

Olch AJ, Beumer J, Schwartz HC, Kagan AR (1988) Proposition: that oral hygiene is as important as dose-time factors in the prevention of osteoradionecrosis in the mandible. Endocuriether Hyperther Oncol 4: 11–16

Parsons JT, McCarty PJ, Rao PV, Mendenhall WM, Million RR (1990) On the definition of local control. Int J Radiat Oncol Biol Phys 18: 705–706

Pernot M, Malissard L, Aletti P, Hoffstetter S, Forcard JJ, Bey P (1990a) Ir 192 brachytherapy in the management of 147 T2N0 oral tongue carcinoma treated with irradiation alone. Int J Radiat Oncol Biol Phys 19 [Suppl]: 139

Pernot M, Malissard L, Hoffstetter S, Carolus JM, Forcard JJ, Kozminiski P, Bey P (1990b) Palato-tonsillar lesions: treatment of 269 cases with associated external irradiation and brachytherapy. 15th Interstitial Cancer Congress, Suppl, Part II: 116, 798

Pierquin B, Mazeron JJ, Grimard L (1991) Interstitial radiotherapy of oral cavity and oropharynx carcinomas (Paris technique). In: Sauer R (ed) Interventional radiation therapy techniques – brachytherapy. Springer, Berlin Heidelberg New York, pp 133–144

Puthawala AA, Syed AMN, Neblett D, McNamara C (1981) The role of afterloading iridium (Ir-192) implant in the management of carcinoma of the tongue. Int J Radiat Oncol Biol Phys 7: 407–412

Puthawala AA, Syed AMN, Eads DL, Neblett D, Gillin L, Gates TC (1985) Limited external irradiation and interstitial 192-iridium implant in the treatment of squamous cell carcinoma of the tonsillar region. Int J Radiat Oncol Biol Phys 11: 1595–1602

Puthawala AA, Syed AMN, Eads DL, Gillin L, Gates TC (1987) Limited external beam and interstitial 192-iridium irradiation in the treatment of carcinoma of the base of the tongue: a ten year experience. Int J Radiat Oncol Biol Phys 14: 839–848

Puthawala AA, Syed AMN, Rafie S, McNamara C (1990) Interstitial hyperthermia and interstitial irradiation (thermoendocurietherapy) in the treatment of recurrent and/or persistent head and neck cancers. Endocuriether Hyperthermia Oncol 6: 203–210

Saunders MI, Dische S, Hong A, Grosch E, Fermont DC, Ashford RFU, Maher EJ (1989) Continuous hyperfractionated accelerated radiotherapy in locally advanced carcinoma of the head and neck region. Int J Radiat Oncol Biol Phys 17: 1287–1293

Schramm VL, Myers EN, Sigler BA (1980) Surgical management of early epidermoid carcinoma of the anterior floor of the mouth. Laryngoscope 90: 207–215

Seegenschmiedt MH, Sauer R (1992) The current role of interstitial thermo-radiotherapy Strahlenther. Onkol. 168: 119–140

Seegenschmiedt MH, Sauer R, Brady LW, Karlsson UL (1991) Techniques and clinical experience of interstitial thermoradiotherapy. In: Sauer R (ed) Interventional radiation therapy techniques – brachytherapy. Springer Berlin Heidelberg New York, pp 345–357

Skolyszewski J, Korzenlowski S, Reinfoss M (1980) The reirradiation of recurrences of head and neck cancer. Br J Radiol 53: 407–410

Son YH, Ariyan S, Sasaki CL, Goodwin WJ, Kacinski BM, August D, Ponn RB (1989a) Intraoperative iodine-125 brachytherapy in the management of advanced or recurrent head and neck and thoracic-abdominal tumors. Endocuriether Hyperther Oncol 5: 9–19

Spanos WJ, Shukovsky LJ, Fletcher GH (1976) Time, dose, and tumor volume relationships in irradiation of squamous cell carcinomas of the base of the tongue. Cancer 37: 2591–2599

Stell PM, Rawson NSB (1990) Adjuvant chemotherapy in head and neck cancer. Br J Cancer 61: 779–787

Suit HD (1982) Potential for improving survival rates for the cancer patient by increasing the efficacy of treatment of the primary. Cancer 50: 1227–1234

Syed AMN, Feder BH (1977) Technique of afterloading interstitial implants. Radiol Clin North Am 46: 458–475
Syed AMN, Fedge BH, George FW (1977) Persistent carcinoma of the oropharynx and oral cavity retreated by afterloading interstitial 192-iridium implant. Cancer 39: 2443–2450
Syed AMN, Feder BH, George FW. III, Neblett D (1978) Iridium 192 afterloaded implant in the retreatment of head and neck cancers. Br J Radiol 51: 814–820
Vikram B, Strong EW, Shah JP, Spiro RH, Gerold F, Sessions RB, Hilaris BS (1985) A non-looping afterloading technique for base of tongue implants: results in the first 20 patients. Int J Radiat Oncol Biol Phys 11: 1853–1855
Vikram B, Strong EW, Shah JP, Spiro RH, Gerold F, Sessions RB, Hilaris BS (1986) Intraoperative radiotherapy in patients with recurrent head and neck cancer. Am J Surg 150: 485–487
Wang CC (1989) Radiotherapeutic management and results of T1N0, T2N0 carcinoma of the oral tongue: evaluation of boost techniques. Int J Radiat Oncol Biol Phys 17: 287–291
Wang CC (1990) How essential is interstitial radiation therapy to curability of head and neck cancer? Int J Radiat Oncol Biol Phys 18: 1529–1530
Wazer DE, Schmidt-Ullrich R, Keisch M, Karmody CS, Koch W (1989) The role of combined composite resection and irradiation in the management of carcinoma of the oral cavity and oropharynx. Strahlenther Onkol 165: 18–22
Wendt CD, Peters LJ, Delclos L et al. (1990a) Primary radiotherapy in the treatment of stage I and II oral tongue cancers: importance of the proportion of therapy delivered with interstitial therapy. Int J Radiat Oncol Biol Phys 18: 1287–1292
Wendt TG, Wustrow TPU, Schalhorn A (1990b) Ergebnisse der simultanen Radio-Chemotherapie bei fortgeschrittenen Kopf-Hals-Tumoren. Strahlenther Onkol 166: 569–579
White D, Byers RM (1980) What is the preferred initial method of treatment for squamous carcinoma of the tongue? Am J Surg 140: 553–555
Whitehurst JO, Droulias CA (1977) Surgical treatment of squamous cell carcinoma of the oral tongue. Factors influencing survival. Arch Otolaryngol 103: 212–215
Wilson GD, McNally NJ, Dische S, Saunders M, Des Rochers C, Lewis A, Bennet MH (1988) Measurement of cell kinetics in human tumours in vivo using bromodeoxyuridine incorporation and flow cytometry Br J Cancer 58: 423–431
Yam JH, Gu XZ (1983) Radiation therapy of recurrent nasopharyngeal carcinoma. Acta Radiol Oncol 22: 23–28
Yco MS, Cruickshank JC (1986) Treatment of stage I carcinoma of the anterior floor of the mouth. Arch Otolaryngol Head Neck Surg 112: 1085–1089

22 Clinical Rationale for Interstitial Thermoradiotherapy of Gynecological Tumors: Review of Clinical Results and Own Experiences with Continuous Mild Hyperthermia

A. Martinez, D. Gersten, and P. Corry

CONTENTS

22.1 Introduction

In gynecological malignancies, external beam treatments in combination with intracavitary treatment with applications such as the Fletcher–Suit, Henschke, Bleodorm, Delclos, Chassagne and others have been utilized. To a lesser degree, interstitial treatments (radium implants) combined with external beam therapy have been used for advanced vaginal and female urethral lesions. Unfortunately, the local control rates reported in all these patients with bulky pelvic disease have been disappointingly low (Chau 1963; Grabstald et al. 1966; Fletcher 1980; Prempree et al. 1980; Perez et al. 1983). The most likely explanations for these low control rates are: (a) inability to deliver a high dose of irradiation to rather large volumes of tumorous tissues; (b) inadequate tumor coverage (target volume) by either the intracavitary application or radium needles, and (c) tumor dose inhomogeneity within the treated volume.

In an attempt to improve on tumor control for large pelvic tumors, transperineal interstitial–intracavitary applicators such as the Martinez Universal Perineal Interstitial Template (MUPIT) (Martinez et al. 1984, 1985a, b) and the Syed-Neblett parametrial butterflies (Feder et al. 1978; Fleming et al. 1980) of the afterloading type were developed. They are based on similar principles, i.e., improving target volume coverage and dose distribution. However, there are several crucial design differences between the MUPIT and the Syed-Neblett templates, and there are also differences in respect of dosimetric considerations. For the purpose of this chapter, some of the classic works will be cited as well as some of the most recent publications utilizing standard therapy, i.e., external beam irradiation and when feasible intracavitary or radium implants; these studies will be compared with series using interstitial transperineal boost implants.

A. Martinez, M.D., F.A.C.R.; D. Gersten, P. Corry, Ph.D.; Department of Radiation Oncology, Division of Brachytherapy and Research, William Beaumont Hospital, 3601 West Thirteen Mile Road, Royal Oak, MI 48072, USA

22.2 Intracavitary/Interstitial Experience

22.2.1 Results of Intracavitary Irradiation

In 1979, Van Nagell et al. reported on 103 patients with stage IIIB (locally advanced) cervical cancer. Stage of disease, cell type, lesion size, and malignant cells within vascular spaces were all shown to be prognostically significant. Fifty-three percent of the patients demonstrated persistence of tumor at completion of therapy or developed a local recurrence.

Perez et al. (1980) reported a retrospective analysis with emphasis on the patterns of failure. Looking specifically at 212 patients with stage III disease, 25% of the pelvic failures were central (cervix and vagina) and the remainder (75%) occurred in the parametrial area. This pattern of recurrence emphasizes the difficulty in controlling the disease with conventional intracavitary applicators.

Montana et al. (1986) reviewed 203 patients with stage III epidermoid carcinoma of the cervix treated with radiation therapy with curative intent. The disease-free survival at 5 years was 33%. Eighty-eight patients were treated with external beam therapy only, while 115 received external beam therapy and brachytherapy. The disease-free survival was better for combination therapy but this difference was not sustained beyond 5 years. One hundred and eighty patients developed recurrence within the irradiated field for a locoregional recurrence rate of 53%. Twenty-seven patients (13%) developed complications. Distant metastasis alone was seen in 12% of the patients. However, when distant metastasis is combined with locoregional failure, the incidence rose to 27% overall.

A total of 518 patients with stage III cancer of the cervix were collected from the VAN NAGELL et al.; PEREZ et al.; and MONTANA et al. series. The overall local recurrence rate following external beam and intracavitary irradiation was 48%. However, the combined distant metastatic failure was only 15.3%. This represents the state of the art with conventional therapy from recent series with current technology.

It is clear that local control remains a very important statistical problem. However, for the patient and for the treating physician uncontrolled pelvic disease is not a statistical problem but a clinical nightmare – a challenge that must be taken very seriously. In an effort to improve on this major therapeutic dilemma, interstitial – intracavitary templates, such as the MUPIT and the Syed-Neblett applicators, were designed. We shall now review the pertinent data on locally advanced cervical and vaginal–urethral carcinomas treated using transperineal afterloading templates.

22.2.2 *Results Achieved with Interstitial Transperineal Templates*

Brachytherapy has long been recognized as an excellent way of delivering a high dose of irradiation to a rather limited volume. It was on this basis that the concept of the afterloading interstitial perineal template was developed around 1974. Independently, Martinez at Stanford University and Syed at the University of Southern California began to explore this concept in depth. Today, the resultant technique is widely used. We will review the papers published on the subject.

22.2.2.1 Cervix

FEDER et al. in 1978 published a preliminary report on 35 patients with stage IIB–IIIB cancer of the cervix who had been treated with external beam therapy and transperineal parametrial butterfly implants. They stated, "Although our complication rate is relatively low and results today are very encouraging, it is much too early to report long term survivals". In 1985 ARISTIZABAL et al. reported a cooperative study between the University of Arizona in Tucson and the University of Valle in Cali, Colombia, South America. This series comprised 41 patients with bulky stage IIB disease and 77 with stage IIIB disease, for a total of 118 patients treated. With a minimum follow-up of 24 months, overall pelvic control rate was 75%. Of most interest was the fact that the pelvic control rate was similar regardless of stage, tumor size, degree of parametrial involvement, fixation to one or both pelvic side walls, and extent of vaginal involvement. On the other hand, a high incidence of local failure was observed in patients with bilateral hydronephrosis (75%), barrel-shaped tumors (60%), or frozen pelvis (57%). The incidence of serious radiation side-effects was markedly decreased from 33% to 21% by modifications in implant geometry and reduction of the total milligram hours. In addition, the severity of the complications was also reduced; thus the percentage with grade 3 complications declined from 80% to 35%. In 1985, MARTINEZ et al. published their experience with the combination of external beam irradiation and the MUPIT. A total of 104 patients were treated for locally advanced malignancies of the cervix, vagina, female urethra, and anorectal regions. This represents the combined experience of Stanford University and the Mayo Clinic. Thirty-seven patients had bulky stage IIB or IIIB cervical cancer. Six patients (17%) developed a local recurrence. The complication rate was 5.4%. Only the target tumor volume is treated by the implant. No attempt is made to implant the pelvic lymph nodes.

GADDIS et al. (1983) published an update of the preliminary report by FEDER et al. (1978), using the Syed-Neblett cervical template. They reported the results in 84 women with primary squamous cell carcinoma of the cervix at the Los Angeles County University of Southern California Medical Center. Fifty-one patients with stages IIB–IIIB were treated with external beam irradiation and a Syed-Neblett transperineal implant. Seventeen of these patients (31%) developed a local recurrence. Eight (16%) developed non-tumor-related rectovaginal or vesicovaginal fistulas. Severe or grade III non-fistulous, delayed adverse effects (proctosigmoiditis, cystitis, vault necrosis) occurred in an additional six patients. AMPUERO et al. (1983) reported on 24 patients with advanced disease or poor vaginal anatomy who were selected for this modality of external beam irradiation and Syed-Neblett transperineal template. Nine patients (38%) failed locally. Most distressing is the high complication rate of 29% in stages IIB–IIIB. Twenty-two percent of the patients developed severe rectal stricture or rectovaginal fistula necessitating diverting colostomy.

Even though the local control rates reported by GADDIS et al. and AMPUERO et al. are slightly lower than in the other series, they are much better than would be expected from external beam and intracavitary irradiation. Unfortunately, the complication rate in these two studies is much higher than in the others. From the ARTISTIZABAL et al. (1985) study, one can see that meticulous attention to the dosimetry of the template and early correlation with complications can decrease the number and severity of complications when using the Syed-Neblett template. If one adds all the patients treated with interstitial transperineal boost, a total of 230 patients are compiled. The local recurrence rate was 27%. This represents a 50% reduction in locoregional recurrence when compared to external beam and intracavitary irradiation. The overall complication rate of 18% is no different than that reported by the Patterns of Care Study.

22.2.2.2 Vagina/Urethra

PEREZ et al. (1977) updated the experience in respect of patients treated by radiotherapy for all stages of vaginal carcinoma. Once again, it is clear that the local control rate for locally advanced cases is suboptimal. FLEMING et al. in 1980 provided a preliminary report of an afterloading iridium-192 interstitial–intracavitary technique used in the treatment of carcinoma of the vagina (stage I through III) at U.S.C. Medical Center. Of the 13 patients treated, five (38%) developed a pelvic failure and three developed a posttreatment complication. MARTINEZ et al. (1985a) updated the vaginal–urethral series. Of 25 patients treated with curative intent at Stanford University Hospital and Mayo Clinic, five (20%) developed a local recurrence. No additional major complications were seen.

22.2.3 Summary of Intracavitary/Interstitial Experience

In summary, for patients with locally advanced cervical, vaginal, and urethral carcinoma the use of transperineal interstitial template brachytherapy in conjunction with external beam therapy has significantly increased the local control rates when compared to standard intracavitary and external beam irradiation. Complications of these large volume implants appear to be at acceptable levels. However, despite this improvement, close to 30% of the patients still developed a pelvic failure. For this reason, we were interested in exploring other modalities and, after careful investigation, our group decided on testing brachytherapy with hyperthermia.

22.3 Hyperthermia

22.3.1 General Considerations

Interest in hyperthermia, elevated temperatures in the range 41°C–50°C, has been increasing steadily over the past decade. This interest has been stimulated in part by a compelling biological rationale and in part by limited progress on some other fronts. During this time many phase I, II, and III clinical trials have been conducted. Their conclusions are as follows:

1. When used as a single agent, locoregional hyperthermia is of limited, short-term palliative benefit.
2. When combined with suboptimal radiation therapy, hyperthermia doubles the complete response rate from approximately 25% to 50% and the duration of response is increased. This improvement appears to be independent of tumor cell type.
3. Whether or not hyperthermia will improve local control and cure rates in conjunction with definitive radiation therapy remains unanswered.
4. Locoregional hyperthermia does not increase the acute and chronic toxicities associated with radiotherapy or chemotherapy.

One obvious situation where hyperthermia can be effectively applied is in conjunction with conventional brachytherapy. Such combination therapy has been undertaken in the past primarily using microwave technology, where multiple antennae are placed intratumorally into plastic catheters previously inserted for this purpose (PEREZ and EMAMI 1985; COUGLIN and STROHBEHN 1989).

Another situation where hyperthermia can and has been applied (KONG et al. 1986; VORA et al. 1987) is for implants that involve stainless steel needles to contain the radioactive material. This technique is usually implemented with template guidance. It is the development of this latter type of technology that we have pursued and describe in this chapter. If an electric field is applied to these needles, they behave as electrodes and the electric current passing between them causes power deposition and temperature elevation in the intervening tissues. If the frequency of the applied electric field is sufficiently high, for example, greater than 20 kHz, no sensation of shock is experienced by the patient. An additional advantage of this approach is that hyperthermia can be added with potentially little increase in the complexity of the procedures, other than the introduction of catheters for thermometry devices.

In the past, we have experienced difficulties in applying this form of technology clinically. While power could be introduced easily, the available electronic power drivers afforded only rudimentary control of the spatial power deposition pattern. In every case, the treatment-limiting factor was treatment-induced power level-associated pain, occasionally in the face of heavy narcotic analgesia and sedation. Indeed, this experience was typical of the state of the art for locoregional hyperthermic treatment of deep-seated lesions. Recent clinical trials have shown that the heating of nonsuperficial tumors to above 42°C is not only technically very difficult but can lead to substantial acute toxicities, primarily local pain.

KAPP et al. (1988) reporting on the experience at Stanford University, could not obtain average temperatures beyond the range of 40–42°C in deep-seated tumors although the goal temperature was 43°C. Virtually identical conclusions were reached by SAPOZINK et al. (1988) reporting on the University of Utah experience and by SHIMM et al. (1988) from the University of Arizona. CORRY et al. (1988) reported similar results for the M.D. Anderson Hospital experience, and also observed that increasing the number of intratumoral temperature points further reduced the estimate of tumor heating adequacy.

In all of the above reports, treatment-associated pain was reported by 80%–90% of patients and was the primary limiting factor in 40%–45%. These observations clearly pointed out the need for better systems for hyperthermia induction that are capable of real-time dynamically alterable power deposition patterns to control and elevate temperatures in all parts of the tumor. Another complicating factor is that many deep-seated tumors involve major nervous structures that are irritated by temperatures above 42°C, resulting in a severe but poorly described pain sensation. On the other hand, temperatures below 42°C are much less of an irritant. In all of the above studies, the target intratumoral temperatures were 43°–45°C since for treatment times of the order of 1 h this is the temperature range thought to be needed for therapeutic efficacy. The data cited above also demonstrated that while 43°–45°C was not achievable with current technology, 40°–42°C was achievable, in many cases with significantly decreased pain.

For some time it has been thought that these lower temperatures are ineffective. However, recent data from our laboratories published by ARMOUR et al. (1991, 1992) and by LING and ROBINSON (1988) suggest that this may not be the case. ARMOUR et al.'s data for protracted heat exposures with continuous low dose rate irradiation demonstrated a thermal enhancement ratio (TER) of 2. The sensitization by simultaneous heating and low dose rate brachytherapy occurred even though thermotolerance developed during extended incubation at 41°C (ARMOUR et al. 1991). Extended exposures at lower temperatures may thus be a useful alternative for sensitizing radiation killing in large volume and/or recurrent tumors.

In our laboratory, these regimens of continuous mild hyperthermia (40°–42°C) were substantially more effective than the more conventional pulses of 1 h of hyperthermia at ≥ 43°C before and after the protracted low dose rate radiation course (TER of 1.1) (ARMOUR et al. 1991). Since all of our template-guided needle implant brachytherapy cases are confined to a hospital bed for 48–72 h and we routinely use continually connected remote afterloading, all of the above observations suggested that the protracted hyperthermia might be a very efficacious approach.

22.3.2 *System Development*

We began by applying the commercially available Oncotherm LCF-2032 interstitial hyperthermia system to template-guided implants using the MUPIT developed by MARTINEZ et al. (1984). We quickly realized that the limited operational characteristics of this system precluded the use of large implants. In addition, because of the rudimentary interface, dynamic alteration of the power deposition during therapy and afterloading techniques was also precluded. It quickly became apparent that if this type of application was to become feasible, more advanced and flexible equipment was essential.

The characteristics which we considered to be required for a truly useful clinical system were the following:

1. Compatibility with simultaneous remote afterloading
2. Dynamic alteration of the power deposition pattern at all times during therapy
3. Fully automated control and data acquisition
4. Minimum setup complexity
5. Portability and usability in the patient's hospital room
6. Expansibility for future application to segmented electrodes for three-dimensional power deposition control.

Consideration of these characteristics showed that for most real implants, literally hundreds of electrical connections are required: a minimum of twice the combination for the next neighbor condition. It was clear that the concept of paired connection of electrodes must be eliminated to make application practical. To accomplish this we devised an electronic version of the MUPIT template which we affectionately refer to as the HUPIT.

While the development of this type of template solved the interfacing and afterloading compatibility problems, there were no existing electronic systems that could be modified or adapted to drive it. In designing a new system that was capable of routing power anywhere into the template, we found that it was simpler to fabricate an ideal system. Constraints that would limit power deposition to next neighbor needles substantially increased the hardware complexity. The easiest and most flexible approach was to dedicate a microprocessor to generating and multiplexing the RF power into the template and to have all constraints in the appropriate software. This system as implemented can channel the power generated by four DC/RF converters into any of the potential 1770 connections that would result from a 60-needle implant. Although 60-needle implants are rarely if ever done, the system must have the capability of connecting all positions in the template.

The design can accommodate up to 240 electrode positions to permit future expansion to segmented needles for power deposition control in the third dimension.

22.3.3 Preliminary Clinical Results

The preliminary results of our clinical trial investigating interstitial hyperthermia in combination with brachytherapy were presented at the Sixth International Congress on Hyperthermic Oncology in Tucson, Arizona in April 1992. Twenty-five patients have been treated according to the protocol, 20 of whom had recurrent pelvic malignancies. The initial seven patients received only two hyperthermia exposures at the beginning and at the end of the continuous low dose rate implant. Having gained confidence with the RF generator and since all patients were treated with the remote afterloader, the next nine patients received three acute hyperthermia treatments at the beginning, in the middle, and at the end of brachytherapy. After this satisfactory experience as far as patient tolerance to treatment was concerned, we began the final phase of the trial combining continuous mild hyperthermia at 41°C and remote afterloading continuous low dose rate brachytherapy. Nine patients have been treated with this combined simultaneous modality. Six of the nine had large recurrent tumors and the other three had very large primaries for which conventional therapy was judged to have low probability of control. Table 22.1 summarizes the results of the acute heat

Table 22.1. Results of acute heat exposures (2–4 h at 43°C, BMF) plus brachytherapy (15–40 Gy)

Response category	Number of patients	Follow-up	Mean tumor volume (cm^3)
CR	5 (31.3%)	> 1 year	56 (36, 36, 48, 80, 100)
PR	6 (37.4%)	> 1 year	182 (9, 9, 120, 180, 275, 500)
NR	5 (31.3%)	> 1 year	263 (156, 180, 240, 336, 405)

BMF, before, in the middle of, and after radiation; CR, complete response; PR, partial response; NR, no response

Table 22.2. Results of continuous hyperthermia (48–72 h at 41°C) plus brachytherapy (15–40 Gy)

Response category	Number of patients	Follow-up	Mean tumor volume (cm^3)
CR	6 (66.7%)	> 6 mo	293 (180, 210, 288, 294, 336, 450)
PR(BN)	1 (11.1%)	4 mo	150 (150)
PR	2 (22.2%)	2, 4 mo	286 (180, 392)

CR, complete response; PR, partial response; PR(BN), biopsy negative

exposures and Table 22.2 the results of the continuous hyperthermia exposure.

22.3.4 Discussion

Although it is premature to assess the long-term clinical utility and efficacy of our system, we are pleased with the initial clinical results. The majority of the difficulties associated with the previously impossibly complex setup procedures have been resolved through the use of the electronic template and the unique RF driving system. Real-time dynamic alteration of the power deposition patterns permitted us to ameliorate previously limiting pain toxicities and allowed us to shift additional power to cold spots within the tumor.

The time multiplexing parameters were adjusted to determine the maximum instantaneous spatial peak power levels that were tolerated. These manipulations showed that with a 55% reduction in the instantaneous level, the treatment was well tolerated in the sensitive area. This observation graphically illustrated a significant drawback of the system described here. It continues to be necessary to resort to temporal multiplexing of the power generation capabilities among the various electrode combinations in order to effect dynamic alteration of the power deposition pattern. At the present time, we have a second generation system under construction which will completely eliminate all pairing of electrodes and time multiplexing. We have calculated that this will result in a sixfold reduction in the instantaneous power levels for most tumors.

Little has been discussed concerning the computer software that was developed to run and control this system. With literally hundreds of potential power deposition elements and more than one hundred temperature measurements per minute, to permit responsive, quick, and dynamic control, these programs are understandably complex. Some operator intervention was necessary during the heat-up phase to steady-state temperatures, which lasted 15–20 min. In addition, it was necessary to intervene to optimize the temperature distributions and to minimize pain. Nevertheless, once optimized, after 30–45 min, the system was capable of continuous unattended operation. This is a prerequisite to the institution of protracted simultaneous combined brachytherapy and hyperthermia.

In summary, the conclusions of our limited experience with thermal brachytherapy can be divided into (a) technical conclusions and (b) clinical conclusions. Under technical conclusions, we can state that the system is technically reliable and provides adequate power deposition into the tissues, allowing heating of larger volumes in the range 150–450 cm^3. The new RF generator significantly decreases the setup time when compared with the commercially available generators, and it is user friendly. Within the clinical conclusions, one can say that when acute short duration hyperthermia was used, only small lesions with a mean volume of 56 cm^3 achieved a complete clinical response (31.3% of the patients treated). With continuous hyperthermia, the complete clinical response rate was doubled to 67% despite the large tumor sizes (mean volume of 293 cm^3). The remaining 33% of the patients responded to continuous hyperthermia but it was a partial response of short duration. The final conclusion is that more patients and longer follow-up are needed to solidify this exciting preliminary experience.

Acknowledgments. Special thanks are due to all of the members of the Brachytherapy and Research Teams. Development of the hyperthermia system was supported in part by grant CA-44550 from the U.S. National Cancer Institute. We are grateful to Ms. Glenda Noble, C.P.S., for the typing of this manuscript.

References

Ampuero F, et al. (1987) The Syed-Neblett interstitial template in locally advanced gynaecologic malignancies. Int J Radiat Oncol Biol Phys 9: 1987

Armour E, Wang Z, Corry P, Martinez A (1991) Sensitization of rat 9L gliosarcoma cells to low dose rate irradiation by long duration 41°C hyperthermia. Cancer Res 51: 3088–3095

Armour E, Wang Z, Corry P, Martinez A (1992) Equivalence of continuous and pulse simulated low dose rate irradiation in 9L gliosarcoma cells at 37° and 41°C. Int J Radiat Oncol Biol Phys 22: 109–114

Aristizabal et al. (1985) Interstitial parametrial irradiation in cancer of the cervix, stages IIB–IIIB: analysis of pelvic control and complications. Int J Endocurie/Hyperthermia Oncol 1: 41

Chau PM (1983) Radiotherapeutic management of malignant tumours of the vagina. AJR 89: 502

Corry PM, Jabboury K, Kong JS, Armour EP, McGraw JF, Leduc T (1988) Phase I evaluation of equipment for hyperthermic treatment of cancer. Int J Hyperthermia 4: 53–74

Couglin CT, Strohbehn JW (1989) Interstitial thermoradiotherapy. Radiol Clin North Am 27: 577–588

Feder B et al. (1978) Treatment of extensive carcinoma of the cervix with the "transperineal parametrial butterfly". Int J Radiat Oncol Biol Phys 4: 735

Fleming P, et al. (1980) Description of an afterloading 192 iridium interstitial intracavitary technique in the treatment of carcinoma of the vagina. Obstet Gynecol 55: 525

Fletcher GH (1980) Textbook of radiotherapy, 3rd edn. Lea & Fiebiger, Philadelphia

Gaddis O et al. (1983) Treatment of cervical carcinoma employing a template for transperineal interstitial 192 iridium brachytherapy. Int J Radiat Oncol Biol Phys 9: 819

Grabstald H et al. (1966) Cancer of the female urethra. JAMA 197: 835

Kapp DS, Fessenden P, Samulski TV, Bagshaw MA, Cox RS, Lee ER (1988) Stanford University institutional report: Phase I Evaluation of equipment for hyperthermic treatment of cancer. Int J Hyperthermia 4: 75–116

Kong JS, Corry PM, Saul PB (1986) Hyperthermia in the treatment of gynecologic cancers. In: Freeman Gershenson (eds) Diagnosis and treatment strategies for gynecologic cancers. The University of Texas Press, Austin

Ling CC, Robinson E (1988) Moderator hyperthermia and low dose rate radiation. Radiat Res 114: 379–384

Martinez A et al. (1983) Interstitial therapy of perineal and gynaecological malignancies. Int J Radiat Oncol Biol Phys 9: 409

Martinez A et al. (1984) A multiple-site perineal applicator (MUPIT) for treatment of prostatic, anorectal, and gynaecologic malignancies. Int J Radiat Oncol Biol Phys 10: 297

Martinez A et al. (1985a) Combination of external beam irradiation and multiple-site perineal applicator (MUPIT) for treatment of locally advanced or recurrent prostatic, anorectal, and gynaecological malignancies. Int J Radiat Oncol Biol Phys 11: 391

Martinez A et al. (1985b) Pelvic lymphadenectomy combined with transperineal interstitial implantation of 192 iridium and external beam radiotherapy for locally advanced prostatic carcinoma: a technical description. Int J Radiat Oncol Biol Phys 11: 841

Montana G et al. (1986) Carcinoma of the cervix, stage III: results of radiation therapy. Cancer 57: 148

Perez CA, Emami BA (1985) A review of current clinical experience with irradiation and hyperthermia. Endocurietherapy Hyperthermia Oncology 1: 257–277

Perez et al. (1977) Dosimetric considerations in irradiation of carcinoma of the vagina. Int J Radiat Oncol Biol Phys 2: 639

Perez CA et al. (1980) Radiation therapy alone in the treatment of carcinoma of the uterine cervix: analysis of tumour recurrence. Cancer 51: 1393

Perez CA, et al. (1983) Radiation therapy alone in the treatment of carcinoma of the uterine cervix. Cancer 51: 3193

Prempree T et al. (1980) Parametrial implants in the treatment of stage IIB carcinoma of the cervix: II. Analysis of success and failure. Cancer 46: 1485

Sapozink MA, Gibbs FA, Gibbs P, Stewart JR (1988) Phase I evaluation of hyperthermia equipment: University of Utah institutional report. Int J Hyperthermia 4: 117–132

Shimm DS, Cetas TC, Oleson JR, Cassady JR, Sim DA (1988) Clinical evaluation of hyperthermia equipment: The University of Arizona institutional report for the NCI hyperthermia equipment evaluation contract. Int J Hyperthermia 4: 39–52

Van Nagell JR et al. (1979) Therapeutic implications of patterns of recurrence in cancer of the uterine cervix. Cancer 44: 2354

Vora N, Forrel B, Cappil J, Lipsett J, Archambeau JO (1987) Interstitial implant with interstitial hyperthermia. Cancer 50: 2518–2523

23 Clinical Experience of Interstitial Thermoradiotherapy Using Radiofrequency Techniques

C. MARCHAL

CONTENTS

23.1 Introduction

In 1976, DOSS and MCCABE suggested the use of a radiofrequency technique (RF: 0.5–13 MHz) to heat tissues by means of an implanted array of needles. COSSET et al. (1982) proposed the clinical use of rigid metal and plastic tubes (0.5 MHz) while GOFFINET et al. (1990) developed flexible conductive catheters for radiofrequency interstitial hyperthermia (RF-IHT).

On the basis of the same working principle as underlies localized current field (LCF) methods, MARCHAL et al. in 1985 suggested a capacitive interstitial RF technique at 27 MHz whereby the direct contact of the needle and the tissue was replaced by capacitive coupling through the same catheters as were used for brachytherapy. The electrodes had an active length which could be adapted to each clinical situation. The Rotterdam group (DEURLOO et al. 1991) greatly improved the capacitive RF hyperthermia technique using separate generators and matching networks.

The combined use of interstitial irradiation and RF-IHT not only delivers a high radiation dose in a short time to a limited tumor bed, but also spares the adjacent normal tissues. Therefore its use has increased over the past decade (see Table 23.1). However, the radiation dose delivered is highly heterogeneous compared to external beam irradiation. Temperature distributions are rather more uniform than those obtained with external heating and are comparable to those achieved with the other interstitial heating techniques.

C. MARCHAL, M.D., Ph.D., Unité d'hyperthermie, Service de radiothérapie, Centre Alexis Vautrin, Avenue de Bourgogne, F-54511 Vandoeuvre les Nancy, France

23.2 Overview of the Main Pilot Studies Using Radiofrequency Interstitial Hyperthermia in Cancer Therapy

An incomplete list of groups currently working with RF-IHT is given in Table 23.1. It can be seen that recent updated reports are not available from most of these groups. Only phase I–II studies have been published concerning the feasibility of an original method or the evaluation of new commercial material.

Radiofrequency interstitial heating is mostly performed under general anesthesia to avoid patient discomfort and pain during the treatment but also to make possible convenient heating using the stainless steel needles implanted as guides for the brachytherapy technique. Therefore most of the hyperthermia sessions are delivered *before* brachytherapy.

When RF-IHT is combined with brachytherapy a therapeutic gain (therapeutic enhancement ratio) of about 1.3–1.5 can be achieved (JANORAY et al. 1985; JONES et al. 1989), and treatments delivering a complete dose of brachytherapy are to be preferred. In contrast, most clinical trials have delivered a low dose of interstitial irradiation: the mean is about 30 Gy, which corresponds to an expected maximal biological effect of only 39–45 Gy equivalent dose.

Table 23.2 summarizes the main clinical results published using RF-IHT. A total of 338 evaluable lesions were treated with different RF-IHT techniques. The toxicity in terms of burns and necrosis is about 25%, with some variations from one group

Table 23.1. Institutions currently using radiofrequency interstitial hyperthermia

Institution	Principal investigators	Material used	Frequencies	Patients treated (total)	Last report
Stanford University (Stanford, USA)	R. GOFFINET	Flexible interstitial/ brachytherapy catheter	0.5 MHz	10	1990
City of Hope (Durate, USA)	N.L. VORA B. FORELL	Needles	0.5 MHz	79	1989
The University of Arizona (Tucson, USA)	S.A. ARISTIZABAL R. OLESON R. MANNING T.C. CETAS	Needles	0.5 MHz	64 17	1984 1988
Mallinckdrodt Institute (San Francisco)	B. EMAMI	Needles	0.5 MHz	9	1987
French Multistudy Group (IGR, Lyon, Dijon, France)	J.M. COSSET J.P. GERARD J.M. ARDIET J.C. HORIOT	Needles	0.5 MHz	96	1988
Curie Institute (Paris, France)	A. FOURQUET D. PONVERT	Needles	0.5 MHz	11	1990
Center Alexis Vautrin (Nancy, France)	C. MARCHAL M. PERNOT S. HOFFSTETTER	Insulated electrodes	27 MHz	5	1986
The Dr. Daniel Den Hoed Cancer Center (Rotterdam, The Netherlands)	A.G. VISSER P.C. LEVENDAG	Insulated electrodes	27 MHz	11	1992
Shiga University (Shiga, Japan)	E. YABUMOTO	Needles	8 MHz	14	1988
William Beaumont Hospital (Royal Oak, USA)	A. MARTINEZ J.C. BORREGO P. CORRY	Needles	0.5 MHz	13	1990

Table 23.2. Clinical experience with RF-IHT

Authors	Evaluable lesions	CR (%)	PR (%)	Interstitial radiation dose (Gy)	Toxicity (%)	Follow-up (months)
OLESON et al. (1984)	52	38	42	–	21	3–18
COSSET et al. (1985)	29	66	14	30	25	2
LINARES et al. (1986)	10	30	70	20–40	40	–
MARCHAL et al. (1985)	5	60	40	20–60	20	2–36
EMAMI et al. (1987)	9	55	11	20–60	25	6–48
GAUTHERIE (1988)	96	61	14	15–60	26	> 2
VORA et al. (1989)	78	53	19	20–30	17	1–13
YABUMOTO et al. (1989)	14	57	14	12–45	31	3–13
GOFFINET et al. (1990)	10	100	0	20–43	10	–
FOURQUET et al. (1990)	11	82	0	20	27	–
BORREGO et al. (1990)	13	46	–	20–35	50	2–20
LEVENDAG et al. (1992)	11	54	0	20–66	10	1–36
Total	338	59	20	15–66	25	2–48

CR, complete response; PR, partial response

to another. The overall complete response rate is 59% and the partial response rate is 20% with brachytherapy doses ranging from 15 to 66 Gy; however, most of the tumors were preirradiated by external beam irradiation and primary tumors actually received a total dose of 60 Gy and recurrences 40 Gy.

With the aim of reducing toxicity, CORRY et al. (1990) have developed a new radiofrequency generator and a new coverplate applicator named HUPIT (hyperthermia universal perineal template) which can be linked up to the microselectron LDR system and to the RF generator. From their preliminary clinical experience, BORREGO et al. (1990) reported that "this electronic template permits unlimited two-dimensional control of power deposition within the tumor by effectively generating power to 1670 electrode pairs. This new design has a significant impact on patient comfort, staff set-up time and treatment interrupt time."

23.3 Clinical Experience According to Tumor Site

23.3.1 Tumors of the Pelvis

As regards gynecological tumors, RF-IHT has mainly been used in the primary treatment of cervical carcinomas of stage IIIA or IIIB, uterine adenocarcinomas, and tumors of the vagina, but it has also been employed for pelvic recurrences of gynecological tumors.

Of the 87 lesions found in the literature and detailed with precision (see Table 23.3), 49% showed complete regression with an acceptable toxicity evaluated at ca. 20%.

For large perineal implantations, as in the case of cervical tumors or recurrences of gynecological cancers, perfect identification of each pair of electrodes is needed. Up to 40 needles may be implanted with a lot of technical difficulties due to converging or diverging electrodes inducing undesired hot spots.

23.3.2 Colorectal Tumors

For rectal cancers six to ten needles are usually required with different template immobilization systems. The method has proved simple to use and reproducible.

An excellent tumor response rate of close to 75% is also described for these tumors (Table 23.4), but severe toxicity is seen in a few cases, often in previously irradiated sites which required surgery.

23.3.3 Tumors of the Breast

The implanted sites are usually superficial with typical arrays of 8–12 needles in two parallel planes, with special templates for immobilization. Heating is performed under general anesthesia before iridium-192 loading. Excellent temperature uniformity is usually achieved, though toxicity is observed in a surprisingly large number of cases (between 20% and 29%).

As shown in Tables 23.5 and 23.6, the efficacy of combined RF-IHT and brachytherapy is excellent for both primary tumors of the breast and recurrences (complete responses having been achieved in 88% and 79% of cases, respectively), but very few patients have been treated as yet.

Table 23.3. RF-IHT for gynecological tumors

Authors	No. of lesions (Patients)	General anesthesia	Average tep.	Burns	Duration of IHT	Radiation does (Gy)	CR	PR
VORA et al. (1989)	20 (20)	Yes	43°–44°C	4/20	30 min to 1 h	30–40	10/20 (50%)	–
OLESON et al. (1984)	36 (36)	Yes	–	–	1 h	26	–	–
GAUTHERIE (1988)	23 (23)	Yes	44°C	4/23	1 h	20–40	11/23 (48%)	–
BORREGO et al. (1990)	8 (8)	Yes	41.5°–43 °C	Pain (62%)	2 × 1 h	20–35	–	
Total	87	Yes	41.5°–44 °C	20%	30 min–2 h	20–40	49%	

IHT, interstitial hyperthermia; CR, complete response; PR, partial response

Table 23.4. RF-IHT for colorectal tumors

Authors	No. of lesions (Patients)	General anesthesia	Average tep.	Burns	Duration of IHT	Radiation does (Gy)	CR	PR
Vora et al. (1989)	18 (8)	Yes	43°–44 °C	?	30 min to 1 h	30–40	?	–
Oleson et al. (1984)	9 (9)	Yes	–	–	1 h	26	–	–
Gautherie (1988)	16 (16)	Yes	44°C	3/16	1 h	20–40	75%	–
Borrego et al. (1990)	5 (5)	Yes	41.5°–43 °C	Pain (62%)	2 × 1 h	20–35	?	
Total	48	Yes	41.5°–44 °C	19%	30 min–2 h	20–40	75%	

See Table 23.3 for abbreviations

Table 23.5. RF-IHT for primary tumors of the breast

Authors	No. of lesions (Patients)	General anesthesia	Average tep.	Burns	Duration of IHT	Radiation does (Gy)	CR	PR
Fourquet (1990)	11 (11)	Yes	44.2°C	3/11 (27%)	1 h	20	9/11 (82%)	0 (0%)
Oleson et al. (1984)	2 (2)	Yes	–	–	1 h	–	–	–
Vora et al. (1989)	15 (15)	Yes	42°–43 °C	2/14 (14%)	30 min to 1 h	15–30	13/14 (93%)	1/14 (7%)
Total	28	Yes	42°–44.2 °C	20%	30–60 min	15–30	88%	7%

See Table 23.3 for abbreviations

Table 23.6. RF-IHT results in recurrent tumors of the breast

Authors	No. of lesions (Patients)	General anesthesia	Average tep.	Burns	Duration of IHT	Radiation does (Gy)	CR	PR
Vora et al. (1989)	9 (9)	Yes	43°–44 °C	–	30 min to 1 h	20–40	–	–
Gautherie (1988)	14 (14)	Yes	44°C	4/14 (29%)	1 h	20–40	11/14 (79%)	3/14 (21%)
Total	23	Yes	43°–44 °C	29%	30–60 min	20–40	79%	21%

See Table 23.3 for abbreviations

23.3.4 Head and Neck Tumors

The literature contains few details on the use of RF–IHT for head and neck tumors. Base of tongue cancers are well vascularized and many technical difficulties are encountered using the LCF technique. Surprisingly high temperature inhomogeneities observed in fairly "good" implantations have been related to the high perfusion rate in some tumors and healthy tissues. Nevertheless, the complete tumor response rate is ca. 65% when RF-IHT is combined with a total dose of radiation. Patient tolerance can be a problem with the use of rigid needles requiring parallel implantations and therefore most of the treatments reported have been performed under general anesthesia.

Table 23.7. RF-IHT for head and neck tumors

Authors	No. of lesions (Patients)	General anesthesia	Average tep.	Burns	Duration of IHT	Radiation does (Gy)	CR	PR
VORA et al. (1989)	9/9	Yes	43°–44 °C	–	30 min to 1 h	30 40	–	–
OLESON et al. (1984)	9/9	Yes	–	–	1 h	26	–	–
GAUTHERIE (1988)	35/35	Yes	44°C	?	1 h	20–40	75%	–
LEVENDAG et al. (1992)	11/11	No	41°–47 °C	Pain (45%)	1 h	20–66	54%	0%
Total	64				30–60 min	20–66	65%	0%

See Table 23.3 for abbreviations

23.4 Conclusions

Radiofrequency interstitial hyperthermia, and especially the LCF technique, has proved to be efficient for inducing therapeutic temperatures with an acceptable though significant toxicity of ca. 25% (see Table 23.2). This toxicity is partly due to the risk of creating hot spots near the tip of converging planes of needles. Therefore we regard it as likely that the use of flexible electrodes as proposed by GOFFINET et al. (1990) will increase this risk whereas multiplexing the RF power in a lot of parallel needles, as proposed by CORRY et al. (1990) with the HUPIT system, should improve the set-up and patient tolerance.

With the LCF technique, the treatments are mainly conducted under general anesthesia, thus raising the risk of uncontrollable hot spots. New capacitive RF techniques are promising in that standard catheters and conventional brachytherapy implantations can be used.

References

Aristizabal SA, Oleson JR (1984) Combined interstitial irradiation and localized current field hyperthermia: results and conclusions from clinical studies. Cancer Res 44: 4757s–4760s

Astrahan MA, Norman A (1982) A localized current field hyperthermia system for use with Ir-192 interstitial implants. Med Phys 9: 419–424

Bicher HA, Wolfstein RW, Fingerhut AG, Frey HA, Lewinsky BS (1984) An effective fractionation regime for interstitial thermoradiotherapy: preliminary clinical results. In: Overgaard J (ed) Hyperthermic oncology. 1. Taylor and Francis, London, pp 575–578

Borrego JC, et al. (1990) Combined interstitial thermoradiotherapy for advanced or recurrent pelvic neoplasia. Int J Radiat Oncol Biol Phys 19 [suppl 1]: 209

Brezovich IA, Young JH (1981) Hyperthermia with implanted electrodes. Med Phys 9: 79–84

Brezovich IA, Atkinson WJ, Lilly MB (1984) Local hyperthermia with interstitial techniques. Cancer Res 44: 4652s–4756s

Cetas TC, Hevezi JM, Manning MR, Ozimek EJ (1982) Dosimetry of interstitial thermoradiotherapy. Natl Cancer Inst Monogr 61: 505–507

Corry PM (1990) Simultaneous hyperthermia and brachytherapy with remote afterloading. In: Martinez AA et al. (eds) Brachytherapy HDR & LDR. Nucletron, Columbia, pp 193–204

Cosset JM, Brule JM, Salama AM, Damia E, Dutreix J (1982) Low frequency (0.5 MHz) contact and interstitial techniques for clinical hyperthermia. In: Biomedical Thermology. Alan R. Liss, New York, pp 649–657

Cosset JM, Dutreix J, Dufour J, Janoray P, Damia E, Haie C, Clarke D (1984a) Combined interstitial hyperthermia and brachytherapy: the Institut Gustave Roussy experience. In: Overgaard J (ed) Hyperthermic oncology vol 1, Taylor and Francis, London, pp 587–590

Cosset JM, Dutreix J, Dufour J, Janoray P, Damia E, Haie C, Clarke D (1984b) Combined interstitial hyperthermia and brachytherapy: Institut Gustave Roussy technique and preliminary results. Int J Radiat Oncol Biol Phys 10: 307–312

Cosset JM, Dutreix J, Haie C, Gerbaulet A, Janoray P, Dewars JA (1985) Interstitial thermoradiotherapy: a technical and clinical study of 29 implantations performed at the Institut Gustave Roussy. Int J Hyperthermia 1: 3–13

Cosset JM (1990) Interstitial hyperthermia. In: Gautherie M (ed) Clinical thermology: interstitial, endocavitary and perfusional hyperthermia. Methods and clinical trials. Springer Berlin Heidelberg New York, pp 1–42

Coughlin CT, Strohbehn JW (1989) Interstitial thermoradiotherapy. Radiol Clin North Am 27: 577–588

Deurloo IKK, Vissert AG, Morawska M, van Geel CA, van Rhoon, Levendag PC (1991) Application of a capacitive-coupling interstitial hyperthermia system at 27 MHz: study of different applicator configurations. Phys Med Biol 36: 119–132

Doss JD (1975) Use of RF fields to produce hyperthermia in animal tumors. Proceedings of international symposium on cancer therapy by hyperthermia and radiation. ARC, Washington DC, pp 226–227

Doss JD, McCabe A (1976) A technique for localized heating in tissue: an adjunct to tumor therapy. Med Instrumentation 10: 16–20

Dutreix J, Cosset JM, Salama M, Brule JM, Damia E (1982) Experimental studies of various heating procedures for clinical application of localized hyperthermia. In: Biomedical thermology. Alan R Liss, New York, pp 585–596

Emami B, Marks J, Perez C, Nussbaum G, Leybovich L (1984) Treatment of human tumors with interstitial irradiation and hyperthermia. In: Overgaard J (ed) Hyperthermic oncology vol 1. Taylor and Francis, London, pp 583–586

Emami B, Perez C, Leybovich L, Straube W, Vongerichten D (1987) Interstitial thermoradiotherapy in treatment of malignant tumours. Int J Hyperthermia 3: 107–118

Frazier OH, Corry PM (1984) Induction of hyperthermia using implanted electrodes. Cancer Res 44: 4854s–4866s

Gautherie M (1988) Clinical evaluation of the minerve hyperthermia system: synthesis. Transfer and Valuation of Prototype process

Gautherie M (1989) Interstitial hyperthermia: state of the art and prospects. Proceedings of the 5th international symposium on hyperthermic oncology, Kyoto, pp 63–68

Gérard JP, Romestaing P, Ardiet JM, Delaroche G, Montbarbon X, Sentenac I, Cosset JM (1991) Interstitial hyperthermia: general overview and preliminary results. In: Urano and Douple (eds) Hyperthermia and oncology, vol 3. Springer, Berlin Heidelberg New York, pp 221–230

Jones EL, Lyons BE, Douple EB, Dain BJ (1989) Thermal enhancement of low-dose irradiation in a murine tumour system. Int J Hyperthermia 5: 509–524

Levendag PC (1992) Interstitial radiation and/or interstitial hyperthermia in advanced and/or recurrent cancers in the head and neck: a pilot study. Hyperthermia Bulletin n°10

Linares LA, Nori D, Brenner H (1986) Interstitial hyperthermia and brachytherapy: a preliminary report. Endocurietherapy/Hyperthermia Oncology 2: 39–44

Manning MR, Cetas TC, Miller RC, Oleson JR, Connor WG, Gerner EW (1982) Clinical hyperthermia: results of a phase I trial employing hyperthermia alone or in combination with external beam or interstitial radiotherapy. Cancer 49: 205–216

Marchal C, Hoffstetter S, Bey P, Pernot M, Gaulard ML (1985) Development of a new interstitial method of heating which can be used with conventional afterloading brachytherapy techniques using Ir 192. Strahlentherapie 161: 523–557

Marchal C, Nadi M, Hoffstetter S, Bey P, Pernot M, Prieur G (1989) Practical method of heating operating at 27.12 MHz. Int J Hyperthermia 5: 451–466

Marchal C, Pernot M, Hoffstetter S, Bey P (1992) Clinical experience with different interstitial hyperthermia techniques. In: Handl-Zelle L (eds) Interstitial Hyperthermia. Springer Berlin Heidelberg New York, pp 207–228

Merrick HW, Andrew JM, Woldenberg LS, Ahuja RK, Dobelbower RR (1987) Intraoperative interstitial hyperthermia in conjunction with intraoperative radiation therapy in a radiation-resistant carcinoma of the abdomen: report on the feasibility of a new technique. J Surg Oncol 36: 48–51

Nadi M, Tosser AJ, Marchal C (1987) New interstitial hyperthermia using insulated wires at 27, 12 MHz. In: Proceed IEEE/Ninth Annual Conf of the EMBS, 13–16 Nov 1987, Boston, MA

Nadi M, Marchal C, Tosser A, Roussey J, Gaulard ML (1988) New interstitial hyperthermia technique at 27 MHz. Innov Tech Biol Med 9: 105–115

Oleson JR, Manning MR, Heusinkveld RS, Aristizabel SA, Cetas TC, Connor WG (1984) A review of the University of Arizona. Human clinical experience. Front Radiat Ther Oncol 136–143

Perez CA, Emami B (1989) Clinical trials with local (external and interstitial) irradiation and hyperthermia. Current and future perspectives. Radiol Clin North Am. 27: 525–541

Puthawala AA, Nisard Syed AM, Sheikh Khalid MA, Rafie S, McNamara CS (1985) Interstitial hyperthermia for recurrent malignancies. Endocuriether/Hyperthermia Oncology 1: 125–131

Satoh T, Stauffer PR (1988) Implantable helical coil microwave antenna for interstitial hyperthermia. Int J Hyperthermia 4: 497–512

Seegenschmiedt MH, Brady LW, Sauer R (1990) Interstitial thermoradiotherapy: review on technical and clinical aspects. Am J Clin Oncol 13: 352–363

Strohbehn JW (1983) Temperature distributions from interstitial RF electrode hyperthermia systems: theoretical predictions. Int J Radiat Oncol Biol Phys 9: 1655–1667

Visser AG, Deurloo IKK, Van Rhoon GC, Levendag PC (1991) Evaluation of a capacitive coupling interstitial system. Selectron Brachytherapy J 5: 114–119

Vora NL, Forell B, Luk KH (1989) Interstitial thermoradiotherapy (IT) in recurrent and advanced malignant tumors. Seven years of experience. Proceeding of the 5th international symposium on hyperthermic oncology, Kyoto, pp 588–590.

Yabumoto E, Suyama S, Show K, Yamazaki I (1989) A phase I clinical trial of radiofrequency interstitial hyperthermia combined with external radiotherapy. Proceedings of the 5th international symposium on hyperthermic oncology, Kyoto, pp 591–593

24 Clinical Experience of Interstitial Thermoradiotherapy Using Microwave Techniques

M.H. Seegenschmiedt

CONTENTS

24.1 Introduction

The first interstitial procedure for local hyperthermia (HT) was described by James Doss in 1975 at the First International Symposium on Cancer Therapy by Hyperthermia and Radiation in Washington D.C.: "I want to talk ... about a modality for the use of electromagnetic energy which is really quite different from (external) microwaves. It has a disadvantage – that is, the technique ... is usually very invasive ..." (Doss 1975). At that time the use of "external" heating techniques was preferred by most groups involved in clinical hyperthermia research. Although Doss proposed a specific radiofrequency (RF) technique (Doss and McCabe 1976), the idea of placing a heating source directly inside the human body or even the tumor itself stimulated researchers worldwide to invent and implement other internal heating techniques. Interstitial HT (IHT), however, is just one type of "internal" thermotherapy by which energy is supplied directly to the tumor tissue in situ; other internal heating techniques include (a) endocavitary HT using applicators introduced into natural body cavities (Roos, this volume, Chap. 10), (b) perfusional HT by means of extracorporeal blood perfusion, and (c) intraoperative HT using different HT technologies during a surgical procedure.

The basis for clinical implementation was well prepared by the available brachytherapy techniques for different malignancies including head and neck, brain, gynecological, and urological tumors. Moreover, several radiobiological studies indicated the potential of radiosensitization when combining heat and low dose irradiation (Ben-Hur et al. 1974; Gerner et al. 1983; Harisiadis et al. 1978; Miller et al. 1978; Moorthy et al. 1980, 1984; Sapozink et al. 1983; Jones et al. 1986, 1989). Thus, it seemed logical to combine these two invasive treatment modalities either sequentially or simultaneously. The only problem in the mid 1970s was to design an effective and compatible interstitial heating system.

While several clinical centers started to use resistive heating by means of low current field radiofrequency IHT as proposed by Doss (Astrahan 1982; Emami et al. 1984; Joseph et al. 1981; Lilly et al. 1983; Vora et al. 1982; Yabumoto and Suyama 1985) or with a slightly modified technique (Brezovich et al. 1984; Cosset et al. 1982, 1984), other groups preferred to investigate radiative heating by means of microwave (MW) antennas operating at a frequency range of 300–2450 MHz (Arcangeli et al. 1982; Bicher et al. 1985a, b; Coughlin et al. 1983; Emami et al. 1984; Puthawala et al. 1985; Strohbehn et al. 1979, 1984; Trembly et al. 1982; Turner 1986).

As has been shown in previous chapters of this volume (Visser et al., Chap. 5; Hand, Chap. 6), the basic physical concepts of resistive heating are completely different from those which govern

M.H. Seegenschmiedt, M.D., Strahlentherapeutische Klinik, Universität Erlangen-Nürnberg, Universitätsstraße 27, W-8520 Erlangen, Germany radiative heating by microwaves; their underlying physical principles and impact on clinical applications have also been extensively reviewed in the past (Cosset et al. 1985, 1986; Emami et al. 1984; Gautherie 1989; Gautherie et al. 1989; Seegenschmiedt et al. 1990b; Seegenschmiedt and Sauer 1989, 1992; Strohbehn 1987).

24.2 Technical Aspects of Clinical Importance

Since technical details of interstitial MW techniques are well described in a previous chapter of this volume (Hand, Chap. 6), only those technical aspects will be emphasized which greatly influence the clinical practice of MW-IHT.

24.2.1 Clinical Advantages of MW Technology

Microwave uses *radiative heating* emitted from semirigid or flexible coaxial antennas connected to high frequency (300–2450 MHz) power generators. This has several clinical advantages:

1. Significant energy absorption can be achieved away from the immediate environment of the implanted MW antenna; this allows a generous spacing between the MW antennas of 1.2–1.5 or even 2 cm. MW antennas are well suited for many intracavitary approaches when used in a single line, but they are also suitable for all multiarray interstitial implants. Their heating performance is less vulnerable to locally high tissue perfusion. All established brachytherapy guidelines can be routinely applied, without modification of the MW-IHT technology.

2. The semirigid or flexible applicator design offers considerable advantages compared to other IHT techniques; it allows adaptation to many clinical situations where the *bending* of afterloading probes is essentially required, e.g., looping techniques for some head and neck, tumors and for esophageal, bronchial, and bile duct tumors and for other intracavitary approaches to tumors in the small pelvis (cervix and corpus uteri, rectum, prostate, etc.). Multiple-antenna arrays do not require strict parallelism and equidistance between the implanted antennas. Moreover, depending upon the specific clinical demands, different designs of antennas, generators, and interfaces have been developed.

3. At all applied frequencies, MW antennas do not require direct contact to the tissue to be heated and therefore can be easily inserted into the plastic afterloading catheters which are usually implanted for various brachytherapy methods. It can be shown theoretically and practically that a thin layer of insulation between tissue and antenna can even improve the latter's radiative ability (Strohbehn 1987; James et al. 1989).

4. Unlike with other IHT techniques, all patients can be treated fully awake and in direct verbal contact to the operator, thereby avoiding unnecessary toxicity and allowing excellent treatment toxicity screening. There are two main factors which should guarantee excellent treatment control: (a) the possibility of large spacing between the heating probes allows use of additional open catheters for invasive thermometry and thereby the acquisition of truly interstitial thermometry data as compared with thermometry data retrieved at or in the immediate vicinity of the heating sources; (b) power deposition of all MW antennas can be individually controlled using different generators and power output channels.

24.2.2 Clinical Disadvantages of MW Technology

1. The ideally ellipsoidal power deposition pattern of MW antennas in tissue is not completely predictable and depends upon various other parameters: frequency of operation, dielectric properties of surrounding catheters (plastic coating), insertion depth, and tissue type (Chan et al. 1989; James et al. 1989; Mechling and Strohbehn 1986; Mechling et al. 1992; Stauffer et al. 1989; Strohbehn 1987). As the "active" antenna length, (i.e., the 50% iso-SAR profile) is inversely related to the operating frequency, usually small lesions should be treated with higher frequencies (2450 MHz) and large lesions with lower frequencies (433 MHz).

2. The radial and longitudinal heating patterns of coaxial dipole MW antennas are relatively heterogeneous: (a) the longitudinal heating length is limited to about 5–6 cm for 915 MHz MW antennas, (b) at tissue interfaces power deposition is heterogeneous, including constructive and destructive interference eventually creating "hot" and "cold spots," and (c) at the antenna tip a cold spot is described for most antenna designs (Trembly 1985; Turner 1986).

24.2.3 Compatible Invasive Thermometry

The heterogeneous energy deposition possible with MW devices and variations in blood perfusion can induce steep thermal gradients as high as 1°C–2°C per millimeter within the treatment volume. This necessitates precise invasive thermometry for all current IHT technologies, unless noninvasive approaches are available. The relevant thermometric devices have been well characterized previously (CETAS 1982; HAND, this volume, Chap. 11; SAMULSKI 1988); however, only expensive high resistive nonperturbing thermistors or fiberoptic thermometry systems are compatible with MW techniques.

The minimum number of thermometric probes required in clinical practice strictly depends on the size of the implant; the recommended locations for invasive thermometry include: (a) the center of the implant, (b) the center of each subarray of three (triangle) or four (square) heat sources, (c) the periphery of the implant, and (d) the surrounding normal tissue. Thus, in nearly all instances at least two to six thermometry catheters have to be employed (EMAMI et al. 1991; SEEGENSCHMIEDT et al. 1989a). An additional perpendicular thermometric probe in the central plane of the tumor is advisable, if this is feasible. Stationary multiple-sensor probes or automatically mapped single-sensor probes are recommended (ENGLER et al. 1987); however, most clinical users of commercial equipment can only perform manual mapping, consisting of repeated incremental movements of one or multiple sensors along the implanted catheter track.

For clinical analysis, two different invasive thermometry methods should be carefully distinguished: (a) thermometry *inside MW antennas*, and (b) thermometry *inside nonheated catheters*. The advantage of the first method is the indication of maximum temperatures, possibly allowing prevention of treatment toxicity. An important drawback, however, is the possible presence of artifacts, e.g., due to self-heating and thermal conduction smearing (ASTRAHAN et al. 1988). Even if reliable thermometry is obtained, the measurements concern only regions close to the heat sources, with significantly higher temperatures being recorded than in the interstitial regions between the heat sources. In contrast, the second method i.e., thermometry inside nonheated catheters, has the advantage of sampling truly interstitial data without major artifacts. However, the possible underestimation of high temperatures close to the heat source surface can be hazardous, too, especially when patients are treated under general anesthesia.

24.3 General Clinical Experience with MW-IHT

24.3.1 *Rationale of Trials*

Over the past decade various clinical groups have reported their clinical experiences, which in most instances had characterization of heating equipment, feasibility, efficacy, and treatment toxicity as primary study goals. The clinical rationale for using MW-IHT in combination with brachytherapy and/or external beam radiation therapy (RT), may be summarized as follows: (a) conventional methods are unable to achieve sufficient local control; (b) the improved local control may result in a higher cure rate or better prevention of morbidity; (c) improved tumor effects can be obtained with less toxicity and patient discomfort; (d) organ preservation can be offered instead of mutilating surgery; and (e) no other effective treatment alternatives are available. Thus, in particular advanced primary and recurrent local malignancies of the head and neck, breast, pelvis (gynecological, urogenital, anal, and colorectal tumors), extremities, and brain with a poor overall prognosis are suitable candidates for this investigative treatment approach (KAPP 1986; OVERGAARD 1989).

Interstitial HT has been primarily used in specialized institutions which already have had long-term clinical experience with brachytherapy. Nearly all studies have been conducted as nonrandomized phase 1–2 trials; in most instances patients were treated who presented with implantable primary, recurrent, or metastatic tumors; almost all were treated with palliative intention, since they had failed all previous treatments.

24.3.2 *Treatment Prescription*

The published data on clinical trials of MW-IHT demonstrate wide variation in respect of many aspects of treatment: the applied interstitial RT dose (15–50 Gy, 25–75 cGy/h dose rate), the (additional) external beam RT dose (20–60 Gy), the number of applied IHT sessions (up to eight), the sequencing of the IHT and IRT treatments, the fractionation between subsequent IHT sessions, the "thermal dose" prescription, the therapeutic temperature levels to be considered effective, and the overall treatment time or time at steady-state temperature. Despite these variations and the unfavorable patient selection, all these series have demonstrated encouraging results.

24.3.2.1 Treatment Schedule

A variety of IHT-IRT treatment schedules have been employed. They may be divided into two groups: (a) IHT plus IRT with *one* IHT session either before or after IRT, and (b) IRT combined with *two* IHT sessions, one before and one after IRT. In addition, various combinations of IHT with external beam RT have been reported: (a) IHT combined only with external beam RT, (b) IHT combined with interstitial and external beam RT, and (c) IHT combined with external HT and other different external beam and/or interstitial RT approaches (MITTAL et al. 1990; TUPCHONG et al. 1988). Some clinical groups have also used two interstitial implants separated by 2–4 weeks, the interstitial RT being combined with two IHT sessions on each occasion (PUTHAWALA et al. 1985).

24.3.2.2 "Thermal Dose" Prescription

The prescribed IHT treatment has varied in several respects: total treatment time, time at the prescribed temperature, and whether the thermal level of treatment is based on one thermometry probe (that registering the minimum or maximum temperature) or all thermometry probes (the mean temperature being used as the point of reference). The treatment goals have usually ranged from 41°C for 30 min (VORA et al. 1982) to 43.5°C for up to 60 min (GAUTHERIE et al. 1989) or 44°C for 45 min (COSSET et al. 1985). Another approach has applied the "thermal dose" concept of SAPARETO and DEWEY (1984), prescribing an IHT treatment of 20 min equivalent 43°C (thermal equivalent minutes = TEM) (DUNLOP et al. 1986). In some recent studies employing moderate continuous IHT, temperatures of 41°C have been maintained for up to 72 h simultaneously with low dose IRT (GARCIA et al. 1992), pulsed high dose IRT (ARMOUR et al. 1992), or BCNU systemic chemotherapy (MARCHOSKY et al. 1992).

24.3.2.3 Survey on Trial Design

The different designs of published clinical trials are summarized in Table 24.1, including the IHT treatment parameters, the sequencing of IHT and RT, the number of implants, and the prescribed RT dose. In contrast to RF-IHT series, in most MW-IHT studies patients have been treated without general anesthesia, and only mild sedation and analgesic medication have been applied. Due to the use of plastic afterloading tubes, many groups have also been able to perform two MW-IHT sessions, one before and one after interstitial RT. The application of IHT-IRT in preirradiated lesions has in general forced the radiation oncologist to significantly reduce the concurrent RT dose: the cumulative RT does, i.e., the previous and the concurrent interstitial or external dose, has not exceeded 100–110 Gy.

24.3.3 Tumor Response

The clinical experience with MW-IHT is summarized in Table 24.2. Taking the studies together, a very high overall response rate is seen in the 333 patients: 206(62%) achieved a complete response (CR), 88(26%) a partial response (PR), and 34 (10%) no response (NR) or tumor progression as the initial response. Five patients (2%) were not evaluable. The follow-up period ranged from 1 to 65 months, but was often not reported. The overall response rate (CR plus PR) was 294/333 (86%) (AOYAGI et al. 1989; BICHER et al. 1985a, b; COUGHLIN et al. 1991; EMAMI et al. 1984, 1987; INOUE et al. 1989; PETROVICH et al. 1989; PUTHAWALA et al. 1985; RAFLA et al. 1989; SEEGENSCHMIEDT et al. 1990a, b; SEEGENSCHMIEDT and SAUER 1992; STROHBEHN et al. 1984; TUPCHONG et al. 1988).

However, most MW-IHT trials lack more detailed information about the local and/or regional relapse rate. Furthermore, information is missing or incomplete regarding long-term tumor control at a predetermined follow-up or at the final date of the study evaluation; in most instances such control depends on the scope of the study and the selection of patients, who generally have a low overall survival rate. The available data demonstrate large variations, as shown in Table 24.3. For example, PETROVICH et al. reported an overall median survival of only 39 weeks and a 2-year survival of 22% in a group of 44 patients with recurrent tumors (PETROVICH et al. 1989), despite a high initial complete response rate of 64%; in contrast, PUTHAWALA et al. (1985) observed an overall local control rate of 74% at a minimum follow-up period of 12 months. Unfortunately very few groups apply a stringent definition of local control for all patients (PARSONS et al. 1990) or plot survival according to the standardized actuarial method of Kaplan–Meier (PETROVICH et al. 1989; SEEGENSCHMIEDT et al., 1992a, b).

Table 24.1. Design of clinical trials using MW-IHT

Reference	No. of evaluable patients (lesions)	Antenna frequency (MHz)	HT treatment parameters		Sequence (HT/RT)	No. of implants	RT dose
			Temp.	Duration			
STROHBEHN et al. (1984)	6	915	42.5°C	60 min	HT-RT-HT	1	1×30–40 Gy (LDR)
BICHER et al. (1985a)	8	915/300	42°–45°C	60 min	HT-RT/RT/HT-RT	2	2×25 Gy (LDR) 4×2 Gy eRT
PUTHAWALA et al. (1985)	43	915	41.5°–43°C	60 min	HT-RT-HT	1 or 2	2×20–25 Gy (LDR)
EMAMI et al. (1984, 1987)	39	915	42°C	60 min	HT-RT-HT	1	1×20–60 Gy (LDR)
TUPCHONG et al. (1988)	14	915	42°–45°C	60 min	HT+eHT with fractionated RT	1	15×3 Gy eRT (LDR)
RAFLA et al. (1989)	(35)	915/251	42.5°C	60 min	HT-RT-HT	1	1×30–60 Gy (LDR)
AOYAGI et al. (1989)	10	915	42°C		Not specified	1	Not specified
INOUE et al. (1989)	9	251	No data specified		1–3 HT with fractionated RT	1	30–60 Gy eRT (2 Gy single fract.)
PETROVICH et al. (1989)	39 (44)	915/630	42.5°C	45–60 min	HT-RT-HT[a]	1	1×25–50 Gy (LDR)
COUGHLIN et al. (1991)	35	915	42.5°–43°C	60 min	HT-RT-HT	1	1×20–60 Gy (LDR)
SEEGENSCHMIEDT and SAUER (1992)	90	915	41°–44°C	60 min	HT-RT ±HT	1	1×20–30 Gy (LDR) Up to 50 Gy eRT (2 Gy single fract.)

HT, interstitial hyperthermia; RT, interstitial radiotherapy; eHT, external hyperthermia; eRT, external beam RT; LDR, low dose rate
[a] Twenty percent did not receive the second heat treatment

Table 24.2. Survey on clinical results in trials using MW-IHT

Reference	No. of lesions	Clinical response				Toxicity	Follow-up (months)
		CR	PR	NR	Unevaluable		
STROHBEHN et al. (1984)	6	3 (50%)	2 (33%)	1 (17%)	–	1 (17%)	Short
BICHER et al. (1985a)	8	5 (63%)	2 (25%)	1 (13%)	–	1 (13%)	Short
PUTHAWALA et al. (1985)	43	37 (86%)	6 (14%)	0 (0%)	–	9 (21%)	>12
EMAMI et al. (1984, 1987)	39	21 (54%)	9 (23%)	5 (13%)	4	10 (25%)	6–48
TUPCHONG et al. (1988)	14	9 (64%)	2 (14%)	3 (22%)	–	NA	NA
RAFLA et al. (1989)	35	19 (54%)	13 (37%)	3 (9%)	–	8 (23%)	NA
AOYAGI et al. (1989)	10	2 (20%)	4 (40%)	4 (40%)	–	2 (20%)	NA
INOUE et al. (1989)	9	1 (11%)	6 (67%)	1 (11%)	1	1 (11%)	NA
PETROVICH et al. (1989)	44	28 (64%)	15 (34%)	1 (2%)	–	11 (25%)	6–30
COUGHLIN et al. (1991)	35	23 (66%)	4 (11%)	8 (23%)	–	NA	1–62
SEEGENSCHMIEDT and SAUER (1992)	90	58 (64%)	25 (28%)	7 (8%)	–	20 (22%)	4–65
Total experience	333	206 (62%)	88 (26%)	34 (10%)	5	63 (22%)	

CR, complete response; PR, partial response; NR, no response; NA, not available

Table 24.3. Local control after interstitial thermoradiotherapy in trials using MW-IHT

Reference (year) No. of pts	Follow-up (months)	Specific definition of local tumor control	Local relapse	Overall control
PUTHAWALA et al. (1985) 43 pts.	>12	Total regression of visible and palpable tumor at 12 months FU	5/37 CR (14%) at 1 year FU	32/43 (74%) at 1 year FU
EMAMI et al. (1987) 48 pts.	6–48	Best response at any time after treatment: "sustained complete tumor response"	NA	23/48 (48%) at last FU
TUPCHONG et al. (1988) 14 pts.	Short	Stabilization of locoregional disease	3/9 CR (33%)	6/14 (43%) at last FU
RAFLA et al. (1989) 35 pts.	Short	No tumor progression, no tumor recurrence during 6 months FU	NA	19/35 (54%) at last FU
PETROVICH et al. (1989) 44 pts.	6–30	Complete response for >1 month FU	0/28 CR (0%)	NA Overall median survival 39 wks; 2-year survival 22%
SEEGENSCHMIEDT et al. (1992a) 62 pts. (H&N)	4–58	"Sustained complete response" until last FU or patient's death; minimum 12 months' FU	3/32 CR (9%)	29/50 (58%) at 1 year FU; overall median survival 18 mo
SEEGENSCHMIEDT et al. (1992b) 26 pts. (pelvis)	5–65	"Sustained complete response" until last FU or patient's death; minimum 12 months' FU	1/17 CR (6%)	16/26 (62%) at 1 year FU; overall median survival 25 mo

H&N, head and neck tumors; CR, complete response; FU, follow-up; NA, not available

24.3.4 Treatment Toxicity

Generally MW-IHT in conjunction with IRT is well tolerated, with side-effects similar to those observed with IRT alone. When treatment is performed without general anesthesia, 20%–25% of patients may experience locoregional pain, general discomfort, and systemic stress (e.g., hypertension, tachycardia) during application of IHT; this can lead to a poor and ineffective heating performance. Surprisingly, when patients are heated under general anesthesia (as is the case in most trials using

RF-IHT), the complication rate is not increased; nevertheless, general anesthesia should be avoided if clinically possible. The overall complication rate ranges from 11% to 25% and was 22% in the collective experience for MW-IHT (Table 24.2) as compared to 25% in the collective experience for RF-IHT (MARCHAL, this volume, Chap. 23). This rate is quite acceptable considering the often large tumor burden and the extensive pretreatment course in most of these patients.

When analyzing treatment toxicity more carefully, the published data are again seen to vary considerably between the different studies. The relevant details are compiled in Table 24.4. Acute toxicity can occur during the IHT treatment and is usually associated with pain or general distress. Only a few reports have addressed the question of how many patients have had a poor heat treatment owing to subjective tolerance. Our own data show that about 25% of patients suffer acute treatment toxicity (SEEGENSCHMIEDT et al., 1992a, b). In contrast, side-effects which appear shortly after completion of IHT can be regarded as early complications, as distinct from late complications and long-term sequelae, which appear late or persist after IHT. Sometimes reports simply cite an overall complication rate.

Besides the minor complications, including blisters and thermal burns, which usually heal within days or weeks, major complications, such as soft tissue necrosis and rapid tumor necrosis and tissue breakdown, have also been observed occasionally. The latter complications can cause deep necrotic craters and delayed wound healing lasting over

Table 24.4. Acute and late complications after interstitial thermoradiotherapy in trials using MW-IHT

Reference (year)	No. of patients (sites)	Specific description of relevant treatment complications	Overall rate of complications
PUTHAWALA et al. (1985)	*43 total:*	2 (5%) Burns	Early: 4 (9%)
		1 (2%) Soft tissue necrosis	Late: 5 (12%)
	20 H&N	1 (2%) Brachial neuropathy	Overall: 9 (21%)
	13 pelvic	1 (2%) Orocutaneous fistula	
	10 others	5 (12%) Soft tissue necrosis	
EMAMI et al. (1987)	*48 total:*	2 (4%) Delayed wound healing	Overall: 12 (25%)
	29 H&N	6 (12%) Delayed healing of necrotic crater	
	7 pelvis	2 (4%) Cutaneous sinus	
	6 breast	1 (2%) Orocutaneous fistula	
	6 others	1 (2%) Vesicovaginal fistula	
RAFLA et al. (1989)	*35 total:*	2 (6%) Immediate discomfort	Early: 3 (9%)
		1 (3%) Blistering chest wall	Late: NA
	20 H&N	"Many" ulcers, i.e., delayed	Overall: NA
	18 pelvis	healing of necrotic crater	
	7 breast		
PETROVICH et al. (1989)	*44 total:*	6 (14%) Acute erythema	Early: 9 (20%)
		7 (16%) Moist desquamation	Late: 2 (4%)
	23 H&N	2 (4%) Blistering	Overall: 11 (25%)
	5 pelvic	1 (2%) Aspiration pneumonitis	
	9 breast	1 (2%) Soft tissue necrosis	
	8 others	1 (2%) Skin necrosis (ulcer)	
SEEGENSCHMIEDT et al. (1992a)	*90 total:*	14 (23%) Pain limiting sufficient power deposition	Acute: 14 (23%)
			Early: 12 (19%)
	62 H&N	7 (11%) Blistering/mucositis	Late: 7 (11%)
		3 (5%) Ulceration	Overall: 13 (21%)
		2 (3%) Fistula	
		1 (1%) Carotid arterial rupture	
		3 (3%) Arterial bleedings due to local tumor progression	
SEEGENSCHMIEDT et al. (1992b)	*90 total:*	7 (27%) Pain limiting sufficient power deposition	Acute: 7 (27%)
			Early: 8 (31%)
	26 pelvis	4 (15%) Blistering/mucositis	Late: 7 (27%)
		4 (15%) Ulceration	Overall: 8 (31%)
		4 (15%) Fistula	

H&N, head and neck; NA, not available

several months, even with a concomitant complete response. The majority of these complications are the result of rapid tumor necrosis. Soft tissue necrosis and osteoradionecrosis may occur after treatment of floor of mouth and base of tongue tumors; sometimes orocutaneous fistulas result from larger defects. Patients with gynecological and urogenital tumors in the small pelvis are prone to develop vesicovaginal and rectovaginal fistulas, especially when bulky tumors are treated.

The treatment of complications includes careful nursing care, antibiotics, and pain medication if required. Debridement, skin grafts, and plastic surgery may become necessary for management of long-term non-healing defects of the mucosa or skin.

Thermal damage was correlated neither with the number of applied IHT sessions nor with lesion type, lesion site, or prior treatment. In contrast, maximum temperatures above 44°–45°C in the normal or tumor tissue (OLESON et al. 1984; PUTHAWALA et al. 1985; SEEGENSCHMIEDT et al. 1992b) and thermal doses of T_{max}Eq 43°C $\geq$ 160 in an animal trial (DEWHIRST et al. 1984; DEWHIRST and SIM 1986) were more often associated with the development of "thermal" complications. It is important to realize that in all these heavily pretreated malignant lesions, besides the thermal component a radiation component may contribute to the development of treatment complications, but so far no clear conclusions can be drawn in this regard. As long as no uniform criteria are used to report the type and severity of toxicity, comparison between the various studies or between different IHT techniques will not be possible.

24.4 Site-Specific Clinical Experience with MW-IHT

The collective experience of eight major IHT-IRT trials reveals clear differences in the distribution of tumor sites and applied IHT techniques (SEEGENSCHMIEDT and SAUER 1992; SEEGENSCHMIEDT and VERNON, this volume, Chap. 39): Almost two-thirds of IHT interventions (402/619 = 65%) were at sites of superficial and medium depth tumors (head and neck, breast, skin, etc.) and only about one-third (217/619 = 35%) at sites of deep-seated tumors (gynecological, colorectal, and urogenital tumors). Major reasons for the limited use of IHT for deep-seated tumors include: (a) deep-seated tumors require the same high degree of localization as superficial and medium depth lesions, but this is more difficult to achieve; (b) the necessity of externalizing all heating source connections limits the range of clinical applications. Many MW-IHT studies lack data on the specific complete response and complication rates in a specific tumor site; therefore, in the following presentation of site-specific results the complete response and toxicity rates for a specific site are assumed to be equal to the reported values in the overall patient group as drawn from the various studies.

24.4.1 *Head and Neck Tumors*

Of the total of 619 IHT treatments, 220 (36%) were for tumors of the head and neck. Tongue, base of tongue, floor of mouth, tonsillar, and other accessible oropharyngeal malignancies have been successfully treated. These tumors can be easily implanted; several IRT methods have been traditionally used and a large body of clinical experience has been accumulated. While any of the IHT methods can be configured to operate in these tumors, MW-IHT has been preferred due to the typical types of implant performed in this region (free-hand implants, looping techniques, etc.) and the use of plastic afterloading catheters. The estimated cumulative complete response rate for MW-IHT in the head and neck is 63% (94/149) and the toxicity rate about 22% (Table 24.5).

24.4.2 *Breast and Chest Wall Tumors*

Eighty-two (13%) of the total of 619 IHT treatments were applied for uncontrolled local–regional recurrent breast cancer. This disease can result in significant morbidity, including bleeding, ulceration, pain, arm edema, and brachial plexus neuropathy. Usually treatment of the entire chest wall and not merely a small circumscribed area is indicated. Recurrent lesions of < 3 cm diameter require RT doses of at least 60 Gy and larger masses 65–70 Gy (BEDWINEK et al. 1981; DEUTSCH et al. 1986). Although several other technical options provide effective irradiation of breast and chest wall lesions, IRT techniques have also often been used to boost the primary tumor site as an alternative to the application of an external electron boost.

Adding IHT as an adjunct to this treatment approach appears to be reasonable, but in the past

Table 24.5. Results of interstitial thermoradiotherapy with MW techniques for head and neck tumors

Reference (year)	No. of lesions (total pts.)	Follow-up (months)	IHT schedule (°C/min)	RT dose, total (Gy)	Complete response (%)	Toxicity rate (%)
PUTHAWALA et al. (1985)	20 (43)	>12	60 min 41.5°–43.5°C 2×2 IHT	20–25 LDR-IRT 2×IRT	15 (75%)	NA (21%)
EMAMI et al. (1987)	29 (48)	6–48	60 min 42.5°–43°C	20–60 LDR-IRT	NA (54%)	NA (25%)
RAFLA et al. (1989)	15 (35)	Short	60 min 42.5°C	20–65 LDR-IRT	8 (53%)	NA
PETROVICH et al. (1989)	23 (44)	6–30	45–60 min 42.5°C	25–50 LDR-IRT	16 (70%)	NA (20%)
SEEGENSCHMIEDT et al. (1992a)	62 (90)	4–58	45–60 min 41°–44°C	20–40 LDR-IRT, variable ext. RT	39 (63%)	13 (21%)
Total experience	149	Variable	Variable	Variable	≈94 (63%)	≈(22%)

IHT, interstitial hyperthermia; RT, radiation therapy; LDR, low dose rate; IRT, interstitial radiation therapy; NA, not applicable

primarily external HT techniques have been successfully applied (GONZALES GONZALES et al. 1988; KAPP et al. 1991; LINDHOLM et al. 1987; PEREZ et al. 1986; SEEGENSCHMIEDT et al. 1989b; VAN DER ZEE et al. 1988). Since breast and chest wall lesions easily allow and often require the application of a template technique, RF-IHT has been preferred (VORA et al. 1986). Entry and exit points of heating sources require special attention and additional bolus application (SUNDARARMAN et al. 1990). Table 24.6 represents the compiled data of MW-IHT for breast and chest wall tumors. In summary, the estimated cumulative complete response rate is 61% (19/31) and the toxicity rate about 20%.

24.4.3 Pelvic Tumors

Of the 619 IHT treatments, 217 (35%) were applied in the pelvis: 152 (23%) were for gynecological

Table 24.6. Results of interstitial thermoradiotherapy with MW techniques for breast and chest wall tumors

Reference (year)	No. of lesions (total pts.)	Follow-up (months)	IHT schedule (°C/min)	RT dose, total (Gy)	Complete response (%)	Toxicity rate (%)
PUTHAWALA et al. (1985)	8 (43)	>12	60 min 41.5°–43.5°C 2×2 IHT	20–25 LDR-IRT 2×IRT	5 (63%)	NA (21%)
EMAMI et al. (1987)	6 (48)	6–48	60 min 42.5°–43°C	20–60 LDR-IRT	NA (54%)	NA (25%)
RAFLA et al. (1989)	6 (35)	Short	60 min 42.5°C	20–65 LDR-IRT	3 (50%)	NA
PETROVICH et al. (1989)	9 (44)	6–30	45–60 min 42.5°C	25–50 LDR-IRT	7 (78%)	NA (20%)
SEEGENSCHMIEDT and SAUER (1992)	2 (90)	4–58	45–60 min 41°–44°C	20–40 LDR-IRT, variable ext. RT	1 (50%)	– (0%)
Total experience	31	Variable	Variable	Variable	≈19 (61%)	≈(20%)

Abbreviations as in Table 24.5

tumors and 65 (12%) for colorectal tumors, including lesions of the anal canal and the genitourinary tract. Many advanced cancers in the pelvis are primarily unresectable. Smaller tumors also frequently fail within the pelvis following radical surgery and/or full dose external beam and/or intracavitary RT. In general, the survival and quality of life is dismal for patients with recurrences which cannot be locally controlled: besides palliation, the major rationale for the use of interstitial RT and IHT would be to support therapeutic strategies aimed at achieving tumor downstaging or surgical resectability.

The preferred IRT methods in this anatomical region have been endocavitary afterloading and interstitial template techniques using rigid needle implants. Although the needles could be replaced by flexible plastic catheters, the majority of IHT treatments have been performed using RF-IHT (ARISTIZABAL and OLESON 1984; GAUTHERIE et al. 1989; OLESON et al. 1984; VORA et al. 1988, 1989). The advantage of RF needles compared to MW antennas is their fairly homogeneous longitudinal heating pattern, and with appropriate insulation of entry and exit points RF-IHT appears to be the optimal approach for these tumors. However, a small subset of patients have been treated with MW-IHT. The results are summarized in Table 24.7. The estimated cumulative complete response rate for gynecological and colorectal tumors reaches 66% (40/61) and the toxicity rate about 25%. In summary, only confined lesions < 6 cm in diameter which are easily accessible and thus permit a geometrically precise IRT implant are suitable for additional MW-IHT.

24.4.4 Brain Tumors

Despite aggressive surgery, radiation therapy, and multiagent chemotherapy, the clinical outcome for most malignant brain tumors such as high-grade astrocytomas is generally grim and aggressive treatment approaches have been accompanied by significant side-effects and complications (GARFIELD 1986; KORNBLITH and WALKER 1988; NELSON et al. 1986). Interstitial delivery of cytotoxic therapy has a substantial appeal because localized cytotoxic therapy may allow delivery of such high doses to the confined tumor volume as would otherwise be intolerable to the whole brain. Clinical experience has been accumulated with IRT of primary and recurrent astrocytomas (GUTIN et al. 1984). Due to the poor prognostic index, clinical researchers became interested in IHT as an adjunct therapy. Preliminary results revealed the remarkable ability of the brain to withstand implantation of multiple catheters (MARCHOSKY et al. 1990) and overall technical and clinical feasibility. Good patient tolerance was demonstrated, with side-effects limited and reasonable in the normal context of the underlying disease.

While other IHT techniques have been employed (MARCHOSKY et al. 1990; STEA et al. 1990; YABUMOTO and SUYAMA 1985; YABUMOTO et al. 1989), MW-IHT is the preferred heating technique in this location.

Table 24.7. Results of interstitial thermoradiotherapy with MW techniques for gynecological and colorectal pelvic tumors

Reference (year)	No. of lesions (total pts.)	Follow-up (months)	IHT schedule (°C/min)	RT dose total (Gy)	Complete response (%)	Toxicity rate (%)
PUTHAWALA et al. (1985)	13 (43)	>12	60 min 41.5°–43.5°C 2×2 IHT	20–25 LDR-IRT 2×IRT	10 (77%)	NA (21%)
EMAMI et al. (1987)	3 (48)	6–48	60 min 42.5°–43°C	20–60 LDR-IRT	2 (66%)	NA (25%)
RAFLA et al. (1989)	14 (35)	Short	60 min 42.5°C	20–65 LDR-IRT	8 (57%)	NA
PETROVICH et al. (1989)	5 (44)	6–30	45–60 min 42.5°C	25–50 LDR-IRT	3 (60%)	NA (20%)
SEEGENSCHMIEDT et al. (1992b)	26 (90)	5–65	45–60 min 41°–44°C	20–40 LDR-IRT, variable ext. RT	17 (65%)	8 (31%)
Total experience	61	Variable	Variable	Variable	≈40 (66%)	≈(25%)

Abbreviations as in Table 24.5

Table 24.8. Results of interstitial thermoradiotherapy with MW techniques for malignant brain tumors

Reference (year)	No. of lesions (type)	Technique (frequency)	IHT treatment schedule	Adjunct therapy	Response	Toxicity
SAMARAS et al. (1982)	5: Rec. GBM	2450 MHz	30–60 min 3×45°C IHT	(Chemotherapy)	NA	"Minor"
WINTER et al. (1985)	12: AA/GBM	2450 MHz	60 min 2×45°C IHT	(Chemotherapy)	NA	NA
ROBERTS et al. (1986)	6: AAF/GBM	915 MHz	60 min 2×42°–43°C	^{192}Ir LDR IRT 20 Gy plus ERT 60 Gy	Survival 5–16 mo	1 CSF leakage 1 infection
KARLSSON et al. (1989)	3: Rec. GBM	915 MHz	60 min 2×41°–45°C	^{192}Ir LDR IRT 50 Gy	Survival 6–12 mo	1 CSF leakage with infection
SNEED et al. (1991)	49: 26 GBM 16 AAF 7 MET	915 MHz	30 min 42.5°C	^{125}I LDR IRT 48–63 Gy	Median surv. GBM: 11 mo AAF: not yet reached	9 seizures 4 infections 3 neurologic deficits 1 venous thrombosis
Overall results	75	Variable	Variable	Variable	Inconclusive	About one-third

Rec., recurrent; GBM, glioblastoma multiforme; AA, anaplastic astrocytoma; AAF, astrocytoma with anaplastic foci; MET, metastases; other abbreviations as previously defined; ^{192}Ir = iridium-192; ^{125}I = iodine-125

The cumulative experience in respect of 75 patients treated with MW-IHT is summarized in Table 24.8. The estimated toxicity rate ranged between 20% and 50%, but was about one-third in the larger series. However, so far the reported long-term results seem inconclusive (KARLSSON et al. 1989; SAMARAS et al. 1982; SEEGENSCHMIEDT et al. 1987; SNEED et al. 1991; TANAKA et al. 1984; WINTER et al. 1985).

24.4.5 Other Tumor Sites and Clinical Approaches

Special clinical indications for IHT are given and special IHT techniques have been developed for the eye (ASTRAHAN et al. 1987; FINGER et al. 1984, 1989; HANDL-ZELLER, this volume, Chap. 25). During abdominal surgery adjuvant intraoperative RT and IHT have been employed for selected and confined thoracic, pancreatic, bile duct, and colorectal tumors (COLACCHIO et al. 1990; COUGHLIN et al. 1985; FRAZIER and CORRY 1984; MERRICK et al. 1988). In addition, a variety of intraluminal MW-IHT techniques have been developed and clinically applied for esophageal, broncheal, and vaginal tumors (PETROVICH and BAERT, this volume, Chap. 35).

24.5 Prognostic Treatment Factors

Presently only a few series present larger numbers of patients and provide information for careful interpretation of prognostic parameters correlating with initial and long-term tumor control. The scientific value of many other clinical data is compromised by the low rate of patient accrual, the lack of detailed reporting on RT and HT parameters, the insufficient tumor and treatment analysis, and the lack of a sufficiently long follow-up. Historical clinical series are compromised by less developed invasive thermometry and interstitial heating technology.

The first report to address the importance of prognostic factors for treatment outcome concerned a large series of patients treated with RF-IHT at the University of Arizona in Tucson (ARISTIZABAL and OLESON 1984; OLESON et al. 1984). In an evaluation of 64 and 1661 patients, respectively, complete response was significantly ($P < 0.05$) correlated with increasing radiation dose, increasing time-averaged tumor temperature, and decreasing tumor volume. With logistic regression analysis the most significant parameters in predicting tumor response were identified as tumor volume, radiation dose, and *minimum* intratumoral temperature.

Among the various applied HT technologies, MW-IHT proved to achieve the best thermal performance and yielded the highest complete response rate (Aristizabal and Oleson 1984; Oleson et al. 1984).

Lately these prognostic parameters have been confirmed by several other groups: smaller tumor volume, higher (total) RT dose, and those thermal parameters which are associated with a higher time-averaged intratumoral minimum temperature or better "quality of heating" were all correlated with complete response; in some trials complete response was also associated with improved local control (Aristizabal and Oleson et al. 1984; Oleson et al. 1984; Petrovich et al. 1989; Rafla et al. 1989; Seegenschmiedt et al. 1990a, 1992a, b). Table 24.9 summarizes the established prognostic factors in trials involving MW-IHT techniques together with the results of the initial RF-IHT study of the University of Arizona, Tucson (Aristizabal and Oleson et al. 1984; Oleson et al. 1984).

In some trials recurrent and metastatic lesions received significantly lower total RT doses and tumor volumes were considerably larger in these lesions compared to primary and persistent lesions; these different tumor and treatment conditions may explain the significantly different response of different lesion types (Emami et al. 1987; Puthawala et al. 1985; Seegenschmiedt et al. 1992a, b).

Instead of using a time–temperature data matrix, the group from Dartmouth University has proposed a hyperthermia equipment performance (HEP) rating based on the percentage of the tumor area exceeding an index temperature of 43°C over a fixed time period (Paulsen et al. 1985). However, the clinical implementation of this concept in various tumor sites has not yet proved its prognostic value (Coughlin et al. 1991). It has been emphasized that all currently used invasive thermometry techniques are inappropriate for exactly locating and monitoring the whole tumor volume; various parameters, including the number and specific location of thermometry sensors and the spatial and temporal resolution of measurements, greatly influence the thermal data analysis (Corry et al. 1988). Obviously, with the use of more thermometry sensors per implant volume, the probability of recording lower tumor temperatures increases significantly. Unless the standardized hyperthermia data file format (Sapareto and Corry 1989) is adapted for interstitial heating and then uniformly applied by clinical users, interinstitutional comparison of thermometry data and clinical parameters will become very difficult.

Table 24.9. Prognostic factors for complete response in clinical trials using interstitial MW thermoradiotherapy

Reference (year) No. of pts.	Tumor class	Radiation dose	Tumor volume	Thermal parameters	Other factors
Aristizabal and Oleson (1984)[a]	NA	Higher RT dose:	Smaller volume:	high T_{min}.	IHT technique;
Oleson et al. (1984) 64 pts./161 pts.		>60 Gy	not specified	≥ 44°C	high temperature and complications: positive correlation
Puthawala et al. (1985) 43 pts.	NA	NA	NA	NA	High temperature and complications: positive correlation
Emami et al. (1987) 48 pts.	NA	NA	Smaller volume: <4 cm average diameter	At least 1 good HT treatment (≤ 42°C)	CR and local control: positive correlation
Rafla et al. (1989) 35 pts.	NA	Higher RT dose: >60 Gy	Smaller volume: <30 cm^3	NA	Treatment site: pelvis and chest wall: positive correlation
Petrovich et al. (1989) 44 pts.	NA	No correlation	Smaller volume: <150 cm^3	No correlation	Treatment site; CR and local control: no correlation
Seegenschmiedt et al. (1992a, b) 90 pts.	Primary and persistent: positive correlation	Higher RT dose: >50 Gy	Smaller volume: <80 cm^3	T_{min}(av) ≥ 41°C; T_{mean} ≥ 42°C; "thermal quality"	CR and local control: positive correlation

[a] First clinical trial analyzing prognostic factors in which RF-IHT was used

24.6 Future Perspectives

Interstitial MW-IHT and interstitial RT apply the same technical and clinical concepts: (a) to obtain an optimally targeted tumor dose together with adequate normal tissue sparing; (b) to distribute the RT dose homogeneously within the implanted target volume; and (c) to induce a different tumoricidal effect compared to fractionated external beam RT. MW-IHT methods can be easily combined and are fully compatible with nearly all standard free-hand or template brachytherapy techniques. However, MW-IHT is not useful as a single treatment modality, but only as an important adjunct to both external beam and interstitial RT. Its cytotoxic potential is in many respects complementary to radiation effects at both the cellular and the environmental level of the tumor (LEEPER 1985; REINHOLD and ENDRICH 1986; SONG 1984). IHT-IRT is safe and adaptable to various tumors, and it can be applied for all tumors that have been poorly treated by standard strategies (KAPP 1986; OVERGAARD 1989).

Each IHT technique provides specific advantages; in clinical practice the specific method should be carefully selected. MW techniques are less dependent on a strict implantation geometry and therefore can be recommended for head and neck lesions and free-hand implants as well as in all sites where bending of the applicators is an essential requirement; however, with the confined active heating length of MW antennas, the clinical approach is limited to lesions smaller than 5–7 cm in greatest dimension when using conventional coaxial dipole MW antennas operated at 915 MHz. In contrast, all radiofrequency, ferromagnetic seed, or other hot source IHT techniques allow heating of dimensions up to 12 cm or longer, but on the other hand they are all more bound to strict parallelism and equidistance of the implanted heating sources (BREZOVICH et al. 1989; CORRY and BARLOGIE 1982; DEURLOO et al. 1989; SCHREIER et al. 1990; HANDL-ZELLER, this volume, Chap. 25; STEGER et al. 1989; VISSER et al. 1989).

New MW antenna designs have been proposed which can extend their longitudinal power deposition even to the antenna tip, and also provide a more homogeneous axial heating pattern. These designs have incorporated multiple active sections, "sleeves", "chokes", and a helical coil design (LEE et al. 1986; LIN and WANG 1987; ROOS and HUGANDER 1988; SATOH and STAUFFER 1988). Phase-coherent activation of antenna arrays and individual phase shifting to each antenna (TURNER, 1986; WONG et al. 1989) may be other possibilities for future improvements.

Targets of ongoing and future research are as follows:

1. The improvement of the interstitial MW antenna technology (e.g., individual power steering, phase shifting, or multisegment antenna design)
2. Development of improved invasive (e.g., automatic thermal mapping) and additional noninvasive thermometry methods (e.g., integrated microwave radiometry)
3. Prospective thermal modeling and treatment control
4. Implementation of user-friendly computer software (screen and mouse controlled menus, integrated thermal performance analysis)
5. Biological, biomolecular, and physiological studies on radiosensitizing effects of low dose versus high dose RT
6. Assessment of the thermal enhancement ratio for various tumor models addressing thermotolerance and the influence of local metabolic and perfusion characteristics
7. Design of multicenter prospective randomized trials which are controlled for specific tumor types and tumor locations as well as specific IHT technique

The value of IHT needs to be confirmed in well-designed randomized prospective trials which control carefully for pretreatment prognostic factors. Two randomized phase 1–2 studies comparing IRT alone and combined IRT-IHT await final evaluation: the American RTOG 84-19 study and the ESHO 4-86 protocol. Further trials are mandatory as the aforementioned trials have been performed with a low standard of technical and clinical quality assurance compared to the recent RTOG guidelines (EMAMI et al. 1991). Strong emphasis has to be given to these quality assurance procedures in future trials to control for the broad spectrum of possible critical treatment parameters.

References

Aoyagi Y, Kanehira C, Kobori K, Hayakawa Y, Mochizuki S, Harada N (1989) Clinical experience with microwave interstitial hyperthermia. In: Sugahara T, Saito M (ed) Hyperthermic oncology 1988, vol 1, Taylor & Francis, London, pp 601–603

Arcangeli G, Barni E, Cividalli A, Lovisolo G, Nervi C, Mauro F (1982) Hyperthermia by implantable applicators. In: Gautherie M (ed) Biomedical thermology. Alan R. Liss, New York, pp 641–647

Aristizabal SA, Oleson JR (1984) Combined interstitial irradiation and localized current field hyperthermia: results and conclusions from clinical studies. Cancer Res [Suppl] 44: 4757s–4760s

Armour E, Wang Z, Corry PM, Martinez A (1992) Equivalence of continuous and pulsed simulated low dose rate irradiation in 9L gliosarcoma cells at 37°C and 41°C. Int J Radiat Oncol Biol Phys 22: 109–114

Astrahan MA (1982) A localized current field hyperthermia system for use with 192 iridium interstitial implants. Med Phys 9: 419–424

Astrahan MA, Liggett P, Petrovich Z, Luxton G (1987) A 500 kHz localized current field hyperthermia system for use with ophthalmic plaque radiotherapy. Int J Hyperthermia 3: 423–432

Astrahan MA, Luxton G, Sapozink MD, Petrovich Z (1988) The accuracy of temperature measurements from within an interstitial microwave antenna. Int J Hyperthermia 4: 593–608

Bedwinek JM, Fineberg B, Lee J, Ocwieza M (1981) Analysis of failures following local treatment of isolated local regional recurrence of breast cancer. Int J Radiat Oncol Biol Phys 7: 581–585

Ben-Hur E, Elkind MM, Bronk BV (1974) Thermally enhanced radiosensitivity of cultered Chinese hamster cells; inhibition of repair of sublethal damage and enhancement of lethal damage. Radiat Res 58: 38–51

Bicher HI, Moore DW, Wolfstein RS (1985a) A method for interstitial thermoradiotherapy. In: Overgaard J (ed) Hyperthermic oncology 1984, vol 1. Taylor & Francis, London, pp 595–598

Bicher HI, Wolfstein RS, Fingerhut AG, Frey HS, Lewinsky BS (1985b) An effective fractionation regime for interstitial thermoradiotherapy–preliminary clinical results. In: Overgaard J (ed) Hyperthermic oncology 1984, vol 1. Taylor & Francis, London, pp 575–578

Brenner DJ, Hall EJ (1991) Conditions for the equivalence of continuous to pulsed low dose rate brachytherapy. Int J Radiat Oncol Biol Phys 20: 181–190

Brezovich IA, Atkinson WJ, Lilly MB (1984) Local hyperthermia with interstitial techniques. Cancer Res [Suppl] 44: 4752s–5756s

Brezovich IA, Meredith RF, Henderson RA, Brawner WR, Weppelmann B, Salter MM (1989) Hyperthermia with water-perfused catheters. In: Sugahara T, Saito M (eds) Hyperthermic oncology 1988, vol 1. Taylor & Francis, London, pp 809–810

Cetas TC (1982) Invasive thermometry In: Nussbaum G (ed) Physical aspects of hyperthermia. American Institute of Physics, New York, pp 231–265

Chan KW, Chou CK, McDougall JA, Luk KH, Vora NL, Forell BW (1989) Changes in heating patterns of interstitial microwave antenna arrays at different insertion depths. Int J Hyperthermia 5: 499–508

Colacchio TA, Coughlin CT, Taylor J, Douple E, Ryan T, Crichlow RW (1990) Intraoperative radiation therapy and hyperthermia: morbidity and mortality from this combined treatment modality for unresectable intra-abdominal carcinomas. Arch Surg 125: 370–375

Corry PM, Barlogie B (1982) Clinical application of high frequency methods for local hyperthermia. In: Nussbaum GH (ed) Physical aspects of hyperthermia. American Institute of Physics, New York, pp 307–322

Corry PM, Jabboury K, Kong JS, Armour EP, McCraw FJ, LeDuc T (1988) Evaluation of equipment for hyperthermia treatment of cancer. Int J Hyperthermia 4: 53–74

Cosset JM, Brule JM, Salama AM, Damia E, Dutreix J (1982) Low-frequency (0.5 MHz) contact and interstitial techniques for clinical hyperthermia. In: Gautherie M (ed) Biomedical thermology. Alan R. Liss, New York, pp 649–657

Cosset JM, Dutreix J, Dufour J, Janoray P, Damia E, Haie C (1984) Combined interstitial hyperthermia and brachytherapy: Institute Gustave Roussy technique and preliminary results. Int J Radiat Oncol Biol Phys 10: 307–312

Cosset JM, Dutreix J, Haie C, Gerbaulet A, Janoray P, Dewars JA (1985) Interstitial thermoradiotherapy: a technical and clinical study of 29 implantations performed at the Institute Gustave Roussy. Int J Hyperthermia 1: 3–13

Cosset JM, Dutreix J, Haie C, Mabire JP, Damia E (1986) Technical aspects of interstitial hyperthermia. Recent Results Cancer Res 101: 56–60

Coughlin CT, Douple EB, Strohbehn JW, Eaton WL, Trembly BS, Wong TZ (1983) Interstitial hyperthermia in combination with brachytherapy. Radiology 148: 285–288

Coughlin CT, Wong TZ, Strohbehn JW, Colacchio TA, Sutton JE, Belch RZ, Douple EB (1985) Intraoperative interstitial microwave-induced hyperthermia and brachytherapy. Int J Radiat Oncol Biol Phys 11: 1673–1678

Coughlin CT, Ryan TP, Stafford JH (1991) Interstitial thermoradiotherapy: The Dartmouth experience 1981–1990. In: Chapman JD, Dewey WC, Whitmore GF (eds) Radiation research: a twentieth century perspective, vol 1. Academic, San Diego, p 386

Deurloo IKK, Visser AG, Ruifrok ACC, Lakeman RF, van Rhoon GC, Levendag PC (1989) Radiofrequency interstitial hyperthermia: a mulicentric program of quality assessment and clinical trials. In: Sugahara T, Saito M (eds) Hyperthermic oncology 1988, vol 1. Taylor & Francis, London, pp 874–875

Deutsch M, Parsons JA, Mittal BB (1986) Radiation therapy for local-regional recurrent breast carcinoma. Int J Radiat Oncol Biol Phys 12: 2061–2065

Dewhirst MW, Sim DA (1986) Estimation of therapeutic gain in clinical trails involving hyperthermia and radiotherapy. Int J Hyperthermia 2: 165–178

Dewhirst MW, Sim DA, Sapareto S, Connor WG (1984) The importance of minimum tumour temperature in determining early and long-term response of spontaneous pet animal tumours to heat and radiation. Cancer Res [Suppl] 44: 43s–50s

Doss JD (1975) Use of RF fields to produce hyperthermia in animal tumors. In: Robinson JE (ed) Proceedings of the international symposium on cancer therapy by hyperthermia and radiation. American College of Radiology, Washington DC, pp 226–227

Doss JD, McCabe CW (1976) A technique for localized heating in tissue: an adjunct to tumor therapy. Medical Instrumentation 10: 16–21

Dunlop PRC, Hand JW, Dickinson RJ, Field SB (1986) Early experience with combined interstitial hyperthermia and brachytherapy. Br J Radiol 59: 525–527

Emami B, Marks JE, Perez CA, Nussbaum GH, Leybovich L, von Gerichten D (1984) Interstitial thermoradiotherapy in the treatment of recurrent residual malignant tumors. Am J Clin Oncol 6: 699–704

Emami B, Perez CA, Leybovich L, Straube W, von Gerichten D (1987) Interstitial thermoradiotherapy in the treatment of malignant tumours. Int J Hyperthermia 3: 107–118

Emami B, Stauffer P, Dewhirst MW et al. (1991) RTOG quality assurance guidelines for interstitial hyperthermia. Int J Radiat Oncol Biol Phys 20: 1117–1124

Engler MS, Dewhirst MW, Winget JW, Oleson JR (1987) Automated temperature scanning for hyperthermia treatment planning. Int J Radiat Oncol Biol Phys 13: 1377–1382
Finger PT, Packer S, Svitra PP, Paglione R, Chess J, Albert DM (1984) Hyperthermic treatment of intraocular tumors. Arch Ophthalmol 102: 1477–1481
Finger PT, Packer S, Paglione R, Gatz JF, Ho TK, Bosworth JL (1989) Thermoradiotherapy of choroidal melanoma: clinical experience. Ophthalmology 96: 1384–1388
Frazier OH, Corry PM (1984) Induction of hyperthermia using implanted electrodes. Cancer Res [Suppl] 44: 4864s–4866s
Garcia DM, Nussbaum GH, Fathman AE, Drzymala RE, Bleyer M, DeFord JA, Welsh D (1992) Simultaneous chronic LDR interstitial radiotherapy and conductive interstitial hyperthermia in treatment of recurrent prostatic tumors. In: Gerner W (ed) Hyperthermic oncology 1992, vol 1. Taylor & Francis, London, p 386
Garfield J (1986) Recent status and future role of surgery for malignant supratentorial gliomas. Neurosurgery Review 9: 23–25
Gautherie M (1989) Interstitial hyperthermia: state of the art and prospects. In: Sugahara T, Saito M (eds) Hyperthermic oncology 1988, vol 2. Taylor & Francis, London, pp 63–68
Gautherie M, Cosset JM, Gerard JP, Horiot JC, Ardiet JM, El Akoum H, Alperovitch A (1989) Radiofrequency interstitial hyperthermia: a multicentric program of quality assessment and clinical trials. In: Sugahara T, Saito M (eds) Hyperthermic oncology 1988, vol 2. Taylor & Francis, London, pp 711–714
Gerner EW, Oval JH, Manning MR, Sim DA, Bowden GT, Hevezi J (1983) Dose rate dependence of heat radiosensitization. Int J Radiat Oncol Biol Phys 9: 1401–1404
Glicksman AS, Leith JT (1988) Radiobiological considerations of brachytherapy. Oncology 2: 25–30
Gonzalez Gonzalez DG, van Dijk JDP, Blank LECM (1988) Chest wall recurrences of breast cancer: results of combined treatment with radiation and hyperthermia. Radiother Oncol 12: 95–103
Gutin PH, Phillips TL, Wara WM et al. (1984) Brachytherapy of recurrent malignant brain tumors with removable high-activity iodine-125 sources. J Neurosurg 60: 61–68
Hall EJ (1985) The biological basis for endocurietherapy. Endocurietherapy/Hyperthermia Oncology 1: 141–152
Hall EJ (1988) Hyperthermia. In: Hall EJ (ed) Radiobiology for the radiologist. JB Lippincott, Philadelphia, pp 293–329
Handl-Zeller L, Arian-Schad K, Stücklschweiger G (1991) Review on clinical experiences using hot water. Hyperthermia Bulletin 9: 64–67
Harisiadis L, Sung D, Kessaris N, Hall EJ (1978) Hyperthermia and low dose rate irradiation. Radiology 129: 195–198
Inoue T, Masaki N, Ozeki S, Ikeda H, Nishiyama K, Matayoshi Y, Kozuka T (1989) Clinical experience of interstitial hyperthermia combined with external radiation using MA-251 interstitial applicator. In: Sugahara T, Saito M (eds) Hyperthermic oncology 1988, vol 1. Taylor & Francis, London, pp 598–600
James BJ, Strohbehn JW, Mechling JA, Trembly BS (1989) The effect of insertion depth on the theoretical SAR patterns of 915 MHz dipole antenna arrays for hyperthermia. Int J Hyperthermia 5: 733–747
Jones EL, Douple EB, Strohbehn J (1986) Thermal enhancement ratios for single and fractionated dose external beam radiotherapy combined with hyperthermia. In: Orphanoudakis SC (ed) Proceedings of the 12th Northeast Bioengineering Conference. IEEE, New York, pp 58–61
Jones EL, Lyons BE, Douple EB, Dain BJ (1989) Thermal enhancement of low-dose irradiation in a murine tumour system. Int J Hyperthermia 5: 509–524
Joseph CD, Astrahan M, Lipsett J, Archambeau J, Forell B, George FW (1981) Interstitial hyperthermia and interstitial iridium-192 implantation: a technique and preliminary results. Int J Radiat Oncol Biol Phys 9: 827–833
Kapp DS (1986) Site and disease selection for hyperthermia clinical trials. Int J Hyperthermia 2: 139–156
Kapp DS, Barnett TA, Cox RS, Lee ER, Lohrbach A, Fessenden P (1991) Hyperthermia and radiation therapy of local regional recurrent breast cancer: prognostic factors for response and local control of diffuse and nodular tumours. Int J Radiat Oncol Biol Phys 20: 1147–1164
Karlsson UL, Seegenschmiedt MH, Finkelstein S, Black P, Brady LW (1989) Effects of interstitial radiation therapy and hyperthermia on recurrent malignant astrocytoma and normal brain tissue. Radiology 173 (P) : 113
King KWP, Trembly BS, Strohbehn JW (1983) The electromagnetic field of an insulated antenna in a conducting or dielectric medium. IEEE Trans Microwave Theory Tech 31: 574–583
Kornblith PL, Walker M (1988) Chemotherapy for malignant gliomas. J Neurosurg 68: 1–17
Le Bourgeois JP, Convert G, Dufour J (1978) An interstitial device for microwave hyperthermia of human tumors. In: Streffer C (ed) Cancer therapy by hyperthermia and radiation. Urban & Schwarzenberg, Baltimore, pp 122–124
Lee D, O'Neill MJ, Lam K, Rostock R, Lam W (1986) A new design of microwave interstitial applicator for hyperthermia with improved treatment volume. Int J Radiat Oncol Biol Phys 12: 2003–2008
Leeper DB (1985) Molecular and cellular mechanisms of hyperthermia alone or combined with other modalities. In: Overgaard J (ed) Hyperthermic oncology 1984, vol 1. Taylor & Francis, London, pp 9–41
Lilly MB, Brezovich IA, Atkinson W, Chakraborty D, Durant JR, Ingram J, McElvein R (1983) Hyperthermia with implanted electrodes. In vitro and in vivo correlations. Int J Radiat Oncol Biol Phys 9: 373–382
Lin JC, Wang YJ (1987) Interstitial microwave antennas for thermal therapy. Int J Hyperthermia 3: 37–47
Lindholm CE, Kjellen E, Nilsson P, Hertzman S (1987) Microwave-induced hyperthermia and radiotherapy in human superficial tumours: clinical results with a comparative study of combined treatment versus radiotherapy alone. Int J Hyperthermia 3: 393–411
Marchosky JA, Babbs CF, Moran CJ, Fearnot NE, DeFord JA, Welsh DM (1990) Conductive, interstitial hyperthermia: a new modality for treatment of intracranial tumors. In: Bicher HI (ed) Consensus on hyperthermia. Plenum, New York, pp 129–143
Marchosky JA, Welsh DM, Horn BA, Van Amburg AL (1992) Experience with long-duration interstitial hyperthermia and systemic BCNU in the treatment of recurrent malignant brain tumors. In: Gerner W (ed) Hyperthermic oncology 1992, vol 1. Taylor & Francis, London, p 387
Mechling JA, Strohbehn JW (1986) A theoretical comparison of the temperature distributions produced by three interstitial hyperthermia systems. Int J Radiat Oncol Biol Phys 12: 2137–2148

Mechling JA, Strohbehn JW, Ryan TP (1992) Three-dimensional theoretical temperature distributions produced by 915 MHz dipole antenna arrays with varying insertion depths in muscle tissue. Int J Radiat Oncol Biol Phys 22: 131–138

Merrick HW, Milligan AJ, Greenblatt SH, Dobelbower RR (1988) Clinical experience with intraoperative interstitial hyperthermia and intraoperative radiation therapy. In: Abstracts of the 36th annual meeting of the Radiation Research Society, Philadelphia, PA, 16–21 April 1988, p 45

Miller RC, Leith JT, Voemett RC, Gerner EW (1978) Effects of interstitial radiation therapy alone, or in combination with localized hyperthermia on response of a mouse mammary tumor. Radiat Res 19: 175–180

Mittal BB, Sathiaseelan V, Kies MS (1990) Simultaneous localized 915 MHz external and interstitial microwave hyperthermia to heat tumors greater than 3 cm in depth. Int J Radiat Oncol Biol Phys 19: 669–675

Moorthy CR, Hahn EW, Kim JH, Feingold BS, Alifieri AA, Hilaris BS (1980) Improved response of a murine fibrosarcoma to interstitial radiation when combined with hyperthermia. Int J Radiat Oncol Biol Phys 6: 1386–1387

Moorthy CR, Hahn EW, Kim JH, Feingold BS, Alifieri AA, Hilaris BS (1984) Improved response of a murine fibrosarcoma (Meth-A) to interstitial radiation when combined with hyperthermia. Int J Radiat Oncol Biol Phys 10: 2145–2148

Nelson DF, Urtasun RC, Saunders WM, Gutin PH, Sheline GE (1986) Recent and current investigations of radiation therapy of malignant gliomas. Seminars in Oncology 12: 46–55

Neyzari A, Cheung AY (1985) A review of brachyhyperthermia approaches for the treatment of cancer. Endocurietherapy/Hyperthermia Oncology 1: 257–264

Oleson JR, Manning MR, Sim DA, Heusinkveld M, Aristizibal SA, Cetas TC, Hevezi JC, Connor WG (1984) A review of the University of Arizona human clinical hyperthermia experience. Front Radiat Ther Oncol 18: 136–143

Overgaard J (1989) The current and potential role of hyperthermia in radiotherapy. Int J Radiat Oncol Biol Phys 16: 535–549

Parsons JT, McCarty PJ, Rao PV, Mendenhall NB, Million RR (1990) On the definition of local control. Int J Radiat Oncol Biol Phys 18: 705–706

Paulsen KD, Strohbehn JW, Lynch DR (1985) Comparative theoretical performance of two types of regional hyperthermia systems. Int J Radiat Oncol Biol Phys 11: 1659–1671

Perez CA, Kuske RR, Emami B, Fineberg B (1986) Irradiation alone or combined with hyperthermia in the treatment of recurrent carcinoma of the breast in the chest wall: a nonrandomized comparison. Int J Hyperthermia 2: 179–187

Petrovich Z, Langholz B, Lam K, Luxton G, Cohen D, Jepson J, Astrahan M (1989) Interstitial microwave hyperthermia combined with iridium-192 radiotherapy for recurrent tumors. Am J Clin Oncol 12: 264–268

Puthawala AA, Syed AMN, Khalid MA, Rafie S, McNamara CS (1985) Interstitial hyperthermia for recurrent malignancies. Endocurietherapy/Hyperthermia Oncology 1: 125–131

Rafla S, Parikh K, Tchelebi M, Youssef E, Selim N, Bishay S (1989) Recurrent tumors of the head and neck, pelvis, and chest wall: treatment with hyperthermia and brachytherapy. Radiology 172: 845–850

Reinhold HS, Endrich B (1986) Tumour microcirculation as a target for hyperthermia. Int J Hyperthermia 2: 117–137

Roberts DW, Coughlin CT, Wong TZ, Frankin JD, Douple EB, Strohbehn JW (1986) Interstitial hyperthermia and iridium brachytherapy in treatment of malignant glioma. J Neurosurg 64: 581–587

Roos D, Hugander A (1988) Microwave interstitial applicators with improved longitudinal heating patterns. Int J Hyperthermia 4: 609–615

Samaras GM, Salcman M, Cheung AY, Abdo HS, Schepp RS (1982) Microwave-induced hyperthermia: an experimental adjunct for brain tumor therapy. NCI Monographs 61: 477–482

Samulski TV (1988) Current technologies for invasive thermometry. In: Paliwal B, Hetzel F, Dewhirst MW (eds) Biological, physical and clinical aspects of hyperthermia. American Institute of Physics, New York, pp 168–181

Sapareto SA, Corry PM (1989) A proposed standard data file format for hyperthermia treatments. Int J Radiat Oncol Biol Phys 16: 613–627

Sapareto SA, Dewey WC (1984) Thermal dose determination in cancer therapy. Int J Radiat Oncol Biol Phys 10: 787–803

Sapozink MD, Palos B., Goffinet DR, Hahn GM (1983) Combined continuous ultra low dose rate irradiation and radiofrequency hyperthermia in the C3H mouse. Thermal dose determination in cancer therapy. Int J Radiat Oncol Biol Phys 9: 1357–1365

Satoh T, Stauffer PR (1988) Implantable helical coil microwave antenna for interstitial hyperthermia. Int J Hyperthermia 4: 497–512

Schreier K, Budihna M, Lesnicar H et al. (1990) Preliminary studies of interstitial hyperthermia using hot water. Int J Hyperthermia 6: 431–444

Seegenschmiedt MH, Sauer R (1989) Methoden und klinische Ergebnisse der interstitiellen Thermoradiotherapie. Strahlenther Onkol 165: 360–368

Seegenschmiedt MH, Sauer R (1992) The current role of interstitial thermo-radiotherapy. Strahlenther Onkol 168: 119–140

Seegenschmiedt MH, Brady LW, Karlsson UL, Black P, McCormack T (1987) A critical review of interstitial thermoradiotherapy for recurrent malignant astrocytoma: problems and promises. Int J Hyperthermia 3: 589

Seegenschmiedt MH, Sauer R, Herbst M, Thiel H-J, Fietkau R, Brady LW, Karlsson UL (1989a) Interstitial hyperthermia for head and neck tumors: treatment planning and quality assurance (QA). In: Sugahara T, Saito M (eds) Hyperthermic oncology 1988, vol 2. Taylor & Francis, London, pp 524–527

Seegenschmiedt MH, Karlsson UL, Sauer R et al. (1989b) Superficial chest wall recurrences of breast cancer: prognostic treatment factors for combined radiation therapy and hyperthermia. Radiology 173: 551–558

Seegenschmiedt MH, Sauer R, Fietkau R, Brady LW, Karlsson UL (1990a) Primary advanced and local recurrent head and neck tumors: effective management with interstitial thermo-radiotherapy. Radiology 176: 267–274

Seegenschmiedt MH, Brady LW, Sauer R (1990b) Interstitial thermoradiotherapy: review on technical and clinical aspects. Am J Clin Oncol 13: 352–363

Seegenschmiedt MH, Sauer R, Fietkau R, Iro H, Chalal JA, Brady LW (1992a) Interstitial thermal radiation therapy: 5-year experience with head and neck tumors. Radiology 184: 795–804

Seegenschmiedt MH, Sauer R, Miyamoto C, Chalal JA, Brady LW (1992b) Clinical experience with interstitial

thermo-radiotherapy for localized implantable pelvic tumors. Am J Clin Oncol 15: (in press)
Sneed PK, Stauffer PR, Gutin PH et al. (1991) Interstitial irradiation and hyperthermia for the treatment of recurrent malignant brain tumors. Neurosurgery 28: 206–215
Song CW (1984) Effect of local hyperthermia on bloodflow and microenvironment. Cancer Res [Suppl] 44: 4721s–4730s
Stauffer PR, Sneed PK, Suen SA, Satoh T, Matsumoto K, Fike JR, Phillips TL (1989) Comparative thermal dosimetry of interstitial microwave and radiofrequency-LCF hyperthermia. Int J Hyperthermia 5: 307–318
Stea B, Cetas TC, Cassady JR et al. (1990) Interstitial thermoradiotherapy of brain tumors: preliminary results of a phase I clinical trial. Int J Radiat Oncol Biol Phys 19: 1463–1471
Steger AC, Lees WR, Walmsley K, Bown SG (1989) Interstitial laser hyperthermia: a new approach to local destruction of tumours. Br Med J 299: 362–365
Strohbehn JW (1987) Interstitial techniques for hyperthermia. In: Field SB, Franconi C (eds) Physics and technology of hyperthermia. Martinus Nijhoff, Dordrecht, pp 211–240
Strohbehn JW, Bowers ED, Walsh JE, Douple EB (1979) An invasive microwave antenna for locally induced hyperthermia for cancer therapy. J Microwave Power 14: 339–350
Strohbehn JW, Douple EB, Coughlin CT (1984) Interstitial microwave antenna array systems for hyperthermia. Front Radiat Ther Oncol 18: 70–84
Sundararman S, Denman DL, Legoretta RA et al. (1990) The modification of specific absorption rates in interstitial microwave hyperthermia via tissue-equivalent material bolus. Int J Radiat Oncol Biol Phys 19: 667–685
Tanaka R, Yamada N, Kim CH, Saito Y (1985) RF hyperthermia of human malignant brain tumor. In: Overgaard J (ed) Hyperthermic oncology 1984, vol 1. Taylor & Francis, London, pp 747–750
Trembly BS (1985) The effects of driving frequency and antenna length on power deposition within a microwave antenna array used for hyperthermia. IEEE Trans Biomed Eng 32: 152–157
Trembly BS, Strohbehn JW, de Sieyes D, Douple EB (1982) Hyperthermia induction by an array of invasive microwave antennas. NCI Monographs 61: 497–499
Tupchong L, Nerlinger RE, Waterman FM (1988) Combined use of external beam radiation and interstitial heat for advanced recurrent head and neck carcinomas – a new approach. In: Abstracts of the 36th annual meeting of the Radiation Research Society, Philadelphia, PA, 16–21 April 1988, p 42
Turner PF (1986) Interstitial equal-phased arrays for EM hyperthermia. IEEE Trans Microwave Theory Tech 34: 572–578
van der Zee J, Treurniet-Donker AD, The SK et al. (1988) Low dose reirradiation in combination with hyperthermia: a palliative treatment for patients with breast cancer recurring in previously irradiated areas. Int J Radiat Oncol Biol Phys 15: 1407–1413
Visser AG, Deurloo IKK, Levendag PC, Ruifrok ACC, Cornet B, van Rhoon GC (1989) An interstitial hyperthermia system at 27 MHz. Int J Hyperthermia 5: 265–276
Vora NL, Forell B, Joseph C, Lipsett JA, Archambeau J (1982) Interstitial implant with interstitial hyperthermia. Cancer 50: 2518–2523
Vora NL, Shaw S, Forell B et al. (1986) Primary radiation combined with hyperthermia for advanced (stage III–IV) and inflammatory carcinoma of breast. Endocurietherapy/Hyperthermia Oncology 2: 101–106
Vora NL, Luk KH, Forell B et al. (1988) Interstitial local current field hyperthermia for advanced cancers of the cervix. Endocurietherapy/Hyperthermia Oncology 4: 97–106
Vora NL, Forell B, Luk KH, Pezner RD, Desai KR, Lipsett JA, Wong JYA (1989) Interstitial thermoradiotherapy in recurrent and advanced carcinoma of malignant tumors: seven years' experience. In: Sugahara T, Saito M (eds) Hyperthermic oncology 1988, vol 1. Taylor & Francis, London, pp 588–590
Winter A, Laing J, Paglione R, Sterzer F (1985) Microwave hyperthermia for brain tumors. Neurosurgery 17: 387–399
Wong TZ, Ryan TP, Strohbehn JW, Jones KM (1989) A phase-coherent interstitial microwave antenna array hyperthermia system. In: Sugahara T, Saito M (eds) Hyperthermic oncology 1988, vol 1. Taylor & Francis, London, pp 894–895
Yabumoto E, Suyama S (1985) Interstitial radiofrequency hyperthermia in combination with external beam radiotherapy. In: Overgaard J (ed) Hyperthermic oncology 1984, vol 1. Taylor & Francis, London, pp 579–582
Yabumoto E, Suyama S, Show K, Yamazaki T (1989) A phase I clinical trial of radiofrequency interstitial hyperthermia combined with external radiotherapy. In: Sugahara T, Saito M (eds) Hyperthermic oncology 1988, vol 1. Taylor & Francis, London, pp 591–593

25 Clinical Experience of Interstitial Thermoradiotherapy Using Hot Water Perfusion Techniques

L. HANDL-ZELLER

CONTENTS

25.1 Introduction

The aim of hyperthermia (HT) is to increase the efficiency of radiotherapy without raising the toxicity to normal tissue. Keeping this in mind we have developed a heating device which can be easily combined with brachytherapy (BT) implantations. Although external beam irradiation has sometimes been employed in conjunction with interstitial heating, most groups have developed combinations of interstitial hyperthermia (IH) and BT.

Compared to external HT techniques, IH offers several advantages:

1. Two invasive techniques are combined, the only problem being to design a compatible system.
2. Uniform radiation dose and heat distribution can be achieved compared with externally applied HT, without transit through overlying normal tissue.
3. The interstitial technique allows the application of radiation and heat in a defined volume and also spares the adjacent normal tissue.
4. High (HDR) and low dose rate (LDR) irradiation can be administered with HT simultaneously: If preferential tumor heating can be achieved, an improved therapeutic effect is possible with the simultaneous protocol.

L. HANDL-ZELLER, M.D., Universitätsklinik für Strahlentherapie und -biologie, Alserstraße 4, A-1090 Wien, Austria

Our aim was to induce heat directly through hot water tubes (heat conduction) and not through transformation (electromagnetic waves, ultrasound). In this procedure the distribution of heat depends solely on the heat conductivity of the tissue. In interstitial irradiation a homogeneous distribution of the dose can be ensured only by using geometrically exact implants. With spacing of about 1 cm it is possible to distribute the radiation dose homogeneously and also to achieve optimum isotherms. One of the main reasons for the development of the hot water system (Hydrotherm) at the Department of Radiotherapy and Radiobiology in the Vienna University School of Medicine was the safety aspect. Another important factor was the simple operability of the device; in daily routine, constant supervision by a physicist is not necessary. A further reason for developing the method was to achieve the biologically optimal thermal enhancement ratio (TER) by using irradiation and heat simultaneously. Clinically, simultaneous application of IH is possible with LDR, HDR, and external beam irradiation.

25.2 Physical Aspects of Interstitial Hyperthermia

Many basic physical studies have been performed on different methods of IH. Therefore we would like to restrict this discussion to the physical aspects of hot water HT, furthermore keeping it to the absolute minimum required for comparison with other interstitial techniques.

From a physical point of view most heating techniques depend on constant power or constant temperature. Both types of procedure have their limitations, which can cause cold or hot spots if they are not carefully considered. A common problem for all heating techniques is the inhomogeneity of the tumor tissue. Regions of higher blood flow, necroses, etc. cause different thermal conductivity, different thermal flow, and therefore different temperature distribution within the tumor.

25.3 Physical and Technological Aspects of Hot Water Hyperthermia

25.3.1 Physical Aspects

Energy is directly transferred through hot water tubes via conduction and radiation. Through technical improvement (combination of booster and suction pumps) the flow rate in the needles has been increased (2.5–4.0 ml/s). Due to the specially designed coaxial inner needle system there are turbulent conditions and practically no longitudinal temperature gradients within the entire therapeutic zone.

The rate of heat transfer from the hot water needle is:

$$Q = \mathrm{Nu} k_w \, \Pi L (T_w - T_m).$$

The Nusselt number for turbulent conditions is:

$$\mathrm{Nu} = 0.023 \mathrm{Re}^{0.8} \mathrm{Pr}^{0.3}.$$

The Reynolds number is:

$$\mathrm{Re} = \rho_w u_m d_i / \eta_w.$$

In the above,
Nu = the Nusselt number;
Re = the Reynolds number;
Pr = 3.67 = the Prandtl number;
k_w = 0.623 W/m · K = thermal conductivity;
L = tube length;
T_m = tissue temperature;
T_w = water temperature;
ρ_w = 988 kg/mm^3 = density;
η_w = 544 10^{-6} kg/m · s = dynamic viscosity;
u_m = flow rate; and
d_i = internal diameter.

There is an exact cylindrical temperature symmetry radial to the longitudinal axis, in contrast to radiofrequency (RF) and microwave (MW) systems. RF techniques are known to be very sensitive to any deviation between the implanted electrodes. Most of the power tends to concentrate in the area where the distance between the electrodes is closer (Hand 1992).

The problem with MW systems is the nonuniform power deposition along the antennas as well as the dependence of power deposition on depth of insertion. Figure 25.1 illustrates, in a very simplified manner, the influence of tissue inhomogeneities using constant power or constant temperature. (Constant power = electromagnetic sources with low or high frequency, ranging from 0.5 MHz to 2.4 GHz; constant temperature = hot sources comprising ferromagnetic seeds, hot water tubes and hot wire systems.)

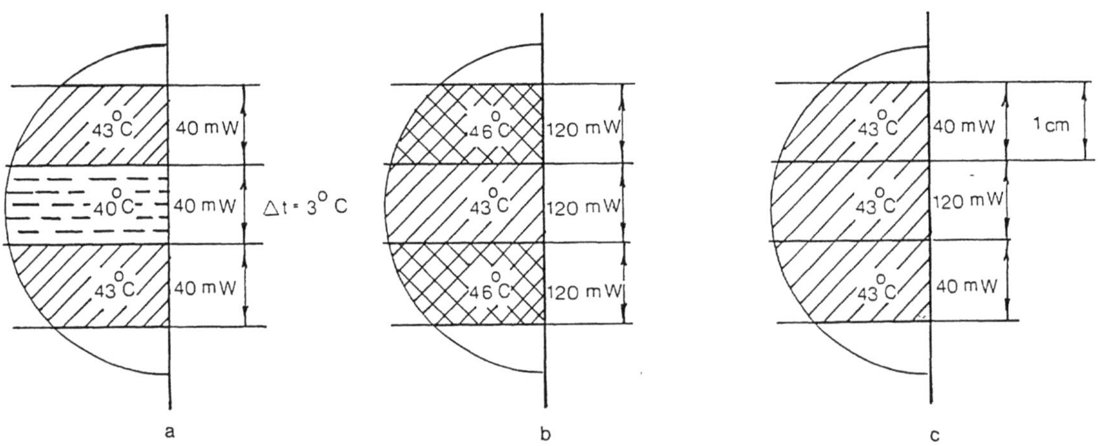

Fig. 25.1 a–c. Simplified illustration of the difference between constant power and constant temperature. **a** With a constant power source at a power input of 40 mW cm^{-1} the areas with normal blood flow reach therapeutic temperatures, whereas regions with high blood flow do not reach therapeutic temperatures. **b** In the case of high blood flow the power has to be raised to achieve therapeutic temperatures. Areas with low blood perfusion are overheated. **c** In contrast to sources of constant power, sources of constant temperature have a kind of inner control. The power deposition is directly dependent on the temperature difference between tissue and needle

The inner control of constant temperature sources not only tries to equalize local temperature minimums but is also one of the great advantages of this method that each needle of a three-dimensional array controls its heat flow by itself. Needles placed in the center automatically provide less power than needles in outer parts of the array. Therefore the control of individual needles is not necessary for achieving a homogeneous temperature distribution. The higher temperature gradient also increases the power input to the tissue at the end of the needles.

Three-dimensional temperature uniformity is calculated as follows:

$$\rho_m c_m \frac{\partial T}{\partial t} = k_m \nabla^2 T - c_b w \,(T - T_b)\,.$$

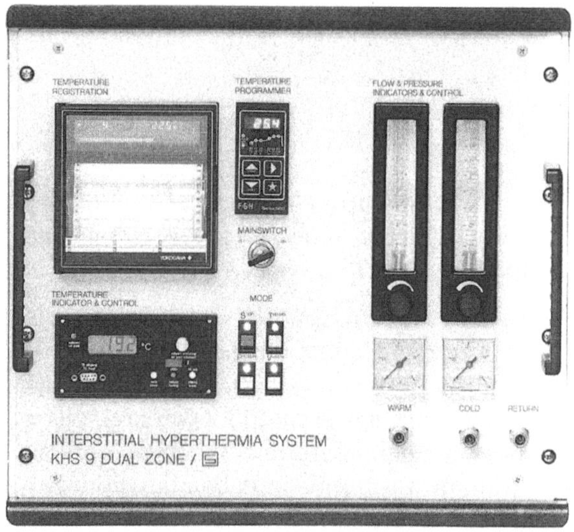

Fig. 25.2. Hydrotherm hyperthermia system

25.3.2 Technological Aspects

The standard hot water IH unit (Hydrotherm) consists of a water reservoir with a precision thermostat including heater and cooler, pressure and suction pumps, a proportional integral differential (PID) device to control water temperature, a manually controlled device for pressure and flow rate, and a manifold to distribute water to the implant (Figs. 25.2, 25.3). The accuracy of the control system is ± 0.1 C for temperature, ± 0.1 bar for pressure, and ± 0.1 ml/s for flow. Open-ended metallic or plastic tubes with an outer diameter (OD) of 1.6 or 1.9 mm are used. They are usually made of a single material. Closed-end metal tubes or plastic catheters, OD 1.6 or 1.9 mm, with a sealed tip are used when the tumor is heated preferentially and the normal tissue is cooled. In these tubes, hot water is brought to the tip through a smaller diameter metal tube inserted into the main tube through its entire length. Hot water from the tip flows backwards into the main tube. Another shorter tube is also inserted which brings cold water into the main tube. This shorter tube can be easily inserted into the outer tube as far as necessary. Hot water returning from the end of the main needle mixes with the cold water at the tip of the shorter inner tube. The mixture flows to the exit, rendering this part of the needle relatively cool.

25.3.2.1 Material for the Implantations

1. Straight plastic tube, open ended for through-flow method.

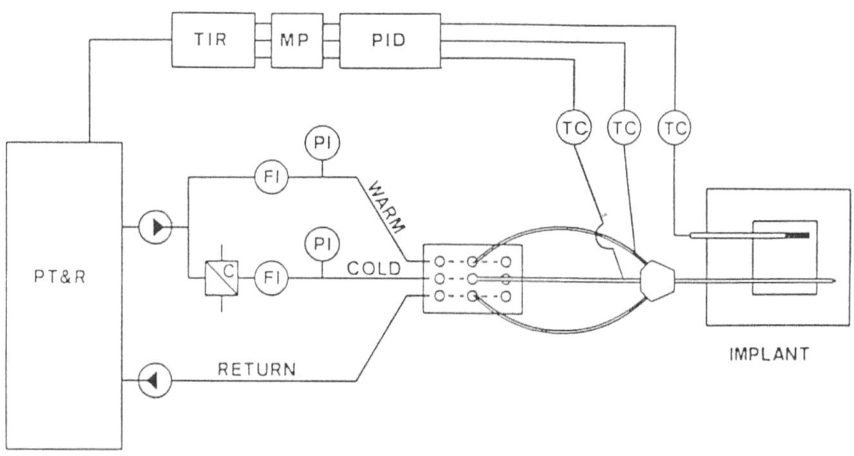

Fig. 25.3. Schematic presentation of the HT unit with the closed-ended counterflow needle and thermoprobe. *MP*, microprocessor; *PID*, controller; *TIR*, temperature indicator and registration; *FI*, flow indicator; *PI*, pressure indicator; *TC*, thermocouple; *PT&R*, precision thermostat and reservoir; C, cooler

2. Straight plastic tube with a closed end, allowing insertion of inner tubes for counterflow and cooling.
3. Plastic loop for throughflow method.
4. Steel catheter, open ended for throughflow method.
5. Steel catheter with a closed end, allowing insertion of inner tubes for counterflow and cooling.

Polyethylene tubes have been used for several years. However, polyethylene tends to absorb fluid and hence the tubes gradually lose their firmness; the resulting problems are well known (e.g., piercing of the wall upon insertion of microwave antennas or iridium wires, leaking in combination with water systems). As these problems do not occur when using polypropylene tubes, we now use this material exclusively.

25.3.2.2 Spacing of the Probes

It is expected of IH systems that they will deliver a homogeneous temperature distribution, even if the needles are spaced far apart and not parallel to each other. Most reports indicate that a gap of 8–12 mm is necessary for adequate distribution of isodoses. Such gaps are also ideal for the application of hot water tubes. Again, it must be emphasized that HT is an adjuvant therapy to irradiation.

25.3.2.3 Temperature Distribution

Homogeneous distribution of temperature for therapeutic purposes can be achieved by using a hot water IH system with a water temperature of 46°C and spacing between tubes of 10 mm. Longitudinally for a 20-cm-long tube the gradient is less than 0.5°C for the throughflow system and less than 0.2°C for the counterflow system. Within the array the temperature gradient around the tubes is 0.2°C/mm. Outside the array the gradient is 0.5°C/mm (Budihna 1992). With an average gradient of 0.2°C/mm within the implant and a spacing of 1 cm temperature uniformity at steady-state conditions is between 0.4°C and 0.7°C.

25.3.2.4 Thermometry

Since there is no electromagnetic interference in hot water HT, thermocouples can be used for temperature measurements. We have used single point as well as multisensor type T thermocouples (manganin–constantan), the thickness of the wire being 50 μm. Temperature registration is by means of standard temperature recorders as well as PC registration systems. The accuracy of these systems is about 0.1°C. Thermocouples are either implanted at significant points or thermal mapping is done under movement in at least two axes.

25.4 Clinical Aspects of Hot Water Hyperthermia

25.4.1 Techniques of Implantation

Basically there is a choice between synthetic tubes and steel needles of various types. Various techniques for implantation have been devised to suit different institutes and their areas of special interest in brachytherapy.

Superficial Lesions. At least two rows of needles are placed in superficial lesions. Synthetic tubes, synthetic needles, or steel needles can be used with the throughflow or counterflow technique. Simultaneous HT and external beam irradiation for superficial lesions was first employed. Figure 25.4 illustrates the technique used at the Oncological Institute in Ljubljana for simultaneous HT and external beam irradiation of superficial lesions.

Head and Neck Tumors. Three major techniques are used in interstitial treatment of head and neck tumors:

1. In manual loading of LDR activity, loop-shaped tubes are used (Fig. 25.5a). This technique is

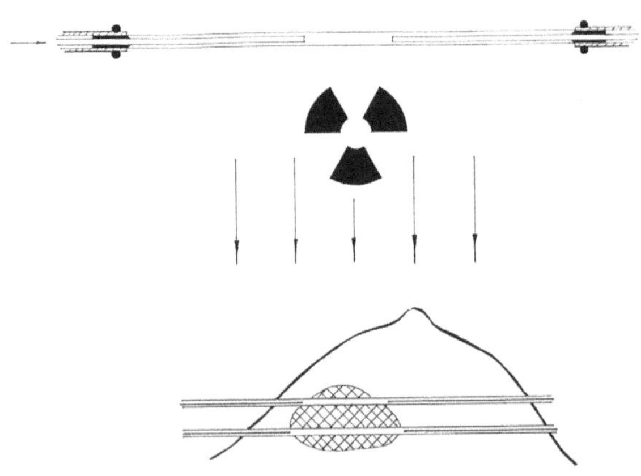

Fig. 25.4. Ljubljana HT technique with cooling of the normal tissue and external beam RT for breast carcinoma

very time consuming but is advantageous because of its ideal adaptability to surrounding anatomical structures. The Alexis Vautrin Center in Nancy, the Leon Berard Center in Lyon, and the Oncological Institute at Ljubljana use this technique in combination with warm water HT by means of the throughflow technique.

2. At the Medical School in Erlangen (FRG), the aforementioned procedure is applied in combination with an LDR afterloading device, with closed-end nylon tubes, employing the counterflow technique (Fig. 25.5b).

3. At the Medical School in Vienna, standard closed-end steel needles with an OD of 1.6 mm are used in combination with an HDR afterloading device employing the counterflow technique (Fig. 25.5c).

Pelvic Tumors. Implants of the type illustrated in Fig. 25.6 are used in rectal, anal, and gynecological tumors. The use of HDR afterloading devices is increasing in this kind of treatment. At the medical schools in Vienna and Graz, standard closed-end steel needles with an OD of 1.6 or 1.9 mm are used with the counterflow technique.

Advanced Breast Carcinomas. The technique developed at the Curie Institute in Paris (Fig. 25.7) entailed the use of polypropylene implants. A cooling system was devised for the application of the technique using the throughflow method. The iridium-192 LDR activities are loaded manually.

The approach developed at the medical school in Düsseldorf (FRG) aimed at preoperative shrinking

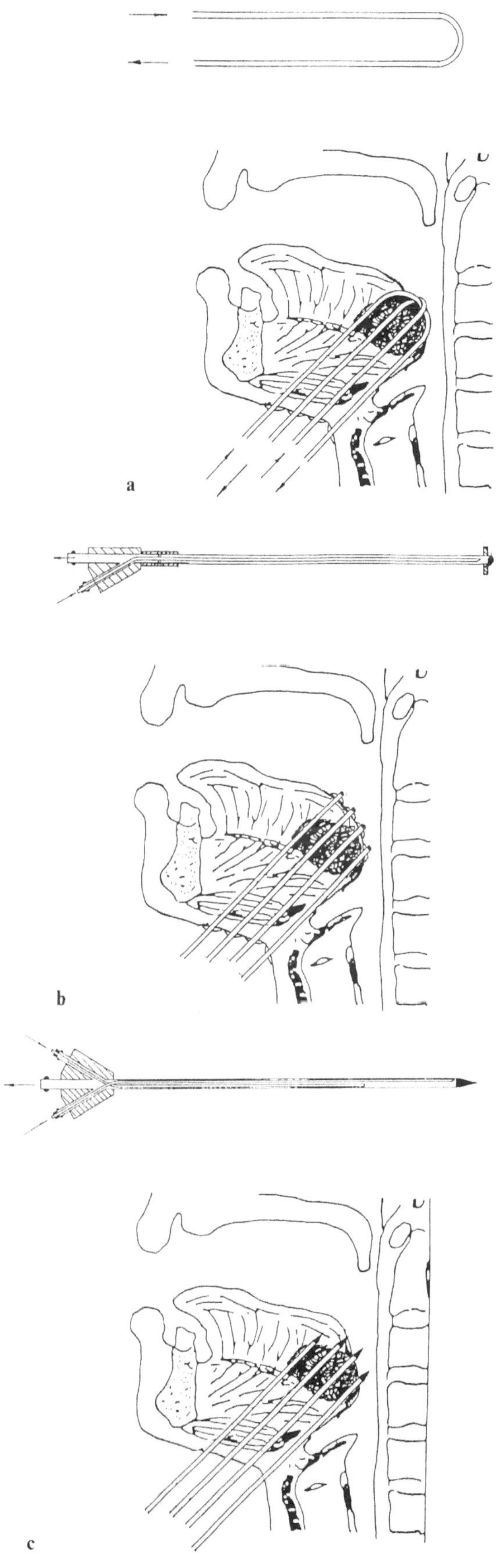

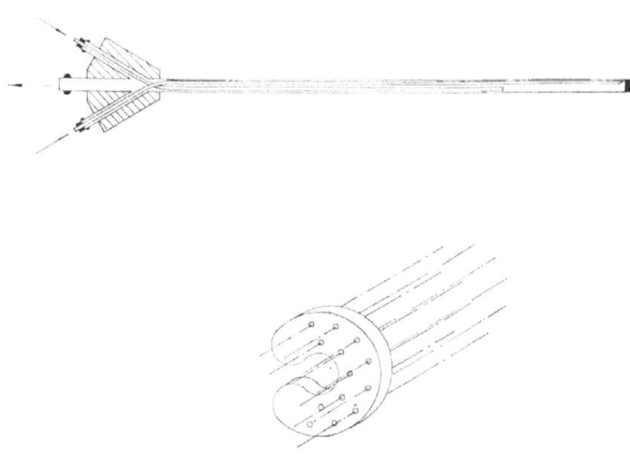

Fig. 25.6. Template technique for pelvic tumors with cooling of normal tissue

Fig. 25.5 a–c. Techniques for base of tongue carcinoma. **a** French loop technique; **b** Erlangen closed-end catheter technique; **c** Viennese technique

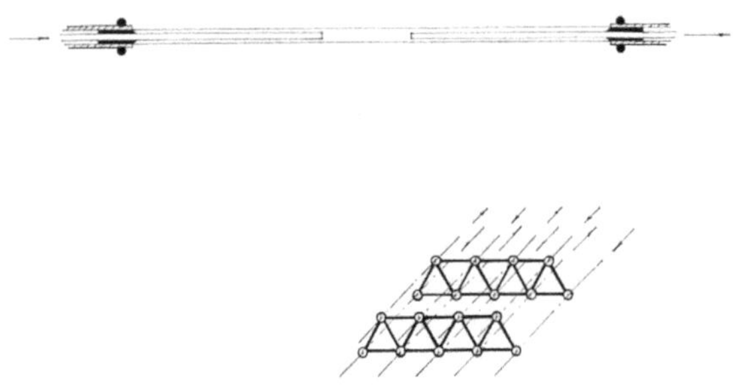

Fig. 25.7. Institute Curie technique with cooling of normal tissue

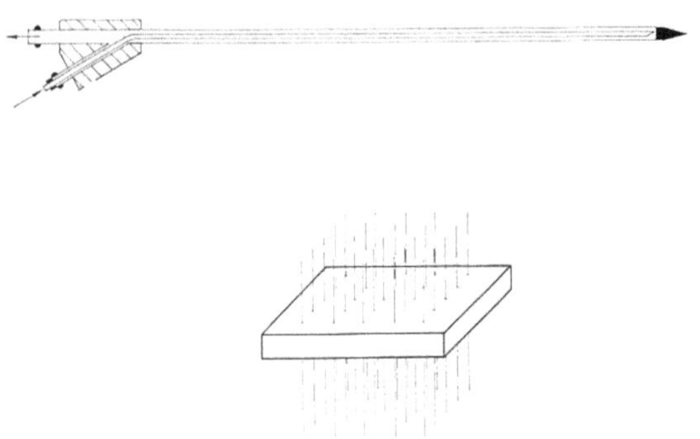

Fig. 25.8. Düsseldorf technique using counterflow needles

of advanced breast tumors. Standard HDR needles are used, employing the counterflow technique (Fig. 25.8).

25.4.2 Simultaneous Application of Radiation and Heat with Hot Water Hyperthermia

A moderate temperature (41°C) HT treatment which causes no measurable effect may enhance the response to ionizing radiation. This sensitizing effect is normally expressed in terms of TER, defined as the ratio of doses of ionizing radiation required to achieve a given level of response in the presence or absence of HT, respectively. The HT strategy used clinically is a sequential treatment which mainly utilizes the hyperthermic cytotoxicity against radioresistant cells. However, an interval between RT and HT reduces the response to the combined treatment. In fact, even a so-called simultaneous treatment with only a small interval between HT and RT reduces the sensitizing effect of heat (OVERGAARD 1989). If up to 30 min is allowed between RT and HT, the effect of such treatment will be dominated by the hyperthermic cytotoxicity, although some radiosensitization may persist in both tumor and normal tissue. Simultaneous application of irradiation and heat results in equal sensitization of tumor and normal tissue (FIELD 1990) and is hence of no therapeutic gain (OVERGAARD 1980) if the tumor is not heated selectively.

Although hyperthermic radiosensitization with simultaneous treatment is able to yield the highest TER, this protocol has been clinically impractical until now for various technical reasons. We believe that a simultaneous thermoradiotherapy with RF or MW is difficult to achieve due to inherent technical problems. The main space in the catheter is needed for the use of antennas and temperature sensors. Hence it appears to us that the combination of HT and RT is not possible with standard size afterloading catheters. Again, with constant heat sources such as ferromagnetic seeds or the hot wire technique the inner space of the catheter is occupied. Our aim was to make possible selective tumor heating with the normal tissue being kept at body temperature. All catheters used by us are those used in standard BT. They are connected via a suitable coupling system to the HT device. In each case a heating tube and a cooling water tube are inserted into the center of the catheter (HANDL-ZELLER et al. 1987; HANDL-ZELLER et al. 1988; HANDL-ZELLER 1992; SCHREIER et al. 1990).

25.4.2.1 Treatment Schedule with LDR Low Dose Rate

In LDR systems the cooling water tube is also the carrier of the radioactive iridium-192 wire (HANDL-ZELLER 1990) (Fig. 25.9). Data in respect of localized HT in combination with LDR irradiation suggest that potentiation of LDR irradiation by a single heat treatment may be maximized if the HT is given either during or simultaneously with the BT (JONES et al. 1989).

25.4.2.2 Treatment Schedule with HDR High Dose Rate

In HDR systems, the water supply which controls the temperature in the specific catheter is switched off by computer control during the time the RT is being applied in the active catheter. The water which has remained in the catheter is first removed by the vacuum pump, then the radiation source is inserted through the same catheter into the correct position under computer control. There are two

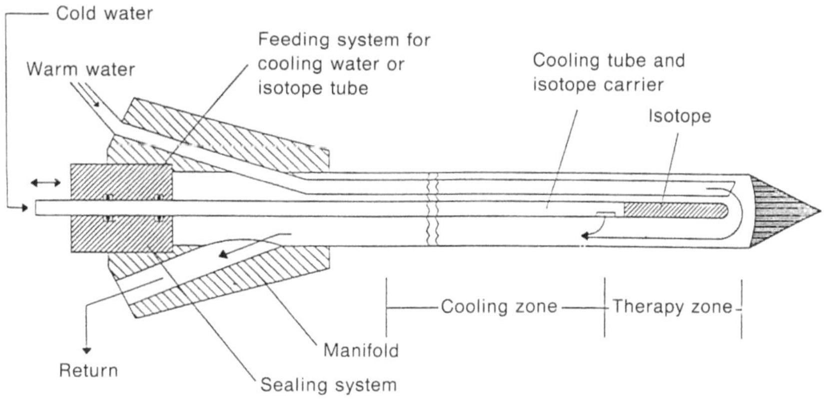

Fig. 25.9. Simultaneous system for LDR

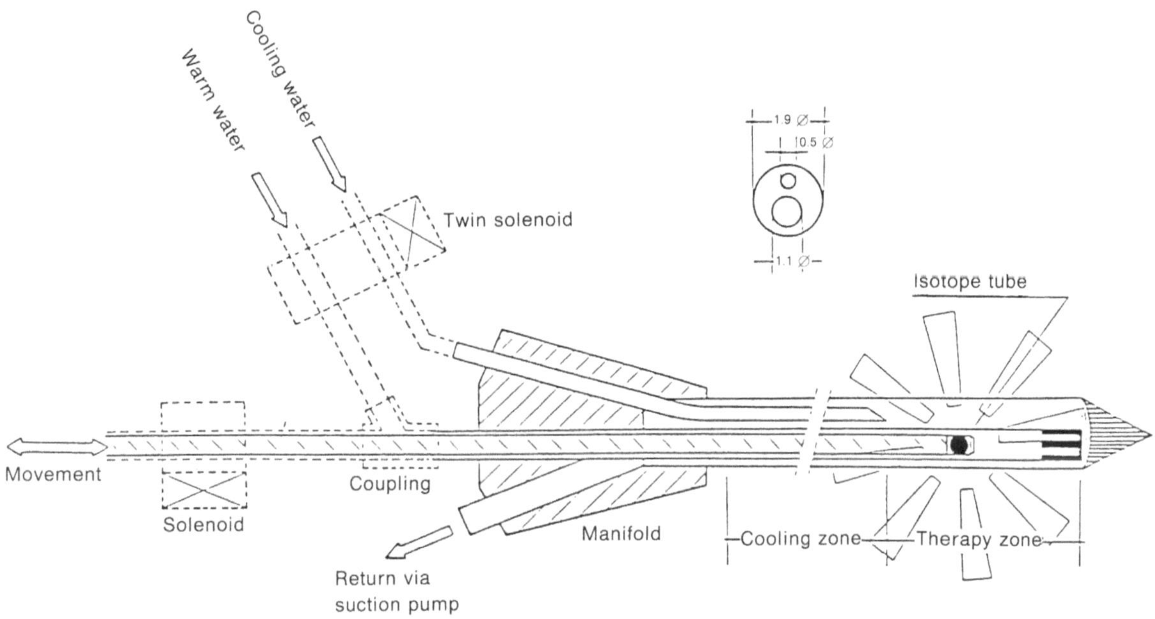

Fig. 25.10. Simultaneous system for HDR

solenoids in the hot water radiation catheter system. The solenoid for the RT remains closed when hot water is flowing. When the RT is to be applied the solenoid for the hot water closes and the RT source enters the tube and supplies the active catheter (Fig. 25.10). The reason for this control system is to ensure that only the active catheter area loses the heat source during RT. All the other catheters continue to provide heat in a three-dimensional manner to the entire tumor volume.

25.5 Clinical Experience

25.5.1 Institutions Using Hot Water Hyperthermia Systems

The institutions using hot water hyperthermia systems are listed in Table 25.1.

25.5.2 Patient and Lesion Characteristics

Since 1986 a total of 154 malignant lesions (127 patients: 52 males, 75 females; age range 38–83 years, mean 57) in the head and neck, breast, pelvic region, or other sites have been treated with combined interstitial hot water thermoradiotherapy. The lesions can be classified into four groups:

1. PT: primary tumor (without previous treatment); $n = 70$ (45%)
2. PTp: primary tumor pretreated (with incomplete surgical treatment + RT and/or chemotherapy); $n = 27$ (17%)

Table 25.1. Institutions using hot water hyperthermia systems

Institution	Physician/physicist
Curie Institute, Paris, France	F. Campana, A. Fourquet, A. Labib, D. Pouvert/G. Gaboriaud
Division of Radiotherapy, University Clinic of Radiology, Graz, Austria	K. Arian-Schad, A. Hackl/H. Leitner, G. Stücklschweiger
University Clinic of Radiotherapy and Radiobiology, Vienna, Austria	L. Handl-Zeller, W. Seitz, C. Stanek/–
Institute of Oncology, Ljubljana, Slovenia	M. Budihna, H. Lesnicar/J. Burger
University Clinic of Radiotherapy, Düsseldorf, Federal Republic of Germany	N. Zamboglou, C. Kolotas/K. Muskalla
Dept. of Radiation Oncology/Physics, University of Alabama, Birmingham, USA	R. Meredith/I. Brezovich
Department of Radiotherapy and Brachytherapy, Alexis-Vautrin Center, Nancy, France	C. Marchal, M. Pernot, S. Hoffstetter/–
Department of Radiotherapy and Brachytherapy, Leon Berard Center, Lyon, France	J. Ardiet/–

3. LRT: Local recurrent tumor (after surgery, after palliative or definitive RT dose, after combined surgery + RT (pre- or postop), or after other modalities; $n = 28$ (18%)

4. ML: metastatic lesion (pretreatment with a variety of treatment modalities); $n = 29$ (20%)

Seventy lesions (45%) were located in the head and neck, 45 (30%) in the breast, 36 (23%) in the pelvic region, and 3 (2%) in other body sites. Body sites treated with hot water HT are listed in Table 25.2b. Most tumor volumes ranged from 40 to 160 cm^3; seven (5%) lesions had extensive tumor volumes exceeding 250 cm^3.

25.5.3 Clinical Results

Table 25.2 summarizes the clinical results obtained in the different centers. HT was administered immediately prior to or both prior to and immediately after the BT. Treatment temperatures ranged from 42.5°C for 45 min to 45°C for 55–60 min. The complete and partial response rates obtained with hot water HT were similar to those reported for RF and MW IH.

In addition to the cases cited in Table 25.2, three female patients with advanced breast carcinoma were treated with interstitial hot water HT with truly simultaneous external beam RT at the Institute of Oncology in Ljubljana. Due to the special treatment conditions this small group is not included in the table. One female patient with previously untreated T3N0M1 breast carcinoma was implanted. After initial therapy with external beam RT to a tumor dose of 12.5 Gy (2.5 Gy daily), mammograms were obtained to establish the tumor size at that phase of treatment. An implant was introduced through the tumor area. For technical reasons only half the tumor could be implanted. The implanted part was treated with truly simultaneous HT and RT (8 Gy, 14 MeV electrons) while the non-implanted part of the tumor was only irradiated. Minimum temperature at steady state was 42.5°C, and total treatment time, 45 min. After 4 weeks of reexamination revealed a 45% regression of the heated and irradiated part, whereas tumor shrinkage of only 75% was observed in the unimplanted tumor part. No obvious tissue damage was observed in the area of skin overlying the implant.

Complications. Considering the advanced nature and the extensive prior treatment of most of the tumors treated, interstitial thermoradiotherapy was very well tolerated. While the average toxicity rates reported with RF and MW systems were 22%–24%, institutions using hot water HT reported a toxicity rate of only 3% on average. These complications included blisters in four patients caused by temperatures accidentally being set at too high a level at the first treatment.

An ulceration in a melanoma in the dorsum of a foot might have been due to radiation overdosage, given the relatively large volume implant for the size of the lesion in conjunction with the thermotoxic effect of the heating procedure.

Table 25.2. a Clinical results achieved using hot water IH systems, as compared with RF and MW IH systems

Authors	No. of evaluable sites	Treatment parameters HT (°C, min)	Sequence	CR %	PR %	NC %	No. uneval	Toxicity %	Follow-up (months)
Hot water:									
Ardiet et al.	2	42.5°–44.5°, 60 min	HT-BT	–	-	–	–	(0)	–
Arian-Schad et al.	10	43°–44.5°, 40 min	BT-HT	40	50	10	–	1 (10)	4–16
Budihna et al.	16	43°–45°, 45–60 min	HT-BT	43	36	21	–	1 (7)	3–56
Campana et al.	8	42.5°–43.5°, 45 min	HT-BT	75	25	0	–	0 (0)	3–24
Handl-Zeller et al.	72	43°–45°, 45–60 min	HT-BT(LDR) BT-HT(HDR)	55	42	3	–	3 (4)	3–56
Marchal et al.	7	42.5°–45°, 60 min	BT-HT	–	-	–	–	(0)	–
Meredith et al.	5	42°–45° 55–60 min	HT-BT-HT	80	20	0	–	(0)	–
Zamboglou et al.	34	43.5°, 60 min	HT-BT	90	10	0	–	(0)	3

Radiofrequency:
A total of 144 patients (59%) achieved CR, 43 patients (18%) PR, 48 patients (20%) NR, 6 patients (3%) were not evaluable.
The overall response rate is 187 & 243 (77%).
Toxicity was 24% in the collective experience. In 11 patients toxicity was not evaluable (Cosset et al. 1985; Ginoves et al. 1986; Emami et al. 1987; Gautherie et al. 1989; Yabumoto et al. 1989; Vora et al. 1989; Levendag et al. 1991)
Microwave:
A total of 95 patients (64%) achieved CR, 35 patients (24%) PR, 10 patients (10%) NR, 4 patients (2%) were not evaluable.
The overall response rate is 130 of 149 (87%) Toxicity was 22% in the collective experience. In 35 patients toxicity was not evaluable (Rafla et al. 1988, Petrovich et al. 1989, Seegenschmiedt et al. 1990, Coughlin et al. 1991).
CR, Complete response; PR, partial response; NC, no change; uneval., Unevaluable; HT, hyperthermia; BT, brachytherapy; LDR, low dose rate; HDR, high dose rate

Table 25.2. b Survey on body sites treated with hot water HT, kind of hot water perfusion technique and type of BT. RT dose: 15–60 Gy

Institution	Breast	Head & Neck	Pelvis gynecological	Pelvis colorectal	Other sites	Prostate	Total	Hot Water Perfusion Technique	Type of BT
Curie Institute, Paris, France	8						8	Through flow-cooled	LDR
Division of Radiotherapy, University Clinic of Radiology, Graz, Austria			2	6	2		10	Counterflow	HDR
University Clinic of Radiotherapy and Radiobiology, Vienna, Austria		43	5	17	1	6	72	Through flow & counterflow	LDR HDR
Institute of Oncology, Ljubljana, Slovenia	3	13					16	Through flow & counterflow	LDR
University Clinic of Radiotherapy, Düsseldorf, Federal Republic of Germany	34						34	Counterflow	HDR
Dept. of Radiation Oncology/Physics, University of Alabama, Birmingham, USA		5					5	Throughflow	HDR
Department of Radiotherapy and Brachytherapy, Alexis-Vautrin, Center, Nancy, France		7					7	Throughflow	LDR
Department of Radiotherapy and Brachytherapy, Leon Berard Center, Lyon, France		2					2	Throughflow	LDR

References

Budihna M, Lesnicar H, Handl-Zeller L, Schreier K (1992) Animal experiments with interstitial water hyperthermia. In: Handl-Zeller L (ed) Interstitial Hyperthermia. Springer, Wien New York pp 155–163

Cosset JM, Dutreix J, Haie C, Gerbaulet A, Janoray P, Dewars JA (1985) Interstitial thermoradiotherapy: a technical and clinical study of 29 implantations performed at the Institute Gustave Roussy. Int J Hyperthermia 1: 3–13

Coughlin CT, Ryan TP, Stafford JH (1991) Interstitial thermoradiotherapy: The Dartmouth experience 1981–1990. In: Chapman JD, Dewey WC, Whitmore GF (eds) Radiation research: A twentieth century perspective, vol 1. Academic Press Inc., San Diego, p 386

Emami B, Perez CA, Leybovich L, Straube W, von Gerichten D (1987) Interstitial thermoradiotherapy in treatment of malignant tumors. Int J Hyperthermia 3: 107–118

Gautherie M, Cosset JM, Gerard JP, Horiot JC, Ardiet JM, El Akoum H, Alperovitch A (1989) Radiofrequency interstitial hyperthermia: a multicentric program of quality assessment and clinical trials. In: Sugahara T, Saito M (eds) Hyperthermic oncology 1988, vol 2. Taylor & Francis, London, pp 711–714

Hahn GM (1992) Brachytherapy and hyperthermia: Biological Rationale. In: Handl-Zeller L (ed) Interstitial Hyperthermia. Springer, Wien New York pp 1–9

Hand JW (1992) Physical Aspects of Interstitial hyperthermia, In: Handl-Zeller L (ed) Interstitial Hyperthermia, Springer, Wien New York, pp 51–75

Handl-Zeller L, Kärcher KH, Schreier K, Handl O (1987) Beitrag zur Optimierung interstitieller Hyperthermiesysteme. Strahlenther Onkol 163: 406–463

Handl-Zeller L, Schreier K, Kärcher KH, Budihna M, Lesnicar H (1988) First clinical experience with the Viennese interstitial two zone hyperthermia system. In: Sugahara T, Saito M (eds) Hypermic oncology, 1988, vol 1. Taylor & Francis, London pp 814–816

Handl-Zeller L (1990) Erhöhung der Thermal Enhancement Ratio durch simultane Applikation von Bestrahlung und Hyperthermie – Technische Möglichkeiten bei interstitieller Applikation. Strahlenther Onkol 166: 643–646

Handl-Zeller L (1992) Simultaneous application of combined interstitial high- or low-dose rate irradiation with hot water hyperthermia. In: Handl-Zeller L (ed) Interstitial Hyperthermia, Springer, Wien New York, pp 165–170.

Jones EL, Lyons BE, Dopule EB, Darin BJ (1989) Thermal enhancement of low dose rate irradiation in a murine tumor system. Int J Hyperthermia 4: 509–523

Levendag PC, Visser AG, Deurloo IK et al. (1991) Interstitial radiation and/or interstitial hyperthermia in advanced and/or recurrent cancers in the head and neck: a pilot study. Hyperthermia Bull 10

Linares LA, Nort D, Brenner H et al. (1986) Interstitial hyperthermia and brachtherapy: a preliminary report. Endocurietherapy/Hyperthermia Oncol 2: 39–44

Oleson JR, Manning MR, Sim DA et al. (1984) A review of the University of Arizona human clinical hyperthermia experience. Front Radiat Ther Oncol 18: 136–143

Overgaard J (1989) The current and potential role of hyperthermia in radiotherapy. Int J Radiat Oncol Biol Phys 3: 535–549

Overgaard J (1989) Simultaneous and sequential hyperthermia and radiation treatment of an experimental tumor and its surrounding normal tissue in vivo. Int J Radiat Oncol Biol Phys 11: 1507–1517

Petrovich Z, Langholz B, Lam K, Luxton G, Cohen D, Jepson J, Astrahan M (1989) Interstitial microwave hyperthermia combined with iridium-192 radiotherapy for recurrent tumours. Am J Clin Oncol 12: 264–268

Puthawala AA, Syed AMN, Khalid MA, Rafie S, McNamara CS (1985) Interstitial hyperthermia for recurrent malignancies. Endocurietherapy/Hyperthermia Oncol 1: 125–131

Rafla SM, Tchelebi E, Youssef E et al. (1988) The treatment of advanced recurrent pelvic tumors by interstitial hyperthermia and brachytherapy – a promising approach. In: Abstracts of the 36th Annual Meeting of the Radiation Research Society, Philadelphia, p 46

Schreier K, Budihna M, Lesnicar H et al. (1990) Preliminary studies of interstitial hyperthermia using hot water. Int J Hyperthermia 2: 431–444

Seegenschmiedt MH, Sauer R, Fietkan R et al. (1990) Primary advanced and local recurrent head and neck tumors: effective management with interstitial thermo-radiotherapy. Radiology 176, pp 267–274.

Seegenschmiedt MH, Brady LW, Sauer R (1990) Interstitial thermoradiotherapy: Review on technical and clinical aspects, Amer J Clin Oncol 13: 352–363

Strohbehn JW, Douple EB, Coughlin CT (1984) Interstitial microwave antenna array systems for hyperthermia. Front Radiat Ther Oncol 18: 70–84

Vora NL, Forell B, Luk KH et al. (1989) Interstitial thermoradiotherapy in recurrent and advanced carcinoma of malignant tumors. In: Sughara T, Saito M (eds) Hyperthermic oncology, 1988, vol 1. Taylor & Francis, London, 1989, pp 588–590

Yabumoto E, Suyama S (1985) Interstitial radiofrequency hyperthermia in combination with external beam radiotherapy. In: Overgaard J (ed) Hyperthermia oncology 1984, vol 1. Taylor & Francis, Philadelphia, pp 579–582

26 Clinical Experience of Interstitial Thermoradiotherapy Using Ferromagnetic Implant Techniques

B. STEA, D.S. SHIMM, and T.C. CETAS

CONTENTS

26.1 Introduction

Interstitial hyperthermia commands much current interest as a method for delivering localized heat treatment to deep-seated as well as superficial tumors. Several interstitial techniques have been developed and used clinically over the past two decades. Interstitial techniques are popular since they can circumvent some problems encountered with non-invasive hyperthermia techniques, such as limited penetration, inefficient and nonuniform power distribution, and excessive heating of adjacent normal tissues. On the other hand, interstitial hyperthermia is an invasive technique and it usually requires general anesthesia. Some patients with bleeding disorders may not be candidates for such an approach. Furthermore, due to the localized nature of the treatment, the resulting temperature distribution may be highly dependent on the blood flow and geometry of the implant. Three major classes of interstitial hyperthermic techniques have been described and developed: interstitial radiofrequency electrodes (IRF), interstitial microwave antennas (IMW), and hot source techniques. Examples of hot source techniques include hot water tubes, electrically heated resistive elements, and ferromagnetic implants (FMIs).

Interstitial hyperthermia has been an area of intensive research at the University of Arizona since 1977 (ARISTIZABAL and OLESON 1984; SHIMM et al. 1990). IRF heating was developed early because of its simplicity and was used extensively until 1986. During the same period, IMW heating was implemented in several institutions and used for a few cases clinically at our institution as well. Both of these methods of interstitial hyperthermia deposit energy at distance from the implanted antenna or electrodes. However, each technique is subject to the limitation that the power deposition pattern is dependent upon tissue properties and therefore susceptible to heterogeneous heating due to altered current paths for IRF or reflections and unpredictable coupling for IMW. Our experience with these techniques has been previously published (SHIMM et al. 1990).

Hot source techniques, including FMI heating, are the most recent addition to the armamentarium available to the radiation oncologist (STEA et al. 1992). With these techniques there is no direct energy deposition into the tissue and therefore heterogeneities in the electrical properties of the tissue do not affect the resulting temperature distributions. The principal advantage of FMI heating is that tissue heating depends only on the implant materials (i.e., the composition of the FMI), the geometry of the implant, and the blood flow within the heated tissue; it is independent of the composition of the implanted volume. This technique is compatible with conventional interstitial brachytherapy techniques since ferromagnetic sources can be afterloaded into the same catheters as are used for interstitial irradiation. With FMI heating, there is little danger of overheating normal tissue since the seeds are the hottest elements, and their temperature is self-limited by their intrinsic design, i.e., by

B. STEA, M.D., Ph.D.; D.S. SHIMM, M.D.; T.C. CETAS, Ph.D.; Department of Radiation Oncology, University of Arizona, 1501 North Campbell Avenue, Tucson, Az 85724, USA the Curie point (the temperature at which ferromagnetism disappears). Another feature of FMI heating is ease of operation; once the ferromagnetic seeds are loaded into the catheters they are heated externally with a magnetic induction coil. The major limitation of FMI heating is that it generally requires a higher density implant than either IMW or IRF heating, because all hot source methods rely upon thermal conduction to heat tissues. Furthermore, once the implant is in place, the only way to change the resultant heating pattern is to use ferromagnetic seeds with a different Curie point.

Finally, an advantage of FMI heating over other hot source techniques is its application to permanent implantation without the need for attendant percutaneous leads (Kobayashi et al. 1991).

The main purpose of this chapter is to present a review of the clinical experience in treating patients with interstitial thermoradiotherapy employing FMI heating and iridium-192 (^{192}Ir).

26.2 Methods and Materials

26.2.1 System Description

Several preliminary reports have been published on FMI heating (Au et al. 1989; Shimm et al. 1991; Stea et al. 1990, 1992). The heating of tissues by implanted ferromagnetic seeds is based upon the absorption of energy by the ferromagnetic seeds from the applied radiofrequency (RF) magnetic field (Haider et al. 1991). The RF magnetic field induces eddy currents within the seeds, and this current in turn heats the seeds resistively. The heated seeds then raise the temperature of the surrounding tissues by thermal conduction. The final temperature achieved in the implanted tissues depends upon the properties of the seeds, the seed spacing, the level of blood flow in the tissue, and finally the strength of the applied magnetic field.

The complete hyperthermia system consists of three different components: the FMIs, the magnetic induction system, and the data acquisition system. The materials used in this study are various alloys of nickel and silicon with Curie points varying from 50° to 80°C (Chen et al. 1988). The most commonly used seeds have Curie points in the range of 50°–65°C. During the initial part of the study, we used seeds that were 1 mm in diameter and 10–12 mm in length which were strung together in heat-shrunk Teflon tubing. More recently, we have been using ferromagnetic materials in the form of multistranded wire bundles. Six of these wires (each 0.45 mm in diameter) are stranded together to form ribbons 1.4 mm in diameter. These are cut to a length sufficient to cover the target volume. The stranded wires have greater power absorption per unit length (Haider et al. 1991). Recently, van Dijk and co-workers (see this volume, Chap. 7) have suggested the use of nickel–palladium alloys. The efficiency of power absorption is somewhat less, but the sharpness of transition from ferromagnetic to nonferromagnetic state is much greater for this type of alloy than for nickel–silicon alloys.

The second component of the FMI heating system is the magnetic induction system. This consists of a generator–amplifier power source connected through a matching network to the induction coil. Four different types of coils are used at the University of Arizona. They differ in the orientation of the induced magnetic field, and therefore their use is matched to the particular orientation of the implant within the body. The primary requirement is that the magnetic vector be within 45° of the implant direction, and that the relative field strength be at least 50%. Typically for our systems the field strength is in the range of 1000–2000 A/m and 85–105 kHz. Figure 26.1 shows a photograph of a coil generally used for extracranial sites. Figure 26.2 shows a smaller coil (aperture 30 cm) used for tumors of the head and neck region, including the brain.

26.2.2 Thermometry

Temperatures were continuously monitored during the heat treatments by means of manganin–constantan thermocouple probes or fluoroptic thermometers with multiple sensors at 1-cm intervals along their length. No significant temperature aberrations were caused by the magnetic field. Temperatures were monitored every 5–10 s using a computerized data acquisition system. The data acquisition system consists of an IBM compatible, 286 based personal computer, interacting with a Hewlett Packard model 3852A Data Acquisition System.

26.2.3 Patient Selection

In 1987 a phase I protocol was activated to treat extracranial tumors with FMIs. To be eligible for the protocol, the patient had to have biopsy-proven

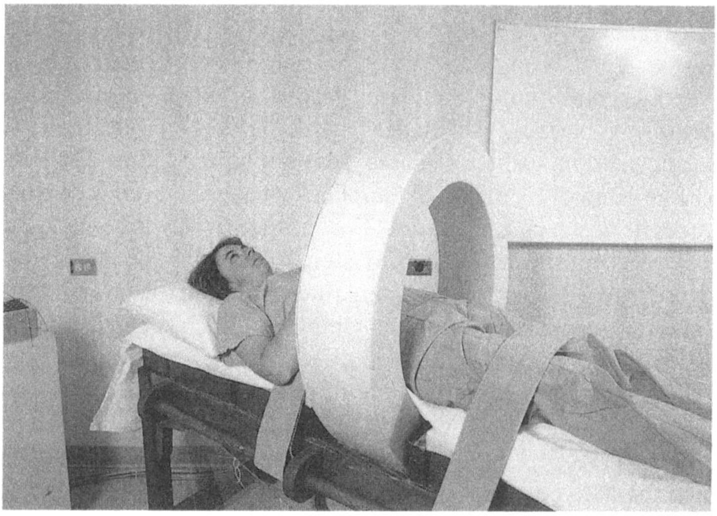

Fig. 26.1. Photograph of "C2" coil. This coil has an aperture of 60 cm (diameter) and generates a magnetic field oriented in the axial direction of a patient lying supine on the couch. It is used for most extracranial tumors

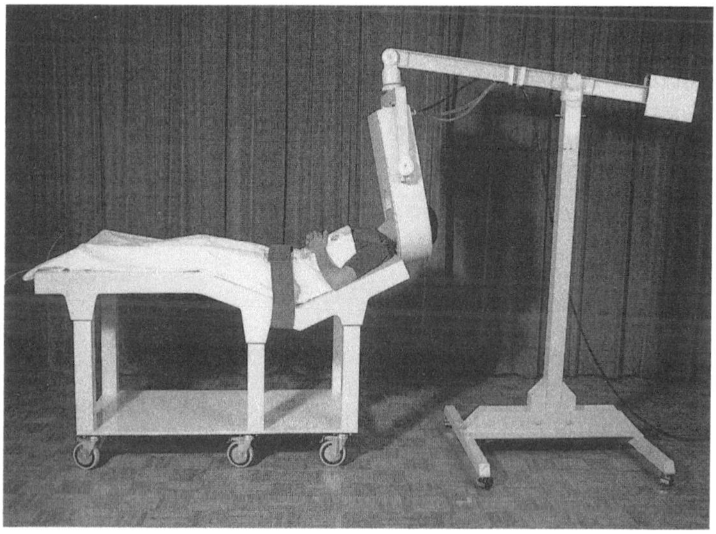

Fig. 26.2. Photograph of a head and neck coil. This coil is designed for head and neck treatments, especially of the brain. It has an aperture of 30 cm and can be oriented as needed

diagnosis of advanced or recurrent carcinoma, sarcoma, or melanoma of the head and neck region, the chest wall, or any pelvic organs. The tumor had to be accessible to implantation with afterloading catheters for ferromagnetic seeds and thermometry probes. The patient was required to have an acceptable general anesthetic risk. Furthermore, the patient had to be at least 18 years of age, have a Karnofsky performance score of 70% or better, have a life expectancy exceeding 3 months, and be able to sign an informed consent.

During the same time, a phase I protocol of interstitial thermoradiotherapy for high grade supratentorial gliomas was also activated at the University of Arizona. To be eligible for this protocol, the patient had to have a biopsy-proven diagnosis of either primary or recurrent anaplastic astrocytoma or glioblastoma multiforme. Tumors located in the posterior fossa or brain stem were excluded, as were multicentric tumors. The tumor volume initially was unrestricted; however, based on our initial experience (see Sect. 26.3), only tumors with a volume of up to 100 cm^3 were heated. The patients had to be 18 years of age, have a life expectancy of at least 3 months, and have a Karnofsky performance status of at least 50 to be eligible for the study. Both protocols had been approved by the University of Arizona Human Subjects Committee, and informed consent was obtained prior to the procedure from all patients.

26.2.4 *Implantation Technique and Treatment Planning*

For extracranial tumors implantation was performed using 14 gauge Teflon Henschke or Flexiguide afterloading catheters. These were implanted either free-hand or by means of templates whenever appropriate (e.g., in the pelvis). For intracranial tumors, implants were performed stereotactically using a Brown-Roberts-Wells stereotactic system modified to accept in-house built templates. Each template allowed the insertion of multiple catheters into the target by specifying the coordinate of only the centrally located catheter (LULU et al. 1990; STEA et al. 1990, 1992a).

Patients received a heat treatment just before the radioactive implant was loaded. Whenever possible a second hyperthermia treatment was given immediately after the removal of the radioactive sources. Each treatment lasted approximately 60 min after plateau temperatures were achieved. The treatments were delivered with the aim of heating the target volumes to temperatures between 42° and 45°C. The time interval between irradiation and hyperthermia was kept between 30 and 60 min.

26.2.5 *Radiation Therapy*

Patients with previously unirradiated tumors received first a course of external beam radiotherapy with doses individualized according to the patient's disease and site (see Sect. 26.3). Two to four weeks after completion of external beam radiation therapy, the patients underwent an interstitial implant with ^{192}Ir. Doses delivered by the implant varied according to the clinical situation (see Sect. 26.3). Patients with recurrent brain tumors after tolerance doses of external beam radiotherapy received only an interstitial implant in conjunction with hyperthermia. Implant dose rates varied between 30 and 80 cGy/h. Computerized dosimetry with display of the isodose lines in multiple planes was carried out to ensure that the chosen isodose lines fully encompassed the tumor volumes.

26.3 Results

26.3.1 *Patient Population and Tumor Characteristics*

A total of 72 patients were treated in two different phase I protocols, one for high grade supratentorial gliomas, and another for extracranial tumors. These two patient populations will be evaluated separately. A total of 44 patients were treated for extracranial tumors at four different institutions (University of Arizona, University of California San Francisco, University of Wisconsin, and City of Hope Medical Center). There were 24 males and 20 females with a median age of 63 years (range 36–88 years). Nineteen patients had head and neck tumors, 11 had gynecological tumors, nine had pelvic tumors, and five had chest wall or breast tumors. Fifty-two percent of the tumors were squamous cell carcinoma, and approximately 30% were adenocarcinoma (Table 26.1). Thirty-eight of the 44 patients had received prior therapy. Twenty-six had received prior radiation with a median dose of 60 Gy (range 39.6–131.5 Gy). The median tumor volume was 30 cm^3 ranging up to 1767 cm^3.

On protocol, patients received a portion of their irradiation by external beam radiotherapy, with a median dose of 40 Gy (range 9–76 Gy). In addition, they received an interstitial implant with ^{192}Ir delivering a median dose of 30 Gy (range 8–52 Gy). Total treatment doses on protocol ranged from 20.25 to 85 Gy, with a median dose of 52.25 Gy. Primary tumors received a median dose of 74.2 Gy, whereas recurrent tumors were treated with a lower median dose of 46.46 Gy.

An additional 28 patients with intracranial tumors were treated on a different phase I protocol. This patient population consisted of 16 males and 12 females with a median age of 44 years (range 21–79 years) and a median Karnofsky score of 90

Table 26.1. Patient population and tumor characteristics for extracranial sites ($n = 44$)

Patients	
Sex	24 males; 20 females
Age	36–88 yrs (median 63 yrs)
Tumors:	
Histology	23 (52%) squamous carcinomas
	13 (30%) adenocarcinomas
	4 (9%) sarcomas
	4 (9%) other
Location	19 (43%) head and neck
	17 (38.6%) pelvis
	5 (11.4%) chest wall/breast
	3 (7%) perineum
Type	15 (34%) advanced primary
	29 (66%) locally recurrent
Prior treatment	26 (59%) radiotherapy
	15 (34%) chemotherapy
	24 (55%) surgery

(range 50–90). Nine patients had anaplastic astrocytoma while 19 had glioblastoma multiforme. Six of these patients were treated at the time of tumor recurrence after having received tolerance doses of external beam radiotherapy, while 22 patients were treated at the time of their initial diagnosis. The latter group first received a course of external beam radiotherapy with a median dose of 48.4 Gy (range 40–54 Gy), followed by an interstitial implant with ^{192}Ir delivering a median dose of 32.67 Gy (range 26–41.4 Gy). Alternatively the patients treated at the time of recurrence received only an interstitial implant with a median dose of 40 Gy (range 13.9–50 Gy). In one patient, interstitial radiation was terminated prematurely at 13.9 Gy due to complications (edema and deterioration of neurological status). The median implant volume for all patients was 55.8 cm^3 and the median number of treatment catheters implanted per tumor was 18 (range 4–33). For brain tumors the source strength and distribution were optimized so that the target boundary (usually located 5–15 mm outside of the contrast-enhancing margin on CT scans) would receive the prescribed dose at a rate of 35–70 cGy/h (STEA et al. 1992b).

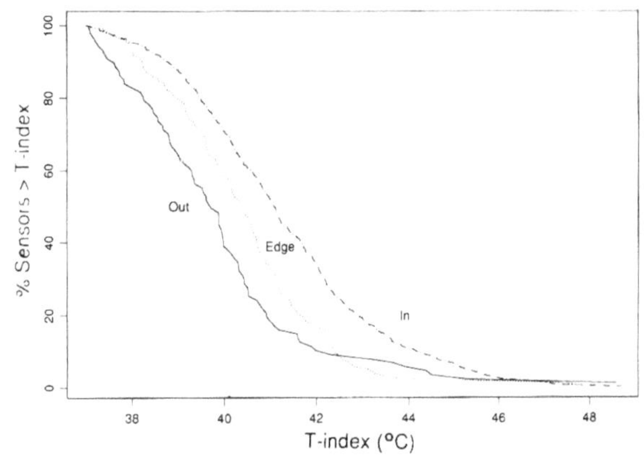

Fig. 26.3. Time-averaged mean temperature distribution for extracranial tumors. Sensors with a known location ($n = 836$) were plotted as a function of their location within the implant. "*In*" refers to sensors located within the implant; "*Edge*" refers to sensors located at the edge of the implant; "*Out*" refers to sensors located outside of the implant (in normal tissue)

26.3.2 Thermal Dosimetry

All 44 patients with extracranial tumors received at least one hyperthermia treatment. Eighteen received a second treatment at the completion of brachytherapy. Data were available for a total of 1471 sensors monitored in 55 heating sessions. The location with respect to the implant was known for 836 of 1471 sensors. The time-averaged mean temperature distribution for the 836 sensors with a known location is shown on Fig. 26.3; this figure shows that the percentage of sensors achieving a temperature exceeding 42°C was 33%, 17%, and 9%, for sensors located within the implant, at the edge, and outside of the implant (within normal tissue), respectively.

Among the 28 patients with high grade gliomas entered on the trial, 26 were able to complete their prescribed treatments. Two patients had partial treatment due to seizures during the hyperthermia treatment. Seventeen patients received a second treatment following removal of the radioactive sources. Eleven patients did not receive a second heat treatment, for the following reasons: seizures during the first treatment, development of edema, and patient anxiety. Thus, a total of 43 full hyperthermia treatments were given to 26 patients. Data were available for 39 heat sessions during which a total of 679 sensors were monitored. Because brain implants were performed stereotactically, accurate reconstruction of the position of each of the sensors with respect to the ferromagnetic seed implant was possible. In order to describe the adequacy of heating for this type of tumor, the sensors were classified according to their location: (a) within the core of the implant, i.e., more than 5 mm inside of the edge of the implant; (b) at the periphery of the implant, i.e., from the edge of the implant to 5 mm within the implant; or (c) outside of the implant, i.e., sensors located in the skull or intervening normal brain tissue. Using this classification, 127 of the 679 sensors were located within the core of the implant, 380 were in the periphery, i.e., in the outermost 5-mm shell of the implant volume, and 172 were located outside of the implant (in normal tissue). The time-averaged mean temperature distribution is plotted in Fig. 26.4. This figure shows that the proportion of sensors exceeding 42°C was 61% in the core of the implant, 35% in the periphery, and only 3.5% in normal tissue.

26.3.3 Clinical Response

Follow-up was available for all patients entered in the two protocols described. Three patients with extracranial tumors were not evaluable due to non-treatment-related death prior to evaluation.

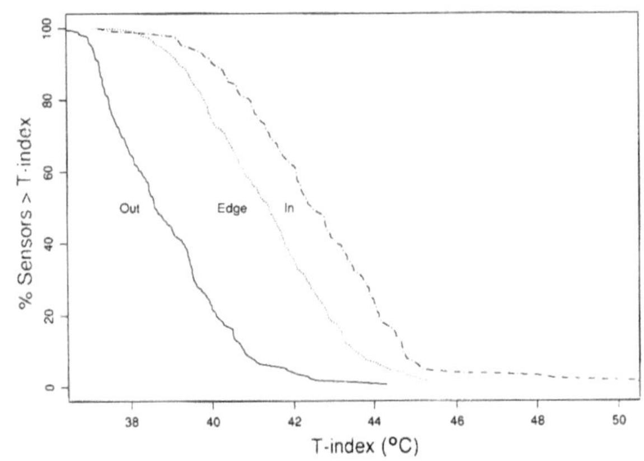

Fig. 26.4. Time-averaged mean temperature distribution for brain tumors plotted as a function of sensor location within the implant. "*In*" refers to sensors located in the core of the implant (i.e., > 5 mm from the edge of the implant); "*Edge*" refers to sensors located in the outer 5-mm shell of the implant; "*Out*" refers to sensors located outside of the implant, in normal tissues

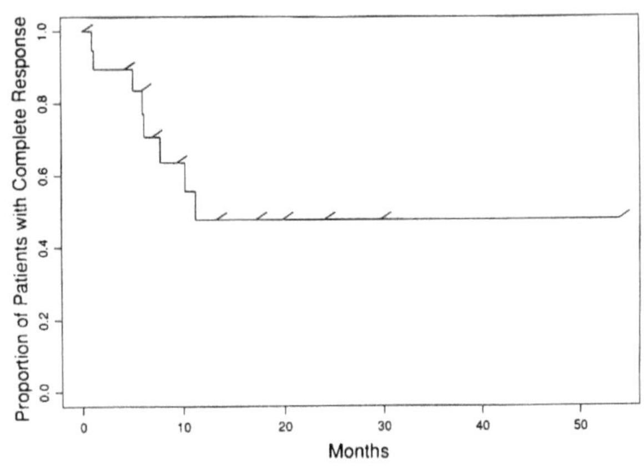

Fig. 26.5. Kaplan–Meier estimates of duration of complete responses ($n = 25$) for extracranial tumors. The *first tick mark* (from the left) represents six patient who had a complete response at their first follow-up; the *second tick mark* (from the left) indicates two patients censored at 4 months of observation

Among the 41 evaluable patients with extracranial tumors, there have been 25 complete responses (61%) and 18 partial responses (32%), for a total response rate of 93%. When analyzed by site, seven of the eight nongynecological pelvic/perineal tumors achieved a complete response, as did 12 of the 18 evaluable head and neck tumors and 7 of the 11 gynecological tumors. There was only one complete response among the four chest wall tumors. When analyzed as a function of tumor size, small tumors had a higher probability of achieving a complete response, with 16 of 20 tumors whose volumes were $\leq 22\ cm^3$ achieving a complete response, vs 8 of 19 tumors whose volumes were $> 22\ cm^3$ ($P = 0.02$). The Kaplan–Meier estimates of the duration of response in this patient population are shown in Fig. 26.5. Despite the advanced nature of the tumors treated in this phase I protocol, 13 patients remain alive between 3 and 53 months after treatment (11 are without evidence of disease and two are alive with disease).

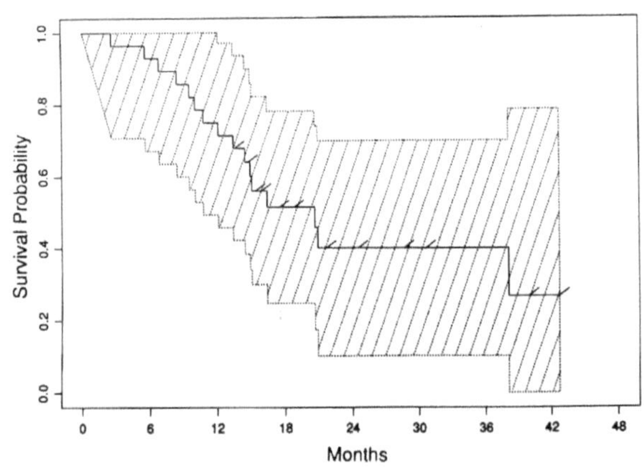

Fig. 26.6. Median survival 20.6 months from diagnosis. Kaplan–Meier estimates of survival from diagnosis for 28 patients with malignant gliomas treated with interstitial thermoradiotherapy. *Tick marks* represent censored patients; the *shaded area* represents the 95% confidence region

For patients with intracranial tumors, survival was used as the ultimate endpoint since CT and MRI cannot distinguish necrosis from recurrent tumor. Sixteen of the 28 patients entered in this protocol have died, with a median survival of 20.6 months from diagnosis (Fig. 26.6). One patient died from complications of treatment; one patient died from a presumed pulmonary embolism, and 14 patients from locally recurrent tumors. More specifically, 11 of the 22 patients treated at the time of their initial diagnosis and only one of the six patients treated at the time of recurrence remain alive. Furthermore, 14 patients underwent reoperation 3–52 weeks after the interstitial radiotherapy. Microscopic examination of the material removed at the time of reoperation revealed massive necrosis in seven of the 14 patients. However, in the remaining seven patients there was evidence of persistent or recurrent glioma within the target volume (six patients) or at the margins of the implant (one patient). Details of this study can be found elsewhere (Stea et al. 1992b).

26.3.4 Patient Tolerance and Toxicity

Among the extracranial tumors, tolerance to treatment was good to excellent. Occasionally a patient required intravenous analgesia with morphine sulfate during the course of hyperthermia. Only 3 of the 44 patients (7%) suffered a toxicity requiring hospitalization and/or surgical intervention. These toxicities consisted of persistent ulceration at known tumor sites, and all occurred in patients with a cumulative dose of radiation above 80 Gy. In one patient, surgical debridement of the ulcer revealed the presence of recurrent tumor. Therefore, it is unclear whether this ulceration resulted from the treatment or rather was associated with the recurrence.

Hyperthermia was generally well tolerated among the patients with brain tumors. In only two cases it was not possible to complete hyperthermia treatment owing to focal seizures. One patient refused a second hyperthermia treatment due to anxiety. Overall there have been 11 minor complications directly associated with hyperthermia. Six patients with a known history of seizure activity had focal seizures. In all cases the seizures lasted only 30–90 s and resolved with the intravenous administration of diazepam. Four patients experienced brain edema and transient worsening of neurological deficits, which responded to conservative medical management with steroids and mannitol. One patient developed a permanent arm weakness postoperatively. There have been three major complications attributable to the surgical implantation of catheters which resolved with appropriate medical or surgical intervention. There was one case of hydrocephalus secondary to edema. One case of pneumocephalus was attributable to failure to suture all the stab wounds on the scalp after removal of the catheters. One case of intracranial hemorrhage occurred at the time of implantation and necessitated surgical evacuation. Finally, one patient with a large tumor (119 cm^3) died 4 days postoperatively of complications from the whole treatment course (STEA et al. 1990).

26.4 Discussion

Although hyperthermia has been shown to increase the response rate over that seen with radiation alone, both in historical series (see OVERGAARD 1989 for review) and in controlled prospective clinical trials (ARCANGELI et al. 1987; VALDAGNI et al. 1988), our ability to control deep-seated tumors has been limited by the availability of equipment that allows heating of deep-seated structures (SHIMM et al. 1988a, b). Interstitial hyperthermia offers the advantage of direct power deposition within the tumor, thus sparing intervening normal tissues. This approach has the theoretical advantage of increasing the therapeutic gain. In this review we have shown that it is possible to heat both intracranial and extracranial tumors. Sixty-one percent of the sensors located in the core of implanted brain tumors achieved a temperature greater than 42°C. For extracranial sites the proportion of sensors in the tumor core achieving a temperature greater than 42°C was only 33.4%. Reasons for such a difference are not apparent. However, all brain tumors were implanted with a template (adhering to very strict geometrical guidelines) and the majority of these implants were done with an intercatheter spacing of 1.2 cm (STEA et al. 1990, 1992b). This resulted in a higher density implant than in extracranial sites, where the majority of the implants were done free-hand and the catheter spacing was quite variable within the implanted volume.

Despite the disappointing thermal parameters, interstitial thermoradiotherapy for extracranial sites has resulted in a high initial response (complete response + partial response = 93%), as well as in an excellent long-term local tumor control (Fig. 26.5). This high level of response has been achieved with a 7% rate of complications, all in patients with high cumulative doses of radiation. Our findings for extracranial sites are similar to those published by other centers using microwave (PUTHAWALA et al. 1985; EMAMI et al. 1987; PETROVICH et al. 1989; SEEGENSCHMIEDT et al. 1992) and/or radiofrequency heating (OLESON et al. 1984; GAUTHERIE 1989; VORA et al. 1989; SHIMM et al. 1990). For intracranial tumors we have used survival as the ultimate end-point of the study, and although this was a phase I study, the median survival for the entire group of 28 patients was 20.6 months from the time of diagnosis. This may not be significantly different from previously reported survival of 8–12 months for brain tumor patients, as shown by the 95% confidence interval in Fig. 26.6, but the trend is encouraging. Results from reoperation of brain tumors showed that approximately half of the operated specimens contained either persistent or recurrent tumor, indicating that either the heat dose or the radiation dose was insufficient to sterilize this type of tumor in 50% of the patients.

Nevertheless, these early results are encouraging, and warrant additional clinical work to establish the efficacy of interstitial hyperthermia both in brain tumors and in extracranial sites.

Acknowledgments. This work was supported by NCI Grants CA 29653 and CA 39468, Cancer Center Core Grant CA 23074, Hyperthermia Program Project Grant 17343, American Cancer Center Grant PDT-310, and Arizona Disease Control Research Commission Grant 8277-000000-1-0-YR-9301. Dr. Stea and Dr. Shimm are recipients of American Cancer Society Clinical Oncology Career Development Awards.

The authors would like to acknowledge the active participation of the following individuals from four institutions in the realization of this study: K. Luk, N. Vora, K.W. Chan, C.K. Chow, and S. Sapareto from City of Hope National Medical Center; T. Phillips, P. Sneed, P. Swift, and P. Stauffer from the University of California San Francisco; R. Steeves, B. Paliwal, and P. Harari from the University of Wisconsin; J.R. Cassady, C. Mack, H. Fosmire, A. Hamilton, J. Kittelson, J.S. Chen, A. Fletcher, B. Lulu, W. Lutz, Y. Contractor, and D. Buechler from the University of Arizona.

References

Arcangeli G, Benassi M, Cividalli A, Lovisolo G, Mauro F (1987) Radiotherapy and hyperthermia: analysis of clinical results and identification of prognostic variables. Cancer 60: 950–956

Aristizabal S, Oleson J (1984) Combined interstitial irradiation and localized current field hyperthermia: results and conclusions from clinical studies. Cancer Res 44: 4757–4760

Au K, Cetas T, Shimm D et al. (1989) Interstitial ferromagnetic hyperthermia and brachytherapy; preliminary results of phase I clinical trial. Endocurietherapy/Hyperthermia Oncol 5: 127–136

Chen J-S, Poirier DR, Damento MA, Demer LJ, Biancaniello F, Cetas TC (1988) Development of Ni-4 wt.% Si thermoseeds for hyperthermia cancer treatment. J Biomed Mater Res 22: 303–319

Emami B, Perez CA, Leybovich L, Straube W, von Gerichten D (1987) Interstitial thermoradiotherapy in treatment of malignant tumors. Int J Hyperthermia 3: 107–118

Gautherie M (1989) Interstitial hyperthermia: state of the art and prospects. In: Sugahara T, Saito M (eds) Hyperthermic oncology 1988, vol 2. Taylor & Francis, London, pp 63–68

Haider S, Cetas TC, Wait J, Chen J-S (1991) Power absorption in ferromagnetic implants from radio frequency magnetic fields and the problem of optimization. IEEE Trans Microwave Theory Tech 39: 1817–1827

Kobayashi T, Kida Y, Tanaka T, Hattori K, Matsui M, Amemiya Y (1991) Interstitial hyperthermia of malignant brain tumors by implant heating system: clinical experience. J Neuro-oncol 10: 153–163

Lulu B, Lutz W, Stea B, Cetas T (1990) Treatment planning of template guided stereotaxic brain implants. Int J Radiat Oncol Phys Biol 18: 951–955

Oleson JR, Manning MR, Sim DA et al. (1984) A review of the University of Arizona human clinical hyperthermia experience. Front Radiat Ther Oncol 18: 136–143

Overgaard J (1989) The current and potential role of hyperthermia in radiotherapy. Int J Radiat Oncol Biol Phys 16: 535–549

Petrovich Z, Langholz B, Lam K, Luxton G, Cohen D, Jepson J, Astrahan M (1989) Interstitial microwave hyperthermia combined with iridium-192 radiotherapy for recurrent tumours. Am J Clin Oncol 12: 264–268

Puthawala AA, Syed AMN, Khalid MA, Rafie S, McNamara CS (1985) Interstitial hyperthermia for recurrent malignancies. Endocurietherapy/Hyperthermia Oncol 1: 125–131

Seegenschmiedt MH, Sauer R, Brady L, Karlsson U (1992) Clinical practice of interstitial microwave hyperthermia combined with iridium-192 brachytherapy. In: Handl-Zeller L (ed) Interstitial hyperthermia. Springer, Wien New York, pp 135–154

Shimm D, Cetas T, Oleson J, Gross E, Buechler D, Fletcher A, Dean S (1988a) Regional hyperthermia for deep seated malignancies using the BSD annular array. Int J Hyperthermia 4: 159–170

Shimm D, Cetas T, Oleson J, Sim D (1988b) Clinical evaluation of hyperthermia equipment. The University of Arizona institutional report for the NCI Hyperthermia Equipment Evaluation Contract. Int J Hyperthermia 4: 39–51

Shimm D, Kittelson J, Oleson J, Aristizabal S, Barlow L, Cetas T (1990) Interstitial thermoradiotherapy: thermal dosimetry and clinical results. Int J Radiat Oncol Biol Phys 18 : 383–387

Shimm D, Kittelson J, Stea B (1991) Interstitial thermoradiotherapy, The University of Arizona experience. In: Urano M, Douple E (eds) Hyperthermia and oncology, vol 3. Zeist, VSP, Utrecht, The Netherlands, pp 181–198

Stea B, Cetas T, Cassady JR et al. (1990) Interstitial thermoradiotherapy of brain tumors: preliminary results of a phase I clinical trail. Int J Radiat Oncol Biol Phys 19: 1463–1471

Stea B, Shimm D, Kittelson J, Cetas T (1992a) Interstitial hyperthermia with ferromagnetic seed implants: preliminary results of a phase I clinical trial. In: Handl-Zeller L (ed) Interstitial hyperthermia. Springer, Wein New York, pp 183–191

Stea B, Kittelson J, Cassady JR et al. (1992b) Treatment of malignant gliomas with interstitial irradiation and hyperthermia. Int J Radiat Oncol Biol Phys 24: 657–668

Valdagni R, Amichetti M, Pani G (1988) Radical radiation alone versus radical radiation plus microwave hyperthermia for N_3 (TNM-UICC) neck nodes: a prospective randomized clinical trial. Int J Radiat Oncol Biol Phys 15 : 13–24

Vora NL, Forell B, Luk KH, Pezner RD, Desai KR, Lipsett JA, Wong JYA (1989) Interstitial thermoradiotherapy in recurrent and advanced malignant tumors: seven years' experience. In: Sugahara T, Saito M (eds) Hyperthermic oncology 1988, vol 1. Taylor & Francis, London, pp 588–590

Part IV
Special Clinical Applications

27 Interstitial Radiation and/or Interstitial Hyperthermia for Advanced and/or Recurrent Cancers in the Head and Neck: a Pilot Study

P.C. LEVENDAG, R.S.J.P. KAATEE, A.G. VISSER, I.K.K. KOLKMAN-DEURLOO, G.C. VAN RHOON, C.A. MEEUWIS, C.A.J.F. VAN GEEL, and C. VAN HOOYE

CONTENTS

27.1 Introduction

Tumors in the head and neck are treated in the majority of cases by surgery and/or radiation therapy (RT). If the primary cancer is irradiated, conceptually a high dose of RT is to be given, particularly if one is dealing with large T3 or T4 tumors. The RT can be given by external beam irradiation (ERT) or interstitial radiation therapy (IRT). In the Dr. Daniel den Hoed Cancer Center (DDHCC), patients with deep-seated advanced and/or recurrent tumors in the head and neck are in some instances treated by a combination of ERT and (subsequent) IRT (LEVENDAG et al. 1992). When using IRT, high tumoricidal doses of RT can be applied while attempting to compromise the surrounding normal tissues as little as possible. Unfortunately, when RT doses in the order of 70–80 Gy are applied, failures do occur even if the RT is tailored to the primary cancer to the greatest extent possible by means of interstitial techniques; moreover, the side-effects of such high doses of RT can be substantial.

With a view to increasing tumor cell kill and decreasing the incidence of side-effects, we embarked on a pilot study in which the IRT is combined with interstitial hyperthermia (IHT); by taking advantage of the additive and/or synergistic effects of hyperthermia, it is hoped that the therapeutic ratio will eventually be improved. The pilot study was initiated in 1988; the main aim of the study was to see whether hyperthermic temperatures (41°–43°C) could be safely achieved in deep-seated tumors when using the 27-MHz capacitive coupling interstitial hyperthermia system that was developed at the DDHCC (VISSER et al. 1989; DEURLOO et al. 1991).

27.2 Materials and Methods

27.2.1 Patient Selection

All newly admitted patients with tumors in the head and neck region are jointly seen by the members of the Rotterdam Head and Neck Cooperative Group once weekly. Patients with advanced and/or recurrent tumors not eligible for standard treatment can enroll in a number of experimental treatment protocols. For example, if brachytherapy is considered (technically) feasible for adequate coverage of the primary and/or regional tumor areas, then a combined modality treatment protocol as part of a nonrandomized pilot study using surgery, ERT and IRT + IHT is an option. This pilot study is now closed for entry, and the present report reviews the available data.

In 11 patients with very advanced and/or recurrent tumors the brachytherapy used for the primary cancer was combined with IHT (Figs. 27.1, 27.2). The total treatment scheme consisted of surgery of the neck ($n = 6$), ERT to the primary tumor and the neck ($n = 9$; 46–50 Gy), and a combination of IRT ($n = 11$; minimum tumor dose 20–66 Gy) plus IHT

P.C. LEVENDAG, M.D.; G.C. VAN RHOON, Ph.D.; C.A.J.F. VAN GEEL, B.Sc.; C. VAN HOOYE, B.Sc.; Department of Radiation Oncology; R.S.J.P. KAATTEE, Ph.D.; A.G. VISSER; I.K.K. KOLKMAN-DEURLOO, Ph.D.; Departments of Clinical Physics and Radiotherapy; C.A. MEEUWIS, Ph.D.; Department of ENT Surgery; Dr. Daniel den Hoed Cancer Center, Groene Hilledijk 301, P.O. Box 5201, NL-3008 AE Rotterdam, The Netherlands

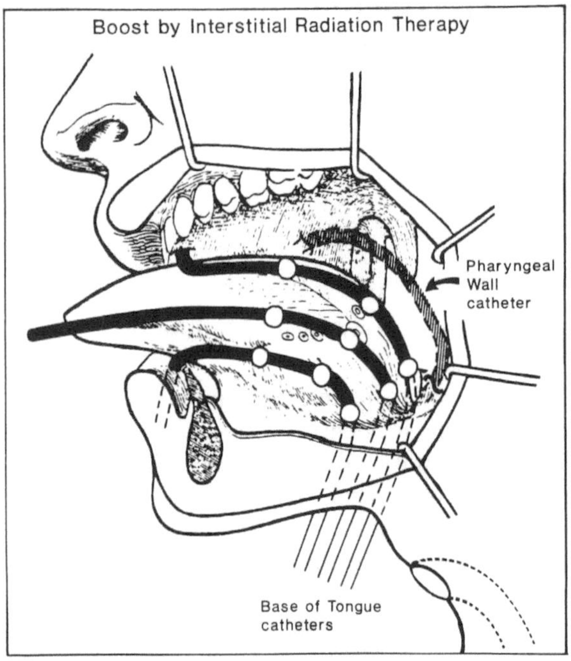

Fig. 27.1. Typical example of patient with base of tongue tumor implanted with standard afterloading catheters

to the primary tumor (Table 27.1). In all patients, the IHT preceded the actual loading of the afterloading catheters with iridium-192 wires (low dose rate irradiation; on average 50 cGy/h) by about 1–2 h. The aim of the feasibility study for IHT was to try to achieve a minimum temperature of 43°C in the tumor without causing any discomfort to the patient. It was specifically stated that the ERT and IRT doses should in no instance be altered, that is lowered, due to the IHT used.

27.2.2 The 27-MHz Capacitive Coupling IHT System

The 27-MHz capacitive coupling IHT system has been described in detail elsewhere (VISSER et al. 1989; DEURLOO et al. 1991). A schematic view of the interstitial hyperthermia system is shown in Fig. 27.3. In short: Each applicator is connected to its own generator (27.12 MHz, maximum output of 10 W, SSB Electronic, FRG) by a coaxial cable. A variable air coil is used for impedance matching. To minimize cross-talk between applicators, isolation transformers are included. The present system consists of 12 generators (Fig. 27.3).

A schematic representation of the applicator is depicted in Fig. 27.4. These applicators are constructed of thin flexible catheters (ID = 0.86 mm, OD = 1.27 mm) partly covered by a conducting paint (Acheson, type Electrodag 1415) (Fig. 27.4). When using this design, the applicators can be easily inserted in standard nylon brachytherapy catheters (ID = 1.5 mm, OD = 2.0 mm).

Due to the "high" frequency (27 MHz) there is an effective capacitive coupling, through the nylon implanted catheter, between the painted segment of the applicator and the surrounding tissue. Electric current can flow to an external groundplane, which is coupled to the tissue through a bag of saline. Through absorption of the electromagnetic energy the tissue is heated. The length and the position of the heated region can be freely chosen. Due to the high impedance associated with the capacitive coupling, the applicators can be seen as current sources (DEURLOO et al. 1991). The current along

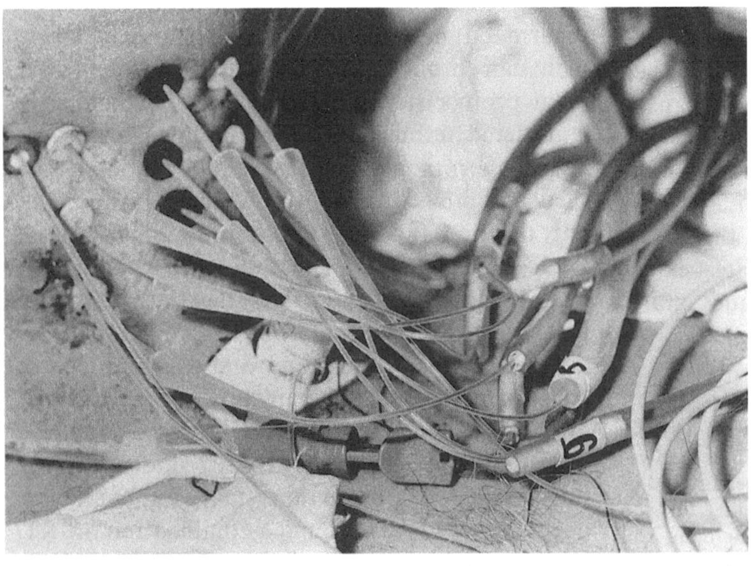

Fig. 27.2. Patient implanted for base of tongue tumor; applicators for interstitial hyperthermia are inserted in implanted afterloading catheters

Table 27.1. Treatment scheme, response, side-effects, and follow-up in the 11 patients with very advanced and/or recurrent tumors who were treated with RT plus IHT

Nr.	Radiation scheme (Gy)	ERT response	Response to total Tx	Side-effects	Last follow-up
1	ERT (50)+IRT (20)	Poor	Unsuccessful palliation	Ulcer/pain	DOD – 5 months
2	ERT (50)+IRT (20)	Good	Complete remission	No	NED – 36 months
3	ERT (50)+IRT (26)	Poor	Complete remission	No	DCU – 21 months
4	ERT (50)+IRT (26)	Good	Complete remission	No	NED – 25 months
5	ERT (50)+IRT (24)	Good	No response	Ulcer/pain	DOD – 19 months
6	ERT (50)+IRT (24)	Fair	No response	Ulcer/fistula/pain	DOD – 19 months
7	ERT (50)+IRT (24)	Good	Complete remission	No	NED – 18 months
8	ERT (46)+IRT (34)	Poor	Complete remission	Ulcer	NED – 20 months
9	IRT (66)		Complete remission	Ulcer pain	NED – 15 months
10	ERT (46)+IRT (28)	Poor	No response	Ulcer/pain	ED – 4 months
11	IRT (55)		Successful palliation	Ulcer	ED – 1 month

Nr., number arbitrarily assigned to patient; ERT, external beam radiation therapy; IRT, interstitial radiation therapy; DOD, dead of disease; NED, no evidence of disease; ED, evidence of disease; DCU, dead – cause unknown

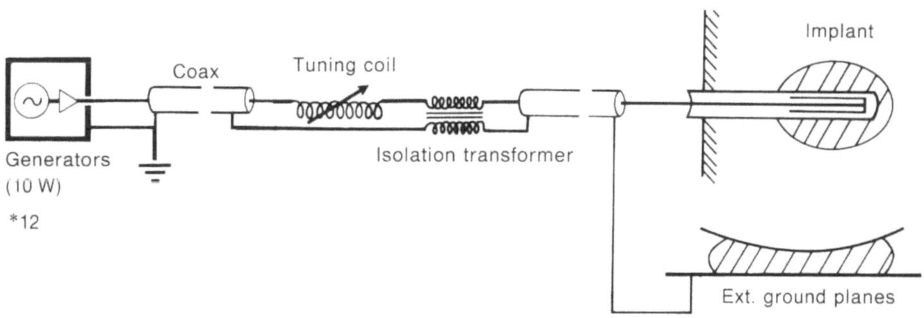

Fig. 27.3. Schematic view of the capacitive coupling IHT system

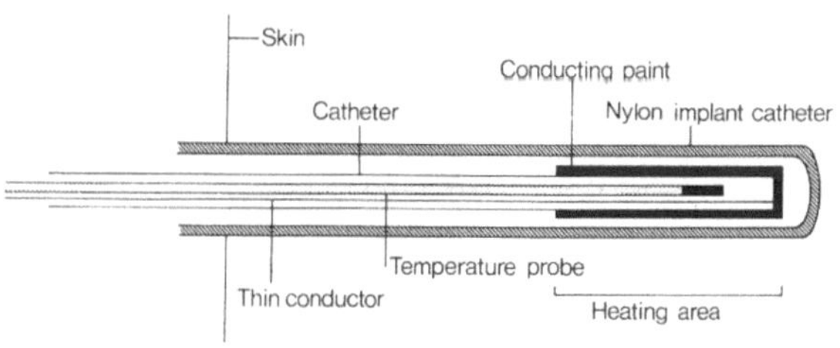

Fig. 27.4. Design of the capacitive coupling interstitial hyperthermia applicator, constructed from a catheter partly covered with a conducting paint. The paint is connected to a coaxial cable by a thin conductor. A thermometry probe can be inserted in the applicator for temperature monitoring

the heated area is less dependent on tissue impedance and thus on applicator configuration. This is in contrast to applicators which are in direct galvanic contact with the tissue. The homogeneous heating pattern along the flexible applicator together with the free choice of length and position of the heating region makes the 27-MHz system quite suitable for irregular implants in head and neck tumors.

27.2.3 Implant Geometry – Spacing

The afterloading catheters are implanted under general anesthesia according to (institutional) standardized treatment techniques used for brachytherapy. The number of applicators per patient in this particular study varied between 6 and 12. Figures 27.1 and 27.2 show a typical example of an implant of a base of tongue tumor. Three "looping" catheters run over the dorsum of the tongue, each with three closed-end catheters attached to it. Usually one extra catheter was implanted for thermometry purposes (three to ten measurement points in one thermometry catheter).

It was anticipated that spacing per se could be a critical parameter for ensuring adequate heating; moreover, large volume implants frequently have an irregular spacing distribution due to anatomical constraints. To arrive at some kind of objective measure to study the influence of spacing, the 'mean spacing" was determined. The mean spacing for this irregular type of implant is determined as follows. In a plane perpendicular to the main direction of the implant, the smallest area which contains all catheters is called S. We define the mean spacing (X) as the square root of S divided by the number of applicators (n). In this respect, not all catheters have equal weight. Each of the catheters is given a specific weight, depending on its position: All catheters whose intersections are lying within the boundary of S have weight 1, while catheters with intersections on the boundary have a lower weight, depending on the angle under which the neighboring intersections are viewed. An example is given in Fig. 27.5. For each patient, X was calculated for two or three planes and then averaged.

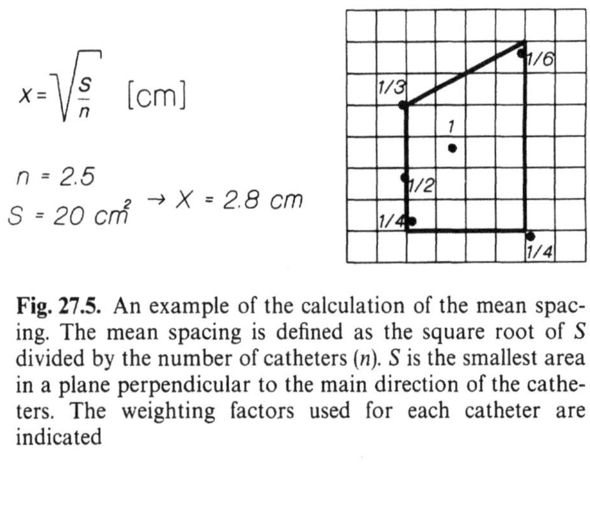

Fig. 27.5. An example of the calculation of the mean spacing. The mean spacing is defined as the square root of S divided by the number of catheters (n). S is the smallest area in a plane perpendicular to the main direction of the catheters. The weighting factors used for each catheter are indicated

27.2.4 Thermometry

During the treatment, at several positions inside the tumor the temperature was measured every 30 s by means of thermocouple probes (except in patients 1 and 2 in whom the temperature was measured every 60 s by means of fiberoptic probes).

Temperature monitoring was performed with a 40 channel data acquisition system (Helios I, Fluke Holland B.V.). Temperatures measured inside the tip of each applicator (applicator temperatures) and temperatures measured inside an (extra) "thermometry" catheter (thermometry temperatures) have been analyzed separately. This ensures that any self-heating artifact in the applicator temperatures will not have influenced the thermal parameters of the thermometry temperatures.

Due to the heating principle, the highest temperatures are found near the applicators. This, together with the fact that care was taken to implant the thermometry catheter in between the applicators, means that temperatures measured inside the applicators and inside the thermometry catheter can be seen as maximum and minimum tumor temperatures respectively. Besides the determination of tumor response and toxicity (Table 27.1), for each patient a number of thermal parameters were calculated. These data are shown in Table 27.2 for the temperatures measured inside the applicators and in Table 27.3 for the temperatures measured in the thermometry catheter. The (Tmean)mean is the average of the time-averaged temperatures measured with each thermocouple. Furthermore, the temperatures achieved in 10%, 50%, and 90% of the measurements (T_{10}, T_{50}, T_{90}) were determined (Tables 27.2, 27.3).

Table 27.2. Thermal parameters for the temperatures measured inside the applicators

Patient Nr.	Number of thermocouples	(Tmean)mean (°C)	SD(mean) (°C)	T_{90} (°C)	T_{50} (°C)	T_{10} (°C)
1	5 (old)	40.9	1.1	–	–	–
	3 (new)	47.3	2.7	–	–	–
2	6	45.6	0.6	43.8	45.6	47.4
3	8	44.1	3.8	37.2	44.2	51.2
4	6	42.3	1.5	39.1	42.3	45.5
5	9	43.3	2.4	40.1	43.3	46.5
6	7	45.7	0.6	43.1	45.7	48.3
7	8	44.8	0.1	44.1	44.8	45.5
8	11	43.5	0.6	41.9	43.5	45.2
9	9	45.2	0.4	43.9	45.2	46.4
10	11	44.7	0.8	41.6	44.7	47.8
11	12	45.0	1.0	42.3	45.0	47.7

(Tmean)mean: the average of the time-averaged temperatures measured within each thermocouple. T_{10}, T_{50}, T_{90}: the temperatures achieved in 10%, 50%, and 90%, respectively, of all measurements inside applicator. SD: standard deviation

Table 27.3. Thermal parameters for the temperatures measured inside the extra thermometry catheter

Patient Nr.	Number of thermocouples	(*T*mean)mean (°C)	SD(mean) (°C)	T_{90} (°C)	T_{50} (°C)	T_{10} (°C)
1	9	37.8	0.3	–	–	–
	9	37.8	0.3	–	–	–
2	4	38.9	2.6	35.9	38.9	41.8
3	5	37.6	1.3	36.0	37.6	39.2
4	6	37.4	0.3	36.7	37.4	38.1
5	0	–	–	–	–	–
6	5	37.1	0.4	36.6	37.1	37.6
7	3	39.5	1.4	37.9	39.5	41.1
8	5	39.6	0.9	38.3	39.6	40.6
9	10	37.3	0.4	36.6	37.3	37.9
10	6	37.7	0.2	37.4	37.7	38.0
11	6	38.3	0.4	37.7	38.3	38.8

(*T*mean)mean: the average of the time-averaged temperatures measured within each thermocouple. T_{10}, T_{50}, T_{90}: the temperatures achieved in 10%, 50%, and 90%, respectively, of all measurements inside thermometry catheters. SD: standard deviation

27.3 Results

27.3.1 Response and Toxicity

For two of the patients, treatment intention was palliation; in one of these two patients the treatment was considered to have been successful (tumor regression and pain reduction). Six of the other nine patients treated with a so-called curative intent showed a complete response (follow-up time: 4–36 months). Regarding side-effects, no complications were observed other than those seen in our clinic when treating patients with advanced cancers by ERT and/or IRT alone (Table 27.1).

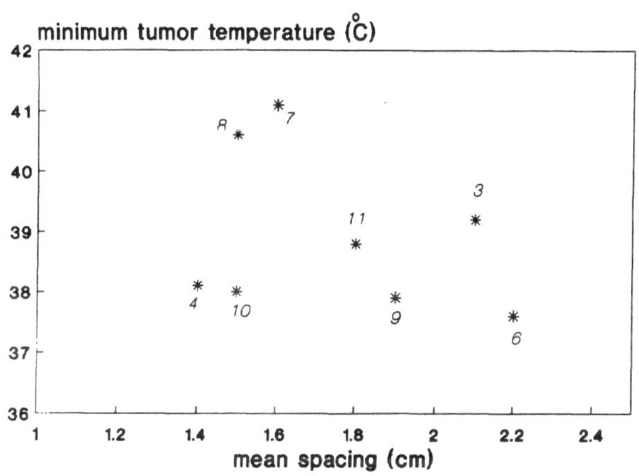

Fig. 27.6. Minimum tumor temperature (T_{10}, inside the extra thermometry catheter) as a function of the mean spacing. In general a smaller spacing gives rise to a higher minimum temperature

27.3.2 Temperature Distribution

(*T*mean)mean inside the applicators varied between 40.9°C and 45.7°C (Table 27.2). Inside the thermometry catheter (*T*mean)mean is considerably lower (37.1°–39.6°C) (Table 27.3). The mean spacings found in the patients were in the range 1.4–2.3 cm. Illustrative for the relation between the spacing and temperature variations inside the tumor are patients 6 and 8, who had a large (2.2 cm) and a small (1.5 cm) mean spacing, respectively. For patient 6 (*T*mean)mean inside the applicators was 45.7°C; inside the thermometry catheter, however, it was only 37.1°C. Patient 8 showed a more homogeneous temperature distribution, that is a (*T*mean)mean inside the applicator of 43.5°C while the (*T*mean)mean in the thermometry catheter was 39.6°C. Figure 27.6 demonstrates the finding that in general the temperature in between the applicators (thermometry temperature) increases with a decreasing spacing. Temperatures in the normal tissues could always be kept at normal (physiological) levels.

27.3.3 Response and Temperature

Although the number of patients is very small and both tumor and radiotherapy regimens varied, the relation between "tumor" temperatures and response to the total treatment was investigated. For complete responders, in general a combination of higher minimum tumor temperatures and

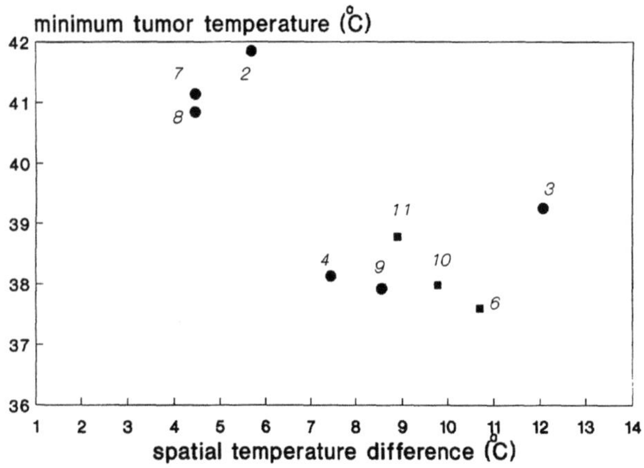

Fig. 27.7. Minimum tumor temperature (T_{10}, inside the extra thermometry catheter) as a function of the spatial temperature differences (T_{10} applicator − T_{10} thermometry) inside the tumor. A *closed circle* denotes a complete response

smaller spatial temperature variations within the tumor was found (Fig. 27.7).

27.4 Discussion

It has to be emphasized that a formal comparison of tumor response in (a) the 11 patients treated with a combination of IRT ± ERT and IHT and (b) patients treated by a conventional treatment regimen (i.e., ERT + IRT) was not the specific aim of this pilot study. However, it might be of relevance to briefly summarize the responses obtained, bearing in mind that the scoring of the (late) side-effects is only feasible with substantial tumor responses and/or follow-up. In 7 of the 11 patients (64%) a satisfactory response was obtained, which seems similar to the results obtained in this poor patient category without the use of IHT. No significant morbidity was observed.

The main goal was to see whether hyperthermic temperatures could be obtained using the 27-MHz IHT system without increasing the morbidity. Frequently we did not obtain adequate minimum temperatures in the tissues, that is thermometry catheters, in between the applicators; moreover, a fairly inhomogeneous temperature distribution was observed. One reason for this inhomogenous temperature distribution is naturally the principle of heating; that is, the power absorption decreases rapidly at greater distances from the applicators. By trying to keep the spacing between the afterloading catheters as small as possible, particularly if one anticipates using IHT during the implantation procedure, it should be possible to obtain a somewhat more homogeneous temperature distribution. In our view, the spacing between the applicators should not exceed 1.5 cm. A second important reason for the inhomogeneity of the temperature distribution has recently been demonstrated to be the high dielectric loss factor of nylon. Because of this dielectric loss, 20%–50% of the elecromagnetic energy is absorbed inside the standard commercially available afterloading catheters for brachytherapy purposes. Use of a catheter material with lower loss would lead to a more advantageous SAR distribution in tissue. Thirdly, there is an effective cooling through blood flow, and large blood vessels will cause cold spots in the tumor. Most of the patients considered had advanced cancers in the base of tongue; this organ (tongue) is particularly known for its high blood flow. High maximum temperatures together with the fact that the patients were not given any analgesic medication during the treatment limited the applicator power and thus the minimum tumor temperature.

The 27-MHz capacitive coupling IHT technique should in theory be suitable for safe and sufficient heating of head and neck tumors. However, unfortunately we were not able to obtain (homogeneous) hyperthermic temperatures in the 11 patients treated for advanced and/or recurrent tumors in the head and neck. By analyzing the data obtained in this small pilot study, we feel confident, however, that things might improve in the future. In collaboration with the Academic Hospital, Utrecht, and Nucletron Corporation, Veenendaal, a 64 channel computer-controlled 27-MHz IHT system has been developed. Furthermore the thermometry system has been improved. At the moment two prototypes are being built and will be available for clinical application in 1992. The improvements of the new system, the use of implantation techniques with smaller separations between the afterloading catheters (sources), and the use of another type of catheter material with a lower loss factor lead us to expect that a more homogeneous temperature distribution will be achievable in the future.

Acknowledgments. This study was supported by a grant from the Dutch Cancer Society (RRTI 91-13) and by gratefully acknowledged donations from the Nijbakker Morra Stichting, the Josephine Nefkens Stichting, and the Maurits and Anna de Kock Stichting.

Material support from Nucletron Corporation Veenendaal is also acknowledged. The excellence in patient care from the members of the Rotterdam Head and Neck Co-operative Group was also much appreciated.

References

Deurloo IKK, Visser AG, Morawski M, Geel CAJF, Levendag PC (1991) Application of a capacitive-coupling interstitial hyperthermia system at 27 MHz: study of different applicator configurations. Phys Med Biol 36: 119–132

Levendag PC, Meeuwis CA, Visser AG (1992) Reirradiation of recurrent head and neck cancers: external and/or interstitial radiation therapy. Radiother Oncol 23: 6–16

Visser AG, Deurloo IKK, Levendag PC, Ruifrok ACC, Cornet B, Rhoon GC (1989) An interstitial hyperthermia system at 27 MHz. Int J Hyperthermia 5: 265–276

28 Interstitial Thermoradiotherapy for Head and Neck Tumors: Results of a Cooperative Phase 1–2 Study

M.H. SEEGENSCHMIEDT, R. SAUER, R. FIETKAU, H. IRO, and L.W. BRADY

CONTENTS

28.1 Introduction

According to the American Cancer Society an estimated 30 500 new cases of and 8350 deaths from oral cancer (buccal cavity and pharynx) occurred in the United States in 1990. About 40% of annual deaths due to oral cancer result from local failure (RUBIN and CARTER 1976). With smoking and use of alcohol expanding worldwide, the incidence of head and neck tumors is still increasing. Standard therapy, including surgery, radiotherapy (RT), or chemotherapy (ChT) alone or in combination, still fails to sufficiently control local, regional, and systemic spread of this malignant disease.

After surgery alone the local relapse rate reaches 20% for T1 and 28% for T2-3 tumors; when no adjuvant therapy is applied, the relapse rate is even higher, reaching 15%–43% for T1-2N0 lesions (WHITEHURST and DROULIAS 1977; LEIPZIG et al. 1982; MARKS et al. 1983; GUERRY et al. 1986; O'BRIEN et al. 1986; NATHANSON et al. 1989). For external beam RT alone the results are unfavorable, with a local relapse rate of 24%–38% for T1, 46%–57% for T2, and about 70% for T3 tumors (FU et al. 1976; LEIPZIG et al. 1982). Interstitial RT (IRT) yields similar results to surgery alone, with local relapse rates of 3%–18% for T1 and 7%–36% for T2 tumors, when favorable patients are selected (FU et al. 1976; INOUE et al. 1978; DECROIX and GHOSSEIN 1981; HAIE et al. 1983; AYGUN et al. 1984; BENK et al. 1990; LEFEBVRE et al. 1990; MAZERON et al. 1990a, b; PERNOT et al. 1990; WENDT et al. 1990). The results achieved with combined IRT and external beam RT are also disappointing: local relapse of 23%–33% for T1, 20%–64% for T2, and 26%–66% for T3 tumors (INOUE et al. 1978; PUTHAWALA et al. 1981; MARKS et al. 1983; AYGUN et al. 1984; MENDENHALL et al. 1989; WANG 1989; BENK et al. 1990; WENDT et al. 1990; NOWAK et al. 1990).

Local and/or regional relapses impair the overall prognosis, although with IRT even local relapses can be salvaged in 59%–75%; long-term survival, however, is still low – only 36%–48% after 2 years and 14%–28% after 5 years (EMAMI and MARKS 1983; MAZERON et al. 1987a, b; PUTHAWALA et al. 1988; LANGLOIS et al. 1988). Therefore the effective control of primary advanced tumors with "high risk" for local or regional relapse (stage T2-3N1-3, grade G2-3, incomplete resection) and locally recurrent tumors (relapse after prior therapy) remains an even greater challenge. Thus the ideal management for primary/recurrent head and neck tumors, which controls primary tumor and lymphatic

M.H. SEEGENSCHMIEDT, M.D.; R. SAUER, M.D.; Professor; R. FIETKAU, M.D.; Strahlentherapeutische Klinik, Universität Erlangen-Nürnberg, Universitätsstraße 27, W-8520 Erlangen, Germany

H. IRO, M.D., Hals-Nasen-Ohren-Klinik der Universität Erlangen-Nürnberg, Waldstraße 1, W-8520 Erlangen, Germany

L.W. BRADY, M.D., Department of Radiation Oncology and Nuclear Medicine, Hahnemann University, Broad & Vine Streets, MS 200, Philadelphia, PA 19102-1198 USA drainage without severe complications, has not yet been found.

Since 1981 our approach for oral cancer has included organ preservation surgery to achieve clear tumor margins, modified neck dissection, and external beam RT with IRT "boost" to the primary tumor site. Whereas the initial results using iodine-125 were poor (THIEL et al. 1987), since 1986 the use of iridium-192 has considerably improved the results: complete response (CR) has been achieved in 60 of 62 primary tumors (96%), with 32 (52%) patients alive with no evidence of disease (NED) after a median follow-up of 27 months; but many complications (soft tissue and osteoradionecrosis) have been observed, and have been associated with IRT doses > 24 Gy (FIETKAU et al. 1991).

In contrast to completely resected lesions, primary or persistent tumors with gross macroscopic residual disease after surgery (tumor resection and/or lymph node dissection) and/or RT as well as locally metastatic or recurrent tumors were treated with RT and IRT in combination with interstitial hyperthermia (IHT) using 915 MHz microwaves. Our initial results have been encouraging (SEEGENSCHMIEDT et al. 1990, 1991). This report summarizes 5 years of clinical experience.

28.2 Material and Methods

28.2.1 Patients and Tumors

Between January 1986 and October 1991, 62 patients with tumors of the head and neck – 24 localized advanced primary (PRIM) and six persistent (PERS) lesions (PRIM/PERS = 30), 28 locally recurrent (REC) lesions and four metastatic (MET) lesions (REC/MET = 32) – were treated in a cooperative phase 1–2 study at the Department of Radiation Oncology of the University of Erlangen-Nürnberg, Germany (N1 = 49 patients) and the Department of Radiation Oncology and Nuclear Medicine, Hahnemann University, Philadelphia, USA (N2 = 13 patients). Eligibility criteria included a Karnofsky index > 70%, an estimated survival > 6 months, medical conditions allowing the use of general anesthesia, and signed informed consent. Potential candidates had localized and implantable macroscopic tumors; they were either ineligible for surgery to the primary tumor site or had macroscopic residual disease after incomplete excision or surgical dissection of cervical lymph nodes, leaving them with a "high risk" for local relapse. Patients with metastases were eligible only if they had symptoms (pain, ulceration, bleeding) but an otherwise good physical condition. All patient and tumor data are summarized in Table 28.1.

PRIM lesions had not received previous RT; PERS lesions still showed macroscopic tumor after completed therapy, whereas all REC/MET lesions were previously treated with different strategies including RT: 28 (45%) had received prior RT doses in the range of 25–75 Gy (mean: 59 Gy). Prior ChT was applied in 29 (47%) and prior surgery in 50 (81%) lesions. The distribution of specific tumor and treatment data for PRIM/PERS lesions versus REC/MET is illustrated in Table 28.2. Significant differences ($P < 0.05$) in favor of PRIM/PERS lesions occurred for volume, RT dose, and survival, whereas thermal parameters showed only a slight nonsignificant advantage for PRIM/PERS lesions.

The assessment of tumor size (with US, CT, or NMR imaging) and pathohistological confirmation preceded IRT and IHT. Tumor size was calculated in three ways:

1. The cuboid volume $V(C) = (a \times b \times c)$
2. The ellipsoidal volume $V(E) = 1/6\pi \times (a \times b \times c)$
3. The averaged tumor diameter $D = 1/3(a+b+c)$, proposed by EMAMI et al. (1987).

The lesions were grouped according to tumor size (Tables 28.1, 28.2). Most lesions were smaller than 80 cm^3 [$V(C)$] and/or 40 cm^3 [$V(E)$]; four lesions (6%) had extensive volumes of more than 150 cm^3 [$V(C)$], 80 cm^3 [$V(E)$], or 6.0 cm diameter respectively.

28.2.2 Interstitial Radiotherapy

Combined IHT-IRT was either delivered as the first treatment step followed by external beam RT after a break of 1–2 weeks or as the second step after completion of RT. Table 28.3 displays our typical treatment schedule. Details of our implantation technique have been reported elsewhere (FIETKAU et al. 1991; SEEGENSCHMIEDT et al. 1990, 1991): free-hand implants (one-end, through-and-through, and looping techniques) were applied encompassing the entire tumor volume with a sufficient safety margin of at least 1 cm; the plastic afterloading tubes were placed 1–1.5 cm apart from each other and in representative planes (HILARIS and HENSCHKE 1985; SEEGENSCHMIEDT et al. 1989).

Table 28.1. Summary of patient and head and neck tumor data

Patients:	Sex:	Males	51 (82%)
		Females	11 (18%)
	Age:	Mean	56.2/range: 6–81 years
		Median	58 years
	Karnofsky:	Mean	90%/range: 70%–100%
Lesions:	Type:	24 (39%)	Advanced primary (PRIM)
		6 (10%)	Primary persistent (PERS)
		28 (45%)	Local recurrent (REC)
		4 (6%)	Local metastatic (MET)
	Location:	26 (42%)	(Base of) Tongue
		17 (27%)	Floor of mouth
		7 (11%)	Oropharynx
		6 (10%)	Neck nodes
		3 (5%)	Larynx
		3 (5%)	Other sites
	Histology:	56 (90%)	Squamous cell carcinoma
		3 (10%)	Adenocarcinoma
		3 (10%)	Soft tissue sarcoma
	Grading:	3 (5%)	G1
		40 (65%)	G2
		19 (31%)	G3
	T stage:	17 (27%)	T2/rT2
		23 (37%)	T3/rT3
		18 (29%)	T4/rT4
		4 (7%)	Unknown T
	Macroscopic volume (*C*):	Mean	61.5 cm^3/range: 8.0–288.0 cm^3
	Macroscopic volume (*E*):	Mean	32.2 cm^3/range: 4.2–150.8 cm^3
	Macroscopic diameter (*D*):	Mean	3.8 cm/range: 2.0–6.7 cm
Pretreatment:		50 (81%)	Biopsy/incomplete resection and/or lymph node dissection
		28 (45%)	Adjuvant radiation therapy
	Prior RT dose :	Mean	59 Gy/range: 25–75 Gy
		29 (47%)	Adjuvant chemotherapy
FU at 12/91:		Mean	21/range: 4–58 months
		Median	18 months

PRIM/PERS lesions were scheduled to receive 70–80 Gy: 50 Gy with external beam RT (photons and/or electrons, conventional fractionation – daily 2 Gy single dose) to the tumor bed and the draining lymph nodes followed by 20–30 Gy local "boost" IRT (iridium-192 at 50 cGy/h). In contrast, previously irradiated REC/MET lesions received reduced or no external beam RT to avoid cumulative doses exceeding 110 Gy per site. When lesions were grouped according to the total (RT + IRT) dose, a significant difference was observed between PRIM/PERS and REC/MET lesions (Table 28.2).

28.2.3 Interstitial Hyperthermia

Details of our IHT technique, clinical practice, and quality assurance (QA) procedures have been reported elsewhere (Seegenschmiedt et al. 1989, 1990, 1991). 915-MHz microwave (MW) IHT was delivered by using miniature antennae and generators from two commercial MW-IHT systems (Clini-Therm Mark VI/XI, Clini-Therm Corporation, Dallas, TX, USA; Lund/Buchler Hyperthermia System 4010, Lund Science, Lund, Sweden). Both systems can simultaneously power up to 16 incoherently driven semiflexible coaxial dipole antennae, which provide a nearly ellipsoidal heating pattern with 6 cm longitudinal (3 cm per lobe) and 1.5 cm axial lengths when measured in the central planes of a static muscle equivalent phantom. Many physical conditions may alter the typical heating pattern, including the coherent/incoherent mode of antenna activation; constructive/destructive interference; antenna insertion depth, which influences the resonance status; antenna

Table 28.2. Distribution of specific tumor and treatment data and different lesion type

Parameter	Advanced primary/ primary persistent	Local recurrent/ local metastatic
Number of sites:	30 (49%)	32 (51%)
1. Tumor stage		
T2/(r) T2	8 (27%)	9 (28%)
T3/(r) T3	12 (40%)	11 (34%)
T4/(r) T4	10 (33%)	8 (25%)
Unknown stage	–	4 (13%)
2. Volume (*C*)		
< 20 cm³	6 (20%)	4 (13%)
20–<40 cm³	11 (37%)	7 (22%)
40–<80 cm³	11 (37%)	6 (19%)
≥80 cm³	2 (7%)	15 (47%)
Mean/range:	40.8/10–120	81.0/8–288
3. Volume (*E*)		
<20 cm³	16 (53%)	11 (34%)
20–<40 cm³	12 (40%)	6 (19%)
≥40 cm³	2 (7%)	18 (57%)
Mean/range:	21.3/5.2–62.8	42.2/4.2–150.8
4. Diameter (*D*)		
<40 mm	26 (87%)	15 (47%)
≥40 mm	4 (13%)	17 (53%)
Mean/range:	3.5/2.2–5.0	4.1/2.0–6.7
5. Total RT dose		
<30 Gy	–	5 (16%)
30–<50 Gy	–	13 (41%)
50–<70 Gy	6 (20%)	6 (19%)
≥70 Gy	24 (80%)	8 (25%)
Mean/range:	73.6/56.8–86	48.6/20.3–84.0
6. HT parameters		
a) $Tmax_{av}$ (°C):		
<42°C	2 (7%)	8 (25%)
42°C–< 43°C	8 (27%)	8 (25%)
43°C–< 44°C	8 (27%)	8 (25%)
≥44°C	8 (27%)	8 (25%)
Mean/range:	43.6/41.2–45.6	43.1/39.1–54.4
b) *T*mean (°C):		
<41°C	4 (13%)	11 (34%)
41°C–<42°C	13 (43%)	11 (34%)
42°C–<43°C	12 (27%)	6 (19%)
≥43°C	1 (3%)	4 (13%)
Mean/range:	41.7/39.8–43.2	41.3/38.7–44.0
c) $Tmin_{av}$ (°C):		
<40°C	5 (17%)	13 (41%)
40°C–<41°C	14 (47%)	12 (37%)
41°C–<42°C	10 (33%)	7 (12%)
≥42°C	1 (3%)	–
Mean/range:	40.6/38.9–42.3	40.0/38.4–41.6
d) Therm. qual. (TQ):		
TQ40°C 100%	23 (77%)	16 (50%)
Mean:	93.6%	75.3%
TQ41°C 100%	9 (30%)	2 (6%)
Mean:	74.9%	49.1%
TQ42°C 100%	1 (3%)	–
Mean:	42.4%	28.7%
TQ43°C 100%	–	–
Mean:	15.7%	13.7%

Table **28.2.** Contd.

Parameter	Advanced primary/ primary persistent	Local recurrent/ local metastatic
7. Survival at 11/91		
Mean	26 months	17 months
Range	4–58 months	4–45 months
Median	22 months	14 months
1-year survival	89%	70%
2-year survival	58%	20%

spacing and distribution; and specific anatomical conditions (e.g., muscle–bone interface) (STAUFFER et al. 1989; JAMES et al. 1989; CHAN et al. 1989; RYAN et al. 1990). The individual antenna distribution was mainly determined by IRT dosimetry guidelines and anatomical constraints.

Our treatment protocol included *two IHT sessions* at 41°–44°C for 45–60 min, one before IRT and one following the removal of the iridium-192 sources. Thirty-five (56%) lesions received IHT twice and 23 (37%) once. Four large lesions received more than two IHT sessions and treatment was continued with external beam RT alone. Ninety-seven IHT sessions were evaluated. Vital signs were monitored during each treatment, with all but one patient (a 6-year-old boy with a sarcoma of the cheek) being awake.

28.2.4 Invasive Thermometry

The integrated thermometric systems, i.e., the gallium–arsenide fiberoptic system (Clini-Therm Mark VI/IX) or the minimally perturbing thermistor system (Lund/Buchler System 4010), were used for invasive thermometry; 16 thermometric probes and 42 sensors are available with a 1-cm spacing between adjacent sensors in the linear array. Sensory arrays were placed near the center and periphery of the tumor, and if possible, in the center of each antenna subarray according to the RTOG quality assurance (QA) guidelines (DEWHIRST et al. 1990; EMAMI et al. 1991). During steady-state, thermal mapping (TM) was performed in at least two perpendicular axes of the target volume. In most of the IHT sessions, SAR (specific absorption rate) calculations at the beginning and thermal washout measurements during and after the completion of IHT were performed. The following thermal parameters were recorded during each IHT session:

1. The minimum mean and best 10-min tumor temperature ($Tmin_{av}$, $Tmin_{10}$).

Table 28.3. Treatment schedule and flow chart of procedures

Diagnostic staging	Tumor location, tumor volume, tumor type, histology, grading
Surgical procedure	Biopsy or incomplete surgery, implantation of afterloading probes
Treatment planning	IRT: orthogonal x-rays, CT scan, isodose distribution planning IHT: antennae and generator setup and specific thermometry sensor setup
Interstitial hyperthermia (IHT)	45–60 min at 41°–44 °C, 1 IHT before and 1 IHT after IRT
Interstitial radiotherapy (IRT)	Iridium-192, 20–30 Gy at 50 cGy/h, total irradiation time about 48–72 h
	Explantation of afterloading probes, 1–2 weeks' break before external beam RT
External beam radiotherapy (RT)	Depending upon prior applied RT dose: Up to 50 Gy photon/electron beam RT, 70–80 Gy total RT (IRT + RT) dose for primary advanced and persistent lesions Up to 110 Gy cumulative RT dose for pre-irradiated recurrent and metastatic lesions
Follow-up examination	Clinical evaluation: 6 and 12 weeks after completion of combined modality treatment Further FU at 6, 12, and every 6 months thereafter

2. The maximum mean and best 10-min tumor temperature ($T\text{max}_{av}$, $T\text{max}_{10}$).
3. The mean tumor temperatures (*T*mean).
4. The thermal equivalent minutes (TEM) according to the "thermal dose" formula (SAPARETO and DEWEY 1984).
5. The thermal quality (TQ), calculated as the ratio of tumor sensors above temperature *T*index to all tumor sensors (TQ40°C, TQ41°C, and TQ42°C).
6. A temperature-time matrix of all tumor sensors with assessment of T_{90}, T_{50}, and T_{20} values (i.e., 90%, 50%, and 20% values of all tumor sensor measurements).

28.2.5 Tumor Response and Statistical Analysis

The evaluation was performed in December 1991, with a median follow-up (FU) of 18 months (mean: 21 months, range 4–58 months). The WHO criteria were applied to define the *local* tumor response: complete remission (CR = total disappearance of tumor), partial remission (PR = more than 50% reduction), no change (NC = 50% or less reduction and 25% or less increase), and progressive disease (PD = more than 25% increase). *Initial response* was analyzed for all 62 lesions at 3 months' FU, whereas *long-term response* was assessed for 50 (81%) lesions at 12 months' FU or longer. Tumor control in long-term analysis was defined as a "sustained complete response" until last FU or the patient's death (EMAMI et al. 1987). Seven patients (11%) have not reached 12 months' FU. Relapse were recorded as occurring within (local) or outside (regional) the treated volume. Acute and long-term complications were graded as "1" for minor complications (superficial blisters, mucositis, erythema) not requiring special care; "2" for those (deep burn, ulceration) requiring long-term medical care, antibiotics, and special dressing; "3" for major complications (tissue breakdown, fistulas) requiring surgical intervention; "4" for fatal complications. The Student *t* and Fisher exact tests (FISHER and YATES 1963) were used as statistical tools. Survival data were assessed with the actuarial method (KAPLAN and MEIER 1958).

28.3 Results

28.3.1 Tumor Response

At 3 months' FU, CR was achieved in 39 (63%), PR in 18 (29%), and NC/PD in 5 (8%) lesions. PRIM/PERS lesions yielded a significantly higher CR, 25/30 (83%), compared to REC/MET lesions, 14/32 (44%) ($P < 0.05$). Fifty of 62 (81%) lesions, including 32/39 (82%) with CR, 15/18 (83%) with PR, and 3/5 (60%) with NC, were available for analysis at 12 months' FU. Twelve (19%) patients have not reached this FU, including five (8%) who are deceased with locally controlled tumor (LC) after initial CR. At 12 months' FU the results are as follows:

1. Of 32 patients with CR, 29 (91%) have achieved local control and are alive; two (6%) patients are alive with local recurrence, and one (3%) is deceased with locoregional relapse. The total local control rate after CR at 12 months' FU is 29/37 (78%), with two lesions being censored

(FU < 12 months). The 2-year survival in this group of patients is 52%.

2. Of 15 patients with PR, ten (67%) are alive at 12 months' FU, including seven (47%) patients with tumors which have very slowly regressed with an unclear residual mass on CT or NMR imaging. Needle biopsies have not revealed viable malignant cells; however, the regressed but residual masses allow no clear distinction between tumor or scarring tissues and these lesions have therefore not been regarded as "local control." The other three (20%) alive patients have developed locoregional progression. Five (33%) patients are deceased, two (13%) from systemic and local disease and three (20%) from intercurrent disease with local control. Three lesions have not yet reached 12 months' FU.

3. Of five lesions with initial NC, two have not reached 12 months' FU and two have progressed rapidly with death at 4 and 6 months. Three patients experienced considerable relief of symptoms (pain); an 81-year-old female died due to intercurrent disease after 16 months' FU with stable tumor locally and considerable symptomatic relief. The 2-year survival for the group of nonresponders (non-CR) is only 10%.

4. The total rate of local control at 12 months' FU is 29/50 (58%) or 36/50 (72%) when including those cases with ongoing tumor regression. PRIM/PERS lesions are significantly better controlled, 20/26 (77%), compared to REC/MET lesions, 9/24 (38%) ($P < 0.05$). We have already pointed out the importance of long-term follow-up to sufficiently analyze local tumor control (SEEGENSCHMIEDT et al. 1990).

The median survival in December 1991 was 18 and the mean survival 21 months (range: 4–58 months) with a significant difference ($P < 0.05$) between PRIM/PERS (median: 22, mean: 26 months, SD ± 15) and REC/MET lesions (median: 14, mean: 17 months, SD ± 11). Although the 1-year survival was not too different (89% for PRIM/PERS versus 70% for REC/MET lesions), at 2 years the survival rate was significantly better for PRIM/PERS lesions (58%) compared to REC/MET lesions (20%) ($P < 0.05$). Kaplan–Meier survival plots are shown for CR versus non-CR patients (Fig. 28.1) and PRIM/PERS lesions versus REC/MET lesions (Fig. 28.2).

28.3.2 Treatment Toxicity

Twelve patients (19%) experienced acute side-effects: grade 1 (mucositis, blister) in seven (11%) and grade 2 (ulceration, fistula, deep burn) in five patients (8%). No grade 3 or 4 toxicities occurred. Pain limited power deposition in 14/62 (23%) patients; this was associated with antennae located too close to bony structures or movement of antennae during the IHT session. Most acute side-effects subsided within 4–6 weeks after completion of therapy and usually required rinsing of the oral cavity with antiseptic fluids or antiseptic dressing of cutaneous defects.

Seven (11%) patients developed long-term side-effects – slowly healing ulcers, fistulas, soft tissue necrosis, and/or osteoradionecrosis – which were handled with systemic or local antibiotics and antiseptic fluids: resolution occurred in a mean period of 6 months (range 4–12 months). Lesions in anatomical regions with compromised blood flow (scar tissue) and lesions biopsied too shortly after completion of IRT-IHT were prone to develop long-term ulcerations and fistulas. Two lesions required

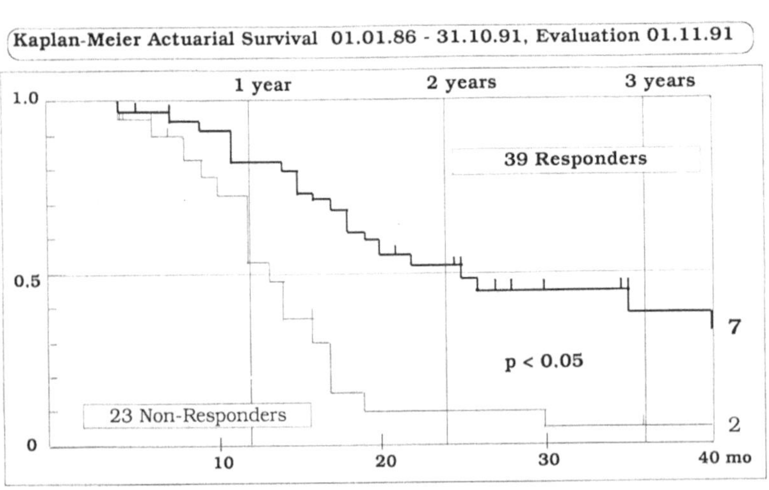

Fig. 28.1. Kaplan–Meier actuarial survival of patients with head and neck tumors treated with interstitial thermal radiation therapy: comparison of survival for 39 complete responders ("*responders*") and 23 partial responders or nonresponders ("*nonresponders*"); *ticks* indicate censored lesions with patients being alive

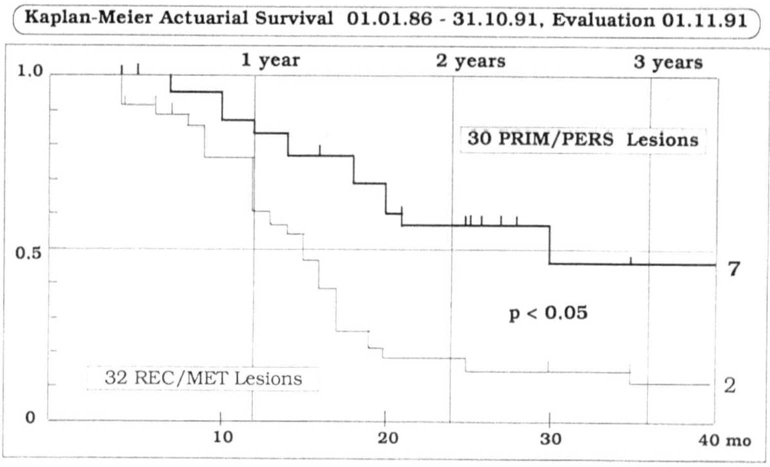

Fig. 28.2. Kaplan–Meier actuarial survival of patients with head and neck tumors treated with interstitial thermal radiation therapy: comparison of survival for 30 advanced primary and persistent lesions (*PRIM/PERS*) and 32 locally recurrent and metastatic lesions (*REC/MET*); *ticks* indicate censored lesions with patients being alive

surgical intervention. One patient with a large N3 metastasis who achieved CR subsequently suffered from a rupture of the carotid artery after 9 months; also three lesions with locally recurring or progressing tumors suffered from repeated arterial bleeds. In this study neither tumor (volume, type of lesion) nor treatment parameters (radiation dose, thermal characteristics) have revealed any prognostic significance for thermal damage.

28.3.3 Local Recurrences

Of the 39 patients with CR at 3 months, three (8%) experienced relapses within the treated volume at 4–10 months; six (15%) had a regional relapse outside the treated volume at 8 14 and 47 months in one instance. The rate of locoregional relapse after CR was 23% (nine patients), with most relapses occurring outside the treated volume and within 12 months' FU. Of the 18 patients with PR at 3 months, five (28%) had renewed local tumor progression. Difference in the relapse rate between PRIM/PERS lesions (two local, one regional) and REC/MET lesions (one local, five regional) were not significant. Patients experiencing local relapse or progression after combined IRT-IHT *usually* had poor tumor and treatment factors. This may explain the early local failure in the treated area (see Table 28.6).

28.3.4 Prognostic Treatment Factors

Tumor factors without prognostic impact were age, sex, tumor location, histology, stage, and tumor grade. Treatment factors lacking prognostic value were dose and duration of IRT, number of IHT sessions, sequence of IHT/IRT/RT, and TEM thermal parameters. In contrast, the following factors had a significant impact on treatment outcome: lesion type, tumor volume, total radiation dose, and thermal parameters including minimum and mean tumor temperatures and thermal quality (TQ) of heating. Except for total radiation dose, these parameters correlated both with the initial tumor response at 3 months *and* the long-term local control at 12 months (Table 28.4).

28.4 Discussion

Clinical implementation of HT as an effective radiosensitizing agent is based on a sound biological (Ben-Hur et al. 1974; Miller et al. 1978; Jones et al. 1989) and physiological rationale (Song 1984; Reinhold and Endrich 1986) and recent improvements of heat delivery and invasive thermometry technology (Cetas 1985); studies in vitro (Overgaard 1981), in vivo (Dewhirst et al. 1984), and in human tumors (Oleson et al. 1988; Overgaard 1989) have revealed an improved tumor control with combined RT-HT. IHT techniques can surpass external HT methods in several respects: (a) application of a higher tumor dose to a confined treatment volume, (b) better sparing of critical surrounding normal tissues, (c) effective heating of accessible deep-seated tumors, (d) extensive temperature data sampling, and (e) better power steering and individual treatment control (Seegenschmiedt et al. 1991; Cosset 1990).

As applied in our treatment concept for unfavorable lesions in the head and neck, IHT-IRT has been shown to be an effective and safe treatment.

Table 28.4. Summary of prognostic tumor and treatment factors

Parameter	Initial response (3 mo) ($n=62$)			Long-term response (12 mo) ($n=50$)		
	CR ($n=39$)	Non-CR ($n=23$)	*P* value	LC ($n=29$)	Non-LC ($n=21$)	*P* value
Lesion type						
PRIM/PERS	25 (83%)	5 (17%)	<0.005	20 (77%)	6 (23%)	< 0.025
REC/MET	14 (44%)	18 (56%)		9 (38%)	15 (62%)	
Volume (*C*)						
<80 cm^3	35 (78%)	10 (22%)	<0.001	27 (75%)	9 (25%)	<0.001
≥ 80 cm^3	4 (24%)	13 (76%)		2 (14%)	12 (86%)	
Volume (*E*)						
<40 cm^3	35 (78%)	10 (22%)	<0.001	27 (75%)	9 (25%)	<0.001
≥ 40 cm^3	4 (24%)	13 (76%)		2 (14%)	12 (86%)	
Total RT Dose						
<50 Gy	7 (42%)	11 (58%)	<0.05	5 (38%)	8 (62%)	<0.20 (NS)
≥50 Gy	32 (73%)	12 (27%)		24 (65%)	13 (35%)	
<70 Gy	14 (47%)	16 (53%)	<0.025	9 (41%)	13 (59%)	<0.06 (NS)
≥70 Gy	25 (78%)	7 (22%)		20 (71%)	8 (29%)	
HT Parameters						
$T\text{min}_{av} < 41°C$	21 (53%)	19 (47%)	<0.05	17 (47%)	19 (53%)	<0.05
≥41°C	18 (82%)	4 (18%)		12 (86%)	2 (14%)	
*T*mean <42°C	22 (52%)	20 (48%)	<0.05	17 (46%)	20 (54%)	<0.01
≥42°C	17 (85%)	3 (15%)		12 (92%)	1 (8%)	
TQ41°C <75%	15 (44%)	19 (56%)	<0.0025	11 (39%)	17 (61%)	<0.01
≥75%	24 (86%)	4 (14%)		18 (82%)	4 (18%)	

Our results are consistent with other published data regardless of the technique employed, including microwave (Emami et al. 1987; Bicher et al. 1985; Puthawala et al. 1985; Tupchong et al. 1988; Rafla et al. 1989; Aoyagi et al. 1989; Inoue et al. 1989; Petrovich et al. 1989; Coughlin et al. 1991), radiofrequency (Emami et al. 1987; Oleson et al. 1984; Cosset et al. 1985; Linares et al. 1986; Gautherie et al. 1989; Yabumoto et al. 1989; Vora et al. 1989; Levendag et al. 1992), ferromagnetic seed (Au et al. 1989; Shimm et al. 1989), hot water perfusion (Handl-Zeller et al. 1987, 1989), and other undefined IHT techniques (Schreiber et al. 1990). Table 28.5 summarizes currently available data on nearly 700 lesions. When reviewing these studies the following preliminary conclusions can be drawn:

1. Nearly 300 head and neck lesions (about 40%) have been treated.
2. Head and neck lesions have been preferentially treated with microwave techniques, whereas radiofrequency techniques have been more often applied for pelvic and other sites.
3. The cumulative CR rate was 56% (range 10%–74%), and the cumulative total response rate 84% (range 60%–100%).
4. The cumulative toxicity was 20%–25% (range 10%–50%).
5. The most frequently used IHT techniques, MW-IHT and RF-IHT, yield comparable results; other IHT techniques require longer follow-up periods for evaluation.
6. The follow-up periods are extremely variable and range between 1 and 74 months.
7. Besides objective response criteria, many trials report subjective palliation including prevention of bleeding, pain relief, and preservation of normal organ functions.

Despite the impressive number of institutions and patients already involved in the clinical research into IHT-IRT, many reported data are compromised in their scientific value for several reasons:

1. Low number of patients.
2. Lack of detailed reporting on treatment performance characteristics (radiation therapy and thermal performance parameters).

Table 28.5. Results of interstitial thermo-radiotherapy for head and neck tumors

Reference, year	Technique	Lesions H&N/all	Clinical response CR	PR	NC	Toxicity (%)	Follow-up (months)
Oleson et al.1984	RF 0.5 MHz	9/52	20 (38%)	22 (42%)	10 (19%)	21%	3–18
Bicher et al. 1985	MW 915 MHz	1/8	4 (50%)	2 (25%)	2 (25%)	13%	NA
Puthawala et al. 1985	MW 915 MHz	20/43	32 (74%)	11 (26%)	–	21%	>12
Cosset et al. 1985	RF 0.5 MHz	8/29	19 (66%)	4 (14%)	–	25%	>2
Linares et al. 1986	RF 0.5 MHz	0/10	3 (30%)	7 (70%)	–	40%	NA
Emami et al. 1987[a]	RF 0.5 MHz	29/9	5 (56%)	3 (33%)	1 (11%)	25%	6–48
Emami et al. 1987[a]	MW 915 MHz	39	21 (54%)	9 (23%)	5 (13%)	25%	6–48
Handl-Zeller et al. 1987	HW PERF	14/23	4 (17%)	17 (74%)	2 (9%)	9%	1–11
Tupchong et al. 1988	MW 915 MHz	14/14	9 (64%)	2 (14%)	3 (22%)	NA	NA
Rafla et al. 1989	MW 915 MHz	15/35	19 (54%)	13 (37%)	3 (9%)	29%	NA
Gautherie et al. 1989	RF 0.5 MHz	35/96	62 (65%)	15 (16%)	18 (19%)	26%	>2
Yabumoto et al. 1989	RF 8 MHz	5/14	8 (57%)	3 (21%)	3 (21%)	29%	1–49
Vora et al. 1989	RF 0.5 MHz	9/78	43 (55%)	15 (19%)	20 (26%)	17%	6–74
Au et al. 1989	FMS 90 kHz	3/4	2 (50%)	1 (25%)	1 (25%)	50%	1–7
Aoyagi et al. 1989	MW 915 MHz	6/10	2 (20%)	4 (40%)	4 (40%)	20%	NA
Inoue et al. 1989	MW 915 MHz	8/10	1 (10%)	7 (70%)	1 (10%)	10%	1–6
Petrovich et al. 1989	MW 915 MHz	23/44	28 (64%)	15 (34%)	1 (2%)	20%	3–36
Schreiber et al. 1990	MW 915 MHz	11/40	21 (52%)	18 (45%)	1 (3%)	15%	1–30
Coughlin et al. 1991	MW 915 MHz	9/35	23 (66%)	4 (11%)	8 (23%)	NA	1–62
Levendag et al. 1991	RF 27 MHz	11/11	6 (55%)	1 (9%)	4 (36%)	NA	NA
Current study 1991	MW 915 MHz	62/86	54 (63%)	23 (27%)	9 (10%)	21%	4–58
Total experience 1991	Various	292/699 (42%)	386 (55%)	196 (28%)	96 (14%)	20%–25%	1–74

CR, complete response; PR, partial response; NC, no change of disease; NA, data not available; RF, radiofrequency HT; MW, microwave HT; FMS, ferromagnetic seed HT; HW PERF, hot water perfusion HT; a = same study

3. Insufficient analysis of tumor and treatment parameters.
4. Lack of long-term follow-up and reporting of long-term results.
5. In the case of older series, less developed invasive thermometry and IHT technique.

Thus, presently only a few recent series with larger numbers of patients provide information relevant for careful interpretation of our own and general results. Several prognostic parameters correlating with initial and long-term tumor control have been identified in our series; these factors are summarized in Table 28.4.

28.4.1 Impact of Radiation Dose

A dose–response relationship revealing improved tumor response with increasing total RT dose has been reported in other studies (PETROVICH et al. 1989; OLESON et al. 1984; COSSET et al. 1985). In our trial the significantly lower total RT dose for REC/MET lesions (mean 48.6 Gy/range 20.3–84.0 Gy) due to prior RT, compared to PRIM/PERS lesions (mean 73.6 Gy/range 56.8–86.0 Gy), could explain the different response pattern between lesion types. Similiar observations were made in two other trials (EMAMI et al. 1987; PUTHAWALA et al. 1985). In contrast, RT dose was the only parameter which did not have prognostic value for long-term local control at 12 months' FU; at 12 months' FU, lesions receiving RT doses ≥ 50 Gy or ≥ 70 Gy were better controlled (65%/71%) than lesions treated with lower RT doses (38%/41%), but this difference is not statistically significant ($P > 0.05$). The actuarial survival at 2 years suggests a trend, with an 18% survival for the low dose RT group compared to 52% for the high dose RT group but this depends also on lesion type.

28.4.2 Impact of Tumor Volume

Tumor volume has been identified as an important prognostic factor (SEEGENSCHMIEDT et al. 1990; EMAMI et al. 1987; PUTHAWALA et al. 1985; DEWHIRST and SIM 1986). We found both the cuboid $V(C)$ and the ellipsoidal volume $V(E)$ to be useful measures for tumor volume assessment and prognostic evaluation. Tumor volume had a significant impact on initial response and long-term tumor control, with smaller tumors doing better than larger tumors (Table 28.4). Surprisingly, the algorithm to calculate the mean tumor diameter D did not prove to be useful; we observed only a somewhat small range of tumor diameters (2.0–6.7 cm) without a clear breakpoint, which is in contrast to the results of another report (EMAMI et al. 1987). Obviously, insufficient tumor size estimation may result in tumor miss, insufficient implantation, and less favorable power deposition. It is important to realize, that the possible risk zone may be as large as 3 cm from the edge of primary advanced and locally recurrent head and neck tumors (DAVIDSON et al. 1984). Thus implantation quality can influence both the IRT dose distribution and the quality of heating throughout the target volume. A crude estimation of the quality of the implant can be made by calculating the ratio of tumor volume and number of activated heating probes (SEEGENSCHMIEDT et al. 1990); whereas for IRT all implanted probes are used for radiotherapy except for "differential unloading," for microwave IHT techniques several probes may not be available, when they are used for invasive thermometry or are inappropriate due to their short implantation length (< 3 cm) or their proximity to critical structures, e.g., the mandible bone.

For our 915-MHz MW antenna design a breakpoint between 5 and 10 cm^3 per antenna was found, which seems reasonable assuming an effective heating volume (50% iso-SAR) of about 5 cm^3 per antenna for an implantation depth of 5–7 cm (SEEGENSCHMIEDT et al. 1990; STAUFFER et al. 1989; JAMES et al. 1989; CHAN et al. 1989; RYAN et al. 1990). Although we were unable to overcome anatomical constraints, we have applied bolus techniques (absorbing 0.9% saline soaked gauzes or muscle equivalent material) underneath the chin or at other locations to avoid limitations due to short implantation length. Other IHT techniques have been developed which are less sensitive to short or unequal implantation length, like the 27-MHz capacitive RF technique (VISSER et al. 1989). So far other groups have not sufficiently reported on implantation data to support these findings; appropriate QA for IHT, including sufficient tumor coverage, has been recognized as a mandatory requirement (SEEGENSCHMIEDT et al. 1989; DEWHIRST et al. 1990; EMAMI et al. 1991).

28.4.3 Impact of Thermal Parameters

The thermal performance of IHT is of critical importance. Several parameters have been identified to correlate with tumor response in animal and clinical studies (EMAMI et al. 1987; DEWHIRST et al. 1984; COSSET et al. 1985; PUTHAWALA et al. 1985; COUGHLIN et al. 1991; OLESON et al. 1984; DEWHIRST and SIM 1986). In the analysis of OLESON et al., for 161 patients treated with combined RT-HT (including 52 lesions treated with IHT-IRT) the minimum average tumor temperature *T*min(mean) was the single most important factor in predicting tumor response. DEWHIRST and SIM observed that the rate of complete responders was doubled for lesions with a "thermal dose" of *T*min Eq 43°C 1–5 (calculated according to the thermal dose formula) (SAPARETO and DEWEY 1984), whereas lesions with *T*min Eq 43°C < 1 achieved results equal to the RT alone control group. The extrapolation of this "thermal dose" translates into an average minimum temperature of 41.3°C.

Our findings on the thermal quality of HT are supported by other investigators (EMAMI et al. 1987; DEWHIRST et al. 1984; COUGHLIN et al. 1991; OLESON et al. 1984; COSSET et al. 1985; GAUTHERIE et al. 1989). EMAMI et al. found no CR in lesions with *T*min ≤ 42°C compared with a 70% rate of CR for lesions treated with *T*min > 42°C. However, their report lacks further thermometry specifications such as the number of invasive thermometric probes or sensors employed. PAULSEN et al. (1984) have proposed a hyperthermia equipment performance (HEP) rating based on the percentage of tumor area exceeding an index temperature of 43 °C. Excellent and good scores are given if the therapeutic region of 43 °C reaches 75%–100% of all measurements.

The currently used invasive thermometry techniques are still inappropriate for exactly locating and monitoring the whole tumor volume; therefore the number and location of thermometric sensors and the spatial and temporal resolution of thermal mapping can greatly influence the thermal data analysis. CORRY et al. (1988) have pointed out that with the implementation of more thermometric sensors per implant volume, the probability of recording lower tumor temperatures increases significantly. In our study as many tumor sensors as possible (mean: 8, range 4–17) were applied, and *all* tumor sensors were included for the "thermal quality" analysis. Although our findings have revealed lower tumor minimum temperatures than have been reported by others, they suggest that $T\text{min}_{av}$, *T*mean, and TQ41°C ≥ 75% values correlate with both initial response and long-term control. The reasons for our lower temperatures are twofold: (a) invasive thermometry was strictly performed interstitially, i.e., outside the heating sources at locations most likely to record the lowest temperatures within the target volume; (b) multiple tumor sensors were more likely to record lower minimum temperatures. In contrast, most RF techniques are controlled by temperatures measured inside the heat sources, missing a potential minimum temperature.

To increase our knowledge of the thermal distribution during IHT we have recently adopted the concept of "*T* index temperature," whereby the percentage of all measurements within a spatial and temporal thermometric matrix above a certain index temperature is calculated. The results are usually illustrated in sigmoid-shaped curves, from which the 90%, 50%, and 20% values (T_{90}, T_{50}, and T_{20}) are derived for comprehensive thermal data reporting (Figs. 28.3, 28.4).

28.4.4 *Analysis of Recurrences*

Only a few authors have addressed local and regional recurrences after implementation of IHT-IRT (SEEGENSCHMIEDT et al. 1990; COSSET et al. 1985; COSSET 1990). Similar to our findings, COSSET and coworkers (COSSET et al. 1985) have reported a rate of 21% locoregional relapses after CR was reported, with a mean interval between treatment and relapse of 9 months (range 5–13 months). There are two types of relapses: those occurring at the tumor edge and those occurring in the lesion center. The underestimation of the target volume and the reluctance to undertake aggressive retreatment in preirradiated sites can contribute to these local failures (DAVIDSON et al. 1984). Only in one instance have we observed a local relapse in a patient with mainly good prognostic factors (small volume, high RT dose, good thermal performance characteristics); all other instances were compromised by unfavorable tumor or treatment performance factors (Table 28.6).

28.4.5 *Analysis of Treatment Toxicity*

Acute and late treatment toxicity was not increased by the addition of IHT to IRT and RT: IRT by itself has a complication rate of 10%–30% after treatment of primary malignancies and pretreated recurrent lesions. Thermal damage was correlated neither with the number of applied IHT sessions

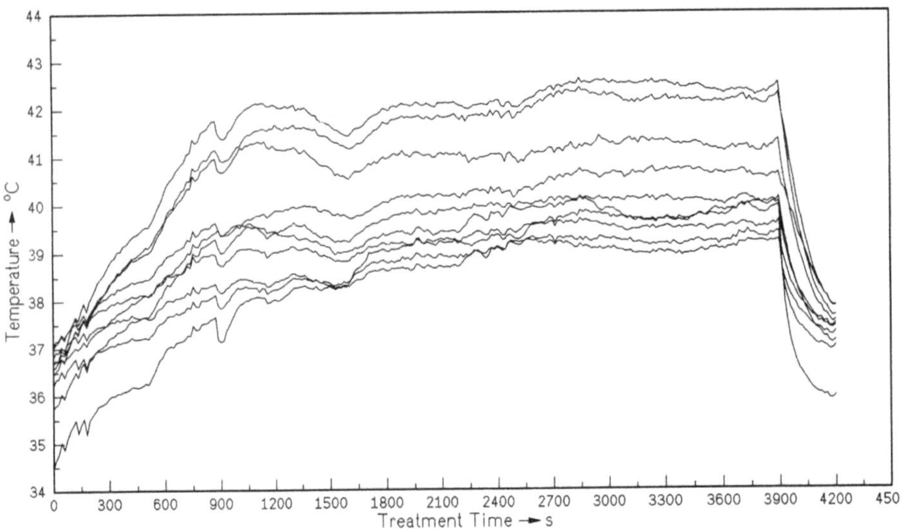

Fig. 28.3. Conventional temperature–time summary plot of an interstitial hyperthermia treatment from a patient with a base of tongue tumor: ten different tumor sensors are represented by individual temperature lines; temperatures are recorded at 15-s intervals for a total treatment time of 70 min (including thermal increment, steady-state, and temperature fall-off at the end of the treatment). Total number of data points measured: 2610.

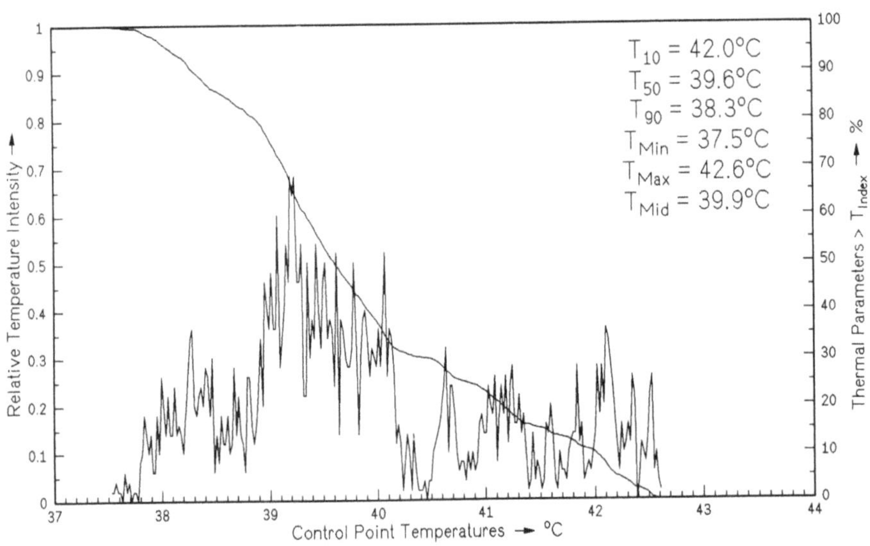

Fig. 28.4. Temperature density and index temperature distribution within the tumor volume of patient and treatment shown in Fig. 28.3: this summary plot includes ten tumor sensors during the whole treatment time of 70 min; the *sigmoid-shaped line* represents the ratio of temperatures above the index temperature, whereas the *scattered line* represents the relative density of measurements at that specific index temperature level

(one vs two or multiple) nor with lesion type or prior treatment. Only maximum temperatures above 44°–45°C in normal or tumor tissue (EMAMI et al. 1987; DEWHIRST et al. 1984; PETROVICH et al. 1989; OLESON et al. 1984) and thermal doses of *T*max Eq 43°C > 160 (DEWHIRST et al. 1984) were associated with thermal damage. When we reviewed our series, we were unable to find any prognostic factor correlated with thermal injury. However, we support the opinion that for H&N treatment oral hygiene is as important as dose–time factors in the prevention of soft tissue and osteoradionecrosis (OLCH et al. 1988). Generally we recommend staying within a "narrow window" of > 41°C minimum and < 45°C maximum temperature to yield effective but nontoxic heating.

Table 28.6. Treatment parameters of patients developing in-field recurrences after combined IHT-IRT

Case Nr, prior RT dose, treatment initiation	Initial response	Type	Volume (cm^3)	Antenna spacing	RT dose (Gy)	Tmin (°C)	TQ 41°C (%)
#1 : 55 Gy 10/87	PR	REC	11	Medium	42	40.1	67
#2 : 75 Gy 01/88	PR	REC	63	Wide	30	40.6	66
#3 : 50 Gy 12/88	CR	PRIM	25	Narrow	71	41.1	100
#4 : 45 Gy 4/89	CR	REC	59	Medium	84	39.3	33
#5 : 54 Gy 3/90	PR	REC	22	Narrow	60	41.0	66
#6 : 51 Gy 4/90	CR	PERS	8	Narrow	78	40.2	50
#7 : 55 Gy 10/90	PR	PERS	44	Wide	72	40.3	40
#8 : 53 Gy 11/90	PR	REC	42	Wide	45	40.3	60

28.5 Conclusions

Interstitial hyperthermia is a safe treatment option adaptable to various H&N tumors and fully compatible with standard free-hand or template brachytherapy techniques. It can be used for malignant lesions that have been suboptimally treated in the past by conventional treatment modalities: implantable locally recurrent, locally metastatic, and selected primary advanced and persistent tumors of the head and neck, but also genitourinary tumors of the pelvis, brain tumors, and tumors of many other sites (KAPP 1986).

Each IHT technique has specific advantages and disadvantages. Microwave techniques are less dependent on a strict implantation geometry; this type of implementation is recommended in the head and neck region, but the confined active heating length of microwave antennae is limited to lesions smaller than 7 cm in greatest dimension. In contrast, radiofrequency, ferromagnetic seed, or hot water perfusion IHT techniques may allow heating dimensions up to 12 cm or more, but they are more bound to strict parallelism and equidistance of the implanted heating sources.

We are aware of all the expenses of IHT-IRT in terms of the materials, time, and personnel involved. A dedicated team is required comprising an ENT surgeon, a radiation oncologist, a physicist, and a nurse; they must have great technical and clinical expertise and achieve a high level of cooperation. This may limit the availability of IHT-IRT to a few clinical sites. Nevertheless, further basic research and technological developments will influence the clinical acceptance of adjuvant and palliative IHT-IRT in various confined malignancies.

Acknowledgments. The authors thank Ulf L. Karlsson, MD, Department of Radiotherapy, University of New Mexico, Albuquerque, NM, USA (former associate professor and attending at the Department of Radiation Oncology, Hahnemann University, Philadelphia, PA, USA); Curtis Miyamoto, MD, senior instructor, Richard Tobin, service engineer, and William Kempin, BS, hyperthermia technologist, Department of Radiation Oncology, Hahnemann University, Philadelphia, PA, USA; Jürgen Erb, Dipl. Phys., Gerhard Grabenbauer, MD, Marianne Kettner, RTT, Rosemarie Rössler, RTT, Ralf Seidel, cand. med., and Gunther Klautke, cand. med., Department of Radiation Oncology, University Erlangen-Nürnberg, for their unfailingly dedicated and skillful clinical, technical, and computer assistance, thorough data management, and diligent patient care.

This work was supported by two grants: Deutsche Krebshilfe e.V. (Dr. Mildred Scheel Stiftung) Grant #300-402-521/6; Deutsche Forschungsgemeinschaft (DFG) Grant #Fi371/2-1.

References

Aoyagi Y, Kanehira C, Kobori K, Hayakawa Y, Mochizuki S, Harada N (1989) Clinical experience with microwave interstitial hyperthermia. In: Sugahara T, Saito M (eds) Hyperthermic oncology 1988, vol 1. Taylor & Francis, London, pp 601–603

Au KS, Cetas TC, Shimm DS et al. (1989) Interstitial ferromagnetic hyperthermia and brachytherapy: preliminary report of a phase I clinical trial. Endocurietherapy/Hyperthermia Oncol 5: 127–136

Aygun C, Salazar OM, Sewchand W, Amornmarn R, Prempree T (1984) Carcinoma of the floor of the mouth: a 20-year experience. Int J Radiat Oncol Biol Phys 10: 619–626

Ben-Hur E, Elkind MM, Bronk BV (1974) Thermally enhanced radiosensitivity of cultured Chinese hamster cells; inhibition of repair of sublethal damage and enhancement of lethal damage. Radiat Res 58: 38–51

Benk V, Mazeron JJ, Grimard L et al. (1990) Comparison of curietherapy versus external irradiation combined with curietherapy in stage II squamous cell carcinomas of the mobile tongue. Radiother Oncol 18: 339–347

Bicher HI, Moore DW, Wolfstein RS (1985) A method for interstitial thermoradiotherapy. In: Overgaard J (ed) Hyperthermic oncology 1984, vol 1. Taylor & Francis, London, pp 575–578

Cetas TC (1985) Thermometry and thermal dosimetry. In: Overgaard J (ed) Hyperthermic oncology 1984, vol 1. Taylor & Francis, London, pp 9–41

Chan KW, Chou CK, McDougall JA, Luk KH, Vora NL,

Forell BW (1989) Changes in heating patterns of interstitial microwave antenna arrays at different insertion depths. Int J Hyperthermia 5: 499–508
Corry PM, Jabboury K, Kong JS, Armour EP, McCraw FJ, LeDuc T (1988) Evaluation of equipment for hyperthermia treatment of cancer. Int J Hyperthermia 4: 53–74
Cosset JM (1990) Interstitial hyperthermia. In: Gautherie M (ed) Interstitial, endocavitary and perfusional hyperthermia. Methods and clinical trials. Springer, Berlin Heidelberg New York, pp 1–41
Cosset JM, Dutreix J, Haie C, Gerbaulet A, Janoray P, Dewars JA (1985) Interstitial thermoradiotherapy: a technical and clinical study of 29 implantations performed at the Institute Gustave Roussy. Int J Hyperthermia 1: 3–13
Coughlin CT, Ryan TP, Stafford JH et al. (1991) Interstitial thermoradiotherapy: the Dartmouth experience 1981–1990. In: Chapman JD, Dewey WC, Whitmore GF (eds) Radiation research: a twentieth-century perspective, vol I. Academic, San Diego, P31 02 WP: 386 (abstr)
Davidson TM, Nahum AM, Hagighi P, Astarita RA, Saltzstein SL, Seagren S (1984) The biology of head and neck cancer: detection and control by parallel histologic sections. Arch Otolaryngol 110: 193–196
Decroix Y, Ghossein N (1981) Experience of the Curie Institute in treatment of cancer of the mobile tongue. Cancer 47: 496–508
Dewhirst MW, Sim DA (1986) Estimation of therapeutic gain in clinical trials involving hyperthermia and radiotherapy. Int J Hyperthermia 2: 165–178
Dewhirst MW, Sim DA, Sapareto S, Connor WG (1984) The importance of minimum tumour temperature in determining early and long-term response of spontaneous pet animal tumours to heat and radiation. Cancer Res [Suppl] 44: 43s–50s
Dewhirst MW, Phillips TL, Samulski TV et al. (1990) RTOG quality assurance guidelines for clinical trials using hyperthermia. Int J Radiat Oncol Biol Phys 18: 1249–1259
Emami B, Marks J (1983) Retreatment of recurrent carcinoma of the head and neck by afterloading interstitial 192 Ir implant. Am J Clin Oncol 6: 1345–1347
Emami B, Perez CA, Konefal J et al. (1987) Interstitial thermoradiotherapy in treatment of malignant tumors. Int J Hyperthermia 3: 107–118
Emami B, Stauffer P, Prionas S et al. (1991) Quality assurance guidelines for interstitial hyperthermia (an RTOG document). Int J Radiat Oncol Biol Phys 20: 1117–1124
Fietkau R, Weidenbecher M, Spitzer W, Sauer R (1991) Temporary and permanent brachycurie therapy in advanced head and neck cancer – the Erlangen experience. In: Sauer R (ed) Interventional radiation therapy: techniques – brachytherapy. Springer, Berlin Heidelberg New York, pp 159–169
Fisher RA, Yates F (1963) Statistical tables for biological, agricultural and medical research. Oliver and Boyd, Edinburgh, p 47 (Table IV)
Fu KK, Lichter A, Galante M (1976) An analysis of treatment results and the sites and causes of failures. Int J Radiat Oncol Biol Phys 1: 829–837
Gautherie M, Cosset JM, Gerard JP et al. (1989) Radiofrequency interstitial hyperthermia: a multicentric program of quality assessment and clinical trials. In: Sugahara T, Saito M (eds) Hyperthermic oncology 1988, vol 2. Taylor & Francis, London, pp 711–714
Guerry TL, Silverman S, Dedo HH (1986) Carbon dioxide laser resection of superficial oral carcinoma: indications, technique, and results. Ann Otol Rhinol Laryngol 95: 547–555
Haie C, Gerbaulet A, Wibault P, Chassagne D, Marandas P (1983) Resultates de la curietherapie et de l'association radiotherapie transcutanee-curietherapie dans 155 cas de cancer de la langue mobile. Actualités de carcinologie cervico-faciale 9: 53–57
Handl-Zeller L, Kärcher KH, Lesnicar H, Budihna M, Schreier K (1987) Newly developed liquid heated interstitial hyperthermia system KHS-9/W18 (abstract). Int J Hyperthermia 3: 567
Handl-Zeller L, Schreier K, Kärcher KH, Budihna M, Lesnicar H (1989) First clinical experience with the Viennese interstitial two-zone hyperthermia system. In: Sugahara T, Saito M (eds), Hyperthermic oncology 1988, vol 1. Taylor & Francis, London, pp 814–816
Hilaris BS, Henschke UK (1985) General principles and techniques of interstitial brachytherapy. In: Hilaris BS (ed) Handbook of interstitial brachytherapy. Publishing Sciences Group, Acton, MA, pp 61–86
Inoue T, Hori S, Miyata Y et al. (1978) Dose and dose rate in 192 Ir interstitial irradiation for carcinoma of the tongue. Acta Radiol Oncol 17 (Fasc 1) : 27–32
Inoue T, Masaki N, Ozeki S et al. (1989) Clinical experience of interstitial hyperthermia combined with external radiation using MA-251 interstitial applicator. In: Sugahara T, Saito M (eds) Hyperthermic oncology 1988, vol 1. Taylor & Francis, London, pp 598–600
James BJ, Strohbehn JW, Mechling JA, Trembly BS (1989) The effect of insertion depth on the theoretical SAR patterns of 915 MHz dipole antenna arrays for hyperthermia. Int J Hyperthermia 5: 733–747
Jones EL, Lyons BE, Douple EB, Dain BJ (1989) Thermal enhancement of low dose irradiation in a murine tumour system. Int J Hyperthermia 5: 509–524
Kaplan EL, Meier P (1958) Nonparametric estimation from incomplete observations. J Am Stat Assoc 53: 457–481
Kapp DS (1986) Site and disease selection for hyperthermia clinical trials. Int J Hyperthermia 2: 139–156
Langlois D, Hoffstetter S, Malissard L, Pernot M, Taghian A (1988) Salvage irradiation of oropharynx and mobile tongue with 192-iridium brachytherapy in Centre Alexis Vautrin. Int J Radiat Oncol Biol Phys 14: 849–853
Lefebvre LJ, Coche-Dequeant B, Castelain B, Prevost B, Buisset E, van Ton J (1990) Interstitial brachytherapy and early tongue squamous cell carcinoma management. Head Neck 12: 232–236
Leipzig B, Cummings CW, Chung CT, Johnson JT, Sagerman RH (1982) Carcinoma of the anterior tongue. Ann Otol 91: 94–97
Levendag PC, Visser AG, Deurloo IKK et al. (1992) Interstitial radiation and/or interstitial hyperthermia in advanced and/or recurrent cancers in the head and neck: a pilot study. Abstracts from the COMAC-BME workshop on interstitial and intracavitary hyperthermia 1991. Hyperthermia Bull 9: 70–76
Linares LA, Nort D, Brenner H et al. (1986) Interstitial hyperthermia and brachytherapy: a preliminary report. Endocurietherapy/Hyperthermia Oncol 2: 39–44
Marks JE, Lee F, Smith PG, Ogura JH (1983) Floor of the mouth cancer: patient selection and treatment results. Laryngoscope 93: 475–480
Mazeron JJ, Langlois D, Glaubiger D et al. (1987a) Salvage irradiation of oropharyngeal cancers using iridium 192 wire implants: 5 year results of 70 cases. Int J Radiat Oncol Biol Phys 13: 957–962
Mazeron JJ, Marinello G, Crook J et al. (1987b) Definitive radiation treatment for early stage carcinoma of the soft

palate and uvula: the indications for iridium 192 implantation. Int J Radiat Oncol Biol Phys 13: 1829–1837
Mazeron JJ, Crook JM, Marinello G, Walop W, Pierquin B (1990a) Prognostic factors of local outcome for T1, T2 carcinomas of oral tongue treated by iridium 192 implantation. Int J Radiat Oncol Biol 19: 281–285
Mazeron JJ, Grimard L, Raynal M et al. (1990b) Iridium-192 curietherapy for T1 and T2 epidermoid carcinomas of the floor of the mouth. Int J Radiat Oncol Biol Phys 18: 1299–1306
Mendenhall WM, Parsons JT, Stringer SP, Cassisi NJ, Million RR (1989) T2 oral tongue carcinoma treated with radiotherapy: analysis of local control and complications. Radiother Oncol 16: 275–281
Miller RC, Leith JT, Voemett RC, Gerner EW (1978) Effects of interstitial radiation therapy alone, or in combination with localized hyperthermia on response of a mouse mammary tumour. Radiat Res 19: 175–180
Nathanson A, Agren K, Lind MG et al. (1989) Evaluation of some prognostic factors in small squamous cells carcinoma of the mobile tongue: a multicenter study in Sweden. Head Neck 11: 387–392
Nowak PJCM, Levendag PC, Visser AG (1990) Brachytherapy failure analysis of floor of mouth and oral tongue. Endocurietherapy Hyperthermia Oncol 6: 1–9
O'Brien CJ, Lahr CJ, Soong SJ et al. (1986) Surgical treatment of early-stage carcinoma of the oral tongue – would adjuvant treatment be beneficial? Head Neck Surg 8: 401–408
Olch AJ, Beumer J, Schwartz HC, Kagan AR (1988) Proposition: that oral hygiene is as important as dose-time factors in the prevention of osteoradionecrosis in the mandible. Endocurietherapy Hyperthermia Oncol 4: 11–16
Oleson JR, Manning MR, Sim DA et al. (1984) A review of the University of Arizona human clinical hyperthermia experience. Front Radiat Ther Oncol 18: 136–143
Oleson JR, Calderwood SK, Coughlin CT et al. (1988) Biological and clinical aspects of hyperthermia in cancer therapy. Am J Clin Oncol 11: 368–380
Overgaard J (1981) Fractionated radiation and hyperthermia: experimental and clinical studies. Cancer 48: 116–123
Overgaard J (1989) The current and potential role of hyperthermia in radiotherapy. Int J Radiat Oncol Biol Phys 16: 535–549
Paulsen KD, Strohbehn JW, Lynch DR (1984) Theoretical temperature distributions produced by an annular phased array-type systemin CT-based patient models. Radiat Res 100: 536–552
Pernot M, Malissard L, Aletti P, Hoffstetter S, Forcard JJ, Bey P (1990) Ir-192 brachytherapy in the management of 147 T2N0 oral tongue carcinoma treated with irradiation alone. Int J Radiat Oncol Biol Phys 19 [Suppl]: 139
Petrovich Z, Langholz B, Lam K et al. (1989) Interstitial microwave hyperthermia combined with iridium-192 radiotherapy for recurrent tumours. Am J Clin Oncol 12: 264–268
Puthawala AA, Syed AMN, Neblett D, McNamara C (1981) The role of afterloading iridium (Ir-192) implant in the management of carcinoma of the tongue. Int J Radiat Oncol Biol Phys 7: 407–412
Puthawala AA, Syed AMN, Khalid MA, Rafie S, McNamara CS (1985) Interstitial hyperthermia for recurrent malignancies. Endocurietherapy/Hyperthermia Oncol 1: 125–131
Puthawala AA, Syed AMN, Eads DL, Gillin L, Gates TC (1988) Limited external beam and interstitial 192-iridium irradiation in the treatment of carcinoma of the base of tongue: a ten year experience. Int J Radiat Oncol Biol Phys 14: 839–848
Rafla S, Parikh K, Tchelebi M, Youssef E, Selim H, Bishay S (1989) Recurrent tumors of the head and neck, pelvis and chest wall: treatment with hyperthermia and brachytherapy. Radiology 172: 845–850
Reinhold HS, Endrich B (1986) Tumour microcirculation as a target for hyperthermia. Int J Hyperthermia 2: 117–137
Rubin P, Carter SK (1976) Combination of radiation therapy and chemotherapy: a logical basis for their clinical use. CA 26: 274–292
Ryan TP, Mechling JA, Strohbehn JW (1990) Absorbed power deposition for various insertion depths for 915 MHz interstitial dipole antenna arrays: experiment versus theory. Int J Radiat Oncol Biol Phys 19: 377–387
Sapareto SA, Dewey WC (1984) Thermal dose determination in cancer therapy. Int J Radiat Oncol Biol Phys 10: 787–800
Schreiber DP, Overett TK, Schneider MJ (1990) Interstitial brachytherapy and hyperthermia. In: Abstracts of papers for the 38th annual meeting of the Radiation Research Society, 10th annual meeting of the North American Hyperthermia Group, New Orleans, LO (USA), 7–12 April 1990, Cza-2: 120 (abstract)
Seegenschmiedt MH, Sauer R, Herbst M et al. (1989) Interstitial hyperthermia for H&N: treatment planning and quality assurance (QA). In: Sugahara T, Saito M (eds) Hyperthermic oncology 1988, vol 2. Taylor & Francis, London, pp 524–527
Seegenschmiedt MH, Sauer R, Fietkau R, Karlsson UL, Brady LW (1990) Primary advanced and local recurrent head and neck tumors: effective management with interstitial thermal radiation therapy. Radiology 176: 267–274
Seegenschmiedt MH, Sauer R, Brady LW, Karlsson UL (1991) Techniques and clinical experience of interstitial thermoradiotherapy. In: Sauer R (ed) Interventional radiation therapy: techniques – brachytherapy. Springer, Berlin Heidelberg New York, pp 159–169
Shimm D, Stea B, Cetas T et al. (1989) Clinical results of interstitial hyperthermia using thermally regulating ferromagnetic seeds. In: Sugahara T, Saito M (eds) Hyperthermic oncology 1988, vol 2. Taylor & Francis, London, pp 536–539
Song CW (1984) Effect of local hyperthermia on bloodflow and microenvironment. Cancer Res [Suppl] 44: 4721s–4730s
Stauffer PR, Sneed PK, Suen SA et al. (1989) Comparative thermal dosimetry of interstitial microwave and radiofrequency-LCF hyperthermia. Int J Hyperthermia 5: 307–318
Syed AMN, Feder FW, Neblett D (1978) Iridium-192 afterloaded implant in the retreatment of head and neck cancers. Br J Radiol 51: 814–820
Thiel HJ, Müller R, Weidenbecher M, Sauer R (1987) Interstitielle Brachycurietherapie von HNO-Tumoren. In: Sauer R, Schwab W (eds) Kombinationstherapie der Oro- und Hypopharynxkarzinome. Urban & Schwarzenberg, Munich, pp 69–89
Tupchong L, Nerlinger RE, Waterman FM (1988) Combined use of interstitial hyperthermia and external beam radiation therapy in advanced head & neck cancer. In: Abstracts of papers for the 36th annual meeting of the Radiation Research Society, 8th annual meeting of the North American Hyperthermia Group, Philadelphia, PA (USA), 16–21 April 1988, Ce-7: 42 (abstract)

Visser AG, Deurloo IKK, Levendag PC, Ruifrok ACC, Cornet B, van Rhoon GC (1989) An interstitial hyperthermia system at 27 MHz. Int J Hyperthermia 5: 265–276
Vora NL, Forell B, Luk KH et al. (1989) Interstitial thermoradiotherapy in recurrent and advanced carcinoma of malignant tumors: seven years' experience. In: Sugahara T, Saito M (eds) Hyperthermia oncology 1988, vol 1. Taylor & Francis, London, pp 588–590
Wang CC (1989) Radiotherapeutic management and results of T1N0, T2N0 carcinoma of the oral tongue: evaluation of boost techniques. Int J Radiat Oncol Biol Phys 17: 287–291
Wendt CG, Peters LJ, Delclos L et al. (1990) Primary radiotherapy in the treatment of stage I and II oral tongue cancers: importance of the proportion of therapy delivered with interstitial therapy. Int J Radiat Oncol Biol Phys 18: 1287–1292
Whitehurst JO, Droulias CA (1977) Surgical treatment of squamous cell carcinoma of the oral tongue. Factors influencing survival. Arch Otolaryngol 103: 212–215
Yabumoto E, Suyama S, Show K, Yamazaki T (1989) A phase I clinical trial of radiofrequency interstitial hyperthermia combined with external radiotherapy. In: Sugahara T, Saito M (eds) Hyperthermic oncology 1988, vol 1. Taylor & Francis, London, pp 591–593

29 Interstitial Thermoradiotherapy for Pelvic Tumors: The City of Hope Experience

N.L. VORA and K.H. LUK

CONTENTS

29.1 Introduction

Interstitial techniques for radiation implants as primary or boost treatments have been practiced successfully by radiation oncologists for many years. When hyperthermia was found to be cytotoxic and synergistic with radiation, this modality was quickly combined with interstitial radioactive implantations. At the City of Hope National Medical Center, clinical trials with interstitial thermoradiotherapy commenced in 1984.

Clinically there are three common methods of producing interstitial hyperthermia, namely, the local current field (LCF) technique, the microwave (MW) technique, and the induction technique employing ferromagnetic seeds (FMS). At the City of Hope, we used the LCF technique to treat pelvic tumors until 1990, thereafter turning to the FMS technique.

So far, we have reported clinical trials at our institution which were phase I–II studies for feasibility and toxicity. The results have been encouraging. At this time, we are also participating in the Radiation Therapy Oncology Group phase III protocol which compares interstitial radiation alone versus interstitial thermoradiotherapy. The study was stratified according to tumor type as well as previous radiotherapy.

We present here our updated material in the treatment of pelvic tumors with interstitial thermoradiotherapy.

29.2 Materials and Methods

29.2.1 Patient Population

The largest component of the patient population who underwent interstitial thermoradiotherapy were those with advanced carcinoma of the cervix. In general they were patients with stage IIIB with tumor extension to the pelvic side wall. Occasionally patients with bulky stage IIB were recruited into the clinical study. Patients with bulky recurrent disease after initial attempts at curative surgery or curative radiation therapy certainly might benefit from this treatment combination.

The other type of pelvic tumor for which interstitial thermoradiotherapy was employed was recurrent rectal cancer, usually after surgery, or after surgery and radiation therapy. Since many of these patients needed to receive chemotherapy because of contemporary findings of metastases, they were not eligible for this study.

Table 29.1 details the patient characteristics in this report. Interstitial thermoradiotherapy was employed in a total of 42 patients with pelvic tumors, but two of the patients did not undergo the planned second implant and therefore were excluded from analysis.

29.2.2 Local Current Field Technique

Doss and McCABE (1976) were credited with the first published paper describing the LCF technique, used for localized heating in tissue. By applying a

N.L. VORA, M.D., Division of Radiation Oncology, City of Hope National Medical Center, 1500 E. Duarte Road, Duarte, CA 91010, USA
K.H. LUK, M.D., FACR, Department of Radiation Oncology, Good Samaritan Regional Medical Center, 1111 E. McDowell Road, Phoenix, AZ 85006, USA

Table 29.1. Patient characteristics

Patients entered	40
Female: male	38:2
Age in years (mean ± SD)	55.8 ± 13.6
Range	25–75
Follow-up time	19.6 ± 21.4
Range	3–98
Diagnoses	
Anal ca.	1 (2.5%)
Bladder ca.	1 (2.5%)
Breast ca.	1 (2.5%)
Cervical ca.	32 (80.0%)
Colon ca.	1 (2.5%)
Endometrial ca.	2 (5.0%)
Rectal ca.	2 (5.0%)
Stage	
2B	6 (15.0%)
3A	2 (5.0%)
3B	15 (37.5%)
4	3 (7.5%)
4A	1 (2.5%)
Recurrent	13 (32.5%)
Grade	
1	3 (7.5%)
2	13 (32.5%)
3	24 (60.0%)
Prior radiation treatment	
Yes	12 (30.0%)
No	28 (70.0%)
Response	
No	19 (47.5%)
Complete	19 (47.5%)
Partial	2 (5.0%)

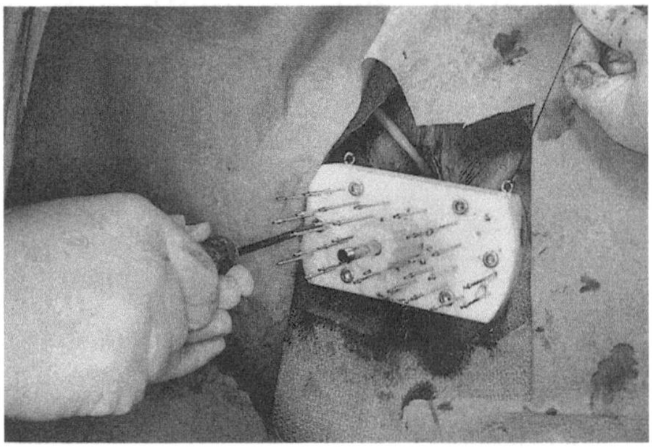

Fig. 29.1. Vaginal template with needles

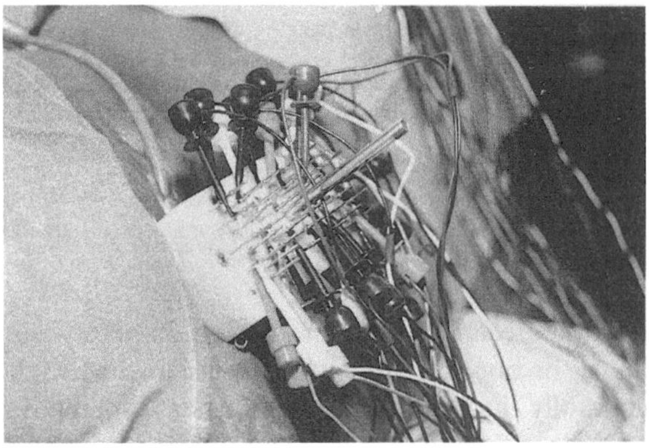

Fig. 29.2. Technique for LCF hyperthermia

voltage between two planes of needle electrodes, electric currents flow through the intervening tissues. Heat is generated by the resistivity of the tissues. Thermometry provides temperature data, as well as feedback control of the power of the radiofrequency generator.

Astrahan and George (1980) described interstitial hyperthermia equipment utilizing 0.5 MHz radiofrequency current, and this was the prototype equipment used at the City of Hope National Medical Center for phase I and II clinical trials. Standard interstitial brachytherapy techniques were modified for interstitial hyperthermia. Seventeen gauge hollow steel needles were implanted into the tumor as electrode pairs for LCF hyperthermia, after which they acted as guides for insertion of nylon tubings for afterloading of radioisotopes (Figs. 29.1, 29.2).

The initial prototype machine at the City of Hope was replaced in 1985 by a system manufactured by Oncotherm Corporation which could record up to 32 data points in 20 sensors and displayed these temperatures on a video display terminal simultaneously. Feedback control of the power as well as the current dwell time across the treatment needle pairs could be adjusted by the computer automatically according to the determination of a reference probe. This unit was used until 1990, when the company become insolvent and could no longer provide service support.

29.2.3 Ferromagnetic Heating Technique

Burton et al. (1971) used thermally self-regulating implants for the production of brain lesions. This technique was also applicable for delivering thermal energy to deep-seated tumors (Brezovich and Atkinson 1984; Stauffer et al. 1984a, b). When exposed to a magnetic field, the ferromagnetic implants absorb energy and become heated, but when a critical temperature (Curie point) is reached, the implant becomes paramagnetic and very little heat is produced. The surrounding tissues are heated by thermal conduction. The influence of blood flow and tissue inhomogeneities of the tumor, which may affect the temperature distribution, as seen in other heating methods, can be compensated by the self-regulating characteristics of the implants, with maintenance of a temperature close to the Curie point.

At the City of Hope, a shielded room was built to accommodate this treatment method. The room consisted of metallic panels on all six sides. The door was made with a locking system, and a window was covered with copper mesh screen in order to provide visual and voice contact with the patient.

An RF generator (ENI Company) capable of providing 8 kW power at about 100 kHz was used. Three coils were available for generating magnetic fields along the X, Y, and Z axes to treat different parts of the body. The coils and matching network were designed by Dr. Thomas Cetas of the University of Arizona. A coil is tuned to resonance with capacitors and transformers matched to the 50-ohm generator. During the treatment, about 300–500 A of RF current flows between the coil and the capacitors, resulting in resistive loss. In order to maintain a safe operating temperature, the coil is cooled with chilled water while the capacitors and matching transformer are oil cooled.

The thermometry and data acquisition system was built by Mr. Kwok Chan of our group. Fifty-six thermocouples, some in linear arrays of up to seven sensors, may be inserted into a tumor, and the temperatures recorded by a microcomputer. Mr. Chan also wrote the computer software for this system. Identical systems were built for the University of Arizona and the University of California, San Francisco.

Large metallic objects can be heated as a result of induced eddy current circulation when placed in intense magnetic fields. Therefore the metal parts of the templates had to be substituted with plastic equivalent parts. We worked with our supplier to modify a Syed–Neblett template to be used for ferromagnetic implant heatings. Implant spacing is dependent on the seeds' Curie point temperatures and is typically 1–1.5 cm. It is possible to mix or to exchange seeds of different Curie points during a treatment session. Preplanning is most desirable to optimize a heat treatment.

29.2.4 Treatment Protocol

29.2.4.1 Radiation Dosage

Whenever possible, patients were first treated with external beam radiation therapy to the whole pelvis. This helped to improve the geometry of the tumors for implant in many instances. For previously untreated patients, the external beam dose was in the range of 45–50 Gy, and the total brachytherapy dose (usually with two implants separated by 2 weeks) was 30–45 Gy. In the group which had previously received radiation, the dose of external beam radiation and the implant dose were determined by the previous irradiation. Figures 29.3 and 29.4 a, b show typical simulation film for whole pelvic external radiation field and typical interstitial implant.

29.2.4.2 Heat Dosage

Patients were heated for 30 min prior to 1989 and then for 60 min at 43°C in the majority of the treatment volume as determined by multiple point temperature measurements with thermocouples. Hyperthermia was delivered before the implant was loaded with iridium isotope ribbons. "Heat-up" and "cool-down" phases of the treatments were

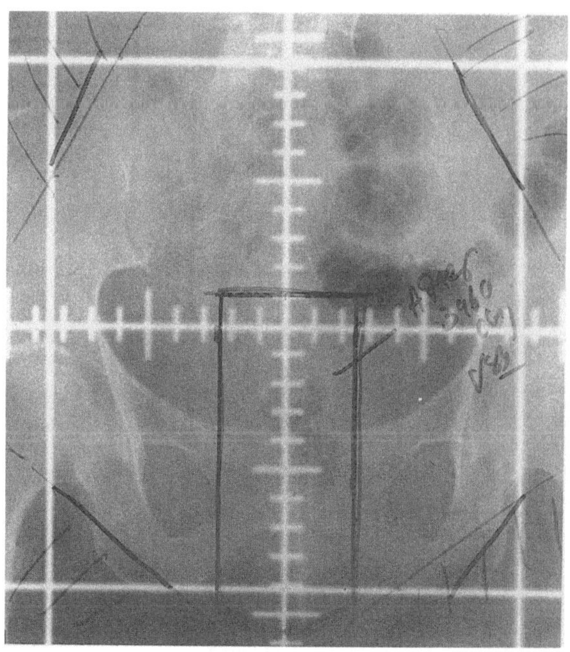

Fig. 29.3. Simulator film for whole pelvic external radiation field

also carefully recorded with our computer systems as described above. Whenever possible, patients received two hyperthermia sessions together with the two implants separated by 2–3 weeks.

29.2.4.3 Other Parameters

All participants in this study gave their full informed consent, and confirmation of pathology was obtained in each case. As far as possible, patients are followed up regularly. Follow-up data include photography, measurements, and radiological tests as indicated.

29.2.4.4 Statistical Methods

For analyses comparing two groups, chi-square tests were used for categorical variables, and Student's t-tests were applied to continuous variables. The variables examined were age, sex, race, diagnoses, stage, prior radiation treatment, hyperthermia time, total radiation dose, and average number of needles used.

Univariate Cox regression analyses were used to determine which of the above prognostic factors were predictive of the recurrence of disease, and to estimate the relative risk of recurrence of disease. Stepwise Cox regression was used to determine which prognostic variables were the most suitable independent predictors of relapse time.

29.3 Results

Table 29.2 presents the relationship between prognostic factors and response. In summary, significant associations were found between response and age, race, prior radiation treatment, and total radiation dose. Patients who had either complete or partial responses were older than those without responses ($P = 0.026$). Non-Caucasian ethnic groups had significantly higher response rates than Caucasians ($P = 0.013$) (Fig. 29.3). Patients who had had prior radiation treatment had a significantly lower response rate than those who had not (Fig. 29.4). Patients who received a higher radiation dose had a significantly higher response rate than those who did not ($P = 0.033$).

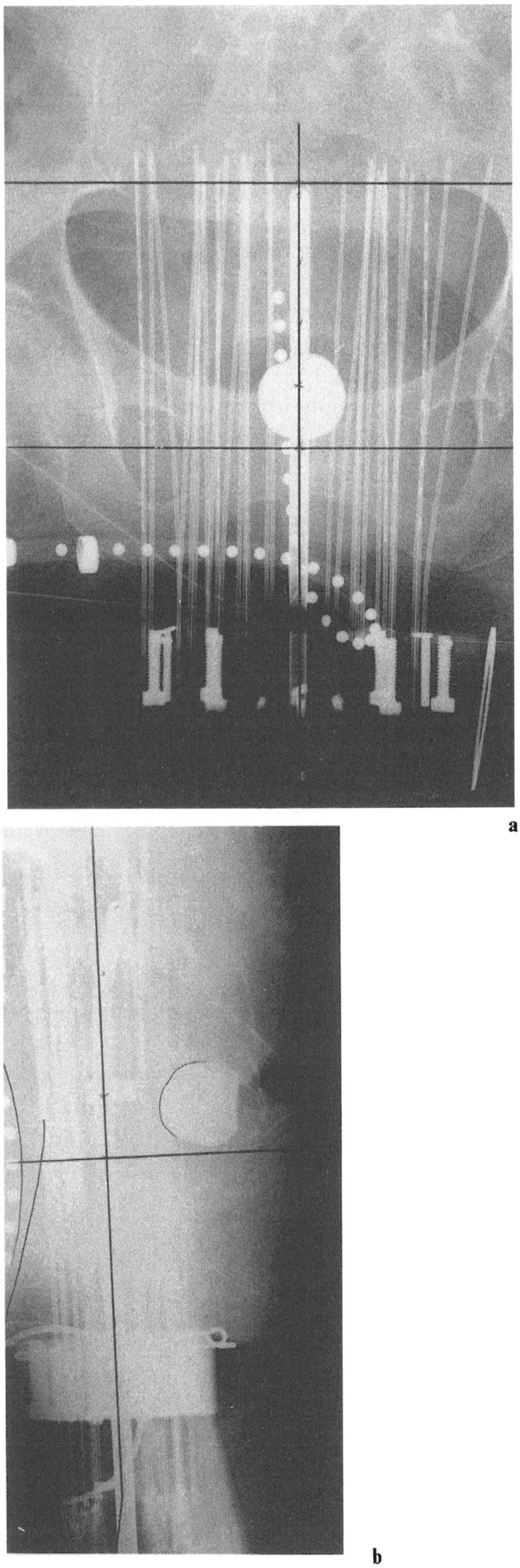
a
b

Fig. 29.4 a, b. Anteroposterior and lateral X-ray localization film for a typical interstitial implant

Table 29.2. Relationship between response and prognostic factors

	Response (CR + PR) (n = 21)	No response (n = 19)	P value
Age	60.2 ± 11.9	50.8 ± 13.8	0.026
Sex (female)	19 (90%)	21 (100%)	0.488
Race			
Caucasian	5	13	
Hispanic	10	5	
Others	6	1	0.013
Diagnoses			
Anal ca.	1	0	
Bladder ca.	0	1	
Breast ca.	1	0	
Cervical ca.	17	15	
Colon ca.	0	1	
Endometrial ca.	1	1	
Rectal ca.	1	1	
Stage			
2B	5	1	
3A	1	1	
3B	8	7	
4	2	1	
4A	1	0	
Recurrent	4	9	
Grade			
1	2	1	
2	7	6	
3	12	12	0.856
Prior radiation treatment			
Yes	3	9	
No	18	10	0.038
Hyperthermia time			
30 min	13	14	
60 min	8	5	0.427
Total radiation dose			
(External + Imp 1 + Imp 2)/100	80.86 ± 17.18	65.96 ± 24.92	0.033
Average no. of needles	32.26 ± 12.22	33.95 ± 8.07	0.614

CR, complete response; PR, partial response; Imp, implant

An interesting observation is that longer hyperthermia treatment times have not resulted in improved control of disease. Comparing 30 min versus 60 min of heating time per session, i.e., 60 vs 120 min total heating time, the difference in results was not statistically significant ($P = 0.427$).

Table 29.3 presents the univariate Cox regression results. Nineteen patients (47.5%) experienced local recurrence, and 21 (52.5%) remained disease-free. The risk of recurrence was significantly higher for Caucasian ($P = 0.008$) and younger patients ($P = 0.015$). Thus, Caucasians had an approximately 3.5 times higher risk of relapse than non-Caucasians, and there was a 1.3 times higher failure rate for a decrement of 5 years of age. Stage (recurrence vs no recurrence) and prior radiation treatment approached statistical significance for failure of control of disease ($P = 0.063$ and $P = 0.064$, respectively).

Table 29.3. Univariate Cox regression analysis of prognostic factors associated with the recurrence of disease

Prognostic factor	Relative risk	P value
Age	0.955	0.015
Race	3.460	0.008
Hyperthermia time	0.683	0.461
Stage	2.299	0.063
Prior radiation treatment	2.289	0.064
Hyperthermia time	0.528	0.174
Total radiation dose	0.986	0.115
Average no. of needles	1.007	0.699

Race = 1 if Caucasian, 0 if non-Caucasian; stage = 1 if recurrent, 0 otherwise; hyperthermia time = 0 if 30 min, 1 if 60 min

Table 29.4 showed the relative risks and the P values for the significant variables yielded by the stepwise Cox regression analysis. This analysis identified which prognostic factors were the most

Table 29.4. Stepwise Cox regression analysis of prognostic factors associated with the recurrence of disease

Prognostic factor	Step entered	Relative risk	*P* value
Race	1	5.351	< 0.001
Age	2	0.932	0.001
Stage	3	3.150	0.019

Race = 1 if Caucasian, 0 if non-Caucasian; stage = 1 if recurrent, 0 otherwise

suitable independent predictors of the recurrence of disease. Significant independent predictors of relapse included race, age, and the stage of the disease. Caucasian patients had a 5.4 times higher rate of relapse than non-Caucasian patients after controlling for other prognostic factors such as age and the stage of the disease. There was a 1.4 times higher recurrence rate for a decrement of 5 years of age after controlling for other prognostic factors. Patients with recurrent disease had a 3.2 times higher relapse rate than those with nonrecurrent disease.

Three patients have developed serious grade 4 complications. They include two patients with rectovaginal fistulas and one patient with vesicovaginal fistula. Less serious complications such as proctitis and cystitis occurred in most of the patients but resolved within 4–6 weeks.

29.4 Discussion

29.4.1 Comparison Between the Two Techniques

29.4.1.1 LCF Technique

Implant geometry and local blood flow are the two important factors for good heat delivery. For LCF hyperthermia, the needles need to be as parallel as possible. When the needles converge towards each other at the tip, more power will be deposited at that region, producing a hot spot. Conversely, cold spots can occur where needles diverge. With superficial implants, e.g., breast or limb, it is possible in some situations to use bridge templates to ensure that the needles are indeed parallel. In other clinical situations, e.g., pelvic tumors, parallel implants are difficult to accomplish.

Spacing between needles is also important in the heat distribution. Since current density is highest near the needles, tissue heating depends a lot on thermal conduction. Wide separation will create cold regions between the needles or planes.

Blood flow is perhaps the dominant factor in heat distribution in tissues. The quantity of blood vessel in a given locale certainly influences the degree of heat loss from that region. In addition, vasodilatation and increased blood flow rate can also effectively cool the tissues.

Clinicians have to make judgments as to how to compensate for inhomogeneous heating. From the engineering point of view, temperature manipulations can be made either by altering the power of the RF generator and the voltage across the needles, or by changing the "dwell time" during which the voltage is applied.

A number of technical improvements have been made in the last few years in the development of the LCF unit. Multiple sensors can be built into a thermocouple probe so that up to five-point measurements can be made. The aggregate temperature information can give an excellent representation of the temperature distribution across a plane or volume of tissue. Research in the direction of improving axial heating along the implanted heating needle or catheter was started by Prionas et al. (1984).

Local current field electrodes require connections to a separate power generator. In the case of a large implant, the number of these connectors can be cumbersome for the physicians and physicists. Dr. Peter Corry has designed a circuit board template which eliminates this problem.

One drawback of LCF hyperthermia is the inconvenience of using rigid steel needles, which preclude multiple heating sessions with the same implant. In our patients with pelvic tumors, usually two implants spaced 2–3 weeks apart were done and the hyperthermia treatment would be delivered with each implant.

29.4.1.2 FMS Technique

Ferromagnetic seeds or wires can be implanted either directly into a tumor or with an afterloading technique. An externally applied magnetic induction field created by a concentric coil placed around a patient creates eddy currents in the implanted seed. Each seed then becomes a heating element to the tissue next to it, and heating of a tumor volume is achieved by thermal conduction. The seeds need not be as parallel as LCF electrodes; however, each seed must be implanted about 20°–30° of the magnetic field.

Each seed is self-regulating, with the highest temperature not exceeding the Curie point of the particular alloy characteristics. In practice, the Curie point heating is not always utilized since the desired temperature can be reached. There are no wire connections. There are no fat heating problems since heating is independent of tissue characteristics. There can be more customization of the heating volume because the lengths of seeds or wires can be cut to fit the size of the tumor, thereby minimizing the heating of normal tissues.

There are certain limitations of FMS. An RF room is mandatory with existing coil configurations. The facility needed is expensive for the current system design and setup. In addition, the efficiency of this system is low: It requires a chilled water cooling system, which is expensive. The seed materials are also quite expensive and labor intensive in production and calibration. Quality assurance is very important and demands significant time and effort to ensure the same Curie point temperatures and transition slopes.

29.4.2 *Local Control, Survival, and Complications*

The initial pilot study in 15 patients with various types of cancer was reported by Vora et al. (1982), who stated that 11/16 lesions (68%) achieved complete response and that normal tissue complications were minimal. Results of LCF treatments at the City of Hope National Medical Center were updated by Vora et al. (1988). Most of the patients had advanced primary breast and cervical cancers which were considered uncontrollable by conventional methods. The complete response rate in primary carcinoma of the cervix was 64.2% (9/14), with follow-up times between 6 and 47 months.

This report provides follow-up data out to 100 months. Figures 29.5 and 29.6 have essentially identical curves indicating disease-free probabilities of those patients with recurrent disease or prior radiation treatments. The long-term probability of local control (cure?) of the favorable categories is about 60%.

Our complication rates are acceptable. Considering the advanced stages of disease being treated and the aggressiveness of our treatment approaches, it is not surprising that fistulas occurred in at least three patients or that there were some reversible grade 1 and 2 side-effects.

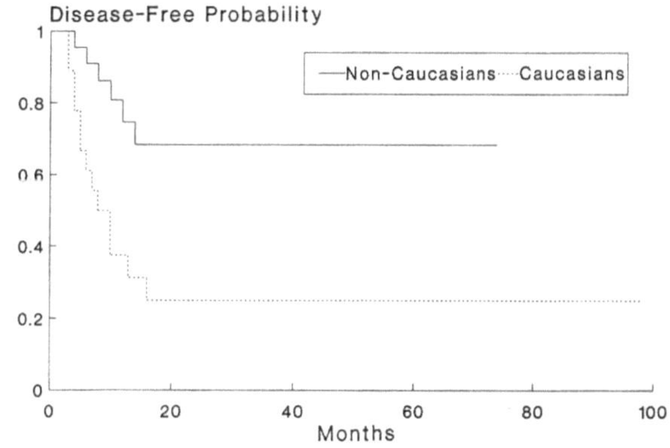

Fig. 29.5. Time to the recurrence of disease according to race (Caucasians vs non-Caucasians)

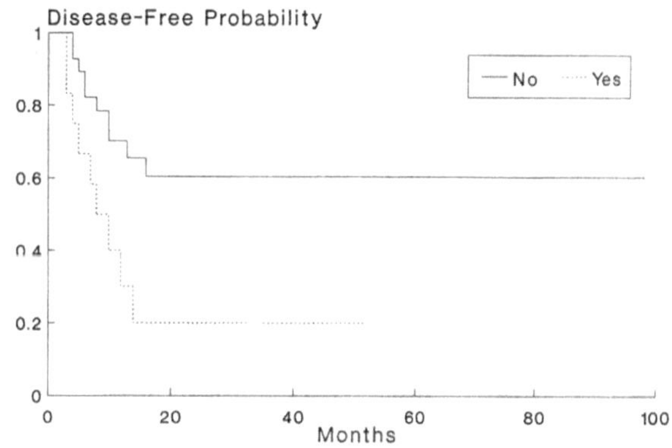

Fig. 29.6. Time to the recurrence of disease according to prior radiation treatment (no vs yes)

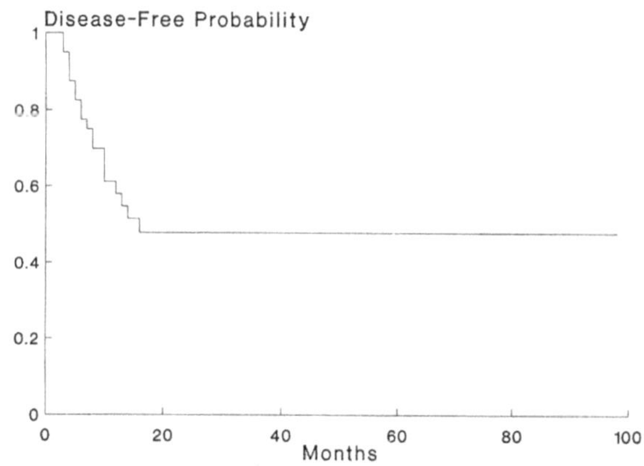

Fig. 29.7. Time to the recurrence of disease

These results are sufficiently encouraging to warrant direct comparison with standard brachytherapy. In fact, as mentioned earlier, we are participating in the RTOG phase III randomized study, and hopefully in another year we will have meaningful information to confirm the usefulness of interstitial hyperthermia in the discussed settings.

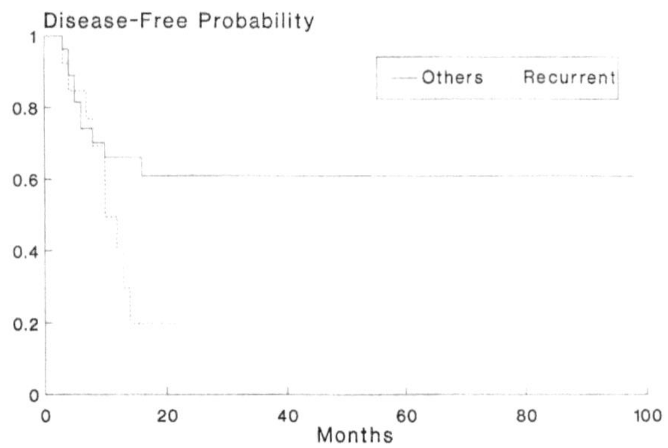

Fig. 29.8. Time to the recurrence of disease according to stage (recurrent vs others)

The results of analysis of heating time e.g., 30 min vs 60 min have resulted in same local control and should be taken as preliminary information, since the numbers of patients studied are small. Data in recent literature regarding fractionation studies of external superficial hyperthermia seem to indicate no difference in outcome according to number of fractions used, e.g., two versus six. However, caution should be exercised in the interpretation of these data, since many factors are likely to be involved. Until we have very accurate temperature measurements and satisfactory control of heat delivery, it is not possible to discern differences (or lack of differences) very easily. It appears that the total time of heating or total number of fractions may not be as important as few fractions of therapeutic homogenous heating.

Acknowledgment. The authors gratefully acknowledge the contribution of Dr. Chul Ahn of the Biostatistics Department.

References

Astrahan MA, George FW II (1980) A temperature regulating circuit for experimental localized current field hyperthermia systems. Med Phys 7: 362–364

Atkinson WJ, Brezovich IA, Chakraborty DP et al. (1984) Usable frequencies in hyperthermia with thermal seeds. IEEE Trans Biomed Eng 31: 70–75

Brezovich IA, Atkinson WJ (1984) Temperature distributions in tumor models heated by self-regulating nickle-copper alloy thermoseeds. Med Phys 11: 145–152

Brezovich IA, Atkinson WJ, Lilly MB et al. (1984) Local hyperthermia with interstitial techniques. Cancer Res [Suppl] 44: 4752s–4756s

Burton CV, Hill M, Walker AE et al. (1971) The RF thermal seed – a thermally self-regulating implant for the production of brain lesions. IEEE Trans Biomed Eng 18: 104–109

Corry P, Martinez A, Armour PE et al. Simultaneous hyperthermia and brachytherapy with remote afterloading. Proceedings brachytherapy meeting. Remote afterloading state-of-the-art. May 4–6, 1989

Doss JD, McCabe CW (1976) A technique for localized heating in tissue: an adjunct to tumor therapy. Med Instrumentation 10: 16–21

Prionas SD, Goffinet DR, Samulski TV et al. (1984) Characterization of an interstitial hyperthermia RF system utilizing flexible electrodes. Abstract of the 32nd Annual Meeting of the Rad. Res. Soc., Orlando, FL, March 25–29, p 18

Stauffer PR, Thomas CC, Fletcher AM et al. (1984a) Observations in the use of ferromagnetic implants for inducing hyperthermia. IEEE Trans Biomed Eng 31: 76–90

Stauffer PR, Thomas CC, Jones RC et al. (1984b) Magnetic induction heating of ferromagnetic implants for inducing localized hyperthemia in deep-seated tumors. IEEE Trans Biomed Eng 31: 235–251

Vora N, Forell B, Joseph C et al. (1982) Interstitial implant with interstitial hyperthermia. Cancer 50: 2518–2523

Vora N, Shaw S, Forell B et al. (1986) Primary radiation combine with hyperthermia for advanced (Stage III–IV) and inflammatory carcinoma of breast. Endocurietherapy/Hyperthermia Oncol 2: 101–106

Vora N, Luk K, Forell B et al. (1988) Interstitial local current field hyperthermia for advanced cancers of the cervix. Endocurietherapy/Hyperthermia Oncol 4: 97–106

30 Interstitial Thermoradiotherapy for Pelvic Tumors: The Washington University Experience

P.W. GRIGSBY and B. EMAMI

CONTENTS

30.1 Introduction

Hyperthermia has been employed as an adjunct to radiotherapy for many patients with advanced or recurrent disease. Most of the available data concern patients with superficial lesions that are heated with external microwave applicators (PEREZ et al. 1983, 1989). One limitation of these external applicators is the lack of ability to adequately heat lesions that have a tumor thickness of greater than 3 cm. The potential advantages for the use of interstitial hyperthermia for these large lesions are better uniformity of heat within the tumor volume, improved thermometry, and better sparing of normal tissue (COSSET et al. 1984; COUGHLIN et al. 1983; EMAMI et al. 1984; JOSEPH et al. 1981; MANNING et al. 1982; MILLER et al. 1978; VORA et al. 1982).

The purpose of this report is to evaluate response rates, prognostic factors, and complication rates for patients with recurrent pelvic tumors that are accessible to interstitial implantation.

30.2 Materials and Methods

Between October 1982 and December 1989 a total of 63 patients with biopsy-proven malignancies were treated following a prospective phase I/II study at the Radiation Oncology Center, Mallinckrodt Institute of Radiology, Washington University Medical Center, with interstitial hyperthermia and radiotherapy.

Entry criteria for this study were biopsy-proven recurrence in a site previously treated with irradiation and a life expectancy of at least 3 months. Informed consent was obtained after the nature of the study was fully explained.

This report is an analysis of a subset of 14 patients with pelvic tumors. There were five males and nine females with a mean age of 65 years. Table 30.1 summarizes the tumor characteristics by primary site, histology, and maximum diameter of the recurrent lesion. All patients had been treated to the site of recurrent disease with combinations of irradiation, chemotherapy, and surgery (Table 30.2).

Patients were treated to the site of recurrence with interstitial thermoradiotherapy. Two hyperthermia treatments of 60 min each were given. The first hyperthermia treatment was given prior to the insertion of the iridium-192 sources and the second

Table 30.1. Tumor characteristics

Variables	No. of patients	(%)
Treatment site:		
Cervix	5	(36)
Uterus/endometrium	3	(21)
Bladder	2	(14)
Rectum/rectosigmoid	2	(14)
Vagina	1	(7)
Unknown	1	(7)
Histology:		
Squamous cell	7	(50)
Adenocarcinoma	5	(36)
Transitional cell	2	(14)
Average maximum diameter (cm):		
≤2	2	(14)
2.1–4	6	(43)
4.1–6	5	(36)
6.1–8	0	(0)
>8	1	(7)

P.W. GRIGSBY, M.D., Associate Professor; B. EMAMI, M.D.; Radiation Oncology Center, Mallinckrodt Institute of Radiology, Washington University School of Medicine, 510 S. Kingshighway, Box 8224, St. Louis, MO 63110, USA

Table 30.2. Prior therapy

Therapy	No.
RT only	6
Radical resection only	4
Excisional biopsy + RT	1
Radical resection + RT	1
Wide excision + RT + chemo.	1
Radical resection + RT + chemo.	1

was given immediately following the removal of the iridium-192 sources.

Interstitial irradiation was administered using iridium-192 seeds in ribbons or wires. Catheter placement was usually performed with a 1-cm spacing. The mean dose delivered with the interstitial irradiation was 37.12 Gy.

Interstitial microwave hyperthermia was delivered using multiple coaxial antennae (Clini-Therm Corporation, Dallas, Texas) placed into the 16 gauge plastic catheters that were also utilized to deliver the interstitial irradiation. Each antennae was driven at 915 MHz using a continuous wave source (915-MHz Multichannel Generator Mark IX, Clini-Therm Corporation, Dallas, Texas) powered independently with separate coherently driven channels. The mean number of antennae was nine, with a range of 4–18 depending on the volume of tumor. An example of 9 catheters is shown in Fig. 30.1a. Additional catheters for thermometry were placed both centrally and on the lateral margins of the tumor.

The goal of the interstitial hyperthermia was to achieve a minimum tumor temperature of 42.5°–43°C for 60 min (Fig. 30.1b, c). The maximum temperature for each sensor during the steady state was recorded. The location of the maximum temperature was determined by mapping along the catheter track during the initial heating stage. The temperature was recorded every 2 min until the desired temperature equilibrium was achieved. Temperature mapping was performed throughout the tumor volume. The mapping procedure was repeated at 10-min intervals during the treatment.

Interstitial thermoradiotherapy toxicity was scored by the grading system shown in Table 30.3. A toxicity was considered acute if it occurred within 90 days following the start of treatment. Toxicity was considered late if its initial occurrence was greater than 90 days.

Tumor response was evaluated by the criteria shown in Table 30.4. Tumor control was defined as

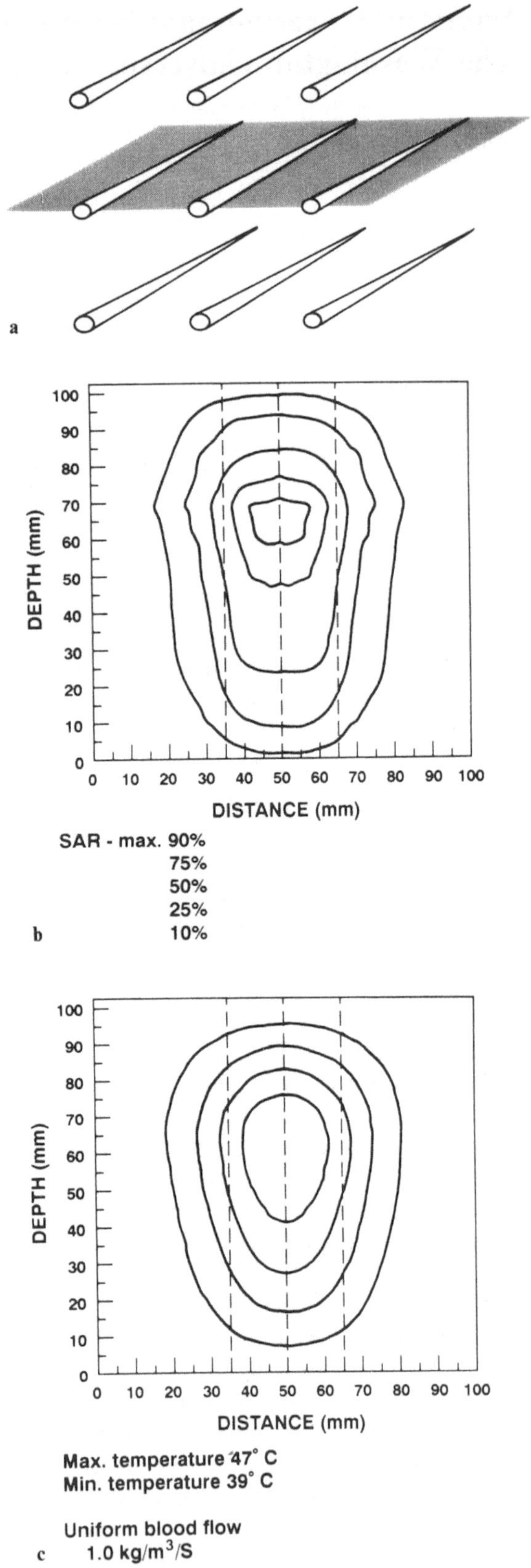

Fig. 30.1. a Array of 9 catheters for interstitial thermoradiotherapy. **b** SAR distribution of the inner plane of catheters in **a**. **c** Temperature distribution of the inner plane of catheters in **a**

Table 30.3. Toxicities score

Grade	No sequelae
Grade I	Mild, self-correcting, sequelae with normal tissue effects noted but only conservative intervention required (superficial blisters, mucositis, etc.)
Grade II	Complications, moderate impairment (deep burn, ulceration, soft tissue necrosis, pain lasting more than 24 h) requiring intensive outpatient care and/or narcotic analgesics
Grade III	Severe complications requiring hospitalization and/or surgical intervention (fistulas, extensive soft tissue, or bone necrosis)
Grade IV	Fatal or life-threatening complications

Table 30.4. Standard response categories used for scoring

Complete response	Total tumor regression for 30 days or longer
Partial response	≥50% tumor regression for 30 days or longer
Stable	No evidence of any response
Progressive disease	Increase in tumor size of ≥25%

"sustained complete response" until the time of last follow-up or until the patients' death.

Survival was calculated from the time of initiation of interstitial thermoradiotherapy by the method of Kaplan and Meier. Equivalency of survival curves was tested using the Wilcoxon–Breslow statistic. Multivariate analysis was performed by the Cox proportional hazards model. All patients were followed for a minimum of 3 months, with a mean follow-up of 13 months. None were lost to follow-up.

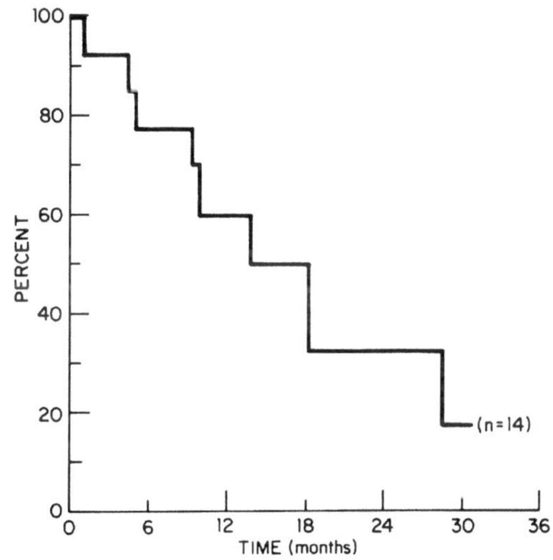

Fig. 30.2. Actuarial overall survival for all patients

30.3 Results

The actuarial overall survival for all patients is shown in Fig. 30.2. The 1- and 2-year survival rates were 61% and 34%, with a median survival of 11 months. All patients who expired did so due to uncontrolled disease at the primary site or distant metastatic disease. Six patients were alive at the time of last follow-up (1 July 1991).

A complete response was obtained in nine patients and this was maintained in five at the time of last follow-up or death as outlined in Table 30.5. The actuarial overall survival was 65% at 1 year for the nine patients achieving a complete response, compared to 50% for those not having a complete response ($P = 0.15$) (Fig. 30.3).

The probability of achieving a complete response at any time was evaluated by univariate and multivariate analysis. Possible prognostic factors that were analyzed included histology, lesion size, prior irradiation dose, interstitial irradiation dose rate, total irradiation dose, maximum temperature, and % sensors with thermal dose ≥ 30 min (Table 30.6). The univariate analysis identified lesion size ($P = 0.05$) and irradiation dose ($P = 0.04$). However, multivariate analysis identified tumor size ($P = 0.01$) and interstitial irradiation dose rate ($P = 0.04$) as significant (Table 30.7).

Acute toxicity occurred in six patients. Severe late toxicity was observed in three patients, with two developing vesicovaginal fistulas and one, an enterovaginal fistula.

Table 30.5. Clinical response and final patient status[a]

Time of evaluation	Clinical response				
	Complete response	Partial response	Stable	Progression	Not evaluable
End of treatment	3	5	4	0	2
Best response	9	2	3	0	0
At last follow-up	5	–	3	5	1

[a] Patient status at last follow-up (1 July 1991): no evidence of disease, $n=4$; alive with disease (any site), $n=2$; dead with disease (any site), $n=8$

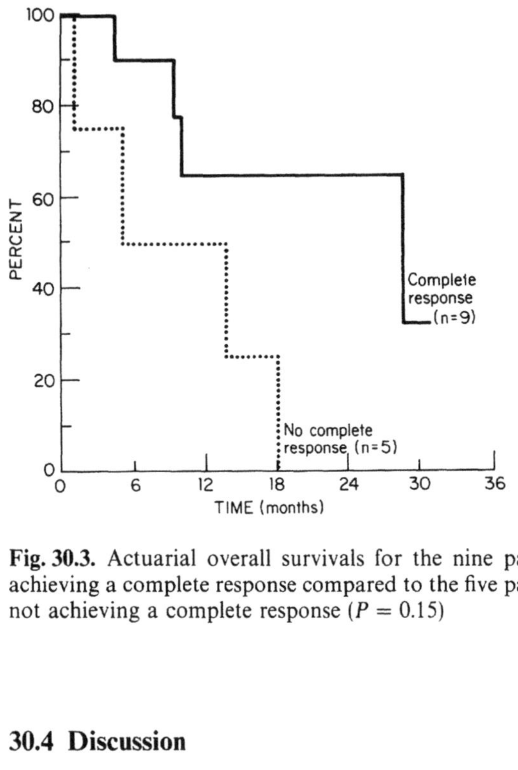

Fig. 30.3. Actuarial overall survivals for the nine patients achieving a complete response compared to the five patients not achieving a complete response ($P = 0.15$)

30.4 Discussion

Reports of patients treated with interstitial thermoradiotherapy include patients with lesions at many different sites. These reports fail to demonstrate a correlation between tumor response and tumor site (Emami et al. 1987; Lam et al. 1988; Petrovich et al. 1989; Phromratanapongse et al. 1990). It may be important to note that the impact of tumor site on the response rate may be correlated with the accessibility of the tumor for implant. Our report is concerned only with patients with recurrent pelvic tumors who would usually undergo interstitial irradiation for recurrence due to accessibility and the restriction of excessive irradiation doses to surrounding normal tissues.

Our analysis identified lesion size and total irradiation dose as significant prognostic factors for complete response. Oleson et al. (1984) and Phromratanapongse et al. (1990) have reported a significant inverse relationship between tumor size and complete response. Lam et al. (1988) and Petrovich et al. (1989) demonstrated that lesions greater than 150 cm^3 were less likely to achieve a complete response than smaller lesions. Several authors have also identified irradiation dose as a significant factor for achieving a complete response (Petrovich et al. 1989; Phromratanapongse et al. 1990). Lam et al. (1988) reported that in sites receiving 30 Gy the complete response rate was 20%, compared to 60% for 40 Gy and 82% for those receiving more than 40 Gy ($P = 0.02$).

We report a relatively high complication rate. However, this must be viewed in light of the site and prior treatment received by the patients. Other authors have reported an overall complication rate of 20%–50%, with a severe complication rate of 5%–20% (Cosset et al. 1985; Petrovich et al. 1989; Phromratanapongse et al. 1990; Vora et al. 1982, 1988). A maximum temperature of 45°C or greater has been reported to correlate with a high complication rate. But, our analysis identified only interstitial irradiation dose rate and lack of control of the lesion as factors associated with the development of complications.

30.5 Conclusion

Interstitial thermoradiotherapy for recurrent pelvic tumors is feasible primarily due to the accessibility of these lesions. We have demonstrated an acceptable complete response rate but with an accompanying high toxicity rate. The value of interstitial thermoradiotherapy over interstitial irradiation alone needs to be tested in a prospective randomized trial. However, our data suggest that total irradiation dose may be more important in achieving a

Table 30.6. Univariate analysis: local control rates at 1 and 2 years following interstitial hyperthermia and radiotherapy

Parameter	Best response #CR/#total	Local controls #LC/#total	LC rates (actuarial) 1 yr	2 yr
Type of lesion:				
New	0/1	0/1	100%	0%
Persistent	1/2	0/2	0%	–[a]
Recurrent	8/11	5/11	55%	55%
Average maximum diameter:				
≤2 cm	2/2	2/2	100%	–
2.1–4 cm	5/6	3/6	67%	67%
4.1–6 cm	2/5	0/5	20%	0%
>6 cm	0/1	0/1	0%	–
Prior RT doses (cGy):				
No RT	4/4	3/4	100%	100%
≤4000	1/1	1/1	–	–
4001–5000	1/3	0/3	0%	–
>5000	3/6	1/6	33%	–
Dose rate interstitial RT (cGy/h):				
31–50	4/9	3/9	44%	–
>50	4/4	2/4	75%	75%
Maximum temperature:				
≤43 °C	0/1	0/1	0%	–
43.1 °–45 °C	6/7	4/7	57%	57%
>45 °C	3/6	1/6	50%	25%
% Sensors with thermal dose ≥30 min:				
≤25%	0/1	0/1	0%	–
26%–50%	2/2	1/2	50%	–
51%–75%	2/2	1/2	50%	–
>75%	5/9	3/9	55%	42%

CR, complete response; LC, local control
[a] No patients in study at this point

Table 30.7. Multivariate analysis: predictors of complete response after interstitial hyperthermia and radiotherapy

Variable	Improvement Chi-square	Improvement P value	Coefficient	Exp. (coeff.)
Tumor size	6.035	0.014	1.0977	3.4925
Dose rate	4.219	0.040	−0.3937	0.6746
Prior RT dose	0.779	0.337	−0.007	0.9993
Total RT dose	0.841	0.359	−0.0009	0.9991

complete response than interstitial hyperthermia as delivered and measured in this study.

References

Cosset JM, Dutreix J, Defour J, Janoray P, Damia E, Haie C, Clarke D (1984) Combined interstitial hyperthermia and brachytherapy: Institute Gustave-Roussy technique and preliminary results. Int J Radiat Oncol Biol Phys 10: 307–312

Cosset JM, Dutreix J, Haie C, Gerbaulelt A, Janoray P, Dewars JA (1985) Interstitial thermoradiotherapy: a technical and clinical study of 29 implantations performed at the Institute Gustave-Roussy. Int J Hyperthermia 1: 3–13

Coughlin CT, Douple EB, Strohbehn JW, Eaton WL, Trembly BS, Wong TZ (1983) Interstitial hyperthermia in combination with brachytherapy. Radiology 148: 285–288

Emami B, Marks JE, Perez CA, Nussbaum GH, Leybovich L, Von Gerichten D (1984) Interstitial thermoradiotherapy in the treatment of recurrent/residual malignant tumors. Am J Clin Oncol 7: 699–704

Emami B, Perez CA, Leybovich L, Straube W, Von Gerichten D (1987) Interstitial thermoradiotherapy in the treatment of malignant tumors. Int J Hyperthermia 3: 107–118

Joseph C, Astrahan M, Lipsett J, Archambeau J, Forell B (1981) Interstitial hyperthermia and interstitial iridium-192 implantation: technique and preliminary results. Int J Radiat Oncol Biol Phys 7: 827–833

Lam K, Astrahan M, Langholz B, Jepson J, Cohen D, Luxton G, Petrovich Z (1988) Interstitial thermoradiotherapy for recurrent or persistent tumours. Int J Hyperthermia 4: 259–266

Manning M, Cetas T, Miller R, Oleson J, Connor W, Gerner E (1982) Clinical hyperthermia: results of a phase I trial employing hyperthermia alone or in combination with external beam or interstitial radiotherapy. Cancer 49: 205–261

Miller RC, Leith JT, Veomett RC, Gerner EW (1978) Effects of interstitial irradiation alone, or in combination with localized hyperthermia on the response of a mouse mammary tumor. J Radiat Res 19: 175–180

Oleson JR, Manning MR, Sim DA et al. (1984) A review of the University of Arizona human clinical hyperthermia experience. Front Radiat Ther Oncol 18: 136–143

Perez CA, Nussbaum GH, Emami B, Von Gerichten D (1983) Clinical results of irradiation combined with local hyperthermia. Cancer 52: 1597–1603

Perez CA, Gillespie B, Pajak T, Hornback NB, Emami B, Rubin P (1989) Quality assurance problems in clinical hyperthermia and their impact on therapeutic outcome: a report by the Radiation Therapy Oncology Group. Int J Radiat Oncol Biol Phys 16: 551–558

Petrovich Z, Langholz B, Lam K, Luxton G, Cohen D, Jepson J, Astrahan M (1989) Interstitial microwave hyperthermia combined with iridium-192 radiotherapy for recurrent tumors. Am J Clin Oncol 12: 264–268

Phromratanapongse P, Seegenschmiedt MH, Karlsson UL, Brady L, Sauer R, Herbst M, Fietkau R (1990) Initial results of phase I/II interstitial thermoradiotherapy for primary advanced and local recurrent tumors. Am J Clin Oncol 13: 259–268

Vora N, Forell B, Joseph C, Lipsett J, Archambeau J (1982) Interstitial implant with interstitial hyperthermia. Cancer 50: 2518–2523

Vora N, Luk KH, Forell B et al. (1988) Interstitial local current field hyperthermia for advanced cancers of the cervix. Endocurietherapy/Hypermia Oncol 4: 97–106

31 Interstitial Thermoradiotherapy for Pelvic Tumors: a Cooperative Phase 1–2 Study

M.H. SEEGENSCHMIEDT, R. SAUER, C. MIYAMOTO, and L.W. BRADY

CONTENTS

31.1 Introduction

Malignancies localized in the pelvis are characterized by an increasing incidence and a high mortality due to local tumor progression. In 1990 the cancer facts and figures of the American Cancer Society indicated an estimated 45 000 new cases of and 7600 deaths from rectal cancer, 46 500 new cases of and 10 000 deaths from uterine (cervix uteri and corpus/endometrium) cancer, 49 000 new cases of and 9700 deaths from bladder cancer, and 106 000 new cases of and 30 000 deaths from prostate cancer (American Cancer Society 1990).

Only if these pelvic malignancies are detected in an early, still localized stage does the 5-year survival rate reach 80%–90%; after the tumors have spread regionally, to involve adjacent organs or lymph nodes, the survival rate decreases to 30%–50%. Theoretically, early detection of cancer could improve the overall survival, but better detection techniques have already been introduced and despite this more than 50% of all pelvic malignancies have spread locally at the time of diagnosis. An alternative means of reducing the relapse and death rates would be improved control of locoregional disease. It has been shown that the number of patients who would potentially benefit from better local control is high, given that the percentage figures for local failure as a major cause of death are 30% for colorectal, 60% for uterine cervix and corpus, 54% for bladder, and 61% for prostate cancer. Improved locoregional treatment of these cancers might be achieved by combined application of hyperthermia (HT), radiotherapy (RT), and/or chemotherapy (ChT) (RUBIN and CARTER 1976; KAPP 1986).

A typical clinical situation for cervical carcinoma may illustrate the current therapeutic dilemma. Analysis of 1054 tumors of the uterine cervix clearly demonstrated that control of the tumor in the pelvis was crucial to survival in all stages (PEREZ et al. 1988). Surgery, external beam RT, or ChT alone or in combination still fail to sufficiently control advanced disease with intrapelvic spread or locoregional recurrence (EVANS et al. 1971; PASASVINICHAI et al. 1978; THOMAS et al. 1984; SPANOS et al. 1987, 1989; THIGPEN et al. 1987; JOBSEN et al. 1989; LAWHEAD et al. 1989; SOMMERS et al. 1989). Interstitial and intracavitary RT may somewhat improve the local control for selected cervical tumors (EVANS et al. 1971; ARISTIZABAL et al. 1983; PUTHAWALA et al. 1985; MARTINEZ et al. 1985; PEREZ et al. 1985; HILARIS and HENSCHKE 1985; SYED et al. 1986; PIERQUIN et al. 1988), but all current treatment approaches are still disappointing. Similar unfavorable therapeutic scenarios hold for most other pelvic malignancies, including rectal, bladder, and prostatic cancer. For this reason, it is necessary to explore other treatment modalities.

M.H. SEEGENSCHMIEDT, M.D.; R. SAUER, M.D., Professor; Strahlentherapeutische Klinik der Universität Erlangen-Nürnberg, Universitätsstraße 27, W-8520 Erlangen, Germany; C. MIYAMOTO, M.D.; L.W. BRADY, M.D.; Department of Radiation Oncology and Nuclear Medicine, Hahnemann University, Broad & Vine Streets, MS 200, Philadelphia, PA 19102-1198, USA

In many in vitro, in vivo, and clinical trials the application of HT as an adjunct to external beam or interstitial RT (IRT) has enhanced the therapeutic ratio, tumor response, and duration of response without increasing treatment toxicity (OVERGAARD 1981, 1985, 1989; LEEPER 1985; DEWHIRST et al. 1982; OLESON et al. 1988). Moreover, thermotherapy is based on a sound biological (OVERGAARD 1981; LEEPER 1985; OLESON et al. 1988) and physiological rationale (SONG 1984, 1989; REINHOLD and ENDRICH 1986). Recent clinical implementations take advantage of newly developed heating (HAND 1990; HYNYNEN 1990) and thermometry devices (CETAS 1985; SAMULSKI 1988).

Compared to external heat delivery, the available interstitial HT (IHT) techniques offer several theoretical and practical advantages: (a) nearly all brachytherapy and "internal" heating methods can be easily combined with each other without major modifications of each technique; (b) even deep-seated implantable tumors can be effectively heated; (c) the power deposition to the tumor site can be precisely confined; (d) a differential and more uniform heating of the target volume is possible, which reduces the toxicity to surrounding normal tissues; (e) the multiple interstitial probes allow three-dimensional thermometry sampling, which can be used for precise feedback control. Recently the technical and clinical quality assurance procedures have reached a high standard, so that multicenter clinical trials now seem warranted.

Our phase 1–2 study aimed to examine the technical and clinical feasibility and efficacy of 915-MHz microwave (MW) IHT in patients with localized primary (PRIM), persistent (PERS), recurrent (REC), and/or metastatic (MET) tumors. Analogous to previous reports on head and neck tumors (SEEGENSCHMIEDT et al. 1990a, this volume, Chap. 28), this report addresses IHT for malignancies in the pelvis, which were managed with the same treatment rationale and clinical approach. Our evaluation includes the assessment of initial and long-term tumor response, acute and late treatment toxicity of the combined treatment regimen, and possibly the identification of prognostic factors.

31.2 Material and Methods

31.2.1 Patient and Tumor Parameters

At the Department of Radiation Oncology of the University of Erlangen-Nürnberg (FRG) and the Department of Radiation Oncology and Nuclear Medicine, Hahnemann University, Philadelphia (USA), a total of 26 patients with localized malignancies in the pelvis, including PRIM, PERS, REC, and MET tumors, were treated in a phase 1–2 study from January 1986 through October 1991. The eligibility criteria of the study included a Karnofsky score $\geq 70\%$, a minimum estimated survival ≥ 6 months, medical conditions allowing the use of general anesthesia, accessible and implantable *localized* tumors, and signed informed consent. The potential candidates had either undergone a surgical dissection of pelvic lymph nodes and/or had been subjected to incomplete tumor excision or had a persistent tumor mass after adjuvant therapy (RT or ChT with or without prior surgery); thus all patients were considered at "high risk" for locoregional relapse within the pelvis. Patients with metastatic disease were eligible only if they presented with severe symptoms (pain, ulceration, bleeding), but were otherwise in good physical condition.

Table 31.1 summarizes all relevant patient, tumor, pretreatment, and follow-up data. The four different tumor classes were defined according to the extent of their prior treatment: (a) all PRIM lesions had undergone incomplete surgery, but previously had not received RT; (b) all PERS lesions presented as macroscopic tumors after a just completed treatment course with either external beam RT or ChT; (c) the REC and MET lesions have been previously treated with various modalities including surgery, interstitial or external beam RT, and ChT. Thus most PRIM/PRES lesions received IHT-IRT in conjunction with the first external beam RT treatment, whereas most REC/MET lesions had received prior external beam RT in the range of 40–90 Gy (mean: 54 Gy)[present in 18 of 26 patients (69%)]. Prior surgery had been applied in 18 (69%) and prior ChT in nine (35%) patients. The specific distribution of tumor and treatment parameters for PRIM/PERS lesions versus REC/MET lesions is illustrated in Table 31.2. PRIM/PERS lesions presented with significantly ($P < 0.05$) smaller tumor volumes and received a significantly ($P < 0.05$) higher radiation dose than REC/MET lesions; however, none of the important thermal performance parameters were significantly different between the two groups.

A complete histopathological workup always preceded IRT and IHT. The tumor extension was assessed clinically and with radiographs, ultrasound, CT, or NMR imaging methods; tumor

Table 31.1. Summary of patient and tumor data

Patients:	Sex:	Females 20 (77%); males 6 (23%)	
	Age:	Mean: 59.2/range: 32–82/median: 58 years	
Lesions:	Tumor class:	3 (12%) primary (PRIM); 7 (27%) persistent (PERS); 10 (38%) recurrent (REC); 6 (23%) metastatic (MET)	
	Tumor site:	8 (31%)	Cervix uteri
		6 (23%)	Colon/rectum
		4 (15%)	Vagina
		3 (12%)	Anal canal
		2 (8%)	Ovaries
	Each	1 (4%)	Urethra, groin, presacral region
	Histology:	13 (50%)	Squamous cell carcinoma
		12 (46%)	Adenocarcinoma
		1 (4%)	Soft tissue sarcoma
	Grading:	2 (8%)	G1
		18 (69%)	G2
		6 (23%)	G3
	T stage:	7 (27%)	T2/rT2
		12 (46%)	T3/rT3
		2 (8%)	T4/rT4
		5 (19%)	Unknown T
	Volume C:	mean: 58.9 cm^3 ± 48.7 (SD)/range: 12.0–240.0 cm^3	
	Diameter D:	mean: 3.8 cm ± 1.0 (SD)/range: 2.3–7.0 cm	
Pretreatment:		18 (69%)	Surgical resection
		18 (69%)	Radiation therapy/prior RT dose: mean: 54 Gy ± 13(SD)/range: 40–90 Gy
		9 (35%)	Adjuvant chemotherapy
Follow up at Dec. 1991:	Overall group: mean: 23 months/range: 5–65 months/median: 25 months		
		PRIM/PERS lesions:	*REC/MET lesions:*
	Mean:	32 months	18 months
	Range:	10–65 months	5–34 months
	Median:	31 months	15 months
	1-y-s:	80%	75%
	2-y-s:	80%	56%

1-y-s, 1-year survival; 2-y-s, 2-year survival

size was calculated as the cuboid volume using the formula $V(C) = a \times b \times c$. The lesions were grouped in four categories according to the tumor size (see Table 31.3). Most tumors were well localized and presented with volumes $\leq 80\ cm^3$; however, three of 26 lesions (12%), including two lesions involving skin and subcutaneous tissue in the groin and presacral region, respectively, had very large volumes of $\geq 150\ cm^3$.

31.2.2 Interstitial Radiotherapy

In some cases (all PRIM lesions) IRT-IHT was applied as the first step in the treatment course after incomplete tumor surgery and/or pelvic lymphadenectomy, and was later followed by external beam RT after a 1- to 2-week break; however, in most instances IRT-IHT was applied as the second step after completion of the external beam RT and/or ChT treatment course (most PERS, REC, and MET lesions); five REC/MET lesions that had previously been irradiated with a dose of 70 Gy received only IRT-IHT without additional external beam RT. While all PRIM/PERS lesions were scheduled to receive 70–80 Gy i.e., 50 Gy with external beam RT to the tumor bed and the draining pelvic lymph nodes (possibly including the para-aortic nodes) and 20–30 Gy as a local "boost" with iridium-192 IRT at 50 cGy/h, all previously irradiated REC/MET lesions similarly received IRT but only reduced or no further external beam RT to avoid a cumulative RT dose of ≥ 100 Gy. Therefore the total (PRT + IRT) dose was significantly ($P < 0.05$) different between PRIM/PERS and REC/MET lesions (Table 31.2).

Table 31.2. Distribution of specific tumor and treatment data and different tumor classes

Parameters	Primary/ persistent 10 (38%)	Recurrent/ metastatic 16 (62%)
1. Volume ($C = a \times b \times c$)		
< 40 cm^3	6 (60%)	4 (25%)
40–<80 cm^3	3 (30%)	6 (38%)
≥ 80 cm^3	1 (10%)	6 (38%)
Mean/range:	40.4/12–108*	81.1/24–240 cm^3
2. Total RT dose (Gy)		
< 50 Gy	1 (10%)	8 (50%)
50–<70 Gy	2 (20%)	8 (50%)
≥ 70 Gy	7 (70%)	–
Mean/range:	73.2/28.8–88.5*	50.8/24.3–65.2 Gy
3. HT parameters		
a) $T\text{max}_{av}$ (°C):		
< 43°C	2 (20%)	3 (19%)
43°C–<44°C	2 (20%)	4 (25%)
≥ 44°C	6 (60%)	9 (56%)
Mean/range:	43.7/40.6–45.1	44.2/41.7–45.3
b) $T\text{mean}$ (°C):		
< 42°C	4 (40%)	7 (44%)
42°C–<43°C	6 (60%)	7 (44%)
≥ 43°C	–	2 (13%)
Mean/range:	42.0/39.7–42.9	42.1/40.4–43.4
c) $T\text{min}_{av}$ (°C):		
< 40°C	1 (10%)	4 (25%)
40°C–<41°C	4 (40%)	8 (50%)
≥ 41°C	5 (50%)	4 (25%)
Mean/range:	40.8/39.0–41.5	40.6/39.2–41.6
d) Therm. qual. (TQ):		
TQ40°C 100%	9 (90%)	11 (69%)
Mean:	93.8%	95.2%
TQ41°C 100%	5 (50%)	5 (31%)
Mean:	86.7%	74.6%
TQ42°C 100%	–	–
Mean:	53.8%	49.6%
TQ43°C 100%	–	–
Mean:	26.0%	31.2%

* Difference statistically significant ($P < 0.05$)

The typical treatment schedule, flow chart of procedures, and quality assurance measures have been reported earlier (Seegenschmiedt et al. 1989, 1990a; Fietkau et al. 1991) and are presented in Chap. 28 of this book. Standard brachytherapy and implantation techniques were applied (Puthawala et al. 1982; Martinez et al. 1985; Perez et al. 1985; Syed et al. 1986; Pierquin et al. 1988).

31.2.3 Interstitial Hyperthermia

Interstitial HT was delivered with two similar commercially available 915-MHz microwave (MW) systems (University of Erlangen-Nürnberg: Lund/Buchler Hyperthermia System 4010, Lund Science AB, Sweden; Hahnemann University Philadelphia: Clini-Therm Mark VI and Mark IX Systems, Clini-Therm Corp., Dallas, Texas, USA). Up to 16 miniature semiflexible coaxial dipole antennae can be simultaneously used and individually powered through four independent "channels" of two generators, each with 200 W power output. Power balancing and individual steering capabilities of each "channel" and simultaneous survey of up to 42 thermometry sensors are controlled either manually or automatically with feedback control by a personal computer. Specific details of our IHT technique, clinical practice, and quality assurance procedures have been reported previously (Seegenschmiedt et al. 1989, 1990a, 1992).

Depending on the target volume, an average of 11–12 (range 4–24) interstitial probes were implanted per lesion; of these an average of 7–8 (range 2–16) were used for heating. The distribution of the inserted MW antennae was determined by well-established IRT guidelines and anatomical conditions, with the exception of some additional probes implanted for invasive thermometry. Figure 31.1 demonstrates a typical plastic template implant in a female for treatment of a perineal and distal rectal recurrence; 12 of the 16 inserted catheters are used to house MW antennae and four are loaded with multipoint thermometry probes.

At a typical insertion depth of 60–70 mm the implemented incoherently driven MW antennae provide a nearly ellipsoidal heating pattern with 50–60 mm longitudinal (30 mm per lobe) and 15–20 mm axial length when tested in an appropriate static muscle equivalent phantom (Chou et al. 1984). However, several physical parameters have been identified which can alter this typical heating pattern: coherent/incoherent mode of activation, constructive/destructive interference, change of insertion depth, spacing and specific distribution of antennae, and individual tissue conditions, e.g., thickness and position of tissue interfaces like fat–muscle and muscle–bone interfaces (Stauffer et al. 1989; James et al. 1989; Chan et al. 1989; Ryan et al. 1990; Cosset 1990).

31.2.4 IHT-IRT Treatment Schedule

In our treatment protocol we prescribed *two IHT sessions* at 41°–44°C for 45–60 min; one IHT session was applied before implantation and one following removal of iridium-192 sources. Of 26

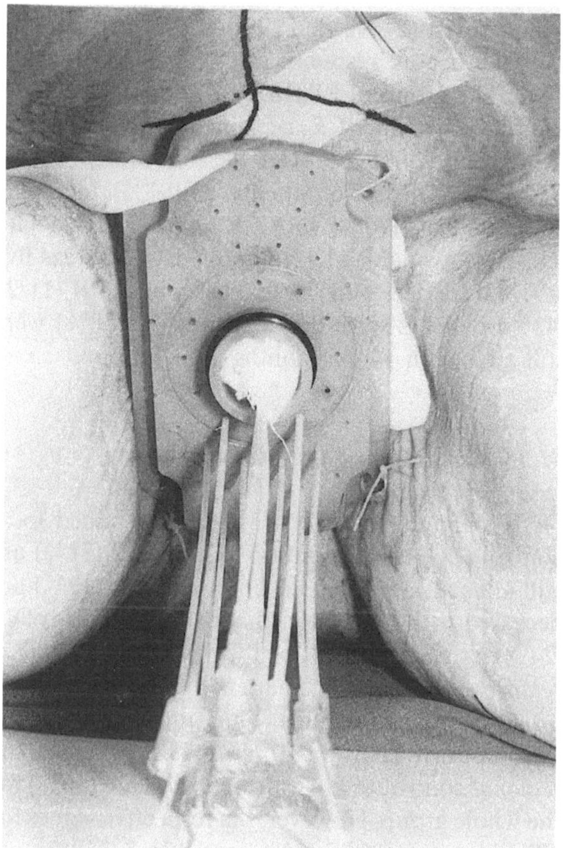

a

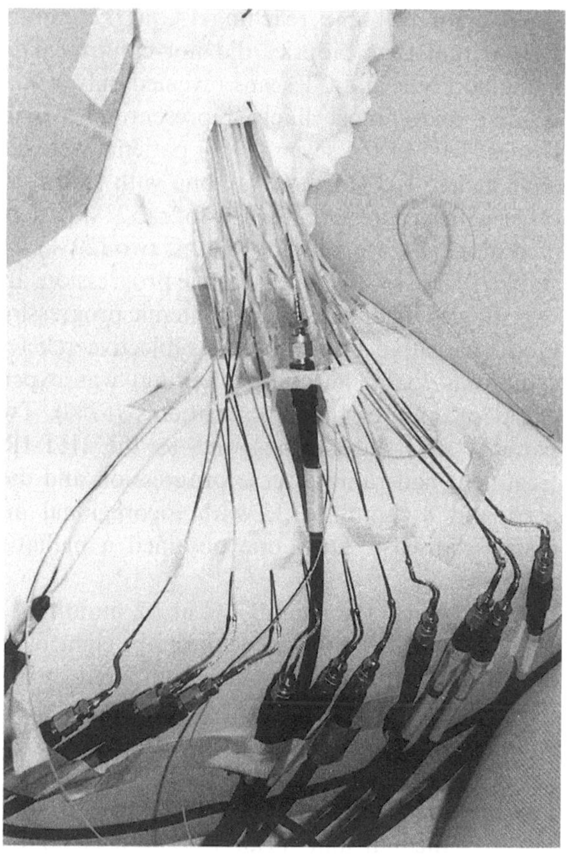

b

lesions, 18 (69%) received IHT twice, but for technical and clinical reasons seven (27%) received only one IHT treatment, either before (five cases) or after (two cases) IRT. One lesion in the presacral region received six IHT sessions combined with external beam RT only. Thus a total of 49 IHT sessions were evaluated. Vital signs (pulse rate, blood pressure, and body temperature) were continuously monitored during IHT treatment, with all patients being treated awake during the whole treatment session.

31.2.5 Invasive Thermometry

Interstitial HT provides a unique opportunity to obtain multiple "invasive" thermometry readings with a close spatial and temporal distribution throughout the treatment. Integrated thermometry systems were used: the gallium–arsenide fiberoptic system (Clini-Therm Mark VI/IX) and the minimally perturbing thermistor system (Lund/Buchler System 4010). Possible limitations and artifacts of these systems have been reviewed by SAMULSKI (1988). Details of our invasive thermometry practice have been reported previously (SEEGENSCHMIEDT et al. 1989, 1990a, 1992): usually our procedures followed all RTOG quality assurance guidelines (DEWHIRST et al. 1990; EMAMI et al. 1991). An average of four to five (range: one to eight) thermometry probes were used for truly interstitial (in between MW antennae) thermometry. An average of seven to eight (range: 3–14) intratumoral sensors and an average of nine (range 3–21) sensors were employed in normal tissue. At least one sensor array was placed close to the tumor center. If possible, during steady-state conditions thermal mapping (TM), SAR (specific absorption rate), and thermal washout measurements were performed.

The following thermal parameters were recorded during each IHT session: (a) the minimum mean and best 10-min (peak) tumor temperature ($T\min_{av}$, $T\min_{10}$); (b) the maximum mean and best 10-min (peak) tumor temperature ($T\max_{av}$, $T\max_{10}$); (c) the overall mean tumor temperatures (Tmean); (d) the thermal equivalent minutes (TEM) (SAPARETO and DEWEY 1984); (e) the thermal quality (TQ), calculated as the ratio of tumor sensors above temperature Tindex to all tumor sensors (TQ40°C,

◀

Fig. 31.1 a, b. Typical plastic template implant for the treatment of perineal and distal rectal recurrence; 12 of the 16 implanted catheters are used to house MW antennae and four are loaded with multipoint thermometry probes

TQ41°C, and TQ – 42°C), and (e) a temperature–time matrix of all tumor sensors during steady state with assessment of T_{90}, T_{50}, and T_{20} values reflecting the 90%, 50%, and 20% values of all tumor sensor measurements. For further analysis only the thermal parameters of the *best IHT session* were considered.

31.2.6 Treatment Endpoints and Statistics

The current evaluation was performed at 31 December 1991, with a median follow-up (FU) of 25 months (mean: 23 months, range 5–65 months). The WHO criteria were applied to define the *local* tumor response: complete remission (CR: total disappearance of tumor), partial remission (PR: more than 50% reduction), no change (NC: 50% or less reduction or 25% or less increase), and progressive disease (PD: more than 25% increase) (World Health Organisation 1979). *Initial response* was analyzed for all 26 lesions at 3 months' FU. *Long-term response* was determined for 21 of 26 (81%) lesions at 12 months' FU or longer. Long-term local tumor control was defined as a "sustained complete response" until the last FU or the patient's death (Emami et al. 1987). Five patients (16%) did not reach 12 months' FU. Tumor recurrences were recorded as occurring within (local) or outside (regional) the treated target volume. Acute side-effects and long-term complications were graded as "0" for no treatment sequelae, "1" for minor complications (superficial blisters, mucositis, erythema) not requiring special medical care, "2" for complications (deep burn, ulceration) requiring medical care of long duration, application of antibiotics, and special dressing of skin or mucosal defects, "3" for major complications (tissue breakdown, fistulas) requiring surgical intervention and "4" for fatal complications. The statistical values were determined with the Student *t* and Fisher exact tests (Fisher and Yates 1963). All survival data were assessed with the actuarial method (Kaplan and Meier 1958). None of the patients were lost to FU.

31.3 Results

31.3.1 Initial Tumor Response

The assessment of initial tumor response at 3 months' FU revealed CR in 17 of 26 (65%) lesions, PR in seven (27%), and NC or PD in two (8%); thus the overall response rate (CR + PR) reached 92%. The group of PRIM/PERS lesions yielded a significantly higher CR, i.e., nine of ten (90%), than the group of REC/MET lesions (8/16: 50%) ($P < 0.05$). Of the 26 patients, 21 (81%), including 16/17 patients (94%) with CR and 5/7 (71%) with PR, were available at 12 months' FU, whereas five (19%) were deceased. At 31 December 1991, 11/26 (42%) patients were deceased and 15 (58%) were still alive with 14–65 months' FU.

31.3.2 Long-Term Tumor Control

Of 17 patients with CR, 15 (88%) sustained local control (LC) at 12 months' FU, and 12 (71%) are still alive at last FU; two other patients (12%) are deceased with LC within the first year. Four of 17 (24%) patients with CR or LC developed a *regional relapse outside*, and one patient (6%) a *local relapse inside* the treated volume. Thus, at the last FU the *local* control rate was 16/26 (62%), whereas the *regional* control rate was lower, at 12/26 (46%) for the whole group. However, the respective values for CR lesions are 16/17 (94%) and 12/17 (71%).

One of seven patients with PR (14%) developed a slow tumor response reaching LC at 12 months' FU; at that time biopsies did not confirm viable malignant cells and CT scans revealed only a small residual mass most likely representing scarring tissues. Two of the seven (29%) patients were still alive at last FU (14 months), one with stable, the other with progressive disease; four (57%) patients died at 11, 14, 16, and 30 months; two (29%) had stable disease locally, but systemic progression, and two showed locoregional and systemic progression. Good palliative response and subjective relief of symptoms (pain, infection, bleeding) was experienced by four of the seven patients (57%). Two patients who did not respond to the IHT-IRT treatment had rapid disease progression and died at 5 and 8 months' FU with locoregional and systemic disease. Only one obtained a palliative response.

In summary, the overall LC at 12 months' FU was 16/26 (62%). LC was achieved in eight of ten (80%) PRIM/PERS lesions as compared to 8/16 (50%) REC/MET lesions ($P < 0.05$), and patients with initial CR ("responders") had a higher LC rate, i.e., 15/17 (88%), than did those with non-CR lesions ("nonresponders") (1/9: 11%) ($P < 0.05$). At last FU median and mean FU were 25 and 23 months (range 5–65 months); the survival difference between CR (median: 31, mean: 29 months, SD ± 14) and non-CR lesions (median: 14, mean: 8 months) was significant (Fig. 31.2). This difference was also observed for PRIM/PERS (median: 31, mean: 33 months, SD ± 17) compared to REC/MET lesions (median: 16, mean: 18 months, SD ± 0.9) (Fig. 31.3)

31.3.3 Treatment Toxicity

Eight of the 26 patients (31%) experienced *acute side-effects*: grade 1 (pain, blister) in four cases (15%), grade 2 (ulceration, fistula, deep burn) in three (15%), and grade 3 (soft tissue breakdown) in one (4%). Pain and adverse side-effects, which limited the power deposition during IHT treatment, were observed in seven (27%) patients; in some instances this was caused by the heating sources being positioned too close to bony structures or by antenna slippage during treatment exposing the skin to higher temperatures. Most acute side-effects subsided within 4–12 weeks after completion of therapy. Seven (27%) patients experienced *long-term complications* including slowly healing ulcers, fistulas of the vesicovaginal and/or rectovaginal wall, and soft tissue necroses which required antibiotic and antiseptic medication and sometimes even surgical debridement: resolution of these treatment sequelae occurred in a mean period of 6 months (range 4–12 months). Two patients received reconstructive surgery; three patients underwent hyperbaric oxygen treatment for 4–10 weeks

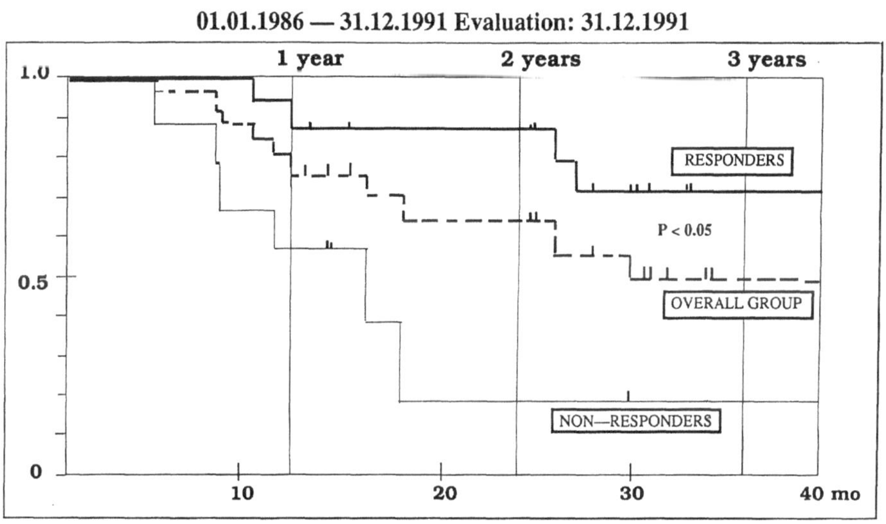

Fig. 31.2. Kaplan-Meier actuarial survival of patients with pelvic tumors treated with IHT-IRT: comparison of 17 complete ("*responders*") versus nine partial or nonresponders ("*nonresponders*"); the *ticks* indicate censored lesions (patients alive in FU)

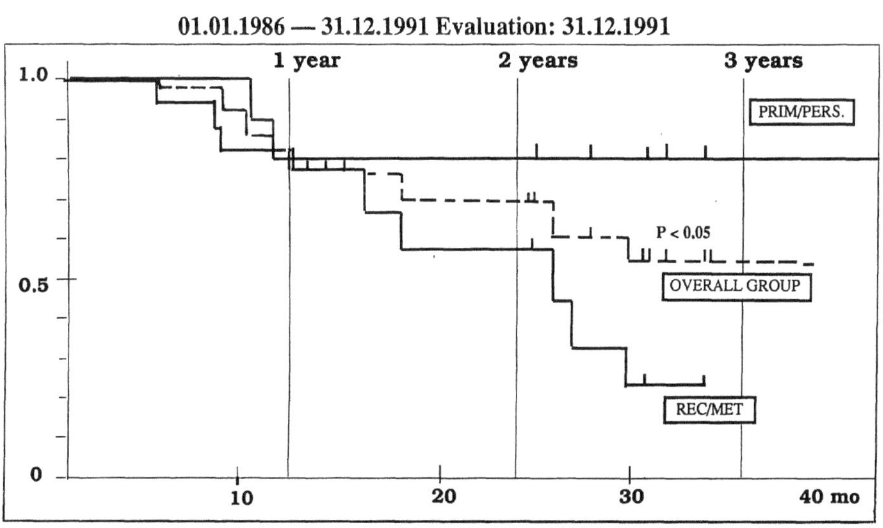

Fig. 31.3. Kaplan-Meier actuarial survival of patients with pelvic tumors treated with IHT-IRT: comparison of ten primary and persistent (*PRIM/PERS*) versus 16 recurrent and metastatic (*REC/MET*) lesions; the *ticks* indicate censored lesions (patients alive in FU)

due to soft tissue necroses. We observed an increased complication rate in lesions which exceeded $T\max_{av} \geq 44°C$ or $T\max_{(10)} \geq 45°C$: complications were noted in respect of six of the 11 lesions (55%) which reached these "high maximum temperatures" but in only two of the remaining 15 (13%) with "lower maximum temperatures." These findings need to be confirmed in a larger series. No other tumor or treatment parameter seemed to have prognostic significance for the development of treatment toxicity.

31.3.4 Prognostic Factors

To analyze prognostic factors, CR ($n_1 = 17/26$ patients) and the long-term LC ($n_2 = 16/21$ patients) were correlated with several tumor and treatment parameters. The following parameters had no prognostic impact; age, sex, tumor location, tumor histology, tumor stage or grade, applied IRT dose, duration of the IRT treatment, number of IHT sessions, sequence of IHT-IRT and external beam RT, and some thermal parameters like thermal equivalent minutes. In contrast, the following parameters seemed to influence initial and long-term tumor control: intial CR ("responders") versus non-CR ("nonresponders"), tumor class (Fig. 31.4), tumor volume (Fig. 31.5), total RT dose (Fig. 31.6), and thermal parameters including minimum tumor temperature (Fig. 31.7) and thermal quality (TQ41°C) of heating (Fig. 31.8). However, due to the small number of patients the analysis mainly indicates statistical trends (Table 31.3).

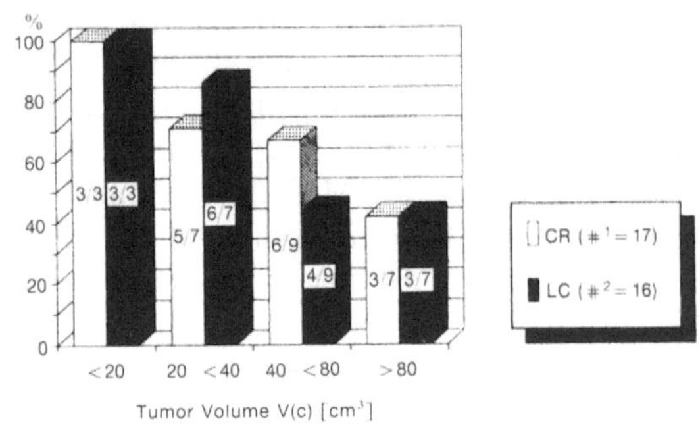

Fig. 31.5. Correlation of complete response (17 patients) and local control (16 patients) with tumor volume $V(C)$ with volumes < 20 cm³ ($n_1 = 3$), 20–< 40 cm³ ($n_2 = 7$), 40–< 80 cm³ ($n_3 = 9$), and ≥ 80 cm³ ($n_4 = 7$). The difference between lesions < 40 cm³ ($n = 10$) versus lesions ≥ 40 cm³ ($n = 16$) has a P value of 0.06

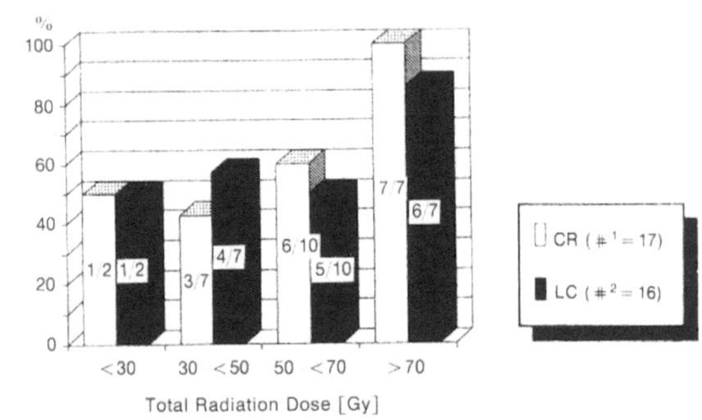

Fig. 31.6. Correlation of complete response (17 patients) and local control (16 patients) with radiation dose with doses < 30 Gy ($n_1 = 2$), 30–< 50 Gy ($n_2 = 7$), 50–< 70 Gy ($n_3 = 10$), and ≥ 70 Gy ($n_4 = 7$). The difference between lesions < 70 Gy ($n = 19$) versus lesions ≥ 70 Gy ($n = 7$) has a P value of 0.06

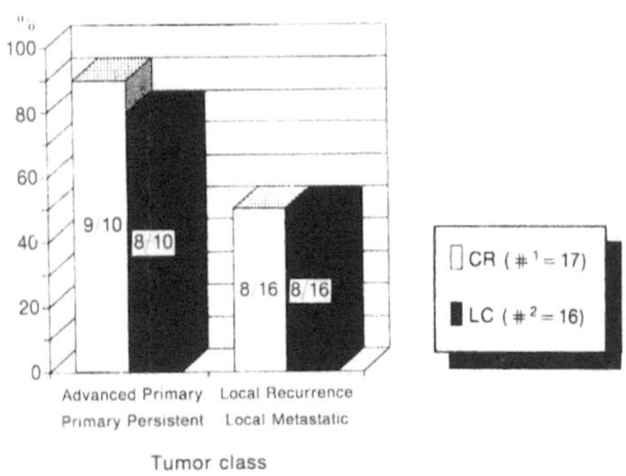

Fig. 31.4. Correlation of complete response (17 patients) and local control (16 patients) with tumor class: differences between primary and persistent tumors ($n_1 = 10$) versus recurrent and metastatic tumors ($n_2 = 16$) are not statistically significant ($P > 0.05$)

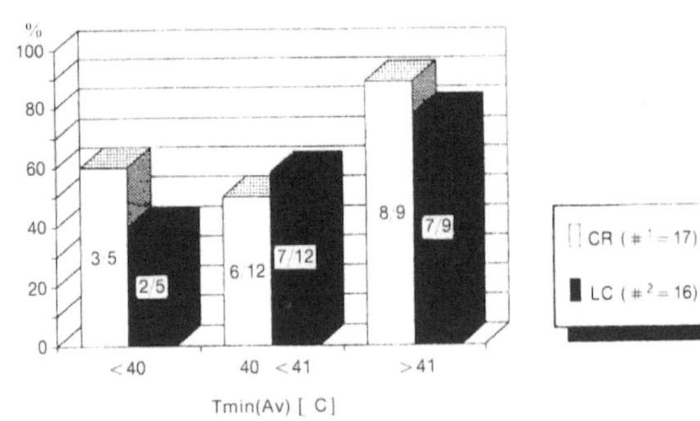

Fig. 31.7. Correlation of complete response (17 patients) and local control (16 patients) with minimum temperature $T\min_{av}$. The differences between lesions reaching $T\min_{av}$ $< 40°C$ ($n_1 = 5$), 40°– $\leq 41°C$ ($n_2 = 12$), and $\geq 41°C$ ($n_3 = 9$) are not significant ($P < 0.08$)

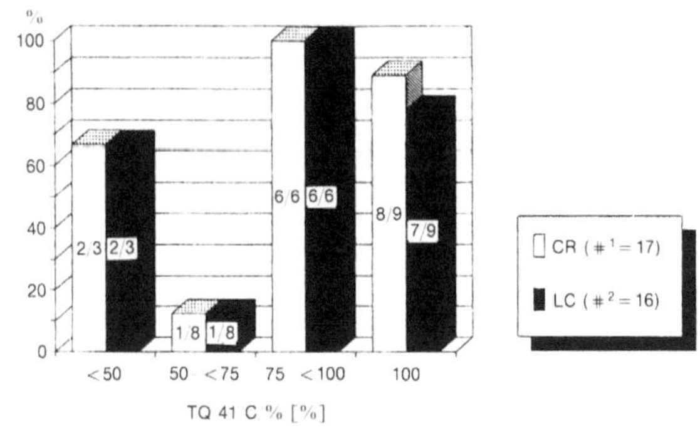

Fig. 31.8. Correlation of complete response (17 patients) and local control (16 patients) with thermal quality of heating TQ41°C, with TQ41°C < 50% ($n_1 = 3$), 50–< 75% ($n_2 = 8$), 75–< 100% ($n_3 = 6$), and 100% ($n_4 = 9$). The difference between lesions < 75% ($n = 11$) versus lesions ≥ 75% ($n = 15$) has prognostic significance ($P = 0.001$)

31.3.5 Locoregional Recurrences

Eight of 26 (31%) patients experienced locoregional recurrences after IHT-IRT treatment: five relapses were located *outside* and three *inside* the treated volume. Four of 17 (24%) patients with an initial CR developed their relapse outside the treated volume at 9, 13, 18, and 30 months' FU, and one (6%) inside it at 22 months' FU. Three of seven (43%) patients with an initial PR experienced renewed tumor progression and/or recurrence at 8 months' FU (outside) and at 16 and 25 months' FU (inside and outside). In the case of tumors of the cervix we observed no relapse, in contrast to colorectal/anal (4/9 = 44%) and vaginal (3/4 = 75%) tumors. A 66-year-old woman with cervical carcinoma developed a second malignancy outside the pelvis (breast carcinoma). PRIM/PERS lesions had a lower relapse rate (1/10 = 10%; regional relapse) than REC/MET lesions (7/16 = 44%; three local and four regional recurrences). The specific patient, tumor, and treatment parameters in respect of locoregional recurrences are summarized in Table 31.4.

31.4 Discussion

31.4.1 Usefulness of IHT Application

Interstitial HT does not represent the only option for the application of heat to pelvic tumors. Several other HT techniques have been developed and clinically applied, including the annular phased array system (APAS) (Petrovich et al. 1989b), scanned focused ultrasound (Shimm et al. 1988), and capacitive radiofrequency HT techniques (Kaheki et al. 1990). These techniques have a specific role in the treatment of large tumors which are not well confined, are deep-seated, or are inaccessible for implantation. Probably due to less effective power deposition, more inhomogeneous heat distribution, and/or insufficient thermometry feedback control, only relatively low tumor temperatures, low CR rates, and a surprisingly high toxicity rate have been reported. In contrast to these reports, we have selected an interstitial heating approach for tumors which were well confined, less than 6–7 cm in diameter, and reasonably accessible for interstitial implantation. In both practical and theoretical terms, IHT techniques are presently more advantageous for these lesions than any external HT technique (Cosset 1990).

It is important to realize that interstitial thermal radiation therapy (IHT-IRT) represents a complex treatment procedure that requires lengthy patient preparation and careful attention to various technical and clinical details. Besides considerable expense as regards material and time, a high degree of

Table 31.3. Distribution of treatment parameters and initial/long-term tumor response and relapse rate

Parameter ($N_{all} = 26$)	Initial Response (3 mo) (CR = 17)	Long-term response (12 mo) (LC = 16)
Tumor Class:		
PRIM/PERS	9/10 (90%)	8/10 (80%)
REC/MET	8/16 (50%)	8/16 (50%)
Volume (C):		
<20 cm^3	3/3 (100%)	3/3 (100%)
20–<40 cm^3	5/7 (71%)	6/7 (86%)
40–<80 cm^3	6/9 (67%)	4/9 (44%)
≥ 80 cm^3	3/7 (43%)	3/7 (43%)
Total RT dose:		
<30 Gy	1/2 (50%)	1/2 (50%)
30–<50 Gy	3/7 (43%)	4/7 (57%)
50–<70 Gy	6/10 (67%)	5/10 (50%)
<70 Gy	7/7 (100%)	6/7 (86%)
HT parameters:		
$T\min_{av} < 40°C$	3/5 (60%)	2/5 (40%)
40°C–<41°	6/12 (50%)	7/12 (58%)
≥41°C	8/9 (89%)	7/9 (78%)
Tmean < 42°C	6/11 (55%)	4/11 (36%)
42°C–<43°	9/13 (69%)	10/13 (77%)
≥43°C	2/2 (100%)	2/2 (100%)
TQ41°C<75%	3/11 (28%)	3/11 (28%)
75%–<100%	6/6 (100%)	6/6 (100%)
=100%	8/9 (89%)	7/9 (78%)
Locoregional relapse distribution:		
PRIM/PERS	1/10 (10%)	Initial CR: 5/7 (29%)
REC/MET:	7/16 (44%)	Initial PR: 3/7 (43%)

Table 31.4. Characteristics of locoregional recurrences after combined IRT-IHT of pelvic tumors[a]

Patient, age (1st IHT)	Lesion site	Initial result	Interval and site of relapse	Lesion type	Volume $V(C)$ (cm^3)	Antenna spacing	RT dose (Gy)	$T\min_{av}$ (°C)	TQ41°C (%)
W.W., 67 yr (05/86)	RECT	CR	22 mo; *inside*	*MET*	*80*	*Wide*	*48*	*39.2*	*30*
C.M., 61 yr (09/86)	RECT	*PR*	25 mo; *inside*	*MET*	24	*Medium*	*48*	*40.8*	*67*
M.P., 76 yr (08/88)	VAG	CR	18 mo; outside	*REC*	34	Small	65	41.5	100
H.M., 43 yr (04/89)	VAG	CR	18 mo; outside	*REC*	*48*	*Medium*	*46*	41.0	100
R.V., 58 yr (06/89)	OVAR	*PR*	16 mo; *inside*	*MET*	*70*	*Wide*	*30*	*39.4*	*40*
K.N., 45 yr (07/89)	VAG	CR	30 mo; outside	*REC*	32	*Medium*	*40*	*40.6*	80
P.J., 78 yr (07/89)	RECT	CR	9 mo; outside	*MET*	*75*	*Wide*	65	41.1	100
K.E., 83 yr (08/89)	RECT	*PR*	8 mo; outside	PERS	*56*	*Medium*	69	*40.1*	*67*

RECT, colorectum; VAG, vagina; OVAR, ovaries; CR, complete remission; PR, partial remission; REC, local recurrence; MET, local metastasis; PERS, persistent lesion; $V(C)$, cuboid volume: $a \times b \times c$; TQ41°C, thermal quality at 41°C
[a] Italicized features represent characteristics which are identified as poor progonostic treatment parameters

team cooperation is required; the team should consist of a specialized (e.g., abdominal, urological, or gynecological) oncological surgeon, a radiation oncologist, a radiation physicist, and a nurse, all with longstanding technical and clinical expertise. Due to technical and clinical limitations already known from interstitial RT, only well implantable and circumscribed tumors of up to 7 cm in diameter can be treated effectively. These restrictions may indeed influence patient and tumor selection criteria and limit the availability of IHT-IRT to a few clinical institutions. Although this selection process in itself may positively influence the treatment outcome, in most clinical studies to date IHT-IRT has been used to achieve palliation in patients with a poor prognosis, a large tumor volume, and worse general performance characteristics as compared to patients treated with adjuvant and conventional treatments. However, the use of IHT-IRT is favored by the promising biological and clinical rationale based on in vitro (Ben-Hur et al. 1974; Overgaard et al. 1981; Jones et al. 1989; Jones, this volume, Chap. 1), in vivo (Dewhirst et al. 1982, 1984; Miller et al. 1978; Jones et al. 1989; Jones, this volume, Chap. 1), and human tumor studies (Oleson et al. 1988; Overgaard et al. 1989).

31.4.2 Previous IHT-IRT Experience

In this study well-localized pelvic malignancies have been effectively and safely treated with IHT-IRT. The results published on IHT-IRT for pelvic tumors are consisent with our data independently of the applied heating technique: microwave (MW)-IHT (Puthawala et al. 1985; Emami et al. 1987; Rafla et al. 1988, 1989; Petrovich et al. 1989a; Phromratanapongse et al. 1990; Coughlin et al. 1991; Grigsby and Emami, this volume, Chap. 30), radiofrequency (RF)-IHT (Aristizabal and Oleson 1984; Oleson et al. 1984; Cosset et al. 1985; Emami et al. 1987; Gautherie et al. 1989; Vora et al. 1988, 1989; Vora and Luk, this volume, Chap. 29), and hot source IHT with ferromagnetic seeds (Shimm et al. 1989; Stea et al., this volume, Chap. 26) or hot water perfusion (Handl-Zeller et al. 1987; Schreier et al. 1990; Stücklschweiger et al. 1991a, b; Handl-Zeller, this volume, Chap. 25).

When reviewing the larger IHT-IRT series which include ≥ 20 patients (Seegenschmiedt and Vernon, this volume, Chap. 40) and experiences with IHT of pelvic tumors, the following conclusions can be drawn:

1. Only one-third (217/619 = 35%) of IHT-IRT treatments have been applied in the pelvis.
2. Pelvic lesions have been preferentially treated with RF-IHT (144/217 = 66%) rather than with MW-IHT (73/217 = 34%).
3. The cumulative CR rate in the pelvis has been about 56% (range 38%–75%), with slightly better results for colorectal (mean: 60%, range 36%–75%) than for gynecological lesions (mean: 53%, range 39%–78%).

4. The cumulative toxicity rate has been approximately 20%–25%.

5. MW-IHT and RF-IHT techniques have achieved a similar response rate.

6. The reported FU periods have been extremely variable and range between 1 and 74 months.

7. Some response criteria that cannot be termed objective have been used for evaluation, e.g., "ongoing/continuous tumor regression," "palliative response (prevention of bleeding, pain relief)," and "preservation of normal organ function."

All important details of IHT-IRT series for 127 gynecological and 78 colorectal/anal tumors are summarized in Tables 31.5 and 31.6, including techniques, treatment parameters, rate of initial response, and treatment toxicity. Unfortunately,

Table 31.5. Interstitial thermoradiotherapy in the pelvis: gynecological tumors

Author, year	No. of lesions (total group)	Technique of IHT	IHT	RT dose, RT type	Clinical response	Complications
Aristizabal and Oleson 1984	36 (64)	0.5-MHz RF-IHT	60 min at 43°C	15–45 Gy LDR	14/36 (39%)	NA (21%)
Puthawala et al. 1985	9 (43)	915-MHz MW-IHT	60 min 41.5°–43.5°C	2× 20–25 Gy LDR	7/9 (78%)	3/9 (33%)
Emami et al. 1987	4 (48)	0.5-MHz RF-IHT	60 min 42.5°–43°C	20–30 Gy LDR	NA (54%)	NA (25%)
Gautherie et al. 1989	23 (96)	0.5-MHz RF-IHT	45 min 43.5°C	40 Gy LDR	11/23 (48%)	NA (16%)
Petrovich et al. 1989a	4 (44)	915-MHz MW-IHT	45–60 min 42.5°C	25–50 Gy LDR	3/4 (75%)	NA (20%)
Vora et al. 1988, 1989	20 (81)	0.5-MHz RF-IHT	30–60 min 42°–43°C	30–40 Gy LDR	10/20 (50%)	1/20 (5%)
Stücklschweiger et al. 1991a, b	5 (20)	HWP-IHT	40 min 42.5 °C	6–8 Gy HDR	NA (50%)	NA
Coughlin et al. 1991	12 (35)	915-MHz MW-IHT	45–60 min 43°C	20–40 Gy LDR	8/12 (66%)	NA
This study	14 (86)	915-MHz MW-IHT	45–60 min 41°–44°C	20–40 Gy LDR	10/14 (71%)	4/14 (29%)
Total experience:	127	RF-IHT: 83	MW-IHT: 39	HWP-IHT: 5	~67 (53%)	~(20%)

RF, radiofrequency; MW, microwaves; HWP, hot water perfusion; LDR low dose rate; HDR, high dose rate; NA, not available

Table 31.6. Interstitial thermo-radiotherapy in the pelvis: colorectal and anal tumors

Author, year	No. of lesions (total group)	Technique of IHT	IHT	RT dose, RT type	Complete response	Complications
Aristizabal and Oleson 1984	11 (64)	0.5-MHz RF-IHT	30–40 min 42°–43°C	15–45 Gy m: 26 Gy	4/11 (36%)	NA (21%)
Puthawala et al. 1985	4 (43)	915-MHz MW-IHT	60 min 41.5°–43.5°C	2× 20–25 Gy LDR	3/4 (75%)	NA (21%)
Emami et al. 1987	3 (48)	0.5-MHz RF-IHT	60 min 42.5°–43°C	20–60 Gy LDR	2/3 (66%)	NA (25%)
Gautherie et al. 1989	16 (96)	0.5-MHz RF-IHT	45 min 43.5°C	40 Gy LDR	12/16 (75%)	NA (16%)
Vora et al. 1989	18 (81)	0.5-MHz RF-IHT	30–60 min 42°–43°C	20–40 Gy LDR	NA (56%)	NA (17%)
Goffinet et al. 1990	5 (10)	RT-IHT	45 min 43°–44°C	20–44 Gy LDR	3/5 (60%)	NA
Stücklschweiger et al. 1991a, b	12 (20)	HWP-IHT	40 min 42.5 °C	6–8 Gy HDR	NA (66%)	NA
This study	9 (86)	915-MHz MW-IHT	45–60 min 41°–44°C	20–40 Gy LDR	5/9 (56%)	2/9 (22%)
Total experience:	78	RF-IHT: 53	MW-IHT: 13	HWP-IHt: 12	~47 (60%)	~(18%)

IHT, interstitial hyperthermia; RF, radiofrequency; MW, Microwaves; HWP, hot water perfusion; NA, not available; numbers in brackets indicate value of total group; LDR, low dose rate; HDR, high dose rate several series are compromised by (a) low patient numbers; (b) lack of detailed reporting on RT and HT treatment characteristics; (c) incomplete anlaysis of patient, tumor, and treatment parameters; (d) lack of information on long-term tumor control and late treatment toxicity; or (e) less developed thermometry and heating technology (in the case of older series).

At the *University of Arizona, Tucson*, 64 tumors including 36 gynecological and 9 colorectal malignancies were treated with RF-IHT (ARISTIZABAL and OLESON 1984; OLESON et al. 1984). IHT was applied for 30 min in one session intraoperatively using 0.5-MHz low current field RF (LCF-RF). Time-averaged intratumor maximum and minimum temperatures were 44.6°C and 41°C, respectively, but it was difficult to achieve minimum tumor temperatures ≥ 41°C. Low dose rate (LDR) iridium-192 IRT was applied 2–3 h after IHT, delivering an RT dose of 15–45 Gy over a period of 24–72 h to a relatively large mean volume of 276 ± 118 cm^3. The overall response rates were CR 38%, PR 39%, and NC 23%. Of 64 patients, eight (13%) experienced severe treatment toxicity. The development of CR was correlated with RT dose, tumor volume, and minimum tumor temperature. When RT doses of ≥ 60 Gy were combined with minimum temperatures ≤ 41°C or when low RT doses were combined with temperatures > 41°C, a high CR rate was achieved. These results have been supported by animal studies conducted at the same clinical institution (DEWHIRST et al. 1982, 1984).

At the *Memorial Cancer Center, Long Beach*, 43 patients were treated for recurrent cancers of various sites, including 13 pelvic tumors – nine gynecological tumors and four rectal tumors (PUTHAWALA et al. 1985). Two LDR iridium-192 treatments applied within 3–4 weeks (each 20–25 Gy) were combined with 915-MHz microwave IHT (60 min at 41.5°–43.5°C). Multiple coaxial MW antennae were placed in flexible plastic tubes. At 6–12 intratumoral points simultaneous multipoint thermometry was performed. With a minimum of 12 months' FU, local control (LC) was observed in 32 (74%) lesions. Five lesions with initial CR relapsed within the first year. In three patients who failed IHT-IRT temperatures could not be raised ≥ 40°C. Early complications were noted in four of the 43 (9%) patients, and five (12%) developed late complications after between 3 and 8 months. Besides temperature, no other prognostic treatment factor was defined.

The large clinical experience at the *City of Hope Medical Center* was updated relatively recently (VORA et al. 1982, 1989). A total of 81 lesions were treated using 0.5-MHz LCF-RF IHT (30–60 min at 42°–43°C) and LDR iridium-192 IRT (20–40 Gy) supplemented by external beam RT (45–50 Gy). Thirty-eight malignancies were located in the pelvis, 20 advanced cancers of the uterine cervix stage IIIA–IV and 18 colorectal/anal tumor recurrences. The overall response rates for 78 evaluable lesions were CR 55%, PR 19%, and NC 26%. Minor and severe toxicity occurred in 13 (17%) patients. Cervical tumors achieved a slightly lower CR, 10/20 (50%), and had a lower toxicity rate, 1/20 (5%), compared to the results of the total group. A large difference was noted between the CR rate achieved in primary (57%) versus retreated (40%) lesions, but no other prognostic factor was found. More specific details and updated results for pelvic lesions are also presented by VORA and LUK in Chap. 29 of this volume.

At *Washington University, St. Louis*, a total of 48 recurrent or persistent tumors were treated with 915-MHz MW-IHT (39 lesions) or 0.5-MHz LCF-RF IHT (nine lesions) (EMAMI et al. 1987). LDR iridium-192 IRT was applied with doses varying between 20 and 60 Gy, depending on the extent of previous RT. IHT was administered in two sessions before and after IRT for 60 min at 42.5°C. Tumor sites included 29 head and neck, six breast, six miscellaneous, and only seven pelvic (four gynecological and three colorectal) lesions. The overall response rates were CR 54%, PR 25%, and NC 13%; four lesions (8%) were unevaluable. Moderate to severe toxicity was noted in 12 lesions (25%). Tumor volume and "satisfactory heating" (temperatures ≥ 42°C within the entire tumor volume) significantly affected the tumor control rate. The updated results of 14 pelvic lesions are also presented in a previous chapter of this volume (GRIGSBY and EMAMI, Chap. 30 of this volume).

The clinical experience at the *University of Southern California, Los Angeles*, consisted of 44 lesions, 23 head and neck, nine breast, four vagina, four skin, and four other tumors (PETROVICH et al. 1989a). These lesions were treated with 915-MHz MW-IHT (45–60 min at 42.5°C) and LDR iridium-192 IRT (25–50 Gy). CR was obtained in 28 (64%) and PR in 15 (34%) sites. Three of four (75%) vaginal carcinomas showed CR. None of the CR patients developed a local relapse. Acute toxicity (moist desquamation, blisters) occurred in nine patients (20%), and serious complications in three

(7%). Tumor volume was the most important factor influencing CR.

The Institute Gustave Roussy, Villejuif, was the first European clinical institution to use IHT (COSSET et al. 1985; COSSET 1990). In the early 1980s a total of 29 lesions were treated using 0.5-MHz LCF-RF IHT (45 min at 44°C) and LDR iridium-192 IRT (30–40 Gy), but only one tumor (a uterine carcinoma) was located in the pelvis. The overall response rates were CR 83% and PR 17%. Four of 23 (17%) patients experienced severe and eight (35%) minor toxicity. In view of the high minimum tumor temperatures of 44°C in 16/25 implantations the high CR rate is of prognostic value, since three of four partial responders achieved only unsatisfactory temperatures < 41°C. Despite exellent thermal data, six (21%) relapses occurred after CR within 5–13 months, partially due to underestimated volume and partially due to a low concurrent RT dose ≤ 30 Gy.

Clinical IHT-IRT data from Villejuif, Lyon, and Dijon have been pooled in a *French collaborative study* (GAUTHERIE et al. 1989). The Minerve 0.5-MHz LCF-RF IHT system was used in all institutions. Overall, 96 patients were treated. Tumor sites included 35 head and neck, 23 gynecological, 16 colorectal or anal, 14 breast and chest wall, and 8 other tumor sites. Tumor volumes were relatively small, ranging between 5 cm^3 and 100 cm^3. The minimal tumor temperature was ≥ 42°C in 90% of all patients. The overall response rates were CR 65%, PR 16%, and NC 19%. The CR rate for gynecological tumors was 11/23 (48%) and for colorectal tumors 12/16 (75%). Minor or moderate side-effects were observed in 25 patients (26%), and severe complications in 15 (16%). Minimum tumor temperature was the only prognostic factor which appeared to impact on tumor control.

31.4.3 Prognostic Factors in IHT-IRT Trials

The aforementioned studies confirm statistical trends and/or prognostic factors correlating with initial and long-term tumor control that have been identified in our series:

1. *Tumor class* had prognostic value in several other trials (VORA et al. 1988, 1989; PHROMRATANAPONGSE et al. 1990). Primary and persistent (PRIM/PERS) tumors achieved significantly better short and long-term tumor control than pretreated recurrent and metastatic (REC/MET) tumors.

2. *Radiation dose* significantly influenced treatment outcome (ARISTIZABAL and OLESON 1984; OLESON et al. 1984; COSSET et al. 1985; COSSET 1990; PHROMRATANAPONGSE et al. 1990; COUGHLIN et al. 1991). Tumors being treated with higher total RT doses achieved significantly better results than those treated with lower RT doses. The decisive breakpoint appears to occur around 50 Gy. In our study, the total RT dose was also a function of lesion type: pretreated REC/MET lesions could only receive significantly lower total RT doses (mean 50.8 Gy, range 24.3–65.2 Gy) compared to previously untreated PRIM/PERS lesions, which usually received full-dose external beam RT (mean 73.2 Gy, range 28.8–88.5 Gy).

3. In several other trials, *tumor volume* was identified as an important prognostic factor (ARISTIZABAL and OLESON 1984; OLESON et al. 1984; COSSET et al. 1985; EMAMI et al. 1987; PETROVICH et al. 1989a; COSSET 1990; PHROMRATANAPONGSE et al. 1990; COUGHLIN et al. 1991): smaller tumors achieved significantly better results than larger tumors. Poor implantation quality, which results in less favorable RT dose distribution and IHT power deposition, is the major reason for the decreased response rate or the increased local relapse rate (COSSET et al. 1985; COSSET 1990). Two methods of anlayzing the implant quality have been proposed (LEVENDAG et al., this volume, Chap. 27; SEEGENSCHMIEDT et al. 1990a. IHT quality assurance criteria, including sufficient tumor coverage, have been recognized as mandatory for all IHT trials (SEEGENSCHMIEDT et al. 1989; DEWHIRST et al. 1990; EMAMI et al. 1991). Some new MW antenna designs help to improve the homogeneity of the power deposition and the effective heating volume (STAUFFER et al. 1989; JAMES et al. 1989; CHAN et al. 1990; RYAN et al. 1990; HAND, this volume, Chap. 6). The major limitations of MW antennae include their fixed SAR distribution and extreme sensitivity to small changes of applicator parameters (insertion depth, spacing and distribution, mode of activation, anatomical conditions). In contrast, multiplexed type LCF-RF (PRIONAS et al. 1989) and capacitive 27-MHz RF techniques (VISSER et al. 1989, this volume, Chap. 5) should allow a better shaping of the power deposition.

4. The prognostic impact of *thermal parameters* has been characterized in animal and clinical studies (DEWHIRST et al. 1982, 1984; ARISTIZABAL and OLESON 1984; OLESON et al. 1984; COSSET et al. 1985; DEWHIRST and SIM 1986; EMAMI et al. 1987; PETROVICH et al. 1989a; GAUTHERIE et al. 1989;

Cosset 1990; Phromratanapongse et al. 1990; Coughlin et al. 1991). The minimum average tumor temperature was the most important factor in predicting human tumor response. Similar to our definition of "thermal quality," other reports have shown the importance of "satisfactory heating" (Paulsen et al. 1984; Emami et al. 1987; Coughlin et al. 1991). However, the number and location of all thermometric sensors and the spatial and temporal thermal mapping resolution can greatly influence the thermal data analysis (Corry et al. 1988). In our study as many tumor probes as possible housing multiple thermometry sensors were implanted and included for thermal analysis. Our relatively low minimum tumor temperatures resulted from invasive thermometry measurements, which were strictly performed *outside* the heating sources at locations most likely to record the lowest temperatures. In contrast, most RF-IHT techniques are powered by feedback control and refer only to maximum temperatures, which are usually measured *inside* the heating sources, thereby missing potential minimum temperatures outside the heating sources.

31.4.4 Treatment Toxicity

The addition of IHT to interstitial and external beam RT does not increase acute and late treatment toxicity: IRT by itself has a complication rate of 10%–30% for primary malignancies and pretreated recurrent lesions. In some trials thermal damage was only correlated with maximum tumor temperatures exceeding 44°–45°C (Dewhirst et al. 1982; Aristizabal and Oleson 1984; Oleson et al. 1984; Cosset et al. 1985; Dewhirst and Sim 1986; Cosset 1990; Phromratanapongse et al. 1990) and/or *T*max Eq 43°C $\geq$ 160 (Dewhirst et al. 1982, 1984; Dewhirst and Sim 1986). In our study, we observed more complications when maximum temperatures exceeded 44°C–45°C. Therefore we recommended that a "narrow thermal treatment window" of at least 41°C minimum but less than 45°C maximum temperature be used in clinical practice.

31.5 Conclusions

The combined use of interstitial RT and HT (IHT-IRT) appears to be more effective than external beam RT, alone or in combination with external HT in the treatment of pelvic neoplasms; the intense and long-term RT from a radioactive implant and the well-localized heat distribution in the tumor bed from implanted heating sources produce a highly effective cytotoxic treatment. Numerous in vitro and in vivo experiments have demonstrated a high thermal enhancement ratio, which confirms the clinical observation that IHT-IRT is an effective and safe treatment in the pelvic, head and neck, and other regions (Kapp 1986; Seegenschmiedt et al. 1990b). It can be used for all localized and implantable malignant lesions that have been suboptimally treated in the past by coventional treatment modalities.

Each IHT technique offers specific advantages and disadvantages; therefore in clinical practice the specific implementation has to be carefully selected: MW-IHT techniques are recommended in the head and neck region, whereas radiofrequency, ferromagnetic seeds, or hot water perfusion IHT techniques may be more suitable for pelvic lesions (Seegenschmiedt et al. 1990b). IHT-IRT offers a reasonable *palliative* approach for recurrent and metastatic lesions. However, it may be more difficult to assess the potential role of *adjuvant* treatment with IHT-IRT, since high local control rates can be obtained with IRT alone. The additional effect of IHT on tumor control has to be proven by prospective randomized multicenter clinical trials comparing IRT with and without IHT. Certainly a large number of patients are required to demonstrate statistically significant differences. Although a first prospective randomized phase 1–2 study involving pelvic lesions awaits final evaluation (Radiation Therapy Oncology Group, Philadelphia; written communication, 1990), further trials are mandatory as these early trials have been performed with a lower technical and clinical quality assurance than recently recommended by the RTOG (Dewhirst et al. 1990; Emami et al. 1991). In the future, new technical and clinical applications of IHT-IRT can be expected for specific tumor types and sites and for implementation of simultaneous LDR, HDR, or pulsed HDR combined with 1-h high temperature IHT or continuous low temperature IHT (Martinez, this volume, Chap. 22).

Acknowledgments. The authors thank Ulf L. Karlsson, M.D., Department of Radiotherapy, University of New Mexico, Albuquerque, NM, USA (former associate professor and attending at the Department of Radiation Oncology, Hahnemann University, Philadelphia, PA, USA); Richard Tobin, service engineer, and William Kempin, BS, hyperthermia technologist, Department of Radiation Oncology, Hahnemann University, Philadelphia, PA, USA;

Jürgen Erb, Dipl. Phys., Marianne Kettner, RTT, Rosemarie Rössler, RTT, Ralf Seidel, cand. med., and Gunter Klautke, cand. med., Department of Radiation Oncology, University Erlangen-Nürnberg, for their unfailingly dedicated and skillful clinical, technical and computer assistance, thorough data management and diligent patient care.

This work was supported by two grants: Deutsche Krebshilfe e.V. (Dr. Mildred Scheel Stiftung) Grant #300-402-521/6; Deutsche Forschungsgemeinschaft (DFG) Grant #Fi 371/2-1.

References

American Cancer Society (1990) Cancer facts and figures-1990

Aristizabal SA, Oleson JR (1984) Combined interstitial irradiation and localized current field hyperthermia: results and conclusions from clinical studies. Cancer Res [Suppl] 44: 4757s–4760s

Aristizabal SA, Surwit EA, Hevezi JM, Heusinkveld RS (1983) Treatment of advanced cancer of the cervix with transperineal interstitial irradiation. Int J Radiat Oncol Biol Phys 9: 1013–1017

Ben-Hur E, Elkind MM, Bronk BV (1974) Thermally enhanced radiosensitivity of cultured Chinese hamster cells; inhibition of repair of sublethal damage and enhancement of lethal damage. Radiat Res 58: 38–51

Cetas TC (1985) Thermometry and thermal dosimetry. In: Overgaard J (ed) Hyperthermic oncology 1984, vol. 1. Taylor & Francis, London, pp 91–112

Chan KW, Chou CK, McDougall JA, Luk KH, Vora NL, Forell BW (1989) Changes in heating patterns of interstitial microwave antenna arrays at different insertion depths. Int J Hyperthermia 5: 499–508

Chou CK, Chen GW, Guy AW, Luk KH (1984) Formulas for preparing phantom muscle tissue at various radiofrequencies. Bioelectromagnetics 5: 435–441

Corry PM, Jabboury K, Kong JS, Armour EP, McCraw FJ, LeDuc T (1988) Evaluation of equipment for hyperthermia treatment of cancer. Int J Hyperthermia 4: 53–74

Cosset JM (1990) Interstitial hyperthermia. In: Gautherie M (ed) Interstitial, endocavitary and perfusional hyperthermia. Methods and clinical trials. Springer, Berlin Heidelberg New York, pp 1–41

Cosset JM, Dutreix J, Haie C, Gerbaulet A, Janoray P, Dewars JA (1985) Interstitial thermoradiotherapy: a technical and clinical study of 29 implantations performed at the Institute Gustave Roussy. Int J Hyperthermia 1: 3–13

Coughlin CT, Ryan TP, Stafford JH et al. (1991) Interstitial thermoradiotherapy: the Dartmouth experience 1981–1990. In: Chapman JD, Dewey WC, Whitmore GF (eds) Radiation research: a twentieth-century perspective, vol I. Academic, San Diego, CA (USA), P31 02 WP: 386 (abstract)

Dewhirst MW, Sim DA (1986) Estimation of therapeutic gain in clinical trials involving hyperthermia and radiotherapy. Int J Hyperthermia 2: 165–178

Dewhirst MW, Connor WG, Sim DA (1982) Preliminary results of phase III trial of spontaneous animal tumors to heat and/or radiation: early normal tissue response and tumor volume influence on initial response. Int J Radiat Oncol Biol Phys 8: 1951–1961

Dewhirst MW, Sim DA, Sapareto S, Connor WG (1984) The importance of minimum tumour temperature in determining early and long-term response of spontaneous pet animal tumours to heat and radiation. Cancer Res [Suppl] 44: 43–50

Dewhirst MW, Phillips TL, Samulski TV et al. (1990) RTOG quality assurance guidelines for clinical trials using hyperthermia. Int J Radiat Oncol Biol Phys 18: 1249–1259

Emami B, Perez CA, Konefal J et al. (1987) Interstitial thermoradiotherapy in treatment of malignant tumors. Int J Hyperthermia 3: 107–118

Emami B, Stauffer P, Dewhirst MW et al. (1991) Quality assurance guidelines for interstitial hyperthermia (an RTOG document). Int J Radiat Oncol Biol Phys 20: 1117–1124

Evans SR Jr, Hilaris BS, Barber HRK (1971) External versus interstitial irradiation in unresectable recurrent cancer of the cervix. Cancer 28: 1284–1288

Fietkau R, Weidenbecher M, Spitzer W, Sauer R (1991) Temporary and permanent brachycurietherapy in advanced head and neck cancer – the Erlangen experience. In: Sauer R (ed) Interventional radiation therapy: techniques – brachytherapy. Springer, Berlin Heidelberg New York, pp 159–169

Fisher RA, Yates F (1963) Statistical tables for biological, agricultural and medical research. Oliver and Boyd, Edinburgh, p 47 (Table IV)

Gautherie M, Cosset JM, Gerard JP et al. (1989) Radiofrequency interstitial hyperthermia: a multicentric program of quality assessment and clinical trials. In: Sugahara T, Saito M (eds) Hyperthermic oncology 1988, vol 2. Taylor & Francis, London, pp 711–714

Goffinet DR, Prionas SD, Kapp DS et al. (1990) Interstitial ^{192}Ir flexible catheter radiofrequency hyperthermia treatments of head and neck and recurrent pelvic carcinomas. Int J Radiat Oncol Biol Phys 18: 199–210

Hand JW (1990) Biophysics and technology of electromagnetic hyperthermia. In: Gautherie M (ed) Methods of external hyperthermic heating. Springer, Berlin Heidelberg New York, pp 1–59

Handl-Zeller L, Kärcher KH, Lesnicar H, Budihna M, Schreier K (1987) Newly developed liquid heated interstitial hyperthermia system KHS-9/W18 (abstract). Int J Hyperthermia 3: 567

Hilaris BS, Henschke UK (1985) General principles and techniques of interstitial brachytherapy. In: Hilaris BS (ed) Handbook of interstitial brachytherapy. Publ Sciences Group Inc., Acton, MA (USA), pp 61–86

Hynynen K (1990) Biophysics and technology of ultrasound hyperthermia. In: Gautherie M (ed) Methods of external hyperthermic heating. Springer, Berlin Heidelberg New York, pp 61–115

James BJ, Strohbehn JW, Mechling JA, Trembly BS (1989) The effect of insertion depth on the theoretical SAR patterns of 915 MHz dipole antenna arrays for hyperthermia. Int J Hyperthermia 5: 733–747

Jobsen JJ, Lee JWH, Cleton FJ, Hermans J (1989) Treatment of locoregional recurrence of carcinoma of the cervix by radiotherapy after primary surgery. Gynecol Oncol 33: 368–371

Jones EL, Lyons BE, Douple EB, Dain BJ (1989) Thermal enhancement of low dose irradiation in a murine tumour system. Int J Hyperthermia 5: 509–524

Kaheki M, Ueda K, Mukojima T et al. (1990) Multi-institutional clinical studies on hyperthermia combined with radiotherapy or chemotherapy in advanced cancer of deep-seated organs. Int J Hyperthermia 6: 719–740

Kaplan EL, Meier P (1958) Nonparametric estimation from incomplete observations. J Am Stat Assoc 53: 457–481
Kapp DS (1986) Site and disease selction for hyperthermia clinical trials. Int J Hyperthermia 2: 139–156
Lawhead RA Jr, Clark DGC, Smith DH et al. (1989) Pelvic exenteration for recurrent or persistent gynecologic malignancies: a ten year review of the Memorial Sloan-Kettering Cancer Center experience (1972–1981). Gynecol Oncol 33: 279–282
Leeper D (1985) Molecular and cellular mechanisms of hyperthermia alone or combined with other modalities. In: Overgaard J (ed) Hyperthermic oncology 1984, vol 1. Taylor & Francis, London, pp 9–41
Martinez AA, Edmundson GK, Cox RS et al. (1985) Combination of external beam irradiation and multiple-site perineal applicator (MUPIT) for treatment of locally advanced or recurrent prostatic, anorectal, and gynecologic malignancies. Int J Radiat Oncol Biol Phys 11: 391–398
Miller RC, Leith JT, Voemett RC, Gerner EW (1978) Effects of interstitial radiation therapy alone, or in combination with localized hyperthermia on response of a mouse mammary tumour. Radiat Res 19: 175–180
Oleson JR, Manning MR, Sim DA et al. (1984) A review of the University of Arizona human clinical hyperthermia experience. Front Radiat Ther Oncol 18: 136–143
Oleson JR, Calderwood SK, Coughlin CT et al. (1988) Biological and clinical aspects of hyperthermia in cancer therapy. Am J Clin Oncol 11: 368–380
Overgaard J (1981) Fractionated radiation and hyperthermia: experimental and clinical studies. Cancer 48: 116–123
Overgaard J (1985) Rationale and problems in the design of clinical studies. In: Overgaard J (ed) Hyperthermia oncology 1984, vol 1. Taylor & Francis, London, pp 325–338
Overgaard J (1989) The current and potential role of hyperthermia in radiotherapy. Int J Radiat Oncol Biol Phys 16: 535–549
Pasasvinichai S, Glassburn JR, Brady LW (1978) Treatment of recurrent carcinoma of the cervix. Int J Radiat Oncol Biol Phys 4: 957–961
Paulsen KD, Strohbehn JW, Lynch DR (1984) Theoretical temperature distributions produced by an annular phased array-type system in CT-based patient models. Radiat Res 100: 536–552
Perez CA, Kuske R, Glasgow GP (1985) Brachytherapy techniques for gynecologic tumors. Endocurietherapy/Hyperthermia Oncol 1: 153–175
Perez CA, Kuske RR, Camel HM et al. (1988) Analysis of pelvic tumor control and impact on survival in carcinoma of the uterine cervix treated with radiotherapy alone. Int J Radiat Oncol Biol Phys 14: 613–621
Petrovich Z, Langholz B, Lam K et al. (1989a) Interstitial microwave hyperthermia combined with iridium-192 radiotherapy for recurrent tumours. Am J Clin Oncol 12: 264–268
Petrovich Z, Langholz B, Gibbs FA et al. (1989b) Regional hyperthermia for advanced tumors: a clinical study of 353 patients. Int J Radiat Oncol Biol Phys 16: 601–607
Phromratanapongse P, Seegenschmiedt MH, Karsson UL et al. (1990) Initial results of phase I/II interstitial thermoradiotherapy for primary advanced and local recurrent tumors. Am J Clin Oncol 13: 259–268
Pierquin B, Marinello G, Mege J-P, Crook J (1988) Intracavitary irradiation of carcinomas of the uterus and cervix: the Creteil method. Int J Radiat Oncol Biol Phys 15: 1465–1473
Prionas SD, Fessenden P, Kapp DS, Goffinet DR, Hahn GM (1989) Interstitial electrodes allowing longitudinal control of SAR distributions. In: Sugahara T, Saito M (eds) Hyperthermic oncology 1988, vol 2. Taylor & Francis, London, pp 707–710
Puthawala A, Syed AMN, Fleming PA, Disaia PJ (1982) Reirradiation with interstitial implant for recurrent pelvic malignancies. Cancer 50: 2810–2814
Puthawala AA, Syed AMN, Khalid MA, Rafie S, McNamara CS (1985) Interstitial hyperthermia for recurrent malignancies. Endocurietherapy/Hyperthermia Oncol 1: 125–131
Rafla S, Tchelebi M, Youssef E, Parikh K, Salloum N (1988) The treatment of advanced recurrent pelvic tumors by interstitial hyperthermia and brachytherapy – a promising approach. Abstracts of papers for the 36th annual meeting of the Radiation Research Society, 8th annual meeting of the North American Hyperthermia Group, Philadelphia, PA (USA), April 16–21, Ch-5: 46 (abstract)
Rafla S, Parikh K, Tchelebi M, Youssef E, Selim H, Bishay S (1989) Recurrent tumors of the head and neck, pelvis and chest wall: treatment with hyperthermia and brachytherapy. Radiology 172: 845–850
Reinhold HS, Endrich B (1986) Tumour microcirculation as a target for hyperthermia. Int J Hyperthermia 2: 117–137
Rubin P, Carter SK (1976) Combination of radiation therapy and chemotherapy: a logical basis for their clinical use. CA 26: 274–292
Ryan TP, Mechlíng JA, Strohbehn JW (1990) Absorbed power deposition for various insertion depths for 915 MHz interstitial dipole antenna arrays: experiment versus theory. Int J Radiat Oncol Biol Phys 19: 377–387
Samulski TV (1988) Current technologies for invasive thermometry. In: Paliwal B, Hetzel F, Dewhirst MW (eds) Biological, physical and clinical aspects of hyperthermia. American Institute of Physics, New York, pp 168–181
Sapareto SA, Dewey WC (1984) Thermal dose determination in cancer therapy. Int J Radiat Oncol Biol Phys 10: 787–800
Schreier K, Budihna M, Lesnicar H et al. (1990) Preliminary studies of interstitial hyperthermia using hot water. Int J Hyperthermia 6: 431–444
Seegenschmiedt MH, Sauer R, Herbst M et al. (1989) Interstitial hyperthermia for H & N tumors: treatment planning and quality assurance (QA). In: Sugahara T, Saito M (eds) Hyperthermic oncology 1988, vol 2. Taylor & Francis, London, pp 524–527
Seegenschmiedt MH, Sauer R, Fietkau R, Karlsson UL, Brady LW (1990a) Primary advanced and local recurrent head and neck tumors: effective management with interstitial thermal radiation therapy. Radiology 176: 267–274
Seegenschmiedt MH, Brady LW, Sauer R (1990b) Interstitial thermoradiotherapy: review on technical and clinical aspects. Am J Clin Oncol 13: 352–363
Seegenschmiedt MH, Sauer R, Brady LW, Karlsson UL (1992) Clinical practice of interstitial microwave hyperthermia combined with iridium-192 brachytherapy. In: Handl-Zeller L (ed) Interstitial hyperthermia. Springer, Wien New York, pp 135–154
Shimm DS, Hynynen KH, Anhalt DP, Roemer RB, Cassady JR (1988) Scanned focussed ultrasound hyperthermia: initial clinical results. Int J Radiat Oncol Biol Phys 15: 1203–1208
Shimm D, Stea B, Cetas T et al. (1989) Clinical results of interstitial hyperthermia using thermally regulating ferromagnetic seeds. In: Sugahara T, Saito M (eds) Hyperthermic oncology 1988, vol 2. Taylor & Francis, London, pp 536–539
Sommers G, Grigsby PW, Perez CA et al. (1989) Outcome of

recurrent cervical carcinoma following definitive irradiation. Gynecol Oncol 35: 150–155

Song CW (1984) Effect of local hyperthermia on bloodflow and microenvironment. Cancer Res [Suppl] 44: 4721s–4730s

Song CW (1989) Physiological and environmental factors in thermal injury of tissues. In: Sugahara T, Saito M (eds) Hyperthermic oncology 1988, vol 2. Taylor & Francis, London, pp 87–92

Spanos W Jr, Wasserman T, Meoz R et al. (1987) Palliation of advanced pelvic malignant disease with large fraction pelvic radiation and misonidazole: final report of RTOG phase I/II study. Int J Radiat Oncol Biol Phys 13: 1479–1482

Spanos W Jr, Guse C, Perez CA et al. (1989) Phase II study of multiple daily fractionations in the palliation of advanced pelvic malignancies: preliminary report of RTOG 8502. Int J Radiat Oncol Biol Phys 17: 659–661

Stauffer PR, Sneed PK, Suen SA et al. (1989) Comparative thermal dosimetry of interstitial microwave and radiofrequency – LCF hyperthermia. Int J Hyperthermia 5: 307–318

Stücklschweiger G, Arian-Schad K, Handl-Zeller L, Leitner H, Poier E, Hackl A (1991a) Interstitielle Ir-192-Afterloadingtherapie mit sequentieller Warmwasser-hyperthermie. Strahlenther Onkol 167: 98–104

Stücklschweiger G, Arian-Schad K, Kapp DS Handl-Zeller L, Hackl A (1991b) Analysis of temperature distributions of interstitial hyperthermia using hot water (abstract). Int J Radiat Oncol Biol Phys 21 [Suppl 1]: 118

Syed AMN, Puthawala AA, Neblett D et al. (1986) Transperineal interstitial-intracavitary "Syed-Neblett" applicator in the treatment of carcinoma of the uterine cervix. Endocurietherapy/Hyperthermia Oncol 2: 1–13

Thigpen T, Vance R, Lambuth B et al. (1987) Chemotherapy for advanced or recurrent gynecologic cancer. Cancer 60: 2104–2116

Thomas G, Dembo A, Beale F et al. (1984) Concurrent radiation, mitomycin C and 5-fluorouracil in poor prognosis carcinoma of cervix: preliminary results of a phase I–II study. Int J Radiat Oncol Biol Phys 10: 1785–1790

Visser AG, Deurloo IKK, Levendag PC, Ruifrok ACC, Cornet B, van Rhoon GC (1989) An interstitial hyperthermia system at 27 MHz. Int J Hyperthermia 5: 265–276

Vora N, Forell B, Joseph C et al. (1982) Interstitial implant with interstitial hyperthermia. Cancer 50: 2518–2523

Vora NL, Luk KH, Forell B et al. (1988) Interstitial local current field hyperthermia for advanced cancers of the cervix. Endocurietherapy/Hyperthermia Oncol 4: 97–106

Vora NL, Forell B, Luk KH et al. (1989) Interstitial thermoradiotherapy in recurrent and advanced carcinoma of malignant tumors: seven years' experience. In: Sugahara T, Saito M (eds) Hyperthermia oncology 1988, vol 1. Taylor & Francis, London, pp 588–590

World Health Organization (WHO) (1979) Handbook for reporting results of cancer treatment. World Health Organization, Geneva, Switzerland

32 Interstitial Thermoradiotherapy for Brain Tumors

P.K. SNEED

CONTENTS

32.1 Introduction

Interstitial radiotherapy (IRT) with removable high activity iodine-125 has been used in the treatment of brain tumors at the University of California, San Francisco since 1979 with promising results. For recurrent tumors treated with implant only, median survival after brain implant was 81 weeks for patients with anaplastic astrocytoma and 54 weeks for those with glioblastoma multiforme (LEIBEL et al. 1989). For primary tumors treated with external beam radiotherapy to 59.4 Gy with hydroxyurea followed by an implant boost, median survival from diagnosis was 157 weeks for patients with anaplastic astrocytoma and 88 weeks for glioblastoma multiforme (GUTIN et al. 1991). However, even with combined external beam and implant doses of 110–120 Gy, malignant gliomas continue to recur or progress most commonly at the primary tumor site or at the margin of the primary tumor.

We hypothesized that adjuvant interstitial hyperthermia (IHT) would improve local control of implanted brain tumors, based on biological rationale provided by in vitro studies (DEWEY et al. 1980) and on encouraging clinical results with external beam radiotherapy and hyperthermia for superficial tumors (OVERGAARD 1990). IHT is easily combined with IRT and makes possible very good heating of implanted tumors (COUGHLIN 1990; EMAMI and PEREZ 1985).

A phase I/II trial of IHT-IRT for recurrent brain tumors was conducted at the University of California, San Francisco from July 1987 to September 1990 (SNEED et al. 1991, 1992), laying the foundation for our ongoing randomized phase II trial in patients with primary glioblastoma multiforme. This chapter describes our treatment methods, presents results of the completed trial, and discusses the potential of brain hyperthermia in the treatment of malignant gliomas.

32.2 Materials and Methods

32.2.1 Patient Selection

In general, tumors considered for brain implantation must be well-circumscribed supratentorial tumors less than 6 cm in diameter, without evidence of subependymal spread or extension across the corpus callosum. Reoperation prior to the brain implant is recommended for steroid-dependent patients in whom the tumor is producing significant mass effect.

Patients included in the IHT-IRT trial for recurrent brain tumors had either malignant gliomas or solitary brain metastases which had recurred or progressed after previous external beam radiotherapy. Our ongoing trial includes adults with newly diagnosed glioblastoma multiforme. These patients receive a 60 Gy implant boost with or without IHT 2 weeks after completing external beam radiation therapy (59.4 Gy at 1.8 Gy per

P.K. SNEED, M.D., Assistant Professor, Department of Radiation Oncology, Room L-75 (Box 0226), University of California, San Francisco, 505 Parnassus Avenue, San Francisco, CA 94143-0226, USA fraction) with oral hydroxyurea (300 mg/m^2 four times daily every Monday, Wednesday, and Friday).

Both protocols were reviewed and approved by the Committee on Human Research at the University of California, San Francisco. Informed consent is obtained in all cases.

32.2.2 Treatment Planning

On the morning of the implant procedure, a Brown-Roberts-Wells stereotactic base ring (Radionics, Burlington, Massachusetts) is fixed to the patient's skull. Axial computed tomography (CT) scans are obtained at 3-mm intervals through the tumor region with a system of graphite localizing rods mounted on the base ring. The magnetic tape from the CT scan is read into a VAX 4000, Model 300 computer (Digital Equipment Corporation, Maynard, Massachusetts).

Using a computer program called BRAIN which was developed at the University of California, San Francisco (Weaver et al. 1990), the target volume is outlined on each CT image 1–2 mm outside the edge of contrast enhancement. Because the same catheters used to house iodine-125 sources must be suitable to heat the tumor with interstitial microwave antennas, they are spaced about 1.2–2 cm apart from each other within 3–5 mm inside the tumor periphery (Fig. 32.1). Additional catheters are planned to house thermometry probes, generally including one at the center of the implant array and one or two at the tumor periphery.

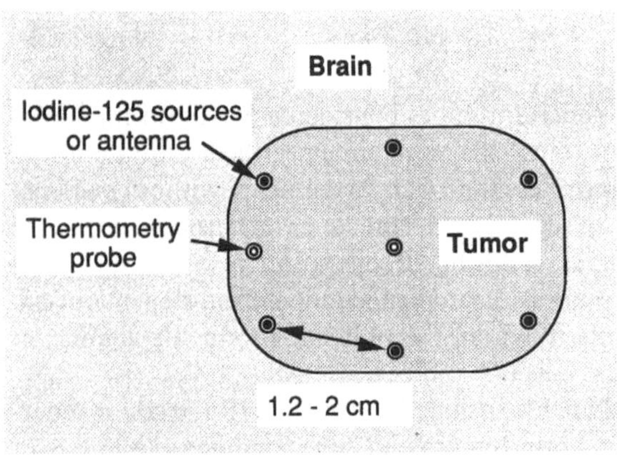

Fig. 32.1. Schematic diagram of an end-on view of a catheter arrangement used for IHT-IRT. Catheters spaced about 1.2–2 cm apart from each other around the periphery of the tumor are used sequentially for both microwave antennas and for iodine-125 sources. Additional thermometry catheters are usually placed at the center and/or edge of the implant array

After a tentative catheter arrangement is determined, tentative iodine-125 source activities and positions within the catheters are chosen. Resulting isodose lines may be viewed in any plane. Adjustments are made until a satisfactory plan is arrived at, closely covering the target volume with the 40–60 cGy/h isodose line while minimizing radiation dose to surrounding normal tissues.

32.2.3 Catheter Implantation

The patient is taken to the operating room after the final plan has been printed along with stereotactic coordinates and angles. For each catheter to be implanted, angles are set on the Brown-Roberts-Wells arc-ring assembly. Local anesthesia is applied at the implant site, a small incision is made in the scalp, a 3.4-mm-diameter twist drill hole is created in the skull, and a purse string suture is placed in the scalp about the catheter entry site. The Gutin Silastic brain catheter (2.16 mm outside diameter) (Radionics, Burlington, Massachusetts) with an inner stylet is inserted to the target depth through the guide in the arc-ring assembly and through the twist drill hole. The catheter is glued to a plastic collar which is then sutured to the scalp and the purse string suture is tightened about the catheter. Burr holes are occasionally used instead of twist drill holes near the sylvian fissure, sagittal sinus, or transverse sinus.

At the conclusion of the implant procedure, smaller nylon catheters (1.47 mm outside diameter) containing dummy sources are inserted into each of the larger brain implant catheters and orthogonal radiographs are taken through a fiducial marker box mounted on the base ring. This allows calculation and display of actual source positions and radiation isodose lines by the BRAIN program, superimposed on the preimplant CT images.

32.2.4 Interstitial Hyperthermia and Interstitial Radiation Therapy

On the morning following the implant procedure, the first IHT treatment is delivered using 915-MHz helical coil microwave antennas, available in a variety of heating lengths (Satoh and Stauffer

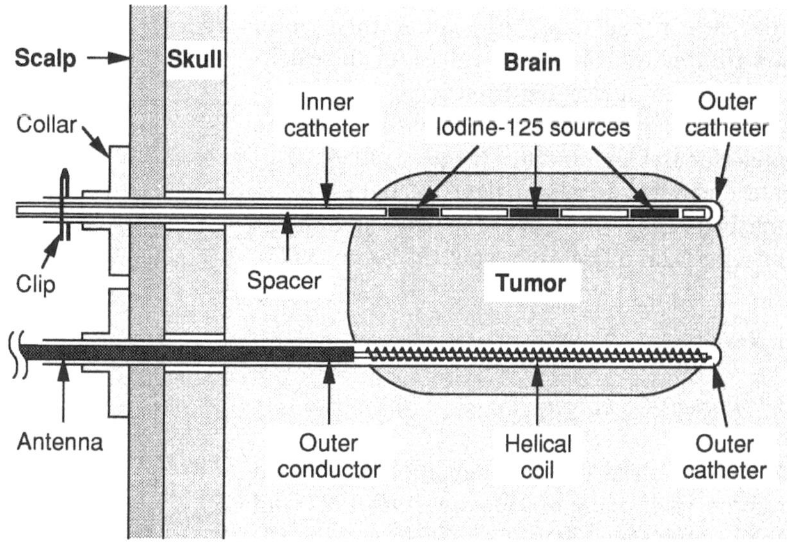

Fig. 32.2. Schematic diagram of a view along two implant catheters. A helical coil microwave antenna is pictured along with the iodine-125 sources for illustrative purposes only, since hyperthermia and interstitial irradiation are given sequentially and not simultaneously, using the same outer brain implant catheters

1988; SATOH et al. 1988) (Fig. 32.2), and an MTS-6200 hyperthermia system (Clini-Therm Corporation, Dallas, Texas). Multisensor fiber optic thermometry probes within dedicated thermometry catheters are mapped at 0.5-cm spatial intervals every 10 min. Our aim is to heat as much of the tumor volume as possible to at least 42.5°C for 30 min at steady state, without incurring neurological changes or normal tissue temperatures above about 43°C. For the first 15 patients, the maximum tumor temperature was limited to 45°C. Since then, maximum tumor temperatures up to 50°C have been permitted.

Within about 20 min after IHT, high activity iodine-125 sources are afterloaded into the brain catheters and fixed in place with surgical clips (Fig. 32.2). Patients wear a lead-lined hat for radiation shielding of medical personnel and visitors during the 4–6 day hospitalization. After a dose of 60 Gy has been delivered, iodine-125 sources are withdrawn and a second IHT treatment is administered. Brain implant catheters are then removed and patients are discharged from the hospital on the following day.

32.2.5 Follow-up Evaluation

Patients are evaluated every 2 months through the Neuro-Oncology service at the University of California, San Francisco with a physical examination and a contrast-enhanced brain CT or gadolinium-enhanced magnetic resonance (MR) scan. Brain scans are reviewed by the Neuroradiology service and scored qualitatively as showing stability, slight decrease, slight increase, definite decrease, or definite increase in the volume of contrast enhancement. A patient with definite increase in the volume of contrast enhancement is scored as having tumor progression unless subsequent reoperation shows only necrosis. Reoperation is generally performed in patients with worsened scans and clinical deterioration and/or increasing steroid requirement, providing confirmation of necrosis and/or tumor progression.

32.2.6 Data Analysis

For each patient treatment, steady-state tumor temperatures are tabulated for 0.5-cm spatial intervals along each thermometry catheter. The percentage of measured steady-state tumor temperatures greater than or equal to specific index temperatures are plotted versus index temperature and fitted with a smooth curve. This allows estimation of T_{50} and T_{90} by interpolation, quantifying the temperatures exceeded by 50% and 90% of the sampled tumor loci, respectively (DEWHIRST et al. 1990; LEOPOLD et al. 1992).

Study endpoints include survival (from the date of the first IHT treatment until death or last follow-up) and freedom from local tumor progression (from the date of IHT until the time of local tumor progression, documented by CT or MR scan changes and often confirmed by reoperation). Actuarial survival and freedom from progression curves are calculated by the product limit method of Kaplan and Meier (KAPLAN and MEIER 1958). Deaths clearly due to a cause other than brain tumor are treated as censored values for the calculation of actuarial freedom from local tumor progression. Actuarial curves are compared using the Mantel-Haenzel log rank test (MANTEL 1966). Univariate and multivariate analyses of data are accomplished using the Cox proportional hazards linear regression model (BRESLOW 1974; COX 1972).

32.3 Results

32.3.1 Patient Characteristics

The IHT-IRT trial for recurrent tumors accrued 49 tumors in 48 patients between June 1987 and September 1990, including 26 glioblastomas (two of which were treated sequentially in one patient), 16 anaplastic astrocytomas, four adenocarcinoma brain metastases, and three melanoma brain metastases. The median patient age was 43 years (range 18–71 and median Karnofsky performance status (KPS) 90 (range 40–90). The volume of contrast enhancement ranged from 1.7 to 78.1 cc (median 17 cc) (SNEED et al. 1992).

All patients had tumor progression after previous external beam radiation therapy given 1 month to 9 years earlier (median 11 months). Three patients had also had previous iodine-125 brain implants and 27 had failed prior chemotherapy. Recurrent tumors were subtotally resected in 24 patients 3–12 weeks prior to thermo-radiotherapy to relieve mass effect (SNEED et al. 1992).

32.3.2 Treatment Delivered

Brachytherapy dose ranged from 47.6 to 63.3 Gy given at 37–70 cGy/h to volumes of 4.7–117.4 cm^3 (median 32.4 cm^3), except that one patient with low KPS was treated with only 32.6 Gy. A total of 3–11 catheters were implanted, including one to eight for antennas (median, four) and one to three for thermometry probes (median, two). A total of 89 IHT treatments were administered. Reasons for cancellation of the second IHT treatment included neurological changes persisting for more than 24 h after the first IHT treatment (six cases), physician preference because of poor KPS (two cases), and implant duration less than 72 h (one case). Four treatment sessions were curtailed due to neurological changes (two cases) or focal motor seizures (two cases) (SNEED et al. 1992).

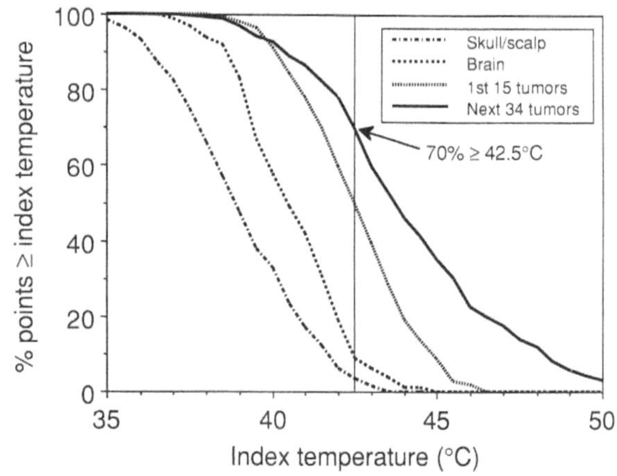

Fig. 32.3. Graph of steady-state temperatures for the best of two IHT sessions (or for the only session) for all 49 tumors, plotting the percentage of monitored points which were greater than or equal to specific index temperatures versus index temperature. For 49 treatments in 49 tumors, 100 points were monitored in normal brain tissue, 198 points in the skull and scalp, 147 points in the first 15 tumors, and 308 points in the next 34 tumors. For the latter group, 70% of the monitored tumor points were ≥ 42.5°C

Through proper selection of antenna heating patterns, IHT was well localized to superficial and deep, small and large tumors. Figure 32.3 shows heating results for the best (or only) treatment for all 49 tumors in terms of the number of steady-state temperatures greater than or equal to specific index temperatures versus index temperature. Only 9% of 100 points in normal brain were ≥ 42.5°C and only 3.5% of 198 points in the skull and scalp were ≥ 42.5°C. For the first 15 tumors, 50% of 147 tumor points were ≥ 42.5°C, whereas for the 34 tumors treated after maximum temperatures up to 50°C were allowed, 70% of 308 tumor points were ≥ 42.5°C. For the best or only treatment, T_{90} temperatures ranged from 38.0° to 45.8°C (median 41.2°C for all 49 tumors, 40.6°C for the first 15 tumors, and 42.0°C for the next 34 tumors).

32.3.3 Toxicity

Most patients experienced no sensation of heating. Complications included reversible neurological changes in 13 patients, nine seizures, two minor scalp infections, one meningitis, one bone flap infection, one deep venous thrombosis with nonfatal pulmonary embolus, and one scalp burn due to inadvertent slippage of an antenna (SNEED et al. 1992). Higher temperatures did not correlate with the occurrence of neurological changes or seizures.

32.3.4 Follow-up and Response

Median follow-up for living patients with anaplastic astrocytoma was 92 weeks (range 34–166 weeks) and median follow-up for living patients with glioblastoma multiforme was 37 weeks (range 11–82 weeks). One patient treated for recurrent brain metastasis is still living with follow-up of 59 weeks (SNEED et al. 1992).

Eighteen patients required reoperation (5–51 weeks after IHT-IRT) for an increasing contrast-enhancing lesion with clinical deterioration and/or an increasing steroid requirement. Tumor cells were seen in all specimens except for two specimens showing only necrosis. Eighteen patients were treated with salvage chemotherapy for tumor progression after IHT-IRT (SNEED et al. 1992).

All failures in glioma patients occurred at the site of the treated brain lesion except for a distant brain failure in one patient and leptomeningeal dissemination in another patient. Interestingly, all three melanoma brain metastases were controlled until death (22–56 weeks). Causes of death included progressive tumor at the treated site (18), melanoma metastases (3), pulmonary embolus 9 and 22 weeks after IHT-IRT (2), and leptomeningeal dissemination of glioblastoma multiforme (1) (SNEED et al. 1992).

Median survival measured from the date of the first IHT treatment was 47 weeks for patients with glioblastoma multiforme and 44 weeks for patients with brain metastases. Median survival has not yet been reached for patients with anaplastic astrocytoma, but is at least 64 weeks, with 81% survival at 1 year (SNEED et al. 1992) (Fig. 32.4).

Mean KPS decreased only slightly after treatment. For patients with follow-up of at least 6 months, the mean KPS was 82 immediately before IHT-IRT ($n = 36$), 75 6 months after treatment ($n = 36$), and 79 12 months after treatment (data available for 20 of 22 living patients). All cases of consistently declining KPS were due to progressive tumor rather than treatment sequelae (SNEED et al. 1992).

32.3.5 Univariate and Multivariate Analyses

Univariate and multivariate analyses were performed for the 41 patients with recurrent gliomas, examining the importance of histology, KPS, age, tumor volume, IRT dose, subsequent reoperation, and, for the best of the two patient treatments,

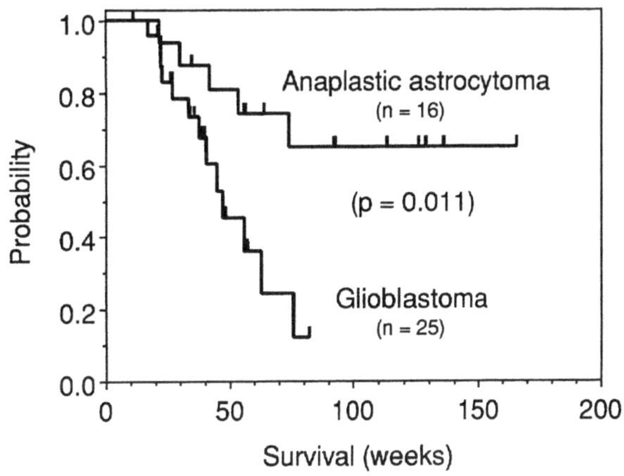

Fig. 32.4. Kaplan–Meier representation of the probability of survival in weeks, measured from the date of IHT-IRT, for patients with recurrent anaplastic astrocytoma and recurrent glioblastoma. *Tick marks* represent censored patients. Median survival has not yet been reached for patients with anaplastic astrocytoma. The median survival was 47 weeks for patients with glioblastoma multiforme

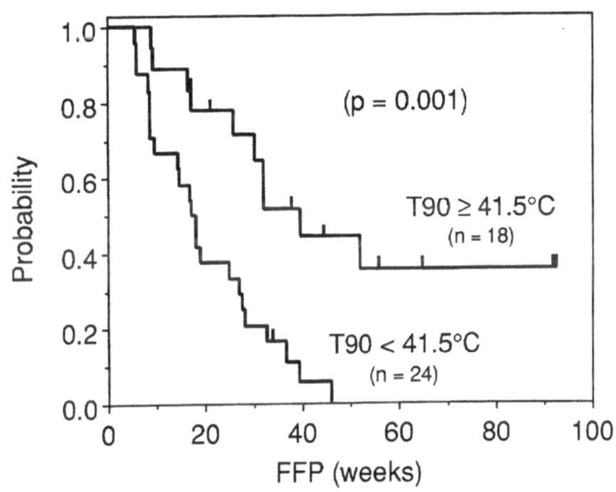

Fig. 32.5. Kaplan-Meier representation of the probability of freedom from local tumor progression (*FFP*) in weeks, measured from the date of IHT-IRT, for patients with recurrent anaplastic astrocytoma and recurrent glioblastoma, showing improved FFP for the 18 tumors which achieved $T_{90} \geq 41.5°C$ in comparison with the 24 tumors with $T_{90} < 41.5°C$ ($P = 0.001$). *Tick marks* represent censored patients

minimum tumor temperature, average tumor temperature, maximum tumor temperature, T_{90}, and T_{50}. Multivariate analyses showed that longer survival correlated with higher KPS ($P = 0.041$) and with anaplastic astrocytoma histological type as opposed to glioblastoma histological type ($P = 0.067$). The only significant parameters correlating with improved freedom from local tumor progression were higher T_{90} ($P = 0.00146$ with $P = 0.64$ for histology and $P = 0.4$ for tumor volume) and higher minimum tumor temperature ($P = 0.0009$ with $P = 0.98$ for histology and $P = 0.4$ for tumor volume) (SNEED et al., to be published).

As shown in Fig. 32.5, actuarial freedom from local tumor progression was significantly better for the 18 recurrent gliomas with $T_{90} \geq 41.5°C$ than for the 24 recurrent gliomas with $T_{90} < 41.5°C$ ($P = 0.001$). There was a trend toward improved actuarial survival for gliomas with $T_{90} \geq 41.5°C$ ($P = 0.083$) and for glioblastomas with $T_{90} \geq 41.5°C$ ($P = 0.093$) in comparison with tumors with $T_{90} < 41.5°C$.

32.4 Discussion

Many different heating methods have been reported for brain hyperthermia (SNEED et al. 1992). Although our center also has the capability to perform IHT with ferromagnetic implants and radiofrequency localized current field electrodes, we prefer microwave antennas for brain hyperthermia because this method requires the fewest implanted catheters.

Our phase I/II study of IHT-IRT for recurrent brain tumors demonstrated the feasibility of this technique. There was little heating of normal tissues outside of the target volume and, for the best treatment for all 49 tumors, 63% of tumor temperatures were $\geq 42.5°C$. The most common reason for failure to achieve a minimum tumor temperature of 41.5°–42.5°C was difficulty in heating the periphery of the tumor. Heating results may be improved by increasing the number of independently controlled antennas used, spacing them 1.2–1.5 cm apart from each other just inside the tumor periphery rather than up to 2 cm apart from each other (Fig. 32.1).

Toxicity was acceptable, with no deaths, no permanent neurological changes, and no increase in the reoperation rate in comparison with the reoperation rate after IRT alone (GUTIN et al. 1991; LEIBEL et al. 1989). However, the frequent occurrence of reversible neurological changes suggests that more aggressive treatment may not be advisable, at least in critical areas of the brain. In some cases, neurological changes during hyperthermia were treatment limiting.

One strategy which may allow delivery of a higher thermal dose without increasing normal brain toxicity is to try low temperature, continuous heating over many hours (ARMOUR et al. 1991; DEFORD et al. 1991). For hyperthermia techniques which allow simultaneous IHT and IRT, there may be an increased thermal enhancement ratio, and hopefully increased therapeutic gain (ARMOUR et al. 1991).

An unresolved issue is that of the appropriate volume to target, given the presence of tumor cells outside of the contrast-enhancing volume on CT or MR (BURGER 1983; KELLY et al. 1987). STEA et al. (1992) are implanting and heating a margin around the contrast-enhancing tumor mass using ferromagnetic implants. We are concerned about possible added toxicity of increasing the target volume for IHT-IRT. As long as the pattern of failure continues to be predominantly local, we prefer to limit the target volume to the contrast-enhancing mass and to rely on external beam radiotherapy with oral hydroxyurea as a radiosensitizer to treat a 3-cm margin around the contrast enhancement. Furthermore, the dose rate from IRT 0.5–1 cm outside the contrast-enhancing rim is approximately 50% of the prescribed dose rate, delivering an additional 30 Gy for our typical implant boost.

The survival of patients with recurrent gliomas treated with IHT-IRT was similar to our previous experience using brachytherapy alone (LEIBEL et al. 1989), but the strong correlation between freedom from local tumor progression and both minimum tumor temperature and T_{90} is evidence for a thermal dose–response relationship and suggests that hyperthermia does have potential to improve local control of malignant gliomas.

Having evaluated feasibility and toxicity in patients with recurrent tumors, we felt that the results warranted a trial in patients with newly diagnosed tumors, where IHT-IRT acts as a boost after external beam radiotherapy. A randomized phase II trial for previously untreated glioblastoma multiforme opened in the fall of 1990 (Northern California Cancer Center protocol 6G-90-2) to evaluate external beam radiation therapy (59.4 Gy at 1.8 Gy per daily fraction) with hydroxyurea (300 mg/m^2 every 6 h on Mondays, Wednesdays, and Fridays) followed by high activity iodine-125 implant boost of 60 Gy with or without IHT. So far 40 patients have been registered on this protocol. No results are available to date, but over the next few years, this trial as well as trials at other institutions should help define the role of IHT-IRT in the treatment of brain tumors.

References

Armour EP, Wang ZH, Corry PM, Martinez A (1991) Sensitization of rat 9L gliosarcoma cells to low dose rate irradiation by long duration 41°C hyperthermia. Cancer Res 51: 3088–3095

Breslow NE (1974) Covariance analysis of censored survival data. Biometrics 30: 89–99

Burger PC (1983) Pathologic anatomy and CT correlations in the glioblastoma multiforme. Appl Neurophysiol 46: 180–187

Coughlin CT (1990) Clinical hyperthermic practice: interstitial heating. In: Field SB, Hand JW (eds) An introduction to the practical aspects of clinical hyperthermia. Taylor & Francis, London, pp 172–184

Cox DR (1972) Regression models and life tables. J R Stat Soc 34: 187–220

DeFord JA, Babbs CF, Patel UH, Bleyer MW, Marchosky JA, Moran CJ (1991) Effective estimation and computer control of minimum tumour temperature during conductive interstitial hyperthermia. Int J Hyperthermia 7: 441–453

Dewey WC, Freeman ML, Raaphorst GP et al. (1980) Cell biology of hyperthermia and radiation. In: Meyn RE, Withers HR (eds) Radiation biology in cancer research. Raven, New York, pp 589–621

Dewhirst MW, Phillips TL, Samulski TV et al. (1990) RTOG quality assurance guidelines for clinical trials using hyperthermia. Int J Radiat Oncol Biol Phys 18: 1249–1259

Emami B, Perez CA (1985) Interstitial thermoradiotherapy: an overview. Endocurietherapy/Hyperthermia Oncol 1: 35–40

Gutin PH, Prados MD, Phillips TL et al. (1991) External irradiation followed by an interstitial high activity iodine-125 implant "boost" in the initial treatment of malignant gliomas: NCOG study 6G-82-2. Int J Radiat Oncol Biol Phys 21: 601–606

Kaplan EL, Meier P (1958) Nonparametric estimation from incomplete observations. J Am Stat Assoc 53: 457–481

Kelly PJ, Daumas-Duport C, Kispert DB, Wall BA, Scheithauer BW, Illig JJ (1987) Imaging-based stereotaxic serial biopsies in untreated intracranial glial neoplasms. J Neurosurg 66: 865–874

Leibel SA, Gutin PH, Wara WM et al. (1989) Survival and quality of life after interstitial implantation of removable high-activity iodine-125 sources for the treatment of patients with recurrent malignant gliomas. Int J Radiat Oncol Biol Phys 17: 1129–1139

Leopold KA, Dewhirst M, Samulski T (1992) Relationships among tumor temperature, treatment time, and histopathological outcome using preoperative hyperthermia with radiation in soft tissue sarcomas. Int J Radiat Oncol Biol Phys 22: 989–998

Mantel M (1966) Evaluation of survival data and two new rank order statistics arising in its consideration. Cancer Chemother Rep 50: 163–170

Overgaard J (1990) The current and potential role of hyperthermia in radiotherapy. Int J Radiat Oncol Biol Phys 16: 535–549

Satoh T, Stauffer PR (1988) Implantable helical coil microwave antenna for interstitial hyperthermia. Int J Hyperthermia 4: 497–512

Satoh T, Stauffer PR, Fike JR (1988) Thermal distribution studies of helical coil microwave antennas for interstitial hyperthermia. Int J Radiat Oncol Biol Phys 15: 1209–1218

Sneed PK, Stauffer PR, Gutin PH et al. (1991) Interstitial irradiation and hyperthermia for the treatment of recurrent malignant brain tumors. Neurosurgery 28: 206–215

Sneed PK, Gutin PH, Stauffer PR et al. (1992) Thermoradiotherapy of recurrent malignant brain tumors. Int J Radiat Oncol Biol Phys 23: 853–861

Stea B, Kittelson J, Cassady JR et al. (1992) Treatment of malignant gliomas with interstitial irradiation and hyperthermia. Int J Radiat Oncol Biol Phys 24: 657–667

Weaver K, Smith V, Lewis JD et al. (1990) A CT-based computerized treatment planning system for I-125 stereotactic brain implants. Int J Radiat Oncol Biol Phys 18: 445–454

33 Intracavitary Thermoradiotherapy for Esophageal Cancer

P. FRITZ, W. HÜRTER, P. SCHRAUBE, F. REINBOLD, W.J. LORENZ, and M. WANNENMACHER

CONTENTS

33.1 Introduction

Curative results in the treatment of esophageal carcinomas have been significantly improved neither by surgery nor by radiotherapy during the past 40 years. Thus the 5-year survival rate is below 10% in both surgically treated and primarily irradiated patients. Survival rates of between 10% and 20% can only be achieved in the subgroup of patients with resectable tumors. This means that surgery is the treatment of choice in cases with potential resectability and lack of metastases. However, only 10%–15% of patients treated surgically undergo potentially curative resection. In the inoperable patients the most effective component in palliative treatment is still radiotherapy. Furthermore, in some cases only radiotherapy offers a chance of cure.

Even after radiation doses of 60 Gy and more, local recurrence rates of approximately 58% have been reported in large series (ISAEV and BEIBUTOV 1988); moreover, 90% of such recurrences occur within the first year after irradiation (WANNENMACHER et al. 1986). In autopsy series, residual disease was found in 78%–93% of cases (MANTRAVADI et al. 1982).

Recent studies on radiation therapy for esophageal cancer indicate that the achievement of local tumor control influences survival and that metastatic spread is not the sole determinant of prognosis (WANNENMACHER et al. 1986; POPLIN et al. 1987; FRITZ et al., to be published). For example, a prospective randomized RTOG study on bronchial carcinoma showed that complete remission had a significant influence on the survival curve (PEREZ 1985). In view of the inadequate local control of esophageal carcinoma, multimodal treatment approaches have been designed to increase the effect of radiotherapy. The most important innovations are (a) simultaneous radio- and chemotherapy, (b) combined external beam and intracavitary radiotherapy, and (c) Nd-YAG laser debulking for initial removal of tumor stenosis. However, the oldest and best known adjuvant for increasing the effect of radiotherapy – hyperthermia – has scarcely been considered for the treatment of esophageal carcinoma.

In comparison with historical reports, most studies of radio-chemotherapy or combined external beam and intracavitary radiotherapy indicate a trend towards improved local remission rates and median survival times. Today it can be expected that treatment approaches which significantly improve local tumor control will also influence early mortality, i.e., survival for the first 2–3 years after treatment.

Local hyperthermia has been performed for about 20 years, leading to the acquisition of extensive data. Almost all comparative studies report an increased remission rate (approx. twice as high) and faster remission when hyperthermia is employed. The toxicity of radiotherapy hardly seems to be influenced by hyperthermia. The high therapeutic ratio of thermoradiotherapy would seem to be advantageous precisely in patients with esophageal carcinomas, who commonly present with other disorders.

P. FRITZ, M.D.; P. SCHRAUBE, M.D.; M. WANNENMACHER, M.D.; Radiologische Universitätsklinik, Abteilung Strahlentherapie, Im Neuenheimer Feld 400, W-6900 Heidelberg, Germany
W. HÜRTER, M.D.; F. REINBOLD, M.D.; W.J. LORENZ, M.D.; Deutsches Krebsforschungszentrum, Im Neuenheimer Feld 280, W-6900 Heidelberg, Germany

33.2 Patients and Methods

33.2.1 Technical Description of the "Endotherm" System

The technically simplest application of hyperthermia for the treatment of esophageal carcinoma is the insertion of an endoluminal hyperthermia applicator. For physical reasons, microwave hyperthermia with a frequency range of between 300 and 1000 MHz seems the most favorable option.

The distribution of the specific absorption rate (SAR) of electromagnetic energy within the target volume is of decisive importance for effective hyperthermia of that area when using high frequency applicators. If the SAR profiles of two interstitial high frequency hyperthermia systems are compared, the advantage of a microwave hyperthermia system over a radiofrequency hyperthermia system is clearly recognizable. In Fig. 33.1 the normalized SAR profile of a 915-MHz microwave antenna and the SAR profile of a 13.56-MHz radiofrequency needle are shown for muscular tissue. The clearly less steep SAR profile of the microwave antenna (Fig. 33.1a) means that it permits a clearly stronger deposition of electromagnetic energy at depth, as a consequence of which a more homogeneous temperature distribution in the tissue can be expected. The high heating of tissue in immediate neighborhood of the applicator surface that occurs with radiofrequency needles is less pronounced when using a microwave antenna. Therefore, no cooling system was designed for our microwave applicators.

The microwave hyperthermia device "Endotherm", developed in cooperation with the German Cancer Research Center (and supported financially by the Krebs- und Scharlachstiftung Mannheim and the Tumorzentrum Heidelberg/Mannheim), operates at 434 MHz and is equipped with various applicators especially for endoluminal hyperthermia. The device has the following components:

1. A 434-MHz generator with continuously adjustable power supply up to 100 W
2. A fiberoptic temperature sensor system with eight probes (Luxtron M 3000)
3. A PC (Hurricane PC-AT/386) for registration of measurement data and regulation of temperature

The power supply can be adjusted manually in the switched-on position. Temperature regulation is achieved by automatic switching off of the generator via the PC as soon as the fluoroptic temperature sensor system measures the chosen threshold temperature at one of the measuring points (maximum number = 8). The threshold temperature is the same for all measuring points, so that the first temperature probe to register the threshold temperature regulates the hyperthermia. By increasing the threshold value the temperatures at the other measuring points can be adjusted to avoid temperatures below 42°C.

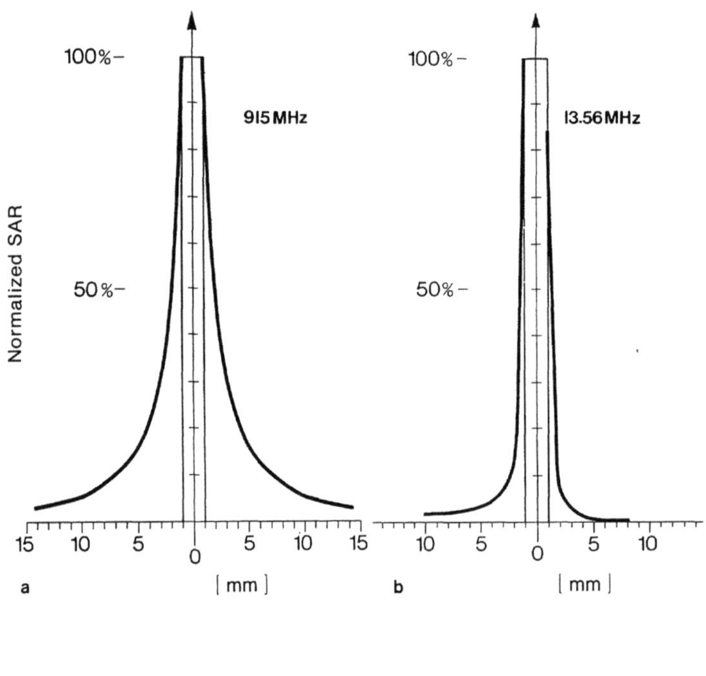

Fig. 33.1a, b. Normalized axial SAR profiles of a 915-MHz microwave antenna and a 13.56-MHz radiofrequency needle

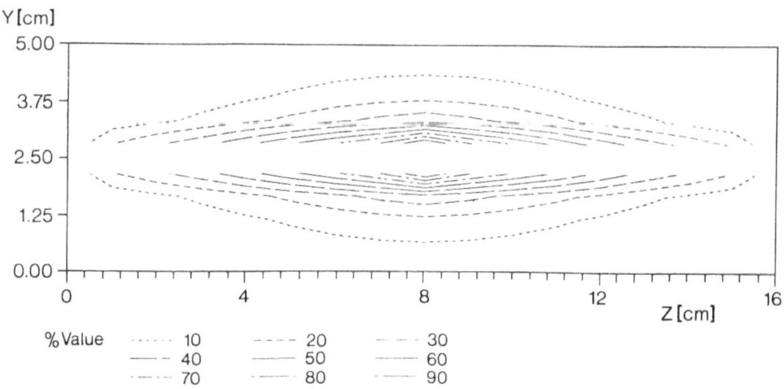

Fig. 33.2. Longitudinal SAR distribution of an esophageal microwave antenna (length: 15 cm; frequency: 434 MHz)

The esophageal antennae are built as flexible dipoles. Two antennae are used with an effective heating length of 10 or 15 cm each (Fig. 33.2). The antennae are inserted into a 7-mm-diameter plastic tube which has been positioned in the esophagus in advance. On the surface of the applicator tube are 8 microchannels in a longitudinal direction, each of which takes a fiberoptic temperature sensor (Fig. 33.3). The measuring points are positioned at intervals of 2 cm in a spiral fashion in the aforementioned microchannels; in accordance with the thickness of the applicator tube, they are generally in contact with the tumor surface or esophageal mucosa. This approach to measuring the tumor surface temperature is the only routinely possible means of temperature control in the case of esophageal carcinomas. Invasive measurement methods, e.g., insertion of a probe into the tumor, would represent a scarcely justifiable risk to the patient.

33.2.2 Treatment Approach

Since 1989 the form of radiotherapy that we have employed for esophageal carcinomas has been combined external beam and intracavitary irradiation. The intracavitary irradiation is performed with an HDR afterloading device (Gammamed IIi) as a boost following conventionally fractionated teletherapy. External reference doses are between 40 and 60 Gy, depending on the treatment plan. The afterloading boost is delivered in 3–4 fractions of 5 Gy, with reference to the surrounding isodose 10 mm lateral to the applicator surface, at intervals of 4–7 days. Since 1990 we have combined the afterloading boost with intraluminal microwave hyperthermia. The same applicator tube is used for intracavitary irradiation and microwave hyperthermia. Immediately after intracavitary irradiation the source guide of the afterloading device is removed from the applicator tube in the esophagus and replaced by a microwave antenna (Fig. 33.4). The hyperthermia is delivered over a period of 30–45 min, with a maximum temperature on the applicator surface of 48°C. For premedication, an anticholinergic neuroleptic drug (Droperidol) is given.

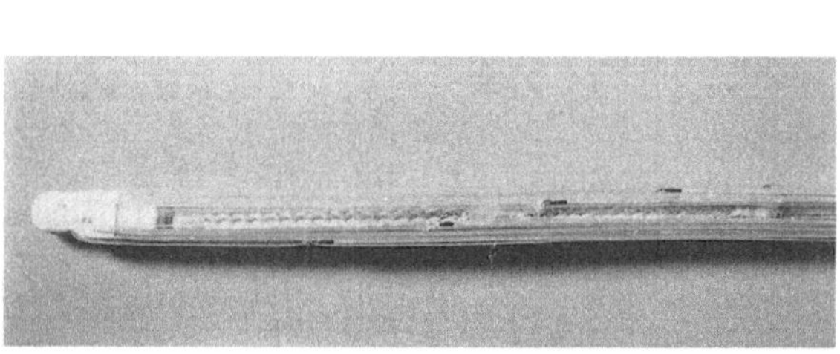

Fig. 33.3. Applicator tube for intracavitary irradiation and hyperthermia with introduced 10-cm microwave antenna. The black points inside the microchannels on the surface of the tube are the temperature probes

The whole treatment plan is adjusted to tumor stage and general condition of the patient (Table 33.1). Afterloading irradiation with hyperthermia alone is only considered for recurrences in the irradiated area or if the patient's general condition is poor (Karnofsky index $\leq 40\%$) (protocol I). For "bulky disease" (tumor length ≥ 10 cm or tumor diameter ≥ 4 cm and/or metastases), simultaneous radio-chemotherapy is carried out (protocol II). When there is insufficient remission of the primary after radio-chemotherapy, an afterloading boost with hyperthermia is carried out (protocol IIb). Patients of advanced age or with a Karnofsky index of between 40% and 60% receive external beam irradiation with 50 Gy as well as an afterloading boost with hyperthermia (protocol III).

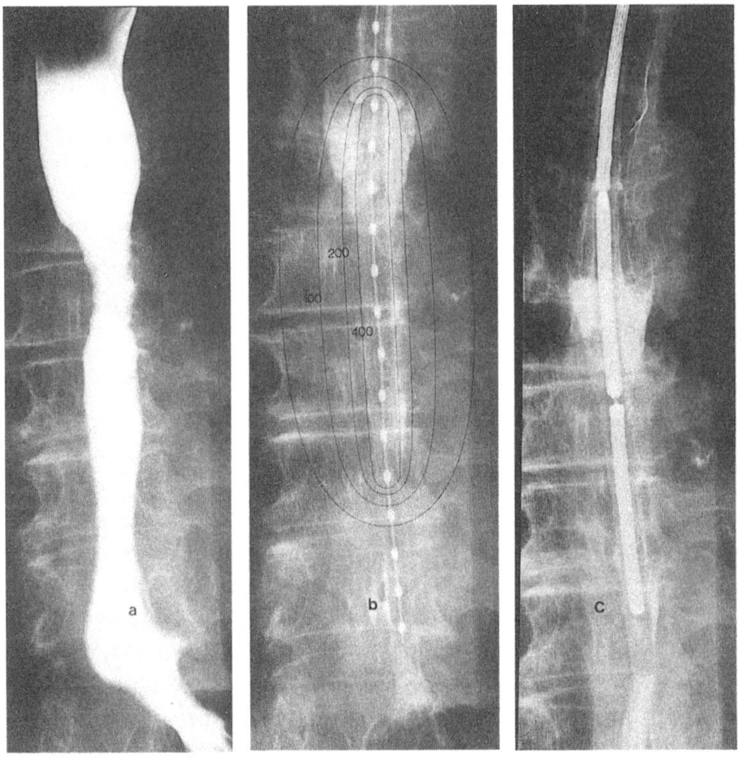

Fig. 33.4. **a** Combined brachy-thermo-radiotherapy for a T2 esophageal carcinoma. **b** Isodose distribution for intracavitary irradiation (100% = 5 Gy). **c** Introduced microwave antenna

In the clincial stage T1-3N0M0 after external beam irradiation with 60 Gy, a local dose increase to 75 Gy is carried out with afterloading and intraluminal hyperthermia (protocol IV). For staging we use the old TNM classification from 1978. The new classification from 1987 is not applicable to inoperable patients because the T stage is based solely on histopathological criteria.

Table 33.1. Heidelberg set of protocols for primary radiotherapy for esophageal cancer

I	*Recurrences after radiotherapy, passage preservation if Karnofsky index ≤ 40%:* N × 3–7 Gy afterloading (AL) with hyperthermia (HT)
II	*"Bulky disease" and/or metastases:* 40 Gy external beam + 2 courses 5-FU/cisplatin (radiochemotherapy)
IIa	≥ 50% remission: additional chemotherapy (4 courses)
IIb	< 50% remission: 4 × 5 Gy AL with HT
III	*All stages and age > 70 years and/or Karnofsky index ≤ 60%:* 50 Gy external beam + 4 × 5 Gy AL with HT
IV	*T1–3N0M0, age < 70 years, and Karnofsky index > 60%:* 60 Gy external beam + 3 × 5 Gy AL with HT

33.3 Results

Up to the closing date of 31 December 1991, 19 patients had been treated in a phase 1 study (Table 33.2). It was shown that in order to achieve a minimum temperature of 42°C on the applicator surface at all measuring points, a threshold temperature of 45° – 48°C was necessary (Fig. 33.5). The power supply to the applicator was about 20–30 W. Hyperthermia was excellently tolerated even with temperature maxima of 48°C. Most of the patients had a clear feeling of warmth retrosternally, but were not in pain. On the closing date eight patients were still alive. Seven patients (37%) achieved complete remission, and of these seven, four had T3

Table 33.2. Thermoradiotherapy for carcinoma of the esophagus: Heidelberg results

Patients:	$n = 19$
Treatment protocol:	I: 1, IIb: 6, III: 7, IV: 5
Follow-up period:	2–20 months (median: 12 months)
T stage (TNM 1978):	T1: 1, T2: 4, T3: 14
Tumor regression:	NC 1/19 (5%), PR 11/19 (58%), CR 7/19 (37%)
Alive at 31 Dec 1991:	8/19 (42%)
NED at 31 Dec 1991:	4/8

NC, no change; PR, partial remission; CR, complete remission

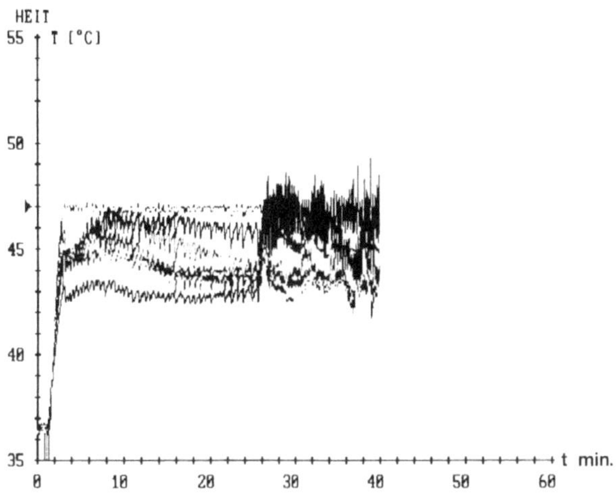

Fig. 33.5. Temperature distribution along the surface of the applicator tube. Each *line* represents a measuring point, the point lying at a distance of 2 cm from each other

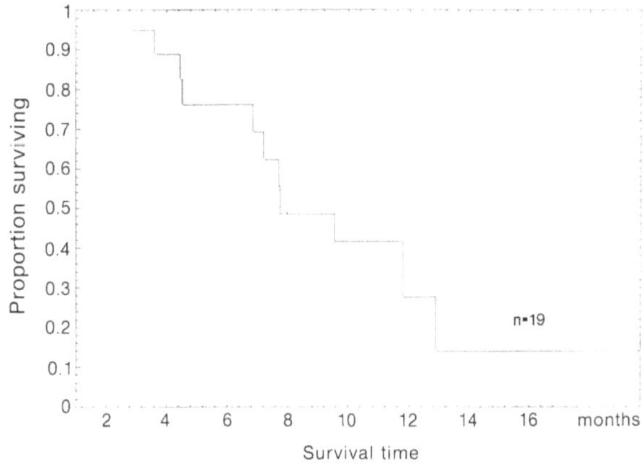

Fig. 33.6. Kaplan–Meier estimation of survival of patients treated with combined hyperthermia and radiotherapy (median survival 235 days)

tumors. All patients with complete remission were free from local relapse up to the day they died or up to the closing date. Additional hyperthermia was not found to increase radiation side-effects.

33.4 Discussion and Literature Review

There are few data in the literature regarding thermoradiotherapy for esophageal carcinoma. Most of the reported studies combined radiotherapy, chemotherapy/radiosensitizer, and hyperthermia. Chemotherapy or radiosensitizer was applied simultaneously with radiotherapy. Hyperthermia was carried out with intraluminal high frequency applicators in combination with external beam irradiation in four to eight sessions (Table 33.3); publications on the combination of hyperthermia with brachytherapy do not exist. The frequency varied between 13, 56 and 2450 MHz. The duration of hyperthermia was at least 30 min. The maximum temperatures were between 42°C and 45°C and always referred to the applicator surface. Invasive temperature measurements have not been carried out routinely.

Presently the most extensive and longest follow-up study is that reported by SUGIMACHI et al. (1986) (Table 33.4). The addition of hyperthermia to radio-chemotherapy improved the results of preoperative as well as primary radiotherapy. SUGIMACHI et al. reported that tumor-free resection specimens were obtained in 22.6% of 62 patients thus treated, in comparison to 12.1% of 116 patients of a control group only treated with

Table 33.3. Carcinoma of the esophagus: methods of thermoradiotherapy

Author	No. of patients	Radiotherapy (Gy)	Chemotherapy	Hyperthermia				
				Reference temperature (°C)	HT time (min)	HT fractions	Frequency (MHz)	Mode
LI et al. (1982)	82	40	0	> 43			2450	Primary
SHA et al. (1984)	42	30–40	0	44–46	30	6–8	2450	Preop.
SUGIMACHI et al. (1986)	62	30	Bleomycin	42–45	30	6	13.56	Preop.
LI and HOU (1987)	32	0	Bleo. + Cispl	45–50	60	6–8	915	Primary
ISAEV and BEIBUTOV (1988)	38	48–51	(Metronidazole)	43	30–45	4	915	Primary
HOU et al. (1989)	34	30	Bleo. + Cispl	43–44	60	6	915	Primary
SUGIMACHI and MATSUDA (1990)	31	30	Bleomycin	42–45	30	6	13.56	Primary

Table 33.4. Carcinoma of the esophagus: results of thermoradiotherapy

Author	No. of Patients	Survival rate (%) 0.5 yr	1 yr	2 yr	5 yr	CR (%)	PR (%)	Tumor-free resected Specimen (%)
LI et al. (1982)	82	86 vs 63[a]	–	–	–	62 vs 58	–	–
SHA et al. (1984)	42	–	90	65	–	–	–	31
SUGIMACHI et al. (1986)	62	–	–	–	43 vs 15[a]	–	–	22.6 vs 12.1[a]
LI and HOU (1987)	32	–	–	–	–	25	41	–
ISAEV and BEIBUTOV (1988)	38	–	95	–	–	65 (72)[b]	–	–
HOU et al. (1989)	34	–	74	44	–	62	32	–
SUGIMACHI and MATSUDA (1990)	31	–	33.2 vs 10.8[a]	15 vs 1.2[a]	–	–	–	–

[a] Irradiation without hyperthermia
[b] With metronizadol

preoperative radio-chemotherapy. SHA et al. (1984) reported 31% tumor-free specimens after preoperative thermoradiotherapy. According to SUGIMACHI et al., postoperative survival rates were also significantly higher in the patients treated with thermo-radio-chemotherapy – 1 year: 65.8% vs 44.9%; 3 years: 43.2% vs 20.4%; 5 years: 43.2% vs 14.7%. In addition, the results of primary radiotherapy for nonresectable tumors were improved through hyperthermia. One-year and 2-year survival rates of 33.2% and 15% were achieved in 31 patients treated with thermo-radio-chemotherapy, as compared with 10.8% and 1.2% in 83 patients treated with radio-chemotherapy (SUGIMACHI and MATSUDA 1990). Also of note are the high complete remission rates reported by LI et al. (1982) ISAEV and BEIBUTOV (1988), and HOU et al. (1989).

The following points favor the use of combined hyperthermia and brachytherapy after external beam irradiation:

1. With both brachytherapy and microwave hyperthermia an effective dose is delivered only in the very close proximity of the applicator, i.e., within 10 mm from the applicator surface. In the case of tumors with a radial thickness exceeding 10 mm, only endoluminal parts can be treated effectively. While this would satisfy the palliative objective of ensuring passage, it would not satisfy the curative objective of definitive local tumor control through a small-volume boost. The preceding external beam irradiation generally substantially reduces the tumor volume and provides optimal conditions for brachytherapy.

2. It has to be taken into consideration that after a course of radiotherapy, hypoxic cell areas, which could not be reoxygenated, may remain. Increased temperature sensitivity of hypoxic cells has been described by numerous authors. Therefore, for hypoxic residual tumor parts, the combined brachy-thermoradiotherapy boost seems especially appropriate.

Presently thermoradiotherapy of the esophageal carcinoma is at the level of phase 1 and 2 studies. As in the case of head and neck tumors, an improvement in local tumor control can be expected. Nevertheless, many questions remain to be answered. There is uncertainty over the optimal number and duration of hyperthermia sessions. It has to be proven that the applicator surface temperature is a suitable parameter for the control of hyperthermia. Finally, standardization of treatment approaches and the technical equipment is a prerequisite for the demonstration of therapeutic benefit by means of phase 3 studies.

References

Fritz P, Schraube P, Oberle J, Wannenmacher M, Friedl P (1992) Perkutan-endokavitäre Strahlenbehandlung der Ösophaguskarzinome. Strahlenther Onkol 168: 154–161
Hou BS, Xiong QB, Li DJ (1989) Thermo-chemo-radiotherapy of esophageal cancer. Cancer 64: 1777–1782
Hürter W, Reinbold F, Lorenz WJ (1991) A dipole antenna for interstitial microwave hyperthermia. IEEE Trans Microwave Theory Tech 39: 6
Isaev IG, Beibutov SM (1988) Strahlentherapie des Ösophaguskarzinoms mit dynamischer Dosisfraktionierung in Kombination mit Metronidazol und lokaler Hyperthermie. Radiobiol Radiother 29: 5–9
Li DJ, Hou BS (1987) Preliminary report on the treatment of esophageal cancer by intraluminal microwave

hyperthermia and chemotherapy. Cancer Treat Rep 71: 1013–1019
Li DJ, Wang CQ, Qin SL, Shao LF (1982) Intraluminal microwave hyperthermia in the combined treatment of esophageal cancer: a preliminary report of 103 patients. Natl Cancer Inst Monogr 61: 419–421
Mantravadi RVP, Lad T, Briele H, Liebner EJ (1982) Carcinoma of the esophagus: sites of failure. Int J Radiat Oncol Biol Phys 8: 1897–1901
Perez CA (1985) Non-small cell carcinoma of the lung: dose-time parameters. Cancer Treat Symp 2: 131
Poplin E, Fleming T, Leichmann L et al. (1987) Combined therapies for squamous-cell carcinoma of the esophagus, a Southwest Oncology Group Study (SWOG 8037). J Clin Oncol 5: 622–628
Sha YH, Li DJ, Qin SL et al. (1984) The combined treatment of esophageal cancer – a clinical pathological study of 42 cases. In: Overgaard JD (ed) Hyperthermic oncology. Taylor & Francis, London, pp 371–374
Sugimachi K, Matsuda H (1990) Experimental and clinical studies of hyperthermia for carcinoma of the esophagus. In: Gautherie M (ed) Interstitial, endocavitary and perfusional hyperthermia. Springer, New York Berlin Heidelberg, pp 59–76
Sugimachi K, Kai H, Matsufuji H et al. (1986) Histopathological evaluation of hyperthermo-chemo-radiotherapy for carcinoma of the esophagus. J Surg Oncol 32: 82–85
Wannenmacher M, Slanina J, Bruggmoser G, Nanko N (1986) Strahlentherapie des Ösophaguskarzinomes – Indikationen, Methodik und erzielbare Ergebnisse. Radiologe 26: 479–489

34 Intracavitary Thermoradiotherapy for Vaginal Carcinoma

B. SORBE, D. ROOS, C. SMED-SÖRENSEN, and B. FRANKENDAL

CONTENTS

34.1 Introduction

Cancer of the vagina has a poor prognosis with regard to both local tumor control and patient survival, the 5-year survival being approximately 38% (PETTERSSON 1985). Probably due to the large proportion of hypoxic cells in these tumors, reduced radiosensitivity is often observed (FLETCHER and SHUKOVSKY 1975). The standard radiotherapy is usually similar to that for cervical carcinoma, with external beam therapy and intracavitary irradiation. Since hyperthermia is known to reduce the survival of hypoxic cells in particular, the local tumor control rate might be expected to increase when hyperthermia is added to radiotherapy. Technical improvements, for example the possibility of using intracavitary microwave antennas (ROOS et al. 1989), have opened up new possibilites of combined intracavitary irradiation and hyperthermia in the treatment of cervical (HAO et al. 1984) and vaginal carcinoma. Thermoradiotherapy was tried by VALDAGNI et al. (1988) in the treatment of cervical cancer recurrences in the vaginal apex using an individualized microwave applicator.

A pilot study was initiated to evaluate intracavitary hyperthermia and intracavitary irradiation using a high dose rate afterloading technique as combination therapy. Previous experience (SORBE et al. 1990) has shown that it is possible to use a vaginal hyperthermia applicator for this purpose. A cooling system was gradually introduced to improve further the efficacy of the vaginal hyperthermia applicator. A more homogeneous temperature distribution and a less steep temperature gradient were thus achieved.

B. SORBE, M.D., Ph.D.; D. ROOS, Ph.D.; C. SMED-SÖRENSEN, M.D.; B. FRANKENDAL, M.D., Ph.D.; Department of Gynecologic Oncology, Örebro Medical Center Hospital, S-701 85 Örebro, Sweden

34.2 Materials and Methods

34.2.1 Hyperthermia

A pen-shaped, 190-mm-long applicator with a diameter of 8 mm was used. The frequency used was 915 MHz, which is the operating frequency of the hyperthermia system used in our treatments (ROOS et al. 1989). Perspex vaginal obturators with 20-mm and 30-mm diameters and measuring 180 mm in length were designed, each with a central or peripheral canal for the insertion of the applicator (Fig. 34.1).

Temperature probes were positioned in Venflon tubes inserted into the vaginal walls. The temperature was recorded at the surface of the applicator, at the center and periphery of the tumor, and at the borders of the risk organs (bladder and rectal walls). Two hyperthermia treatment sessions (after the first and last of the five intracavitary irradiation treatments) were used. The treatment time was 60 min at least 42.5°C measured by thermistors at the periphery of the tumor lesions. The delay time between irradiation and hyperthermia was 30–60 min.

A system with circulating cooling water was developed to obtain a more homogeneous heat distribution. Water channels were milled out at the periphery of the vaginal obturator just beneath its surface and encompassed the whole circumference (symmetrical antenna position) or just a sector of the circumference (asymmetrical antenna position) (Fig. 34.1b). During phantom experiments the importance of various water temperatures and flow

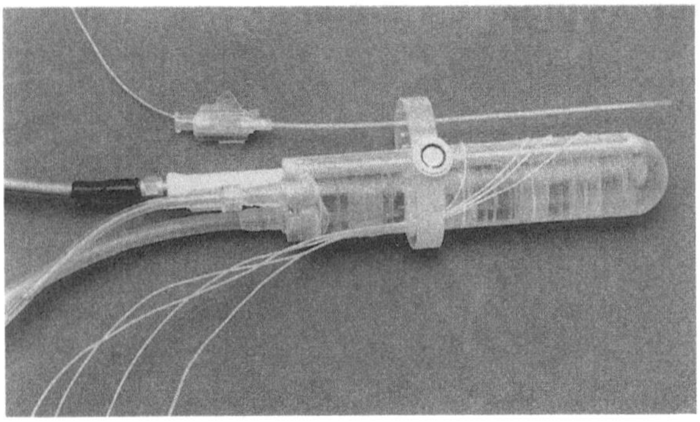

a

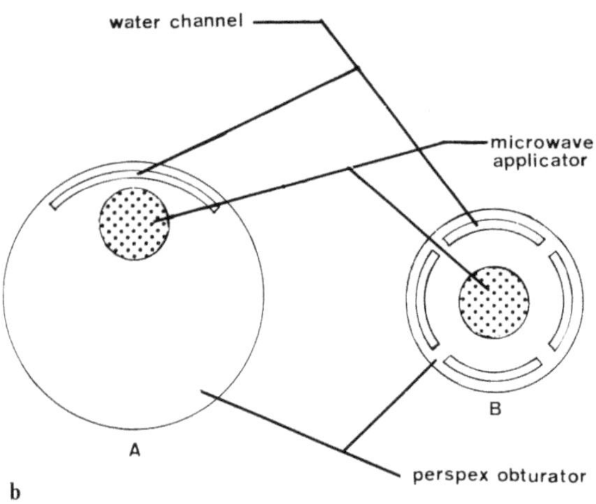

b

Fig. 34.1. a A photograph of the vaginal applicator with the microwave antenna and the water cooling system. A number of thermistor probes fixed to the surface of the Perspex obturator and inserted into a Venflon tube (representing the periphery of the tumor) are also shown. **b** Cross-sectional views of applicators with central (*B*) and peripheral antenna (*A*) positions and built-in cooling channels

rates was explored. The results of these studies showed that it was most convenient to keep the water temperature constant (21°–22°C) and to let the flow rate vary, using a computer-controlled infusion pump (Fig. 34.2). The flow rate varied between 150 and 999 ml/h, depending on the temperature at the surface of the applicator. The cooling is only effective 1–2 mm below the surface of the applicator. The gradient of cooling is much steeper than that of the microwave power gradient, resulting in a more homogeneous heat distribution. Vaginal treatments without cooling are not feasible due to the steep temperature gradient which results in tissue necrosis at the surface of the mucosa when an attempt is made to reach a therapeutic temperature (43°C) at the periphery of the tumor.

34.2.2 Afterloading Radiotherapy

In the vaginal irradiation a remote afterloading technique was used, employing high dose rate cobalt-60 and iridium-192 sources. A straight steel catheter was inserted into the same type of Perspex vaginal obturator as described for the hyperthermia treatments. The irradiation dose was specified at 10 mm from the surface of the obturator. The dose rate was approximately 1 Gy/min and the fraction dose was 6 Gy. The number of fractions was five, given in combination with external beam therapy.

In the primary treatment of the vaginal carcinoma, the external photon beam therapy (10 or 20 MV) was administered to the pelvic tissue, using a "box technique." The dose fraction was 2 Gy, given five times a week for 5 weeks up to a midplane dose of 50 Gy. Intracavitary irradiation alone was used to treat tumor recurrences.

34.2.3 Patient Series

A total of 13 patients (six with primary and seven with recurrent tumors) have been treated so far with a combination of radiotherapy and hyperthermia. The histological types were ten squamous cell carcinomas, two adenocarcinomas, and one sarcoma. The tumors were localized mainly in the lower third of the vagina and in the anterior wall (Table 34.1)

Most primary tumor patients received both external (25 × 2 Gy) and intracavitary (5 × 6 Gy) irradiation, with hyperthermia added in conjunction with the first and last intracavitary irradiation sessions. The patients with recurrent tumors had previously received external pelvic irradiation (40–66 Gy) and were therefore only given additional intracavitary irradiation with a dose of 5–6 Gy per fraction in 2–9 fractions. These patients also received intracavitary hyperthermia after the first and last intracavitary irradiation sessions. The hyperthermia applicator, with temperature probes

Table 34.1. Tumor localization in the vagina

	Upper	Middle	Lower	Total
Posterior	1	2	1	4
Lateral	1	1	2	4
Anterior	–	–	5	5
Total	2	3	8	13

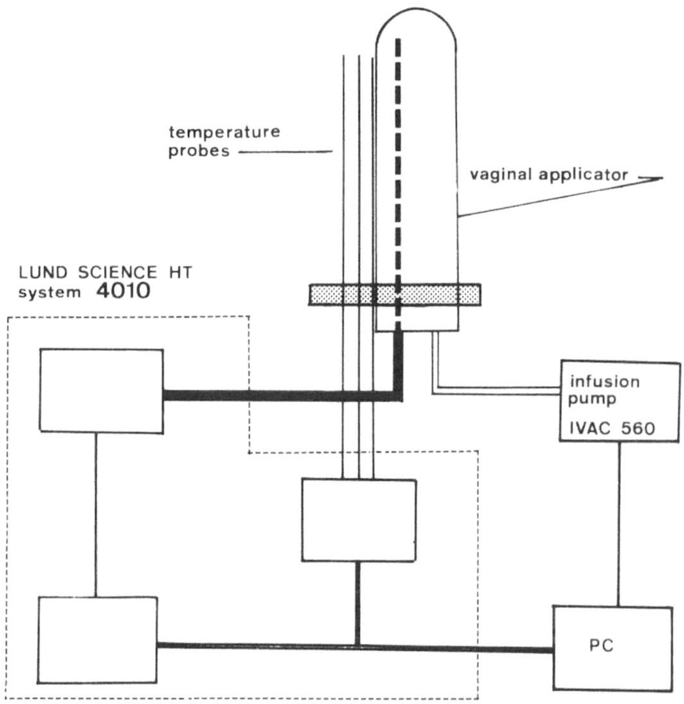

Fig. 34.2. The integrated hyperthermia (Lund Science 4010) and water cooling system. The water flow rate is computer controlled

fixed on its surface, was inserted into the vagina. Two thin catheters were inserted interstitially parallel to the applicator using a template. One catheter was positioned centrally in the tumor and the other at the most distant tumor periphery. These two catheters served as guides for multipoint temperature probes. A total of at least ten points of measurement was obtained in this way (Fig. 34.1a). Both anteroposterior and lateral radiographs were then taken to ensure applicator and catheter positions. The hyperthermia treatment was then started using both microwave heating and cooling by circulating water at room temperature within the applicator. The treatment time was set at 60 min from the moment the tumor periphery temperature reached 43°C. The temperature at the applicator surface was maintained at 43°C by adjusting the rate of flow of the cooling water (Fig. 34.3).

34.3 Results

During the first 10 min of hyperthermia the temperature rise was generally steep and smooth. During the next 5–10 min, a physiological counteraction from tissue circulation started and the generator power had to be increased to 85 W to achieve a measured minimum of 42.5°C at the tumor periphery after 20 min of treatment. During the following 60 min the temperature showed a continuous fluctuation of approximately ± 1.0°C.

Local control was achieved in five of six patients with primary tumors (Table 34.2). In two of these patients distant metastases were diagnosed soon after completion of the primary therapy. In the group with recurrent tumors, two of seven patients showed local control (complete remission) and another three patients showed tumor reductions of

Table 34.2. Results: primary tumors of the vagina

Pat. no.	Diagnosis and stage	RT (Gy) (ext, intracav)	HT (°C/min) (tumor temp/time)	Tumor response	Time (months)
1	Ca vag I	25 × 2, 5 × 6	41.1/51 –	CR	6
2	Ca vag II	25 × 2, 5 × 6	41.4/60, 41.2/58	CR	16
3	Ca vag II	25 × 2, 5 × 6	40.9/70, 41.6/64	CR	17
4	Ca vag II	25 × 2, 5 × 6	40.5/62, 42.9/61	CR	38
5	Ca vag II	25 × 2, 5 × 6	43.8/60, 45.4/75	CR	11
6	Sarc vag III	30 × 2, 3 × 6	46.0/72, 43.2/56	NR	–

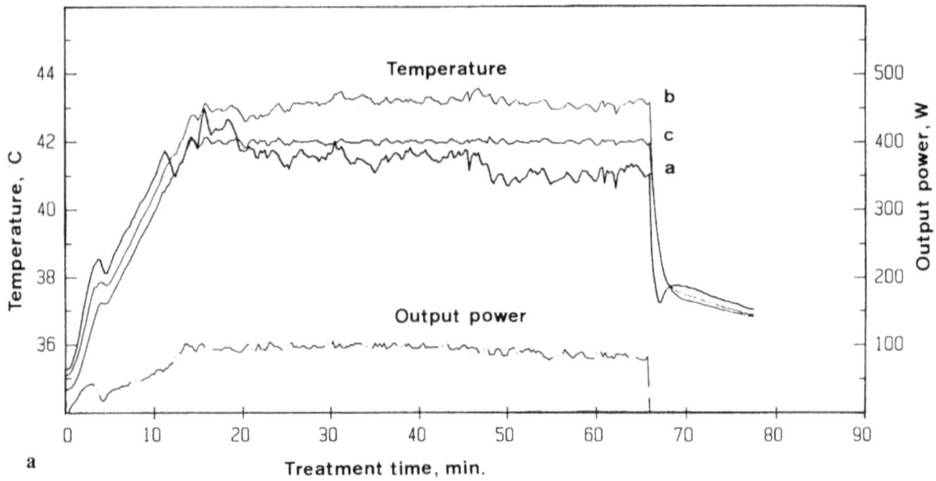

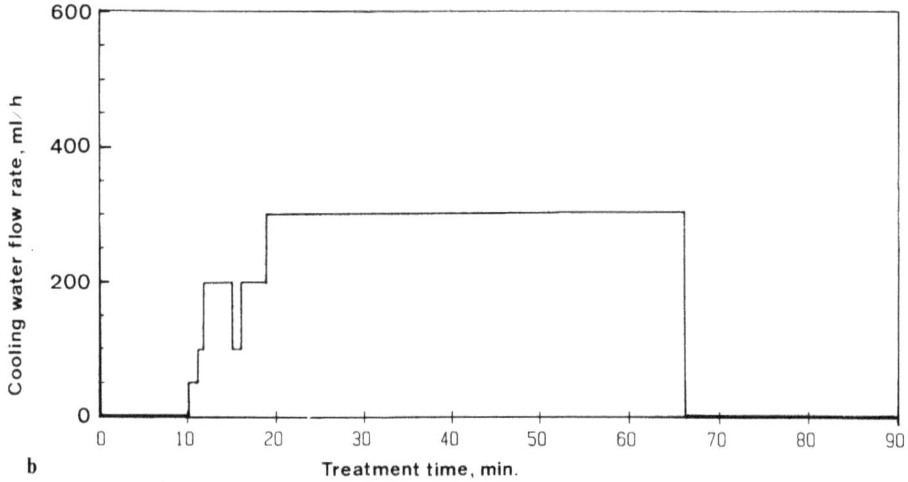

Fig. 34.3. a Temperature recordings from a patient treatment. Central antenna position. The measurements shown on this graph were recorded at the surface of the applicator (*a*), in the center of the tumor lesion (*b*), and at the most distant periphery of the tumor (*c*). A rather homogeneous and constant temperature was achieved within the target volume due to water cooling of the surface of the applicator. **b** Variation of the flow rate (ml/h) of the cooling water during the treatment shown in **a**

more than 50% (partial remission). In two cases no tumor response was recorded (Table 34.3). Tumor responses with regard to primary or secondary tumors are summarized in Table 34.4. In the complete series, four patients are still alive and tumor free (13, 16, 22, and 38 months) and nine patients have died of their tumors.

In seven patients local areas of necrosis developed in the vaginal walls. Fibrosis (two cases) and fistulas (four cases) were also observed. Three of the four cases with fistulas occurred in the group with recurrent tumors and one in a patient with a primary tumor that was not cured locally (Table 34.5).

The mean tumor temperature reached was 41.7°C (range 39.3°–44.6°C). The effective treatment time at steady state varied between 51 and 69 min. The interval between the radiotherapy and the start of hyperthermia averaged 40 min.

The hyperthermia treatments were rather well tolerated. If the surface temperature of the applicator exceeded 43°–44°C, a burning pain and discomfort usually occurred and then some form of anesthesia was needed (general sedation and local anesthesia).

34.4 Conclusions and Discussion

The microwave technique has made it possible to construct hyperthermia applicators with shapes

Table 34.3. Results: recurrent tumors of the vagina

Pat. no.	Diagnosis and stage	RT (Gy) (intracav)	HT (°C/min) (tumor temp/time)	Tumor response	Time (months)
1	Ca colli IIA	9×6	41.2/64, 42.1/58	PR	7
2	Ca colli IIB	4×6	40.8/78, 42.9/53	CR	13
3	Ca colli IIIA	5×6	40.6/55, 38.2/56	CR	6
4	Ca colli IIIB	5×6	43.5/63, 40.4/75	PR	8
5	Ca colli IIIB	4×6	41.1/55, 42.9/56	PR	22
6	Ca colli IIIB	7×5	41.0/53, –	NR	–
7	Ca colli IIIC	2×6	41.7/38, –	NR	–

Table 34.4. Summary of tumor responses

	Primary	Recurrent	Total
CR	5	2	6
PR	0	3	4
NR	1	2	3

Table 34.5. Side-effects associated with hyperthermia/irradiation treatment

Type of reaction	No. of patients
Necrosis of vaginal mucosa	7
Fibrosis (paravaginal tissue)	2
Fistulas (recto-/vesicovaginal)	4
Rectal stenosis and bleeding	1
Hematuria	1

and dimensions similar to those of the catheters and applicators which have long been used in radiotherapy. The design of microwave antennas for hyperthermia involves careful temperature measurements to evaluate the SAR distribution. Tissue-equivalent phantom material was used for this purpose. The temperature distribution will change when a cooling blood circulation is in action. The output power needed was approximately 10 times higher in living tissue, compared with phantom measurements (Sorbe et al. 1990).

Intracavitary hyperthermia reaches the central, and probably most hypoxic and necrotic, part of the tumor and may therefore increase local tumor control when combined with radiotherapy. The risk organs can be protected from excessively high temperatures by positioning multiple thermistor probes in the walls. The most sensitive parts for early reactions after intracavitary hyperthermia, as well as after irradiation, are the vulva, the introitus, and the lower third of the vagina. Regarding the risk of late reactions, the proximal third of the vagina, with its close proximity to the rectal wall and the bladder neck, is of the greatest importance.

The first five patients in this series were treated without cooling of the surface of the applicator. A very steep temperature gradient was then obtained within the target volume with unacceptably high surface temperatures. An increased incidence of patient discomfort (burning pain) during treatment and necrosis of the superficial parts of the vaginal mucosa was recorded. A water cooling system beneath the surface of the obturator was therefore developed and used during the treatment of the last eight patients. The cooling system was fully integrated with the hyperthermia system and computer controlled to keep the surface temperature constant and in the range of 42°–43°C (Fig. 34.1). The most appropriate variable to use for control purposes was found to be the rate of flow of the cooling water (Fig. 34.3b).

Despite the small number of patients treated, we have the impression that the combination of hyperthermia and radiotherapy gives good local control, especially of primary tumors. An advantage of the method is that hyperthermia can be applied in close proximity to the intracavitary irradiation since the practical procedures are similar. A gradual improvement of the technique is in progress and randomized studies should be started in cooperation with other clinics to evaluate further the effect of combined hyperthermia and intracavitary irradiation on vaginal tumors.

References

Fletcher GH, Shukovsky LG (1975) The interplay of radiotherapy and tolerance in the irradiation of human cancers. Radio Electrol 56: 383–390

Hao DZ, Xie MY, Tau HS, Liu YZ, Sun WG (1984) Hyperthermia treatment in carcinoma of the uterine cervix. In: Overgaard J (ed) Hyperthermic oncology, vol 1. Taylor & Francis, Philadelphia, pp 751–752

Pettersson F (ed) (1985) International Federation of Gynecology and Obstetrics (FIGO). Annual report on the results of treatment in gynecological cancer no. 19. Radiumhemmet, Stockholm, p 297

Roos D, Hamnerius Y, Alpsten M, Borghede G, Friberg L-G (1989) Two microwave applicators for intracavitary hyperthermia treatment of cancer colli uteri. Phys Med Biol 34: 1917–1921

Sorbe B, Roos D, Karlsson L (1990) The use of microwave-induced hyperthermia in conjunction with afterloading irradiation of vaginal carcinoma. Acta Oncol 29: 1029–1033

Valdagni R, Amichetti M, Christofretti L (1988) Intracavitary hyperthermia construction and heat patterns of individualized vaginal prototype applicators. Int J Hyperthermia 4: 457–466

35 Intracavitary Thermoradiotherapy for Various Tumor Sites

Z. Petrovich and L.V. Baert

CONTENTS

35.1 Introduction

Interest in clinical studies utilizing adjuvant intracavitary hyperthermia (ICHT) has been stimulated by the high incidence of locoregional tumor recurrence in several common cancers. In spite of major progress in surgery, radiotherapy, and chemotherapy over the past 15 years, approximately one-third of patients with a diagnosis of cancer die as a result of locoregional failure (Kapp 1986). The importance of locoregional tumor control for survival is, as would be expected, widely variable. It has been reported to range from less than 10% in the case of primary brain tumors to 80% or higher for tumors such as carcinoma of the esophagus (Kapp 1986; Isono et al. 1982; Petrovich and Baert 1991; Petrovich et al. 1991). In a study of 638 patients with squamous cell carcinoma of the thoracic esophagus, locoregional tumor recurrence was responsible for the death of 80% of patients (Isono et al. 1982). This high incidence of local tumor recurrence in patients with carcinoma of the esophagus stimulated interest in studies on the use of adjuvant ICHT in this disease (Li et al. 1982, 1987; Petrovich et al. 1988). In a study of 1158 patients with locally advanced tumors treated with adjuvant HT, 261 (22%) received this treatment for carcinoma of the esophagus (Goldobenko et al. 1987). All reports on the use of adjuvant ICHT stress excellent patient tolerance, low morbidity, and improved tumor control, and some also cite better survival (Kuwano et al. 1991; Kochegarov et al. 1981; Berdov and Menteshashvilli 1990).

Z. Petrovich, M.D., Professor and Chairman, Department of Radiation Oncology, University of Southern California, School of Medicine, 1441 Eastlake Avenue, Room. 34, Los Angeles, CA 90033-0804, USA

L.V. Baert, M.D., Professor, Department of Urology, University Hospital K.U.L., Brusselsestraat 69, B-3000 Leuven, Belgium

35.2 Histological Changes

The results obtained from histological studies helped to optimize the ICHT treatment and determined safe treatment temperatures. In the majority of these studies the evaluation of histological changes was performed on animal or human esophagus (Li et al. 1987; Qiu et al. 1982). Mucosal surface temperatures ≤ 46°C were found to be safe while higher temperatures resulted in serious complications (Table 35.1) (Li et al. 1987). Histologically assessed tumor regression and the degree of tumor necrosis were found to be greater in patients treated with radiotherapy (RT) combined with ICHT as compared to those treated with resection only or RT only (Table 35.2) (Qiu et al. 1982). These histological studies on tumor response assessment were in agreement with studies on tumor response performed with radiography (Table 35.3) (Li et al. 1982; Hiraoka et al. 1987).

Histological changes in the prostate following transurethral HT were similar to those reported in the esophageal mucosa (Lauweryns et al. 1991). The intensity of these changes depended on the applied temperature. No histological changes were found in tissue where the temperature was < 39°C (Astrahan et al. 1991a, b; Lauweryns et al. 1991). Additionally, histological changes following ICHT were symmetrical, predictable by the antenna characteristics, and limited to a volume 6–8 mm radially and 4–5 cm longitudinally (Astrahan et al. 1989; Lauweryns et al. 1991; Stawarz et al. 1991). This limited radial power deposition resulting from

Table 35.1. Histological changes in swine esophagus following intracavitary hyperthermia (modified from Li et al. 1987)

Temperature (°C)	Fibrosis		Vasc. abnorm.		Focal necrosis	
	No.	%	No.	%	No.	%
45–46	5	55	1	11	1	11
47	2	40			1	25
48–49	4	40	7	78	3	33

Table 35.2. Histologically assessed tumor regression in patients treated for esophageal cancer (modified from Qiu et al. 1982)

Treatment	None		Mild		Moderate		Marked	
	No.	%	No.	%	No.	%	No.	%
Surgery alone	9	90	1	10				
Radiotherapy (RT)			3	30	5	50	2	20
Intracav. HT (ICHT)			7	70	3	30		
ICHT + RT			1	9	5	45	5	45

Table 35.3. Radiographic assessment of degree of tumor response in esophageal cancer (modified from Li et al. 1982)

Treatment	Poor		Fair		Good		Excellent		Total
	No.	%	No.	%	No.	%	No.	%	
Radiotherapy (RT)	1	4	9	37	12	50	2	8	24
RT + ICHT	3	4	28	34	40	49	11	13	82

the use of intracavitary HT devices is a major limitation in the use of this technique (see this volume, Chap. 10). To some extent this limitation can be offset by repeated application of ICHT. The study of histological changes in the prostate following multiple transurethral HT sessions supports this hypothesis (Lauweryns et al. 1991).

35.3 Treatment Techniques

The optimal number of ICHT treatments is not known. Some investigators reported the need for several ICHT sessions to obtain maximal effectiveness (Baert et al. 1992; Servadio and Leib 1991; Yerushalmi et al. 1982). Other reports, however, have demonstrated the effectiveness of ICHT following a single treatment session (Finger et al. 1989; Petrovich et al. 1992). It is conceivable that tumors with a greater volume may require multiple ICHT treatments while those patients with smaller tumors may benefit from the use of a single treatment.

It is widely believed that tumor temperatures > 41°C are required for a high likelihood of a major response (Perez 1990). In a few sites such as the vagina, tumor temperatures can be routinely measured during ICHT (Li et al. 1984). However, in most patients treated with ICHT direct intratumoral temperature measurements are very difficult to obtain without endangering the patient's well-being (Astrahan et al. 1989; Finger et al. 1989; Liggett et al. 1990; Petrovich et al. 1988). In spite of this limitation, ICHT can be safely administered provided that mucosal surface temperatures are monitored and mapped throughout each treatment session. This is possible because of a predictable and symmetrical power deposition with the highest temperature being recorded on the applicator surface, as seen with the use of virtually all ICHT devices (Astrahan et al. 1987, 1989, 1991b).

35.3.1 Treatment of Gastrointestinal Tumors

Intracavitary hyperthermia has been frequently applied for the treatment of patients with carcinoma of the esophagus. It has been estimated that well over 1000 patients have been treated in various clinical trials (Goldobenko et al. 1987; Kochegarov et al. 1981; Kuwano et al. 1991; Li et al. 1982). A higher incidence of local tumor control has been reported in patients treated with an ICHT-RT combination as compared to those receiving RT alone (Li et al. 1982; Kochegarov et al. 1981).

An important observation was made regarding the dose of irradiation used together with ICHT. A dose of 40 Gy with ICHT had a better antitumor effect than a dose of 60 Gy when given without ICHT (Li et al. 1982; Kochegarov et al. 1982; Qiu et al. 1982). In a prospective randomized trial of 161 patients with locally advanced unresectable carcinoma of the esophagus, the 3-year survival for patients receiving ICHT-RT was 15% versus no survival at 3 years for those treated with RT alone (Kochegarov et al. 1981). A comparison of survival in patients treated with ICHT-RT-chemotherapy (CT) and those receiving RT-CT without ICHT showed 43% 5-year survival in the first group and 15% 5-year survival in the second group ($P < 0.05$) (Sugimachi et al. 1988). A similar survival benefit was noted in patients receiving preoperative ICHT-RT-CT as compared to those receiving preoperative RT-CT only ($P < 0.001$) (Kuwano et al. 1991).

The addition of ICHT to irradiation has been uniformly well tolerated. There was no increase in early or late treatment complications of radiotherapy (Sugimachi et al. 1988; Li et al. 1987; Petrovich et al. 1988). See Chap. 33 for more details on treatment results.

Patients presenting with locally advanced carcinoma of the stomach or biliary tree usually have large tumors making the use of ICHT impractical. Those who may require adjuvant HT usually receive deep, regional treatments rather than ICHT. Consequently, only a few reports on a small number of patients with carcinoma of the stomach or bile ducts are available for review.

Treatment results in four patients who received a combination of ICHT and gastric irradiation were reported from Hiroshima University (Kasiwado et al. 1987). The patients had unresectable recurrent stomach cancer. They received a mean radiation dose of 49.5 Gy and 12 ICHT sessions given twice a week. No details on ICHT instrumentation, treatment techniques, or the treatment temperature were reported. Of the four patients treated, one had a complete response (CR), two had a partial response (PR), and one had no response.

An interesting application for ICHT in a patient with bile duct carcinoma was reported from the City of Hope Medical Center (Wong et al. 1988). The patient was treated with 45 Gy external beam radiotherapy followed by 50 Gy intracavitary iridum-192 radiation. ICHT was given at 915 MHz for 60 min with the temperature controlled on the antenna surface at 43°–45°C. The treatment course was well tolerated and there was a long-term major palliative benefit.

Adenocarcinoma of the rectum treated with radical surgery has at least a 30% incidence of local recurrence and more than half of the patients die with uncontrolled pelvic tumor (Kapp 1986). A study on 28 patients with locally advanced adenocarcinoma of the rectum treated with preoperative ICHT-RT-CT was reported by Mori et al. (1991). RT consisted of pelvic irradiation given at 300-cGy daily fractions for a total of 30 Gy. ICHT was given at 13.6 MHz, twice a week for a total of four sessions. Each treatment was of 40-min duration at a steady state with the temperature controlled on the rectal mucosa at 42°C. Intratumoral temperature was verified interstitially in three patients and was found to be 42°C. ICHT was administered using a water-cooled antenna, 1 h following irradiation. Chemotherapy consisted of Carmoful, 300 mg/day for 10 days. Of the 28 study patients, 23 (82%) had an anterior–posterior resection and five (18%) had a low anterior resection. The treatment course was well tolerated and no unusual or severe toxicity was reported. All 28 patients showed gross tumor regression. Histological examination of surgical specimens showed 14 (50%) patients with no viable tumor cells or few tumor cells; eight (29%) had > 50% tumor necrosis, and six (21%) had < 50% tumor necrosis.

A study of 115 patients with locally advanced (T4N0M0) rectal adenocarcinoma was reported by Berdov and Menteshashvili (1990). All patients received a preoperative course of pelvic irradiation consisting of 40 Gy given in 400-cGy fractions, 3 times per week. ICHT was given at 915 MHz at steady state (42°–43°C) for 60 min, repeated 4–5 times. In seven female patients intratumoral temperatures were measured interstitially through the vagina. The measured intratumoral temperature was 42°C in all seven of the patients. No severe toxicity was reported and there was no difference in the incidence of surgical complications in the 59 patients receiving preoperative ICHT-RT and in the 56 patients receiving preoperative RT alone. A significantly greater incidence of tumor regression was recorded in the 59 patients receiving preoperative ICHT as compared to the 56 patients

Table 35.4. Treatment results in patients with locally advanced rectal carcinoma (modified from BERDOV and MENTESHASHVILI 1990)

Treatment	Degree of regression								Total
	Complete		> 50%		< 50%		None		
	No.	%	No.	%	No.	%	No.	%	
Radiotherapy	1	2	20	34	24	41	14	24	59
RT + HT	9	16	30	54	13	23	4	7	56
	10	9	50	43	37	32	18	16	115

treated with preoperative RT alone ($P < 0.05$) (Table 35.4). The 5-year survival rate was 36% in the ICHT-RT group and 7% in the preoperative RT only group.

35.3.2 Treatment of Genitourinary Tumors

Intracavitary hyperthermia combined with RT and/or CT has been under investigation as an adjuvant therapy in patients with locally advanced tumors of the bladder and prostate. The effect of local failure on survival in patients with these common tumors has not been generally appreciated. In fact, local failure was found to be the cause of death in 54% of fatal cases of carcinoma of the bladder and 61% of fatal cases of adenocarcinoma of the prostate (KAPP 1986). Due to the frequent presence of bulky pelvic tumors and limited power deposition of intracavitary antennas, the use of ICHT is limited to selected patients. The remaining patients with locally advanced prostate and bladder tumors may be satisfactorily managed with deep regional HT combined with pelvic irradiation (PETROVICH et al. 1991; PETROVICH and BAERT 1991). A study of 33 patients with locally advanced bladder cancer treated with ICHT-RT-CT was reported from Yokohama University (KUBOTA et al. 1984). ICHT consisted of bladder irrigations with warmed (42°–43°C) saline solution containing bleomycin 30 µg/ml. A total radiation dose of 35–40 Gy was delivered in 12–16 fractions over 4 weeks. This treatment course was well tolerated without major toxicity. CR was obtained in 14 (42%), PR in ten (30%), and nominal response in nine (28%) patients. The best response rate was obtained in smaller tumors (T1). CR + PR was recorded in 11 (85%) T1 patients while it was seen in 13 (68%) T2 + T3 patients.

The combination of ICHT with CT in locally advanced (T3 + T4) carcinoma of the bladder was reported by the University of Tübingen (BICHLER et al. 1989). ICHT was given with a radiofrequency technique (300–500 KHz). The intratumoral and bladder wall temperatures were measured and controlled at 43°C. CT consisted of intra-arterial infusion of 10 mg mitomycin C, in microspheres. Of the 12 study patients, six were treated with a curative intent. Of these six patients, three showed CR and three, PR; all were long-term survivors. The remaining six patients with more advanced tumors were treated with a palliative intent. PR was obtained in five patients while one showed no response to the treatment.

In the early 1980s a phase I study was reported on the use of ICHT in 15 patients with locally advanced adenocarcinoma of the prostate (YERUSHALMI et al. 1982). The authors used an uncooled transrectal microwave antenna operated at 2450 MHz. A mean of 12 ICHT treatments were given with no details on this therapy being presented. ICHT was administered with RT and/or hormonal therapy. Good treatment tolerance and a lack of major toxicity were noted. Following ICHT, substantial tumor regression was seen in all study patients. Excellent and long-lasting palliative benefit was recorded.

An interesting study on the treatment of 15 patients with locally advanced carcinoma of the prostate was reported by SZMIGIELSKI et al. (1988). The study patients had failed prior treatment and had progressive and symptomatic disease. ICHT alone was administered with a transrectal applicator driven at 2450 MHz. A total of six 30-min treatments were given with the temperature controlled at 43.5°C. ICHT resulted in major objective improvement in eight (53%) patients. It is of interest that two patients showed complete regression of distant skeletal metastases. Cell-mediated immunity studies prior to ICHT showed a significant decrease in the measured parameters as compared to 30 normal control volunteers and 15 benign prostatic hyperplasia (BPH) patients (SZMIGIELSKI et al. 1991). Following ICHT a significant ($P < 0.01$) increase in monitored cell-mediated immune parameters was recorded. This apparent immune stimulation peaked at 2 months and gradually decreased to almost pretreatment levels at 6 months. More work needs to be done to explain these unusual findings.

Intracavitary hyperthermia has been reported to be of major benefit in 44 patients with carcinoma of the prostate (SERVADIO and LEIB 1991). Of the 44 patients treated, 17 (39%) had widespread metastases with severely symptomatic locoregional disease and 27 (61%) had locally advanced inoperable disease. ICHT consisted of six to ten treatments given with a water-cooled transrectal applicator driven at 915 MHz. In addition to ICHT the patients received hormonal therapy and 8 of 27 were treated with 70 Gy pelvic irradiation. Of the 17 patients with metastases treated with palliative intent, 12 (71%) had major objective improvement while six had relief of pelvic pain. Of the 27 patients with locally advanced disease treated with curative intent, all showed subjective or objective improvement. In 11 patients a follow-up prostate biopsy was obtained and it was negative in nine (82%).

In the past 10 years there has been major interest in clinical trials studying the use of transrectal or transurethral HT in the treatment of poor surgical risk, severely symptomatic BPH patients. Multiple phase I studies have been completed and results of phase II trials are currently being analyzed. Major objective and subjective benefit has been consistently reported in more than 70% of the treated patients (PETROVICH and BAERT 1991). This included patients with urinary retention and those with large glands (BAERT et al. 1992; PETROVICH et al. 1992a). A strong correlation between *T*max, *T*average, and the treatment response has also been reported (BAERT et al. 1992). A typical treatment course consisted of five to ten treatments given without sedation or anesthesia. This ICHT was uniformly well tolerated. Acute toxicity was common but mild and no late toxicity has been reported. (PETROVICH and BAERT 1991). The transurethral approach was reported to be more efficient than the transrectal one (STAWARZ et al. 1991; PETROVICH and BAERT 1991). At the present time phase III prospective randomized trials are being conducted to define the role of ICHT in the treatment of BPH.

35.3.3 Treatment of Eye Tumors

Primary tumors of the eye are uncommon but clinically important lesions. Excellent survival and tumor control rates have been reported with the use of episcleral radioactive plaques (PETROVICH et al. 1992). Radiation doses needed for tumor control, however, frequently cause complications resulting in decreased visual acuity or in extreme cases requiring enucleation (PETROVICH et al. 1992c). ICHT in a form of modified episcleral plaque using radiofrequency, microwaves, or ultrasound has been introduced in an attempt to decrease radiation doses while maintaining a high incidence of tumor control (COLEMAN et al. 1986; FINGER et al. 1989; LIGGETT et al. 1990).

The effects of ICHT on normal eye tissues were extensively studied in the laboratory. In the temperature range from 43° to 45°C histopathological changes and changes detected on electroretinography (ERG) were limited to an area exposed to HT (LIGGETT et al. 1990). Additionally, a total recovery of retinal function was recorded. On the other hand temperatures > 46°C resulted in diffuse damage to photoreceptors, as seen on electron microscopy. ERG was extinguished both within and outside of the HT field.

Clinical phase I studies using ICHT combined with episcleral plaque RT demonstrated an excellent treatment tolerance provided that temperature was controlled at ≤ 44°C (FINGER et al. 1989; PETROVICH et al. 1992). Additionally, radiation doses to the tumor apex 30%–50% lower than those usually given without ICHT resulted in the same or better tumor control rates (COLEMAN et al. 1986; FINGER et al. 1989; PETROVICH et al. 1992). Currently at the University of Southern California, a phase II prospective randomized trial of ICHT with episcleral plaque RT is being conducted to establish an optimal radiation dose in patients with choroidal melanomas.

35.4 Summary

Intracavitary hyperthermia combined with external beam radiotherapy and/or brachytherapy is becoming an important HT mode. The application of this HT technique is limited to patients with smaller tumors in accessible sites. Multiple temperature measurements are imperative for all treatments. Intratumoral temperatures should be obtained if the clinical situation permits, i.e., if they can be measured safely. In spite of many optimistic reports including those from large clinical trials showing improved local tumor control and a significant survival advantage over patients treated with radiotherapy alone, more work needs to be done. This work is needed to objectively evaluate the role of ICHT-RT in patients with locally advanced tumors. Many published reports on the use of ICHT lack enough clinical and technical data to permit objective evaluation of treatment results. The addition of chemotherapy or hormonal treatment to irradiation and hyperthermia sharply increases the complexity of this evaluation.

References

Astrahan MA, Liggett PE, Petrovich Z, Luxton G (1987) A 500 kHz localized current field hyperthermia system for use with ophthalmic plaque radiotherapy. Int J Hyperthermia 3: 423–432

Astrahan MA, Sapoznik MD, Luxton G, Kampp T, Petrovich (1989) A technique for combining microwave hyperthermia with intraluminal brachytherapy of the esophagus. Int J Hyperthermia 5: 37–51

Astrahan MA, Ameye F, Oyen R, Willemen P, Baert L, Petrovich Z (1991a) Interstitial temperature measurements during transurethral microwave hyperthermia. J Urol 145: 304–308

Astrahan MA, Imanaka K, Jozsef G, Ameye F, Baert L, Sapoznik MD, Petrovich Z (1991b) Heating characteristics of a helical microwave applicator for transurethral hyperthermia of benign prostatic hyperplasia. Int J Hyperthermia 7: 141–155

Baert L, Ameye F, Pike M, Willeman P, Astrahan MA, Petrovich Z (1992) Transurethral hyperthermia for BPH patients with retention. J Urol 147: 1558–1561

Berdov BA, Menteshashvili GZ (1990) Thermoradiotherapy of patients with locally advanced carcinoma of the rectum. Int J Hyperthermia 6: 881–890

Bichler KH, Fluchter SH, Steimann J, Strohmaier WL (1989) Combination of hyperthermia and cytostatics in the treatment of bladder cancer. Urology 44: 10–14

Coleman DJ, Lizzi FL, Burgess SEP et al. (1986) Ultrasonic hyperthermia and radiation in the management of intraocular malignant melanoma. Am J Ophthalmol 101: 635–642

Finger PT, Packer S, Paglione RW, Gatz JF, Ho TK, Bosworth JL (1989) Thermoradiotherapy of choroidal melanoma. Clinical experience. Ophthalmology 96: 1384–1388

Goldobenko GV, Durnov LA, Knysh VI et al. (1987) Experience in the use of thermoradiotherapy of malignant tumors. Med Radiol 32: 30–35

Hiraoka M, Akuta K, Nishimura Y, Nagata Y, Jo S, Takahashi M, Abe M (1987) Tumor response to thermoradiation therapy: use of CT in evaluation. Radiology 164: 259–262

Isono K, Onoda S, Ishikawa T, Sato H, Nakayama K (1982) Studies on the causes of death from esophageal carninoma. Cancer 49: 2173–2179

Kapp DS (1986) Site and disease selection for hyperthermia clinical trials. Int J Hyperthermia 2: 139–156

Kasiwado K, Sato T, Wadasaki K, Kagemoto M, Hirokawa Y, Haruma K, Katuta S (1987) Experience of radiotherapy combined with thermotherapy to stomach cancer. In: Onoyama Y (ed) Hyperthermic oncology in Japan 1986. Mag Bros, Osaka, Japan, pp 335–336

Kochegarov AA, Maratkhodzhazv NK, Alimorazov SA (1981) Hyperthermia in the combined treatment of esophageal cancer patients. J Sov Oncol 2: 17–22

Kubota Y, Shuin T, Miura T, Nishimura R, Fukushima S, Takai S (1984) Treatment of bladder cancer with a combination of hyperthermia radiation on bleomycin. Cancer 53: 199–202

Kuwano H, Kitamura K, Baba K, Morita M, Matsuda H, Mori M, Sugimachi K (1991) Effects of hyperthermia combined with chemotherapy and irradiation for the treatment of patients with carcinoma of the esophagus. In: Sekiba K (ed) Hyperthermic oncology in Japan 90. Asahi Print, Okayama, Japan, pp 31–32

Lauweryns J, Baert L, Vandenhove J, Petrovich Z (1991) Histopathology of prostatic tissue after transurethral hyperthermia. Int J Hyperthermia 7: 221–230

Li DJ, Wang CQ, Qiu SL, Shao LF (1982) Intraluminal microwave hyperthermia in the combined treatment of esophageal cancer. A preliminary report of 103 patients. Natl Cancer Inst Mongr 61: 419–421

Li DJ, Luk KH, Jiang HB, Chou CK, Hwang CZ (1984) Design and thermometry of an intracavitary microwave applicator suitable for treatment of some vaginal and rectal cancer. Int J Radiat Oncol Biol Phys 10: 2155–2162

Li DJ, Zhou SL, Qiu SL, Qiao SJ (1987) Thermodamage, thermosensitivity and thermotolerance of normal swine esophagus. Int J Hyperthermia 3: 141–151

Liggett PE, Pince KJ, Astrahan MA, Rao N, Petrovich Z (1990) Localized current field hyperthermia: effects on normal ocular tissue. Int J Hyperthermia 6: 517–527

Mori M, Sugimachi K, Matsuda H, Ohno S, Inoue T, Nagamastsu M, Kuwano H (1991) Pre-operative hyperthermochemoradiotherapy for patients with rectal cancer. In: Sekiba K (ed) Hyperthermic oncology in Japan 90. Asahi Print, Okayama, Japan, pp 109–110

Perez CA (1990) International consensus meeting on hyperthermia. Final report. Int J Hyperthermia 6: 837–877

Petrovich Z, Baert L (1991) Hyperthermia in the management of benign and malignant tumors of the prostate. In: Sekiba K (ed) Hyperthermic oncology in Japan 90. Asahi Print, Okayama, Japan, pp 1–10

Petrovich Z, Astrahan MA, Lam K, Tildon T, Luxton G, Jepson J (1988) Intraluminal thermoradiotherapy with teletherapy for carcinoma of the esophagus. Endocurietherapy/Hyperthermia Oncol 4: 155–161

Petrovich Z, Emami B, Kapp DS et al. (1991) Regional hyperthermia in patients with recurrent genitourinary cancer. Am J Clin Oncol 14: 472–477

Petrovich Z, Ameye F, Pike M, Byod S, Baert L (1992) The relationship of response to transurethral hyperthermia and prostate volume in BPH patients Urology 40: 247–251

Petrovich Z, Astrahan MA, Luxton G, Green R, Langholz

B, Liggett PE (1992) Episcleral plaque thermoradiotherapy in patients with chloroidal melanoma. Int J Radiat Oncol Biol Phys 23: 599–603

Petrovich Z, Luxton G, Langholz B, Astrahan MA, Liggett PE (1992) Episcleral plaque radiotherapy in the treatment of uveal melanoma. Int J Radiat Oncol Biol Phys 24: 247–251

Qiu SL, Li DJ, Shao LF, Wang CQ (1982) A pathological study on intraluminal microwave hyperthermia in esophageal cancer. Natl Cancer Inst Monogr 6: 415–417

Servadio C, Leib Z (1991) Local hyperthermia for prostate cancer. Urology 38: 307–309

Stawarz B, Szmigielski S, Ogrodnik J, Astrahan MA, Petrovich Z (1991) A comparison of transurethral and transrectal microwave hyperthermia in poor surgical risk BPH patients. J Urol 146: 353–357

Sugimachi K, Matsuda H, Ohno S, Fukuda A, Matsuoka H, Mori M, Kuwano H (1988) Long term effects of hyperthermia combined with chemotherapy and irradiation for the treatment of patients with carcinoma of the esophagus. Surg Gynecol Obstet 169: 319–323

Szmigielski S, Zielinski H, Stawarz B et al. (1988) Local microwave hyperthermia in treatment of advanced prostatic adenocarcinoma. Urol Res 16: 1–7

Szmigielski S, Sobczynki J, Sokolska G, Stawarz B, Zielinski H, Petrovich Z (1991) Effects of local prostatic hyperthermia on human NK and T-cell function. Int J Hyperthermia 7: 869–880

Wong JYC, Vora NL, Chou CK et al. (1988) Intracavitary hyperthermia and iridium-192 radiotherapy in the treatment of bile duct carcinoma. Int J Radiat Oncol Biol Phys 14: 353–359

Yerushalmi A, Servadio C, Leib Z, Fishelovitz Y, Rokowsky E, Stein JA (1982) Local hyperthermia for treatment of carcinoma of the prostate. A preliminary report. Prostate 3: 623–630

36 Combined Intraoperative Thermoradiotherapy for Abdominal Malignancies: The Dartmouth Experience

T.A. COLACCHIO, T.P. RYAN, C.T. COUGHLIN, E.B. DOUPLE, and J.W. STROHBEHN

CONTENTS

36.1 Introduction

Despite the advances in surgical resection and adjuvant treatment modalities, local recurrence continues to be a significant management problem with intra-abdominal malignancies, in particular for locally advanced colorectal and pancreatic malignancies. The preliminary results for the use of extended surgical resection, external beam radiotherapy, and intraoperative radiotherapy (SHIPLEY et al. 1984; ROLDAN et al. 1988; GUNDERSON et al. 1987, 1988; TUCKSON et al. 1988; ABE et al. 1987; HOEKSTRA et al. 1988; SINDELAR et al. 1988; GOLDSON 1981; TEPPER et al. 1986) for the control of local disease recurrence in colorectal and pancreatic cancers demonstrate that lack of local control continues to be the major cause for failure of this combined modality approach. As a result, it is reasonable to investigate the use of hyperthermia in conjunction with these other modalities in the management of these tumors. Certainly for superficial tumors, clinical studies have shown improved results for combined hyperthermia with radiation therapy when compared with radiation therapy alone (OVERGAARD 1985). A significant cause for delay in the testing and application of this modality has been the lack of adequate technology to effectively heat deep-seated intra-abdominal tumors. Current noninvasive deep-heating devices that deliver heat from the level of the body surface use a variety of techniques to focus power at depth: ultrasound arrays (FESSENDEN et al. 1984), RF capacitive (KATO et al. 1985), focused ultrasound (BEARD et al. 1982; IBBINI and CAIN 1990; OCHELTREE et al. 1984), or scanned, focused ultrasound (LELE 1983; HYNYNEN et al. 1987). In addition, a minimally invasive approach utilizing interstitial microwave arrays has been presented (TREMBLY et al. 1982; RYAN et al. 1990, 1991c). All of these systems present physical and logistical problems which limit their use in the operating room (OR) environment. The opportunity for direct visualization of the tumor volume in the OR makes it possible to use a direct contact, sterilizable superficial applicator capable of various depths of penetration.

The two techniques used for intraoperative hyperthermia have utilized either ultrasound or microwave technology. Interstitial microwave hyperthermia in catheters that are implanted in the tumor during surgery have been previously reported (COUGHLIN et al. 1983, 1985, 1989). The Dartmouth experience with 42 patients in vaginal, bile duct, brain, lung, and pelvic sites utilized arrays of microwave antennas. The number of antennas for interstitial microwave heating ranged from 4 to 15 in this intraoperative implant series. Inherent

T.A. COLACCHIO, M.D., Section of General Surgery, Department of Surgery, Dartmouth-Hitchcock Medical Center, Lebanon, NH 03756, USA; T.P. RYAN, M.S., Section of Radiation Oncology, Dartmouth-Hitchcock Medical Center, Lebanon, NH 03756, USA, *and* Thayer School of Engineering, Dartmouth College, Hanover, NH 03755, USA; C.T. COUGHLIN, M.D., E.B. DOUPLE, M.D., Section of Radiation Oncology, Department of Medicine, Dartmouth-Hitchcock Medical Center, Lebanon, NH 03756, USA; J.W. STROHBEHN, Ph.D.; Thayer School of Engineering, Dartmouth College, Hanover, NH 03755, USA problems included localizing tumor margins along multiple catheters and treatment planning in an array with multiple trajectories and with catheters that may bend during insertion (Coughlin et al. 1985). Since 1986 we have been using ultrasound as a means of administering hyperthermia under direct observation during surgical resection of intra-abdominal tumors.

Unfocused, planar applicators have been used in hyperthermia clinics over the past several years, both in single element (Marmor et al. 1979; Corry et al. 1982; Pounds and Britt 1984; Ryan et al. 1986, 1991a; Richmond et al. 1991) and multi-element (Ryan et al. 1991a, b; Samulski et al. 1990) configurations. The square, multielement applicator described by Underwood et al. (1987) was reported to be heavy and bulky (Samulski et al. 1990) and thus would not be suitable for intra-operative use. For the series of patients reported here, we selected a round, planar applicator because of its ability to accommodate the constraints of the surgical opening and the varying tumor dimensions. In conjunction with continuous temperature monitoring, this system is capable of heating deep-seated intra-abdominal tumors. To determine the feasibility and safety of this system, we designed a phase I trial of combination therapy using intraoperative radiotherapy (IORT) and hyperthermia (IOHT) in the treatment of locally unresectable intra-abdominal carcinomas. We have successfully treated 19 patients with this combination therapy and have reported the morbidity and mortality along with the technical considerations (Colacchio et al. 1990; Ryan et al. 1992).

36.2 Methods and Study Design

36.2.1 Applicator Design

The intraoperative ultrasound applicator had the following specifications:

1. Applicator easily assembles for rapid insertion of 1-, 2-, or 3-MHz elements in the sterile field.
2. Expandable latex membrane to conform to tumor surface.
3. Completely immersible housing with watertight RF connection.
4. Inlet/outlet ports for circulating water located adjacent to RF cable to allow easier placement in deep body cavities.
5. A range of applicator sizes to accommodate 6-, 8-, and 10-cm-diameter elements with a total applicator height of 4 cm.

The applicator went through three stages of development. The third generation design is shown in Fig. 36.1. The applicator shell is machined from a single block of aluminum with recessed threaded water inlet and outlet ports as shown. The RF coaxial cable is fed through a waterproof connector that also serves as a shock cord. The piezoelectric (PZT) crystal (C5800, Valpey-Fisher, Framingham, MA) is air backed and firmly edge clamped to ensure watertightness. A latex covering over the open face insures against blood contamination of the crystal and internal transducer wall. The exterior surface is smoothly polished and coated with a protective sealer to assist in cleanup. The transducer is assembled during surgery with the appropriate ultrasound element to achieve the desired heating depth.

36.2.2 Closed-Volume Circulating System

A closed-volume, sterile water circulation system was assembled for use in the operating room (Fig. 36.2). The attachments to the water inlet and outlet ports self-sealed when disconnected (Genoa Corp., St. Paul, MN), allowing transducers to be interchanged without disturbing the water circulation assembly. The same type of connections were built into each applicator so that it could be filled and then removed. Both water inlet and outlet temperatures were monitored. A bubble trap removed air bubbles that may have occurred due to cavitation. The water circulation system was under temperature control through a heat exchanger in a waterbath whose temperature was also monitored.

36.2.3 Treatment Computer: RF Power and Temperature Control

The RF power system and temperature measurement and control are shown in Fig. 36.3. The system comprises a frequency synthesizer (Wavetek Model 23, San Diego, CA) which, under computer control, allows both amplitude and frequency adjustment over the IEEE-488 bus. RF power is provided by a 400-W amplifier (ENI model AP400, Rochester, NY) that is operated as a fixed gain

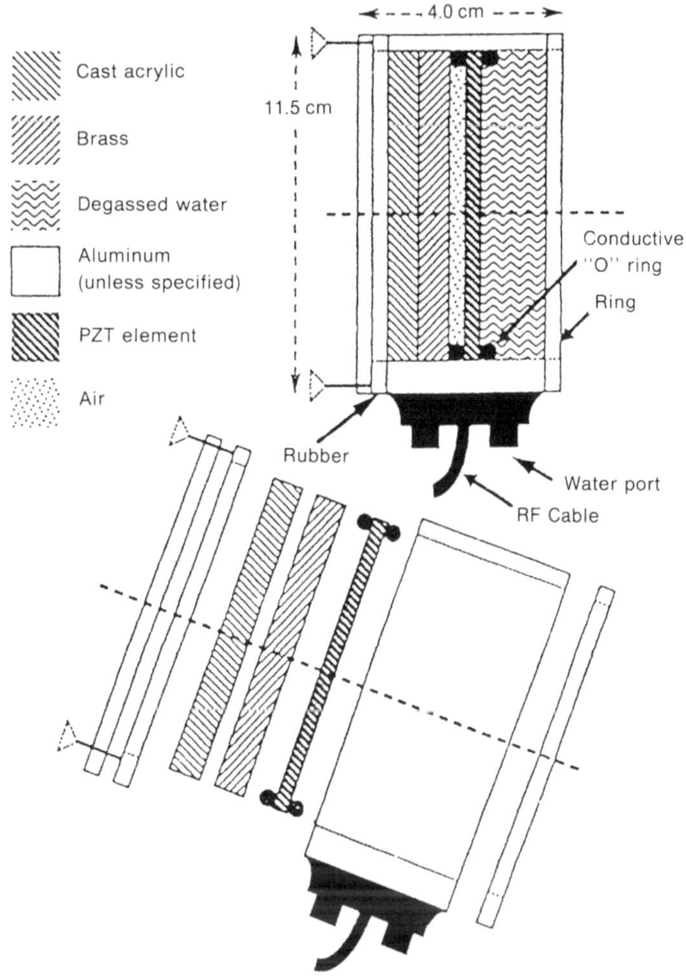

Fig. 36.1. Design of the immersible, intraoperative ultrasound transducer. The 1-, 2-, or 3-MHz ceramic is inserted into the applicator during surgery

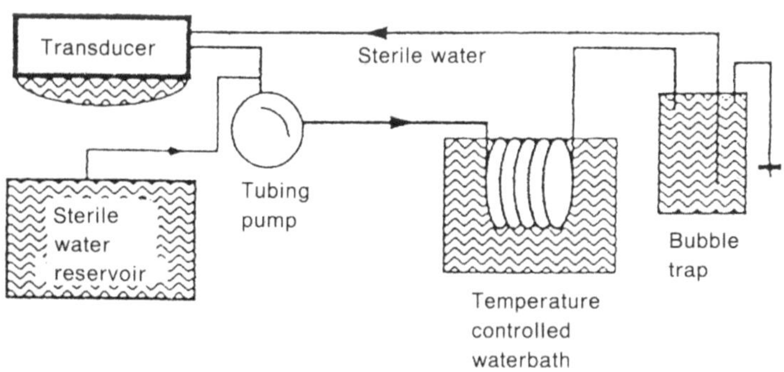

Fig. 36.2. Intraoperative ultrasound sterile, constant volume, circulating water system. Temperature of the degassed, circulating water is controlled for surface cooling

device with the amplitude of the frequency synthesizer providing power control, or as a variable gain device that is directly addressed to provide control of power. The power meter is a digital readout device with a computer interface (Bird model 4385, Cleveland, OH) for data logging.

Thermometry is provided by dual 12 channel thermocouple interfaces (Clini-Therm model 1200, currently out-of-business). These are addressed on dual RS232 ports on the computer. Calibration wells are provided by the manufacturer for a calibration reference. Our quality assurance protocol involves measuring the 24 temperature channels over the range of 0°–100°C and doing a fourth-order curve fit of the thermocouple output to the actual temperature for every channel. The equations for each channel are then programmed into the treatment software. The reference used is a

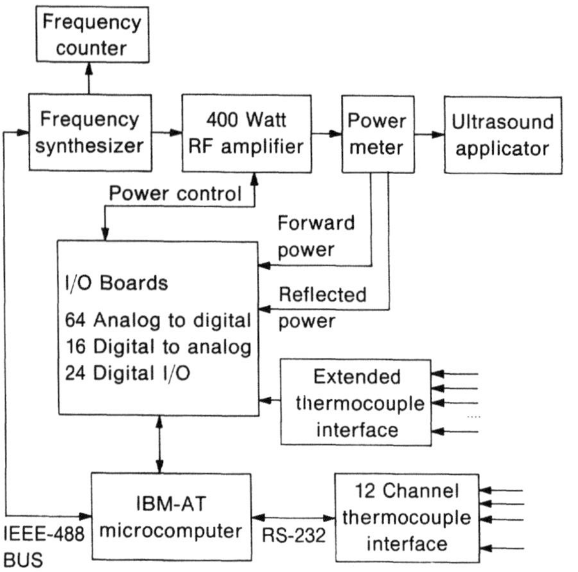

Fig. 36.3. Ultrasound hyperthermia treatment system (Dartmouth ultrasound hyperthermia). Temperature data collection, frequency synthesis, and RF amplifier are all under computer control

precision thermistor (Thermometrics model D774, Edison, NJ) accurate to $\pm 0.002°C$ and NBS traceable. The thermocouple interfaces are placed next to the operating table to simplify connection to the patient.

The RF power and control system reside on a mobile cart to facilitate movement between the hyperthermia suite and the operating room. Since microcomputers frequently have an inherent leakage of 100 mA which is incompatible with patient safety, the instrument cart has its own isolation transformer (Topaz, San Diego, CA) to reduce leakage currents to ≤ 10 mA. The IBM-AT computer controls power and frequency and updates the temperature on the screen every second. All temperature channels are set for a maximum allowable temperature. The treatment-limiting temperature channel blinks on the screen as a reminder that the treatment is constrained by that maximum temperature setting.

36.2.4 Patient Selection

For this phase I trial, we chose to select those patients with recurrent and large unresectable intra-abdominal carcinomas, primarily pancreatic and colorectal. Patients having received previous external beam radiotherapy and those with solid organ metastases were eligible if their expected survival was > 3 months. In addition, we decided to use IOHT only in patients with measurable residual disease (generally greater than 2 cm thick) in which temperature monitoring was feasible, and thereby eliminated those patients with minimal or microscopic disease. As a result of these criteria we have selected out a population of patients with the worst overall prognosis from among those who would be eligible for the future phase II trials of this combination treatment modality. There have been 19 patients treated with combination IORT with IOHT. Ten have had colorectal cancer recurrences, seven have had unresectable primary pancreatic cancers, and, in addition, we have treated one gastric and one endometrial cancer. The patients' demographic, tumor size, treatment, complication, and follow-up data are shown in Tables 36.1–36.3.

Table 36.1. IORT and IOHT for colorectal cancer recurrences

Pt.	Sex	Age	Tumor volume (cm^3)	Metastases[a]	IORT dose (Gy)	Temp. probes	Thermal dose[b] Max.	Thermal dose[b] Min.	F/U (most)	Complications
PP	M	49	360	No	12	3	3955	0	17	None
HR	M	73	729	Yes	17	10	5×10^5	0	11	None
AW	M	63	108	No	17.5	6	2533	29	25	None
JE	M	70	48	Yes	17.5	4	359	1	11	Pelvic abscess
WV	M	60	144	No	17.5	6	463	0	5	None
MS	F	43	188	Yes	17.5	7	1×10^4	37	18	None
WW	M	57	84	No	17.5	6	9486	37	20	Pelvic abscess
JE	M	57	65	No	17.5	12	117	2	16	Osteomyonecrosis
FR	M	70	173	No	15	17	1715	0	8	Increased Nerve paresis
WP	M	77	72	No	15	12	69	0	7	Pelvic abscess

[a] Present at time of treatment
[b] Thermal dose = equivalent minutes at 43 °C

Table 36.2. IORT and IOHT for unresectable primary pancreatic cancers

Pt.	Sex	Age	Tumor volume (cm^3)	Metastases[a]	IORT dose (Gy)	Temp. probes	Thermal dose[b]		F/U (most)	Complications
							Max.	Min.		
BD	M	55	243	No	17.5	6	1599	51	22	None
RF	F	81	71	No	17.5	4	962	147	6	Postop. ileus
BM	F	59	289	No	17.5	4	295	–	0.5	Ischemic bowel
VS	M	61	500	Yes	17.5	6	694	230	3	Postop. ileus
RP	M	49	175	No	15	9	120	0	7	None
VR	F	59	252	Yes	15	14	698	0	0.6	ARDS
PB	F	62	245	Yes	15	11	4214	5	6	None

ARDS, adult respiratory distress syndrome
[a] Present at time of treatment
[b] Thermal dose = equivalent minutes at 43 °C

Table 36.3. IORT and IOHT for cancers other than colorectal and pancreatic cancers

Pt.	Sex	Age	Tumor volume (cm^3)	Metastases[a]	IORT dose (Gy)	Temp. probes	Thermal dose[b]		F/U (most)	Complications
							Max.	Min.		
RM	M	61	361	Yes	15	6	343	122	4	Partial small-bowel obstruction
EE	F	65	320	No	17.5	8	491	0	12	Increased nerve paresis

[a] RM's primary–gastric; EE's primary–endometrial
[b] Present at time of treatment
[c] Thermal dose = equivalent minutes at 43 °C

36.2.5 Surgery

All patients underwent exploratory laparotomy at which time their tumors were exposed and biopsied, and adherent or involved structures overlying or adjacent to the tumor were either resected, retracted, or defunctionalized. The tumors were debulked wherever possible to achieve a maximum diameter of 10 cm and a maximum thickness of 5 cm. The surface of the tumor was thereby exposed and the IORT and IOHT treatments were performed. Following this, the necessary bypasses, resections, etc. were performed and the operation was completed.

36.2.6 Radiotherapy

In early 1986, the decision was made to install a Phillips RT 305 orthovoltage (300 kVp) x-ray machine in one of the operating suites at the Mary Hitchcock Memorial Hospital for the sole purpose of delivering intraoperative radiation therapy. The beam has an HVL (half-value layer) of 3.8 mm Cu which requires relatively little shielding for the room. A full complement of cones were fashioned with both 25 and 30 cm FSD (focal skin distance). Cone diameters range from 4 to 10 cm and have 0°, 15°, or 30° bevel angles. It was felt that tumors with a thickness of up to 5 cm would be satisfactorily treated with 300 kVp x-rays. Generally, the dose of radiation was determined by the thickness of the tumor, i.e., tumors > 2 cm thick received 17.5 Gy while tumors < 2 cm thick received 15 Gy. Treatment times ranged from 15 to 25 min, and there were no tumors which were inaccessible to placement of the IORT cones. A summary of the IORT doses used is shown in Tables 36.1–36.3. Eleven of the 19 IORT/IOHT patients have received either pre- or postoperative external beam radiotherapy (EBRT). Of the remaining eight, five have refused additional therapy and three expired before having recovered sufficiently to begin therapy.

36.2.7 Hyperthermia Treatment

Following IORT, all 19 patients received an intraoperative hyperthermia treatment. This was delivered using either a 6-, or a 10-cm ultrasound transducer with either a 1-, 2-, or 3-MHz piezoelectric crystal. Therapeutic temperatures (> 42°C) were achieved and maintained for 60 min in each IOHT treatment. The power required to attain these temperatures ranged from 70 to 180 W. Thermometry sites were selected in order to monitor the deepest tumor margins, lateral margins, and superficial sites as recommended by the Radiation Therapy Oncology Group (RTOG), which administers multi-institutional trials (Waterman et al. 1991). Any adjacent normal tissue structures that could not be removed from the field were also carefully instrumented with thermocouples. For temperature measurements, custom 21 gauge stainless steel needle thermocouples were fabricated (Sensortek, Clifton, NJ) with 90° bends for precise depth placement. These triple-junction probes had sensors at the tip, halfway between the tip and bend, and 2 mm from the bend for superficial measurements. Flexible, bare-ended microthermocouples were placed superficially or implanted into tissue by placing and removing a 17 gauge needle, leaving the flexible probe in the tissue. The probe was simply pulled out after the treatment. A thermocouple was mounted inside the waterbath to monitor circulating water coolant temperature. The water inlet and outlet temperatures of the transducer were also monitored. Power was switched off briefly every 10 min to record the effects of ultrasound-induced artifacts on the thermocouples.

The number of temperature points within each tumor and the thermal doses for the 19 IOHT patients are shown in Tables 36.1–36.3. A schematic representation of the locations of these points within the tumor volume of two of the patients is shown in Figs. 36.4 and 36.5. In addition, Fig. 36.6 shows a thermal map done of one patient across the center of the tumor, at a depth of 0.5 cm from the surface.

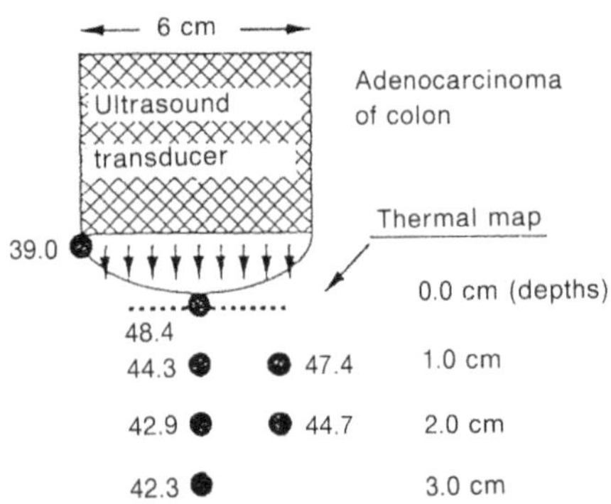

Fig. 36.4. Temperature distribution in a plane orthogonal to the applicator face. A thermal map was made along the *dotted line* and appears in Fig. 36.6. Tumor measured 4 × 4 × 3 cm (deep)

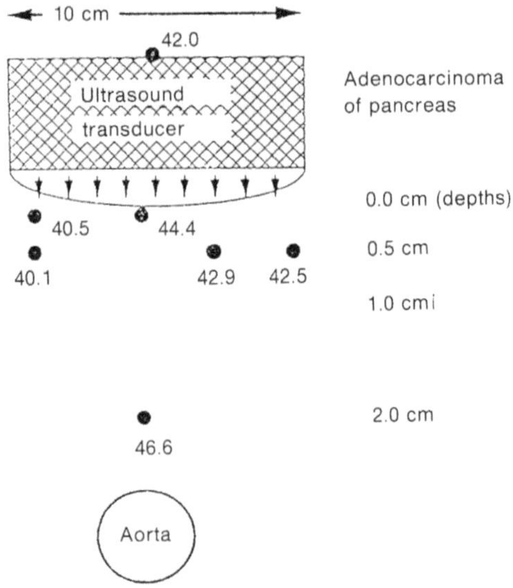

Fig. 36.5. Temperature distribution in a plane orthogonal to the applicator face. Tumor measured 9 × 9 × 3 cm and was in a pancreatic site. Deepest tumor margin along the central axis abutted the aorta

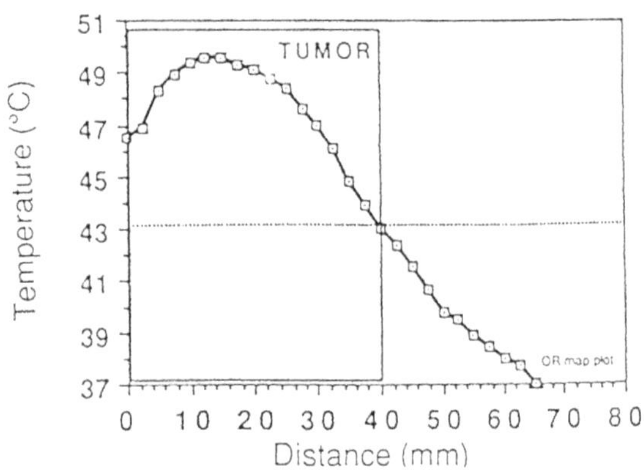

Fig. 36.6. Temperature map through tumor during surgery. This temperature mapping track is pictured in Fig. 36.4. All points in the tumor are ≥ 43°C

36.2.8 Quality Assurance

Quality assurance (QA) is critical in the operating room due to the fact that everything must be calibrated and tested at least 24 hours before surgery. Also, all items are packaged and sterilized and only opened in the sterile field shortly before use. It is imperative that special efforts be made to shorten setup time in the OR so as not to extend the length of surgery. The quality assurance efforts in intraoperative hyperthermia are divided into four categories:

1. Water circulation system. A thorough check for leaks is made before sterilization to prevent system contamination by bodily fluids.

2. Applicator acoustic tests. A nondegradable, acoustic absorbing phantom is used (RYAN et al. 1991b, d), so that applicator performance can be checked and compared to previous measurements. Steady-state temperatures are measured by a fiberoptic probe (Luxtron Corp., Mountain View, CA) that is automatically translated (RYAN et al. 1991e) at 1-mm intervals. As an alternative, a sheet of liquid crystal paper can be held taut and immersed in a water tank. As power is applied to the ultrasound applicator held in the water, the heating pattern is shown as absorption by the sheet induces the temperature-related color changes.

3. Thermometry. Before each treatment, a waterbath is set up with a precision thermistor and all of the clinical thermocouples. The precision thermistor is referenced to an NBS-traceable calibration specification that is accurate to $\pm 0.002°C$. The temperature of the bath is run from 20° to 75°C with data measured every 5 s (roughly every 0.1°C) and recorded and plotted at 0.5°C intervals. Corrections are applied to each channel by a polynomial fit of each channel of measured data to the reference data.

4. Temperature artifacts. To minimize absorption heating artifacts in the ultrasound field, only stainless steel needles are used. Only small diameter (21 gauge) needles are used to minimize scatter and reflection of the field. Also, most of the probes have a right-angle bend and are inserted with the probe axis parallel to the direction of propagation to minimize viscous heating. The temperature artifact is determined for each sensor by briefly interrupting power every 10 min and from a 5-min thermal washout at the end of the treatment. The treatment software was written in-house and can measure temperatures every second during this cooldown period. Artifacts are calculated by analyzing the temperature decay after power off. The linear portion of the decay is extrapolated to the time that power was switched off (WATERMAN 1990).

36.3 Results

36.3.1 Morbidity and Mortality

Despite the fact that this preliminary group of patients has had a dismal overall prognosis, we have been quite heartened and encouraged by the number of partial and complete responses to this therapy which we have seen thus far. The average tumor volume was large, with the mean volumes for the colorectal and pancreatic tumors being 197 cm^3 and 254 cm^3 respectively, and seven patients had solid organ metastases at the time of therapy. The follow-up ranged from 0.5 to 25 months, with the mean follow-up for colorectal and pancreatic patients being 13.8 and 6.4 months respectively. Five patients were still living at the time of this report, and ten had died from progression of their disease.

The morbidity and mortality rates are summarized in Table 36.4. Eleven patients have developed complications for an overall complication rate of 58%. These are summarized in Table 36.5 and include three pelvic abscesses, two cases of prolonged postoperative ileus, one case of partial bowel obstruction not requiring reoperation, and two cases of increased nerve paresis. In both of these latter cases, nerve paresis was demonstrated preoperatively, and they both returned to their baseline deficits within 3 months. In addition, one patient developed osteomyonecrosis of the left lateral abdominal wall 8 months following treatment in association with a regional recurrence. This required debridement and reconstruction. There have been no wound infections, delayed hemorrhages, new permanent neuropathies leading to motor deficits, skin burns, or enteric fistulas in association with the treatment fields.

There have been two postoperative deaths (within 30 days of surgery) in this series, for a mortality of 11%. The first was a patient with pancreatic cancer who developed evidence for progressive

Table 36.4. IORT and IOHT for unresected and gross residual intra-abdominal carcinomas: the Dartmouth experience

Site	No. of cases	Morbidity No. (%)	Mortality No. (%)
Colorectal	10	5 (50)	0
Pancreatic	7	4 (57)	2 (29)
Other	2	2 (100)	0
Total	19	11 (58)	2 (11)

Table 36.5. Complications

Complication	Colorectal	Pancreatic	Other	Total
Adult respiratory distress syndrome	0	1	0	1
Small-bowel ischemia	0	1	0	1
Pelvic abscess	3	0	0	3
Osteomyonecrosis	1	0	0	1
Ileus	0	2	0	2
Partial small-bowel obstruction	0	0	1	1
Increased nerve paresis	1	0	1	2
Total, no. (%)	5 (50)	4 (57)	2 (100)	11 (58)

bowel ischemia along the distribution of the superior mesenteric artery 14 days following surgery, and who was noted to have patent mesenteric vessels at autopsy. The second was a patient with pancreatic cancer who developed progressive respiratory distress beginning 15 days postsurgery and 2 days following initiation of chemotherapy. This progressed to adult respiratory distress syndrome and was thought to be the result of tumor necrosis. She expired from respiratory failure on postoperative day 19.

36.3.2 *Intraoperative Hyperthermia Treatment Analysis*

Right-angled thermocouples made it possible to measure temperatures at exact depths during the intraoperative ultrasound treatments. Figure 36.4 shows the distribution of fixed points in a plane orthogonal to the applicator front face. The applicator housed a 6-cm PZT ceramic operating at 1 MHz. The tumor was 4 cm × 4 cm × 3 cm (deep). The temperature at the tumor margin along a central axis was 42.3°C, with the superficial central tumor temperature averaging 48.4°C at an intensity over the applicator surface of 2.26 W/cm^2 (net forward power/applicator element area). A thermal map was made along the dotted line, and the resulting temperature distribution is shown in Fig. 36.6. The tumor boundaries are demarcated by the box. In most of the tumors in the IOHT series, temperature mapping was not feasible. Figure 36.5 shows another treatment with a tumor of 9 cm × 9 cm × 3 cm (deep), with the aorta underlying the deepest tumor boundary. A 10-cm transducer was used at 1 MHz, and the temperature distribution is shown in the figure.

The results of analysis of the IOHT patients are shown in Table 36.6. A comparison was made with the outpatient series of patients with 64 superficial treatments using the same applicators applied externally. A comparison was also made between fixed position probes and mapping probes which were scanned through the tumor. The average maximum and minimum temperatures sustained throughout the entire 60-min heat treatments were 45.4° and 39.7°C in the Clinic series and 46.6° and 39.8°C in the IOHT series, respectively. The higher maximum temperature in the IOHT series was statistically significant ($P < 0.011$), whereas the minimum temperature difference was not ($P = 0.971$). The overall average of all fixed temperature points was 42.0°C in the Clinic and 43.0°C in the IOHT series. The difference was found to be statistically significant ($P < 0.0002$). All statistical analyses were based on the *t*-test.

Table 36.6. Grand average by series of maximum and minimum temperatures

Series	*T*max (av) °C	SD	Range	*T*min (av) °C	SD	Range	*n*	*T*all (av) °C	SD	*n*
Clinical										
Fixed points	45.4	2.8	39.3–52.2	39.7	1.5	36.2–43.2	64	42	2.6	691
Mapping points	44.7	2.4	40.5–52.9	40	1.5	36.9–43.0	54	41.5	1.9	1457
Intraoperative										
Fixed points	46.6	3.1	43.0–56.0	39.8	1.8	36.0–43.2	19	43	3.2	133

Av, average; max, maximum; min, minimum; SD, standard deviation

Table 36.7. Grand average by series of temperature distribution, power, and tumor volume

Series	T_{90} (°C)	T_{50} (°C)	Percentage points	No. of treatments	Power density	SD	Range (W/cm^2)	Volume (cm^3)	Range	*n*
Clinical										
Fixed points	38.8	41.9	29.6	64	1.14	0.47	0.4–2.6	127	5.4–640	64
Mapping points	39.6	42.1	37.1	64						
Intraoperative										
Fixed points	39.2	42.9	49.6	19	1.65	0.98	0.6–5.0	231	48–1296	19

Table 36.7 extends the comparison to T_{90} and T_{50} analysis. T_{90} is the temperature that 90% of all measured temperatures are greater than or equal to. The T_{90} value is higher in the IOHT series than in the Clinic series (39.2° vs 38.8°C) as is the T_{50} value (42.9° vs 41.9°C). In fact, 50% of all fixed measurement points measured in the IOHT series were ≥ 43°C, while only 30% were ≥ 43°C for the Clinic series.

The average intensity in IOHT was 30% higher than in the Clinic series ($P < 0.003$). Tables 36.6 and 36.7 compare the same values of T_{90}, T_{50}, and average temperatures when mapping points are used as a measure of the Clinic series treatments. Maps were made at 2- or 5-mm intervals in orthogonal hollow needles. The T_{90} was raised slightly when comparing fixed measurement points to mapped points for the Clinic series. This is also demonstrated in Fig. 36.7a, which plots index temperature vs percentage of points ≥ the index temperature. There is good overlap for the two types of analysis.

Figure 36.7b illustrates the difference in distribution between the Clinic and IOHT fixed points. In the IOHT series, by using higher intensity, temperatures were elevated, as compared to the Clinic series.

Temperature artifacts were in the range of 0.1°–0.2°C, which agrees with a larger ultrasound clinical study by Samulski et al. (1990). Additionally, acoustic output of the 1-MHz transducers were within 10% of the RF net forward power readings, as verified by the Hyperthermia Physics Center.

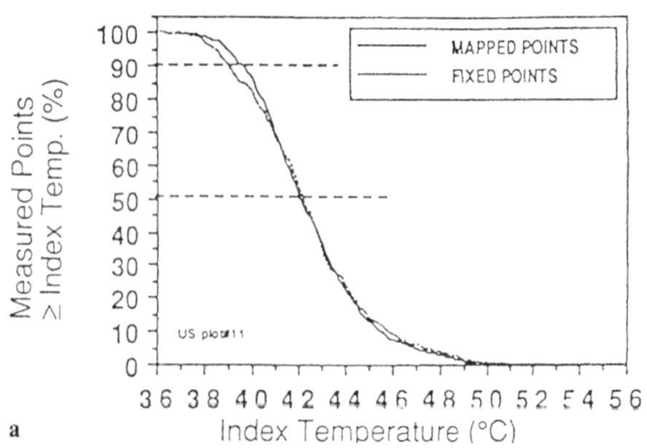

a

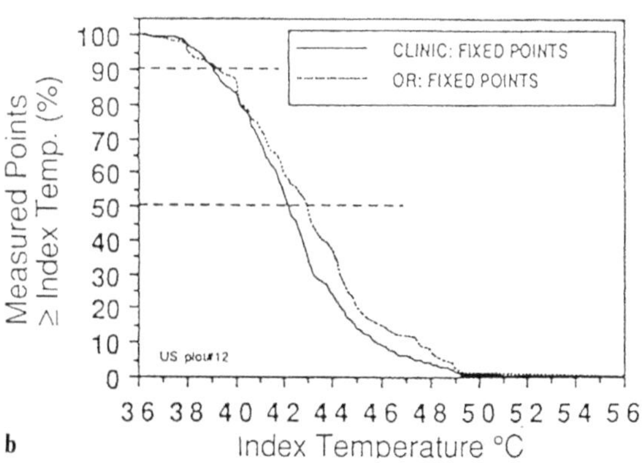

b

Fig. 36.7. a Mapped vs fixed temperature points for 64 treatments in the Clinic series. T_{90} was 39.6° and 38.8°C, respectively, for mapped and fixed points. T_{50} was 42.1° and 41.9°C, respectively. **b** Fixed temperature measurement for Clinic vs IOHT series. T_{90} was 38.8° and 39.2°C, respectively, for Clinic vs IOHT series. T_{50} was 41.9° and 42.5°C, respectively

36.4 Discussion

Locally advanced intra-abdominal carcinomas are significant clinical problems which are relatively resistant to conventional modes of therapy. Some improvement in local control has been made with adjuvant radiotherapy, but normal tissue tolerances make it difficult to deliver sufficient doses of external beam radiotherapy to eradicate residual disease. Intraoperative radiation therapy has allowed the delivery of "boost" doses of radiation to the residual tumor in these cases; however, this has been most successful in patients with only microscopically residual disease. Those patients with gross residual and primarily unresectable disease still have unacceptably high rates of local recurrence despite the use of IORT. This latter situation is particularly suited for the use of hyperthermia in combination with radiation and surgery.

A major difficulty in evaluating a phase I trial of this combination therapy is identifying an appropriate patient group for comparison of morbidity and mortality. There are now several reports on the use of IORT in the management of intra-abdominal (primarily colorectal and pancreatic) carcinomas; however, it is often difficult to identify those patients who had the same disease stage as in this trial (i.e., unresectable grossly residual recurrent and primary disease) in order to make valid comparisons. Tables 36.8 and 36.9 represent a summary of those cases from other published series with their morbidity and mortality data. For unresected and grossly residual colorectal carcinomas, most of the series in Table 36.8 have relatively small numbers of patients ranging from 2 to 11 (SINDELAR et al. 1988; TEPPER et al. 1984, 1986; GUNDERSON et al. 1983, 1988; RICH et al. 1984). The largest series from the Massachusetts General Hospital (TEPPER et al. 1984) did not specify the amount of residual disease which was treated with IORT. In addition, the morbidity and mortality rates are often aggregates which include patients in addition to the specific cases listed. Nevertheless, the morbidity ranges from 13% to 100% with a low mortality of 0%–2%. This is certainly consistent with the 50% morbidity and 0% mortality rates for colorectal cancer patients in this series.

There is somewhat less difficulty in identifying an appropriate group for comparison with pancreatic cancer, since most of the patients treated have unresectable primary disease. As shown in Table 36.9, the complication rate for these patients is generally higher, ranging from 25% to 75% (GUNDERSON et al. 1987; TUCKSON et al. 1988; ABE et al. 1987; HOEKSTRA et al. 1988; SINDELAR et al. 1988; RICH et al. 1984) and this is consistent with the morbidity in this series of 58%. The mortality is also considerably higher and ranges from 1.4% to 24%, and this is not significantly different from the mortality of 29% for the pancreatic cancer patients in this series. Of interest, there was a similar case of small bowel necrosis resulting in a postoperative death reported from the NCI series (HOEKSTRA et al. 1988).

In all OR treatments, at least one temperature averaged $\geq 43.0°C$. With the first few patients, the treatments were power limited since only a 100 W RF generator was available, providing 1.3 W/cm^2 with the largest applicator. A replacement generator capable of 400 W provided more than sufficient intensity at 5.2 W/cm^2. Even at these levels, however, the mechanism of damage is presumed to be thermal (FRIZZELL 1988; BORRELLI et al. 1981), rather than cavitational. The electroacoustic efficiency for PZT elements at 1 MHz is typically around 90% (BENKESER et al. 1989), and our results fall within this range.

During some of the procedures, the applicator was forced into a tight cavity created by the

Table 36.8. IORT for colorectal cancers: unresected and gross residual disease

Institution, year	No. of cases	Morbidity (%)	Mortality (%)
Massachusetts General Hospital, Boston, 1983	4	13[a]	0
Massachusetts General Hospital, 1984	41	32	0
New England Deaconess Hospital, Boston, Mass, 1984	8	25	0
Massachusetts General Hospital, 1986	11	45[a]	0[a]
Mayo Clinic, Rochester, Minn, 1988	2	35[a]	2[a]
National Cancer Institute, Bethesda, Md, 1988	4	100	0

[a] These rates are from a series that includes cases in addition to those reported in this table

Table 36.9. IORT for pancreatic cancers: unresected and gross residual disease

Institution, year	No. of cases	Morbidity (%)	Mortality (%)
New England Deaconess Hospital, Boston, Mass, 1984	15	33	6
Massachusetts General Hospital, Boston, 1987	63	NR	NR
Kyoto (Japan) University Hospital, 1987	69	45	1.4
Mayo Clinic, Rochester, Minn, 1988	44	40	2[a]
National Cancer Institute, Bethesda, Md, 1988	16	25	6
National Cancer Institute, Bethesda, Md, 1988	33	NR	24
Howard University Hospital, Washington, DC, 1988	19	74	16

NR, not reported
[a] This rate is from a series that includes cases in addition to those reported in this table

surgeon and could not be optimally positioned. In other cases, thermal protection of normal tissue structures that could not be removed from the treatment field limited the applied power. Each channel of thermometry was assigned a maximum allowable temperature, and power was automatically adjusted so that this limit was not exceeded.

When pain is removed as a treatment limitation, maximum temperature, T_{90} and T_{50} each increase. This is shown in the comparison between the 19 patient series in the OR and the 43 patient Clinic series (64 treatments) with the same type of applicator. The T_{90} increased from 38.8° to 39.2°, and T_{50} increased from 41.9 to 42.9 for fixed measurement points when comparing the Clinic and IOHT series, respectively.

CORRY et al. (1987) reported that $T_{90} = 41.4$°C and $T_{50} = 45.7$°C for superficial ultrasound in the awake patient. SAMULSKI et al. (1990) reported a series of 147 treatments with $T_{50} = 40.5$°C and $T_{90} = 38.5$°C in which pain rather than temperature was often the limiting factor.

The difficulties in placement of thermometry deep in body cavities were evaluated in the OR and underwent a series of refinements. Initially, microthermocouples were placed in the tumor inside of 17 gauge, open needles. The needles were then slowly withdrawn with the microthermocouples remaining in tissue. The exact final placement was difficult to ascertain with this technique and there was a danger of the thermocouple lead being pulled, thereby dislodging the sensor. The next step was to instrument the same hollow needles with two or three microthermocouples with 1–2 cm separation, which was decided at the time of implant. The final step was to have needle thermocouples custom fabricated with fixed sensor locations and 90° bends. These allowed precise depth penetration and alignment and insured an exact spacing between sensors. The 21 gauge sensors were also much smaller in diameter than the 17 gauge needles used previously. We currently have a selection of right-angled, needle thermocouples with lengths after the bend of 10–60 mm. All of these probes have three sensors, located at the tip, halfway along the bend, and 2 mm before the bend for superficial measurements.

36.5 Conclusions

Intraoperative hyperthermia is a feasible treatment modality which can be used for intra-abdominal malignancies with acceptable rates of morbidity and mortality. Although the T_{90} and T_{50} were greater in the IOHT series than in the Clinic series, the single element applicator is still severely limited in performance even if adequate power is available. In addition, some tumor dimensions exceeded the applicator's capability and thus the 10 cm circular shape was a limitation. Clearly, further equipment development is needed to enable the treatment of larger, complexly shaped intra-abdominal tumors. It appears that a multielement applicator would be the best way to improve performance (CAIN and UMEMURA 1986; RYAN et al. 1991b) in the setting of intraoperative hyperthermia treatments where access to the treatment site is constrained.

In addition, the ability for greater control of power deposition and more precise thermal mapping will enable the inclusion of patients with thinner, more minimal forms of residual disease. These patients are still not adequately treated with IORT alone, but are currently unable to be treated with IOHT. It is this group of patients for whom we have the greatest likelihood for local control and possible cure. Finally, this new technology will enable the performance of phase II and III trials of this combination treatment modality.

References

Abe M, Shibamoto V, Takahashi M, Hanabet, Tobet, Inamoto T (1987) Intraoperative radiotherapy in carcinoma of the stomach and pancreas. World J Surg 11: 459–464

Beard RE, Magin RL, Frizzell LA, Cain CA (1982) An annular focus ultrasonic lens for local hyperthermia treatment of small tumors. Ultrasound Med Biol 8: 177–184

Benkeser PJ, Frizzell LA, Goss SA, Cain CA (1989) Analysis of a multielement ultrasound hyperthermia applicator. IEEE Trans Ultrasonics, Ferroelectrics and Frequency Control 36: 319–325

Borrelli MJ, Bailey KI, Dunn F (1981) Early ultrasonic effects upon mammalian CNS structures (chemical synapses). J Acoust Soc Am 69: 1514–1516

Cain CA, Umemura S-I (1986) Concentric-ring and sector-vortex phased-array applicators for ultrasound hyperthermia. IEEE Trans Microwave Theory Tech 34: 542–551

Colacchio TA, Coughlin CT, Strohbehn JW, Stafford JH, Ryan TP, Douple EB, Crichlow RW (1989) Intraoperative radiation therapy and hyperthermia for unresectable intra-abdominal carcinomas. In: Sugahara T, Saito M (eds) Taylor & Francis, London, pp 561–562

Colacchio TA, Coughlin C, Taylor J, Douple E, Ryan T, Crichlow RW (1990) Intraoperative radiation therapy and hyperthermia. Arch Surg 125: 370–375

Corry PM, Spanos WJ, Tilchen EJ, Barlogie B, Barkley HT, Armour EP (1982) Combined ultrasound and radiation

therapy treatment of human superficial tumors. Radiology 145: 165–169
Corry PM, Jabboury K, Armout EP (1987) Clinical experience with plane-wave ultrasound systems. In: Reeves RA, Paliwal BR (eds) Syllabus, a categorical course in radiation therapy hyperthermia. RSNA, New York, pp 151–158
Coughlin CT, Douple EB, Strohbehn JW, Eaton WL, Trembly BS, Wong TZ (1983) Interstitial microwave-induced hyperthermia in combination with brachytherapy. Radiology 148: 285–288
Coughlin CT, Wong TZ, Strohbehn JW, Colacchio TA, Sutton JE, Belch RZ, Douple EB (1985) Intraoperative interstitial microwave-induced hyperthermia and brachytherapy. Int J Radiat Oncol Biol Phys 11: 1673–1678
Coughlin CT, Strohbehn JW, Ryan TP, Roberts DW, Colacchio TA, Douple EB (1989) Interstitial hyperthermia for deep-seated malignancies. In: Sugahara T, Saito M (eds) Hyperthermic oncology 1988, vol 1. Taylor & Francis, London, pp 596–597
Dickinson RJ (1984) An ultrasound system for local hyperthermia using scanned focused transducers. IEEE Trans Biomed Eng 31: 120–125
Fessenden P, Lee ER, Anderson TL, Strohbehn JW, Meyer JL, Samulski TV, Marmor JB (1984) Experience with a multi-transducer ultrasound system for localized hyperthermia of deep tissues. IEEE Trans Biomed Eng 32: 126–135
Frizzell LA (1988) Threshold dosages for damage to mammalian liver by high intensity focussed ultrasound. IEEE Trans Ultrasonics Ferroelectrics and Frequency Control 35: 578–581
Goldson AL (1981) Past, present and prospects of intraoperative radiotherapy. Semin Oncol 3: 59–64
Gunderson LL, Cohen AC, Dosuretz DD et al. (1983) Residual, unresectable or recurrent colorectal cancer: external beam irradiation and intraoperative electron beam boost +/– resection. Int J Radiat Oncol Biol Phys 9: 1597–1606
Gunderson LL, Martin JK, Kvols LK et al. (1987) Intraoperative and external beam irradiation =/– 5-FU for locally advanced pancreatic cancer. Int J Radiat Oncol Biol Phys 13: 319–329
Gunderson LL, Martin JK, Beart RW et al. (1988) Intraoperative and external beam irradiation for locally advanced colorectal cancer. Ann Surg 207: 52–60
Hoekstra HJ, Restrepo C, Kinsella TJ et al. (1988) Histopathologic effects of intraoperative radiotherapy on pancreas and adjacent tissues: a postmortem analysis. J Surg Oncol 37: 104–108
Hynynen K, Roemer R, Anhalt D, Johnson C, Xu ZX, Swindell W, Cetas T (1987) A scanned, focused, multiple transducer ultrasonic system for localized hyperthermia treatments. Int J Hyperthermia 3: 21–35
Ibbini MS, Cain CA (1990) The concentric-ring array for ultrasound hyperthermia: combined mechanical and electrical scanning. Int J Hyperthermia 6: 401–419
Kato H, Hiraka M, Nakajima T, Ishida T (1985) Deep-heating characteristics of an RF capacitive heating device. Int J Hyperthermia 1: 15–28
Lele PP (1983) Physical aspects and clinical studies with ultrasound hyperthermia. In: Storm FC (ed) Hyperthermia in cancer therapy. Medical Hall, Boston, pp 333–367
Marmor JB, Pounds D, Postic TP, Hahn G (1979) Treatment of superficial human neoplasms for local hyperthermia induced by ultrasound. Cancer 43: 188–197
Ocheltree KB, Benkeser PJ, Frizzell LA, Cain CA (1984) An ultrasonic-phased array applicator for hyperthermia. IEEE Trans Sonics Ultrasonics 31: 526–531
Overgaard J (1985) Rationale and problems in the design of clinical studies. In: Overgaard J (ed) Hyperthermic oncology. Taylor & Francis, London, pp 325–338
Pounds DW, Britt RH (1984) Single ultrasonic crystal techniques for generating uniform temperature distributions in homogeneously perfused tissues. IEEE Trans Sonics Ultrasonics 31: 482–490
Rich TA, Cady B, McDermott et al. (1984) Orthovoltage intraoperative radiotherapy: a new look at an old idea. Int J Radiat Oncol Biol Phys 10: 1957–1965
Richmond RC, Stafford JH, Ryan TP, Mahtani HK, Memoli VA, Taylor JH, Coughlin CT (1991) Platinum levels and clinical responses of tumors treated by cisplatin with and without concurrent hyperthermia: A case study. Int J Hyperthermia 8: 142–156
Roldan GE, Gunderson LL, Nagorney DM et al. (1988) External beam versus intraoperative and external beam irradiation for locally advanced pancreatic cancer. Cancer 61: 1110–1116
Ryan TP, Coughlin CT, Stafford JH, Lyons BE, Strohbehn JW, Douple EB (1986) Temperature analysis of ultrasound-induced hyperthermia in patients with superficial tumors (abstract). North American Hyperthermia Group Annual Meeting, Las Vegas, NV
Ryan TP, Hartov A, Taylor J, Stafford J, Colacchio T (1990) A concentric ring ultrasound applicator for hyperthermia. Proc IEEE Eng Med Biol Soc 1: 270–271
Ryan TP, Colacchio TA, Coughlin CT, Hartov A (1991a) Analysis of hyperthermia treatments: single vs. multiple-element applicators. Proceedings of the International Conference of the IEEE Engineering in Medicine and Biology Society. IEEE Press
Ryan TP, Hartov A, Colacchio TA, Coughlin CT, Stafford JH, Hoopes PJ (1991b) Analysis and testing of a concentric ring applicator for ultrasound hyperthermia with clinical results. Int Hyperthermia 7: 587–603
Ryan TP, Hoopes PJ, Taylor JH, Strohbehn JW, Roberts DW, Douple EB, Coughlin CT (1991c) Experimental brain hyperthermia: techniques for heat delivery and thermometry. Int J Radiat Oncol Biol Phys 20: 739–750
Ryan TP, Wikoff R, Hoopes PJ (1991d) An automated temperature mapping system for use in ultrasound or microwave hyperthermia. J Biomed Eng 13: 348–354
Ryan TP, Colacchio TA, Douple EB, Strohbehn JW, Coughlin CT (1992) Techniques for intraoperative hyperthermia with ultrasound: The Dartmouth experience with 19 patients. Int J Hyperthermia, vol 8. 4: 407–421
Samulski TV, Grant WJ, Oleson JR, Leopold KA, Dewhirst MW, Vallario P, Blivin J (1990) Clinical experience with a multi-element ultrasonic hyperthermia system: analysis of treatment temperatures. Int J Hyperthermia 6: 909–922
Sapozink MD, Cetas T, Corry PM, Egger MJ, Fessenden P (1988) Introduction to hyperthermia device evaluation. Int J Hyperthermia 4: 1–15
Shipley WU, Wood WC, Tepper JE et al. (1984) Intraoperative electron beam irradiation for patients with unresectable pancreatic carcinoma. Ann Surg 200: 289–296
Sindelar WF, Hoekstra HJ, Kinsella TJ et al. (1988) Surgical approaches and techniques in intraoperative radiotherapy for intra-abdominal, retroperitoneal, and pelvic neoplasms. Surgery 103: 247–256
Tepper JE, Gunderson LL, Orlow E et al. (1984) Complications of intraoperative radiotherapy. Int J Radiat Oncol Biol Phys 10: 1831–1839

Tepper JE, Cohen AM, Wood WC et al. (1986) Intraoperative electron beam radiotherapy in the treatment of unresectable rectal cancer. Arch Surg 121: 421–423

Trembly BS, Strohbehn JW, deSieyes DC, Douple EB (1982) Hyperthermia induced by an array of invasive microwave antennas. J Nat Cancer Inst Monogr 61: 497–499

Tuckson W, Goldson AL, Ashayer E et al. (1988) Intraoperative RT for patients with carcinoma of the pancreas. Ann Surg 207: 648–654

Underwood HR, Burdette EC, Ocheltree KB, Magin RL (1987) A multi-element ultrasonic hyperthermia applicator with independent element control. Int J Hyperthermia 3: 257–267

Waterman FM (1990) Determination of the temperature artifact during ultrasound hyperthermia. Int J Hyperthermia 6: 131–142

Waterman FM, Dewhirst MW, Fessenden P et al. (1991) RTOG quality assurance guidelines for clinical trials using hyperthermia administered by ultrasound. Int J Radiat Oncol Biol Phys 20: 1099–1107

Part V
Design and Conduct of Multicenter Clinical Trials

37 Statistical Considerations for the Design and Conduct of Hyperthermia Clinical Trials

C.C. VERNON and M.H. SEEGENSCHMIEDT

CONTENTS

37.1 Introduction

Clinical trials are ideally scientifically of three types – phase I (determination of toxicity and dose), phase II (evaluation of tumour suitability), and phase III (randomised comparison) (OVERGARRD 1984) and all three must be performed before treatment becomes routine clinical practice. While phase III trials may be an effective screening method for many treatments, they may not be so straightforward in the case of hyperthermia, the levels of efficiency of which are difficult to appraise and compare owing to the unpredictability of heating. It may be more correct to refer to extended, but randomised phase II studies in such situations (VAN PUTTEN 1991). Especially for superficial and interstitial (and to a lesser degree for deep) hyperthermia, technology has now advanced to a level that we should be and are now conducting phase II/III studies. It is vital that trials are designed in such a way that the correct question is posed and the answer given in convincing manner. Hyperthermia will need to be acceptable to the patient, and given in such a way that it fits in with present practice of radiotherapy (in terms of economics, time and labour.)

C.C. VERNON, M.A., FRCR, MRC Hyperthermia Clinic, Hammersmith Hospital, Du Cane Road, London W12 OHS, UK
M.H. SEEGENSCHMIEDT, M.D., Strahlentherapeutische Klinik der Universität Erlangen-Nürnberg, Universitätsstraße 27, W-8520 Erlangen, Germany

37.2 Problems

From phase I/II studies we have learnt the problems of protocol design and the types of tumours that can be heated, and have defined Quality Assurance for the treatment. The question of technical feasibility is a major one and problems include not only depth of heating but also homogeneity. Technical knowledge is most advanced for superficial and interstitial techniques, and these techniques are currently the most successful. We also now understand more concerning the number of required treatments (KAPP et al. 1986) and the timing of treatment in relationship to other modalities (OVERGAARD and OVERGAARD 1987) such as radiotherapy and chemotherapy. The problem of dose remains a vexed one and the concept of TID (thermal isoeffect dose) (SAPARETO and DEWY 1984) is a useful but not yet perfected one. Before a trial is commenced certain decisions need to be made, including definition of the population to be studied, treatment methods and scheduling, criteria of success and method of evaluation, the number of patients required, the level of success considered worthwhile, time to be allowed to complete the trial and method of randomisation.

37.3 Size of Trial

The number of patients required and therefore the size of a clinical trial depends on the anticipated clinical differences between the alternative treatments, the level of statistical significance the investigator considers appropriate and the chances of detecting that difference (EVERITT 1989). The null hypothesis assumes that there is no difference between the two treatments and the P value is the probability of obtaining the observed difference or a value more extreme if the null hypothesis is true.

If the trial size is increased, the probability and the power of the study will be increased, while the risk of a type I error (Table 37.1) is reduced (MOULD 1976).

The power function, usually defined in percentage terms and the confidence limits, defines the confidence with which an investigator can claim that a specified treatment benefit has not been overlooked. Sample size and power are also related (Fig. 37.1). The clinical trial outcome may not always measure up to reality perfectly (Table 37.2).

It is possible to calculate the number of patients required based on a known differential between treatments (Table 37.3) (MACHIN 1991), and it can be seen that by altering the differential by only a few per cent, the number of required patients can be changed drastically. An estimation of the expected differential between the two treatments can be made by taking the differential seen in phase I/II studies and dividing it by half! Clinicians are also frequently asked to guess an estimate of the differential that they expected. It is of interest and very hopeful for hyperthermia, that when this was done for a recent phase III trial (VERNON et al. 1989), all of the clinicians (which included some not involved in hyperthermia treatments) thought independently that hyperthermia would improve the response to irradiation (Fig. 37.2). Those "in the know", i.e., the hyperthermists, estimated a higher improvement.

To achieve a statistically significant result is not the same as achieving a clinically convincing result, and the former in itself may not be very useful. To ensure the latter (as well as the former), one must look at the anticipated benefit. If there is an improvement in response when hyperthermia is given, it will need to be of sufficient magnitude to persuade clinicians to change their practice. The smaller the benefit, the larger the trial must be to avoid false positives and false negatives, and therefore the potential patient pool becomes very important. The choice of patients for the trial must ensure a realistic possibility of sufficient numbers, as clinicians always overestimate their possible referrals to studies and there are always a number of

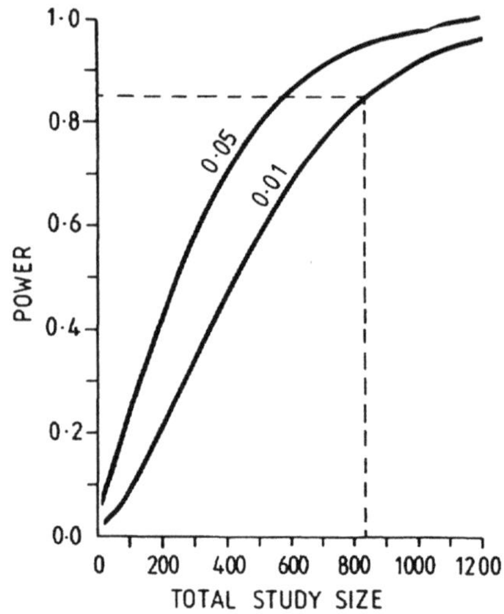

Fig. 37.1. Relationship between sample size and power

Table 37.1. Error types

Error	Definition	Associated risk
Type I	Wrongly rejecting H_0 when H_0 is false	Probability (type I error) = α
Type II	Wrongly accepting H_0 when H_0 is false	Probability (type II error) = β

P value is measurement of the risk of being wrong and interrelates α and β risks

Table 37.2. How perfectly does clinical trial outcome measure up to reality?

1 No difference between teratments	2 Small difference (clinically insignificant)	3 Worthwhile treatment difference
5% of trials conclude treatments differ significant, $P > 0.05$ Direction of difference is fortious	A proportion of trials (more than 50% but less than 80%) declare astatistically significant treatment difference	20% of trials find that the difference between treatments is not statistically significant, $P < 0.05$ Direction of treatment difference is probably reliable nevertheless, and so compute confidence interval

Wrong decisions in columns 1 and 2 are not too serious, but it is important not to miss a worthwhile treatment difference (column 3)

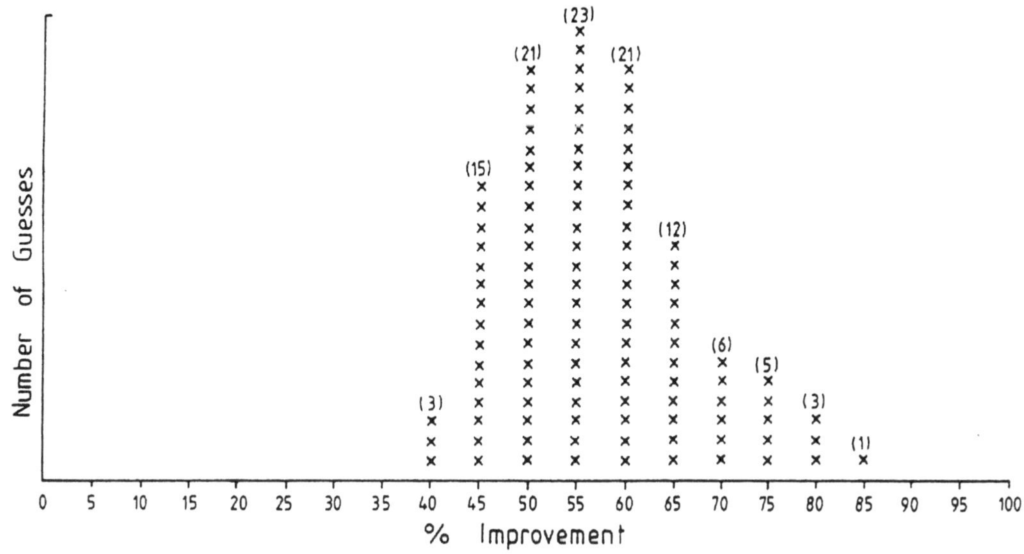

Fig. 37.2. Effect of hyperthermia in improving response to irradiation, as guessed by clinicians (based on VERNON et al. 1989)

Table 37.3. Approximate patient numbers required

Control	Test	Differential	Total number of patients required
20%	35%	15%	250
30%	45%	15%	350
20%	37.5%	17.5%	220
30%	47.5%	17.5%	260
20%	40%	20%	150
30%	50%	20%	180

censored observations. Recently the trend has been to be less restrictive as regards eligibility, to broaden entry criteria to encourage recruitment, and to make studies multicentric to ensure an adequate patient pool. Multicentre studies can be criticised for including possible multifactorial elements, but for hyperthermia this is the only way of achieving sufficient numbers. Properly controlled this does not weaken the trial, but ensures its completion.

37.4 Protocols

All protocols will describe the rationale, background, and objectives of the trials, as well as listing patient selection and exclusion, descriptions of both treatments, toxicity and evaluation, quality assurance, and ethical and statistical considerations. The clinical criteria for trial inclusion must cover patient selection (including likelihood of survival sufficient to make treatment worthwhile and clinical status) and tumour selection (histology, size and location). Hyperthermia practice recognises the existence of prognostic parameters (VALDAGNI et al. 1988), e.g., previous treatments, histology, and tumour site and size, and stratification would allow for this but requires much larger numbers to give a significant result. The simple question of whether hyperthermia adds to the control rate should be addressed first. Once this basic question has been answered, more interesting questions such as scheduling and the addition of hyperthermia to chemotherapy can be tackled.

The non-hyperthermia or control treatment group should be clearly different from the research arm. An example of a good contrast is hyperthermia or no hyperthermia, whereas a bad contrast would be two similar fractionation schedules of hyperthermia which would be unlikely to be markedly different in their efficiency. Both the standard and the research therapy should be given at maximum tolerated and acceptable levels. This ensures that there is minimal criticism of the former as inadequate therapy and that the maximum difference is seen between the two.

Technically the volume, dose and energy of irradiation must be defined as well as the modality, temperature, time fractionation and thermal dose of the heat delivery. The quality assurance procedures for both irradiation and heat must be impeccable and clearly defined in all aspects. They will include calibration and evaluation of the heat delivery and thermometry systems, as now specified in internationally agreed guidelines (HAND et al.

1989), as well as corresponding radiotherapy factors. Ideally there should be visits by a Quality Assurance Committee to ensure that the procedures are adhered to, especially when different techniques and equipment are used in centres in a multicentre study.

Details of timing interim analyses and the level of probability at which the trial would be stopped must be noted. Methods of randomisation should also be noted. Randomisation and collection of data are most satisfactorily handled by a central office. The design of the registration, randomisation, treatment and follow-up forms must be carefully considered and planned, so that these are clear and easy to complete correctly and on time. The collection and completion of forms is a major undertaking and again should be the responsibility of a named person and a central office. Details of publications and named authors as well as organisers and contacts should be noted. To maintain interest and patient recruitment in hyperthermia trials over a period of time, feedback newsletters are very useful.

For a potentially invasive and uncomfortable treatment such as hyperthermia, which is also expensive and labour and time intensive, it is important to include a patient opinion or quality of life form. Any new therapy must be acceptable to the patient.

37.5 Randomisation

Of fundamental importance to the design of any clinical trial is the random allocation of subjects to the alternative treatments. Due to the nature of the disease and the treatment, hyperthermia trials are straight randomisation. Cross-over and sequential trials are not possible. Nor are historical controls acceptable, as the improvement in technology has been so great.

Randomisation (Gore and Altman 1985) is essential to avoid rash decisions based on clinical impressions, to convince the sceptics and to avoid bias. The latter is avoided by close matching of patients, a tough statistician and an independent assessor. Randomisation must always be done by computer as it is essential that the "allocation" is not known before assessing patient eligibility and that the clinician cannot predict the treatment. Blinding is preferable but not possible for hyperthermia trials. In itself randomisation need not be balanced or equal, especially if more information is required from the new treatment arm. One must also be aware of the principle of uncertainty, which is that a clinician should randomise a particular patient to the alternative therapies if he is not convinced that one of them is best for the particular patient. If he is certain that one particular therapy would be most appropriate, then that therapy should be given.

37.6 Results

Recording for evaluation should include survival, timing of tumour regression and control, and normal tissue effects. Side-effects or damage to the most resistant tumour cells and the most sensitive normal tissue must be recorded (both early and late). The most clinically useful response is CR (complete response) with persistent tumour disappearance and control for phase III studies, and there should be a minimum time period noted for this. Recurrence after the combined treatments of hyperthermia and radiotherapy is thought to be both less frequent and less rapid than after radiation alone; thus time to recurrence should be noted. PR (partial response) as an endpoint should be avoided, as should growth delay, which only has a use in phase I/II studies. Radiation and heat damage are different and also occur at different times; therefore it is important to have different scales for assessing the two toxicities. Specific heat-induced complications, e.g., burns and necrosis, should be noted. The use of callipers, photography, CT and radiography by an independent observer for measurement is highly desirable and increases the credibility of a study.

Definitions of response should follow recognised guidelines such as the WHO classification, and by standardising techniques and criteria for measurement, observer variation will be reduced. Despite all these correct attempts at accuracy and independent observations, the endpoint for hyperthermia trials is usually CR and this is a relatively easy and uncontroversial observation to make. One problem in evaluating results from hyperthermia and radiotherapy treatments does exist, however–namely, at the end of a successful treatment, there may remain a measurable "tumour" which represents scar tissue and will remain static over a period of time. Thus "time to failure to progress" as an endpoint also has its attractions. Hyperthermia as used in the majority of these studies is a method of local control only, and the appearance of distant metastases necessitating change of systemic treatment and additionally causing early death, makes long-term follow-up difficult in many of these patients.

37.7 Analysis

For definition of terms, see DALY et al. (1991), or CAMPBELL and MACHIN (1991).

The endpoint for present hyperthermia trials is complete response, rather than survival, which requires different analysis. Frequent interim analyses, i.e., during the course of the trial, should be avoided, so that trials are not terminated early as the smaller number of patients in the interim analysis than in the total proposed study leads to wide confidence intervals, leaving considerable uncertainty about the size of the effect in the clinician's mind.

Some patient data will be lost due to patient withdrawal (for whatever reason) before treatment is complete or before the endpoint (CR or death) is reached. Other data will be lost by failure of follow-up. It is essential to record protocol deviations and reasons for withdrawal, as there may be serious bias if these are eliminated from the final analysis. Likewise, the final analysis should be on the basis of "intention to treat", rather than actual treatment, and all patients should be followed up in the same manner.

The most commonly used test of significance for comparing CR rates between treatments is the chi-square test and associated confidence limits should always be quoted. To investigate the influence of potentially prognostic variables on the CR rate, logistic regression analysis is usually used, and a special computer program is required for this. For this the status of all subjects must be known at a fixed point. Evaluation of the duration of response can be performed with the Kaplan–Meier estimate of the survival curve. Essentially this does not predefine the time interval in terms of weeks or months, but chooses it on the basis of the observed data. The log rank test is used to test differences between the groups, and can be useful where the follow-up period is short. This can be extended to analyse the simultaneous influence of different prognostic factors on the duration of CR by means of a stratification test, but an alternative approach is to use Cox's proportional hazards model (or life table regression model).

37.8 Meta-analysis or Overview

Recently meta-analysis has become popular and this refers to a collection of techniques whereby the results of several independent studies are statistically combined to yield a more powerful overall answer to the question of interest than would the studies separately. It is not a literature review and should include all trials, including negative or unpublished trials, as well as ongoing ones. This may be possible for hyperthermia, especially as there are already many small trials each with no possibility of proving a difference, and recruitment to present trials is slow (MACHIN 1991). Many hyperthermia trials are asking the same basic question: Does the addition of hyperthermia to radiotherapy (or chemotherapy) improve the response rate over the single therapy? The individual doses of radiation and heat should not matter. However, the question of quality control of the hyperthermia treatment would have to be looked at very closely. Meta-analysis should not be regarded as an excuse not to do a phase III randomised trial unless the evidence so collected makes it unnecessary for the trial to procede.

37.9 Ethics

All institutes now demand ethical permission with informed consent (verbal or written) for randomised trials – this is both at a local and at an international level. It is correct that patients should be fully informed about their treatments and any possible side-effects, but the real problem is always that of explaining the randomisation process, especially if they have been referred from other centres for the "new treatment". Because of the sparsity of hyperthermia centres, referral from other centres and non-hyperthermists is common. One way round this is to allow patients to choose whether they wish to have the hyperthermia, or whether they wish to be randomised. Naturally, most patients will opt for non-randomisation when they are told of the minimal side-effects of hyperthermia, which leaves very few for randomisation. The other, much harder way, is only to give hyperthermia after randomisation is agreed on. We (VERNON et al. 1989) have chosen the latter method and made it a little easier by explaining to patients that, if they are randomised to radiotherapy only and this fails, it will be possible to offer them hyperthermia at a later date, either in combination with further low dose radiotherapy or chemotherapy without randomisation. This is easier for patients to accept and we have certainly performed hyperthermia successfully on such patients, following initial randomisation to radiotherapy only. The other advantage to patients who agree to be randomised is that they generally receive better overall care, with more careful assessment and follow-up, than do non-randomised patients.

37.10 The Future

From both animal models and patient studies it has been claimed that hyperthermia has a large beneficial effect, and thus for those who consider it be to an established therapy, randomisation into hyperthermia trials is difficult. In general, hyperthermia is not accepted by all oncologists as a useful adjunct to radiotherapy and chemotherapy, and this implies that hyperthermia is not yet "standard" treatment. Therefore hyperthermia should be regarded as an experimental treatment as there will continue to be considerable uncertainty about its role until more formal proof of its value is established. Certainly at the present there is no proof from scientifically based and randomised studies, and therefore it is unethical not to enter patients into randomised studies. It is essential that all suitable patients are entered into currently ongoing randomised trials, and these should be similar trials so that data can be combined, rather than beginning new and original trials. Because of the difficulty in finding sufficient numbers of suitable patients, trials should be multicentre and preferably international. Hyperthermia has been in usage for a long time and unless we produce a statistically and clinically convincing result soon, there is a bleak future for hyperthermia as funding for it is likely to disappear. Research money in general is becoming more scarce and a good case, now more than ever, needs to be made for research grants. With collaboration, it should be possible to have an answer within a relatively short period of time. The results of these correctly designed and implemented phase III trials are now eagerly awaited, so that hyperthermia can take its rightful place amongst available oncological treatments.

References

Campbell MF, Machin D (1991) Medical statistics: a common sense approach. Wiley, Chichester

Daly LE, Burke GJ, McGilvray J et al. (1991) Interpretation and uses of medical statistics. Blackwell Scientific, Oxford

Everitt BS (1989) Statistical methods for medical investigators. Oxford University Press, Oxford

Gore SM, Altman DG (1985) Statistics in practice, 3rd edn. Devonshire Press for the BMA

Hand JW, Lagendijk JW, Bach Andersen J, Bolomey JC (1989) Quality assurance guidelines for ESHO protocols. Int J Hyperthermia 5: 421–428

Kapp DS, Bagshawe MA, Meyer JL et al. (1986) Hyperthermia as an adjuvant to radiation in the treatment of superficial metastases: a randomised trial if 2 vs 6 treatments. Abstracts of Papers for the 34th Annual Meeting of the Radiation Research Society, p 24

Machin D (1991) Meta-analysis – overview. In: van Dijk J, Lagendijk J, van Rhoon G (eds) Hyperthermia Bulletin #10. Medisch Centrum, Amsterdam

Machin D, Campbell MJ (1987) Statistical tables for the design of clinical trials. Blackwell Scientific, Oxford

Mould RF (1976) Introductory medical statistics. Pitman Medical, London

Overgaard J (1984) Rationale and problems in the design of clinical studies. Hyperthermic Oncol 2: 325–338

Overgaard J, Overgaard M (1987) Hyperthermia as an adjunct to radiotherapy in the treatment of malignant melanomas. Int J Hyperthermia 3: 483–501

Sapareto SA, Dewy WC (1984) Thermal dose determination in cancer therapy. Int J Radiat Oncol Biol Phys 10: 787–800

Valdagni R, Fei-Fei L, Kapp D (1988) Important prognostic factors influencing the outcome of combined radiation and hyperthermia. Int J Radiat Biol Phys 15: 959–972

van Putten WLJ (1991) Randomised phase II and III trials in hyperthermia. In van Dijk J, Lagendijk J, van Rhoon G (eds) Hyperthermia Bulletin #10. Medisch Centrum, Amsterdam

Vernon CC, Field SB, Hand JW (1989) MRC multicentre phase III trial for the use of hyperthermia in the treatment of breast tumours

38 Technical Quality Assurance for Interstitial Hyperthermia

A.G. Visser and R.S.J.P. Kaatee

CONTENTS

38.1 Introduction

Quality assurance guidelines specific for interstitial hyperthermia (IHT) have recently been published by the Radiation Therapy Oncology Group (RTOG) in the United States (Emami et al. 1991). Furthermore, quality assurance guidelines for these specific techniques have been discussed within the framework of the European COMAC-BME Hyperthermia project, during a workshop on Quality Assurance in Hyperthermia held in Sabaudia (Seegenschmiedt and Visser 1991). In this chapter some aspects of equipment performance tests, applicator specification, and guidelines for applicator positioning will be summarized. Because thermometry is covered elsewhere, only the specific problem of temperature measurements with probes inside applicators will be discussed briefly.

38.2 Equipment Performance Checks

For an experimental treatment like (interstitial) hyperthermia it is essential to certify that the equipment intended for clinical use is extensively tested and specified. The specific measurements to evaluate the performance of a heating system are dependent on the technique of IHT used. For example, the tests to be performed on a microwave (MW) system working with an array of coherent coaxial MW antennas are quite different from those to be performed for a hot water circulation system. The following main IHT techniques can be distinguished:

1. Radiative, using MW antennas operating in the range of about 300–2450 MHz; in principle MW antennas have the capability to deposit power at a distance from the applicator, allowing (at least in theory) somewhat larger distances between applicators. Constructive interference between coherently driven antennas can be used to improve the power deposition at depth. Problem areas with MW antennas are the difficulty in varying the length to be heated, the dependence on the insertion depth, and, depending on antenna design, the presence of a "cold tip," i.e., insufficient power deposition at the tip of the antenna.

2. Radiofrequency (RF), using frequencies in the range between 500 kHz and about 27 MHz. The use of frequencies at the lower end of this range, to drive electrodes (e.g., implanted needles) which are in galvanic contact with the tissue volume to be heated, is conceptually the most simple technique for interstitial heating and is often referred to as local current field (LCF) heating. The use of higher frequencies (27 MHz) for interstitial heating is mainly motivated by the utilization of capacitive coupling of electrodes inside nonconductive catheters instead of direct galvanic contact with the surrounding tissue. This technique is therefore designated as capacitive coupling (CC) interstitial hyperthermia.

3. Conductive techniques, which are quite different from the electromagnetic heating methods in the sense that they rely only on thermal conduction to reach hyperthermic temperatures and no power is

A.G. Visser, Ph.D.; R.S.J.P. Kaatee, M.Sc.; Departments of Clinical Physics and Radiotherapy, Dr. Daniel den Hoed Cancer Center, Groene Hilledijk 301, P.O. Box 5201, NL-3008 AE Rotterdam, The Netherlands deposited directly in the tissue. Both the technique using inductively heated ferromagnetic seeds and hot source methods (i.e., hot water circulation systems or hot wire systems) belong to this category.

A number of basic performance checks for hyperthermia equipment in general have been described in AAPM Report 26 (1989). These checks include tests of all generators (for MW and RF techniques), such as:

1. The proper functioning with dummy loads
2. Power linearity with dummy loads
3. Checks of operating frequencies
4. Tests of capability to tolerate impedance mismatches
5. Long-term stability, in terms of both power output and phase

Apart from these basic tests and from general safety and operational checks necessary for all hyperthermia equipment, specific performance evaluation measurements are required for the complete interstitial heating system, i.e., the combination of generators, applicators, thermometry, and data acquisition system. Of course, these specific tests depend on the technique used. In Table 38.1 a number of pretreatment equipment performance tests are summarized for the techniques mentioned above using electromagnetic fields. This table is a modified and augmented version of the table given in the RTOG guidelines (EMAMI et al. 1991).

These checks include selection of applicators (e.g., regarding the length and position of the active heating region) and testing of all selected applicators. If any doubt arises regarding the proper functioning of an applicator or of the associated generator/amplifier, it may be prudent to have a setup available for quick calorimetric efficiency measurements, e.g., for MW antennas, CC applicators, or ferromagnetic seeds.

38.3 IHT Applicator Specification

Careful assessment of the effective iso-SAR (specific absorption rate) contours has to be performed to characterize the specific heating patterns for each individual applicator and, if applicable, in specific applicator arrays as used in clinical applications, e.g., arrays of either two or four parallel applicators at commonly used distances from each other. It should be specified at which reference point the SAR measurements are normalized, i.e., either with respect to the measured maximum temperature elevation above the background (which might be difficult to assess) or with respect to the measured SAR value in a reference point at a defined distance from the applicator, preferably on the perpendicular bisector of the applicator, at a distance of 5 mm from the geometrical center of the applicator.

Possible means of assessing SAR patterns of IHT applicators include:

1. Infrared thermography using the split-phantom technique.
2. Liquid crystal film thermography in transparent phantoms.

Table 38.1. Specific equipment checks to be performed prior to a therapy session (modified from EMAMI et al. 1991)

RF-LCF	RF-CC	Ferromagnetic seeds	Microwave antennas
1. Continuity of leads from generator to electrodes	1. Select type of applicator to be used and required lengths	1. Choose appropriate coil configuration for intended implant seed orientation	1. Check cables and connectors for power loss or reflected power
2. Verify output power of RF generators	2. Verify output of RF generators	2. If seeds with different Curie temperatures are available, choose geometrical distribution	2. Check SAR pattern of antennas at intended insertion depth using catheters (in phantom)
3 Verify parallel implant, equal lengths to be heated; exclude crossed needles from heating	3. Check chosen applicators for impedance matching	3. Determine whether thermometry is needed in regions of expected soft tissue high field	3. For antenna arrays, choose antennas that have similar SAR patterns
4. Check duty cycle heating (if applicable)	4. Check duty cycle heating (if applicable)		4. Choose antenna configurations which match tumor dimensions
			5. Verify power splitting over antennas

3. Thermal mapping in a homogeneous muscle-equivalent phantom using the power–pulse technique. As an example, in the RTOG guidelines it is proposed that MW antennas be tested by turning on the power (about 15 W per antenna) for approximately 30 s and measuring the temperature increase with a multipoint temperature probe inside a catheter parallel to the antenna catheter and at a distance of 5 mm.

Analogous to the specification of the effective field size and penetration depth for external hyperthermia, IHT applicators should be characterized in terms of the effective length and width of iso-SAR contours, the percentage level used (25% or 50%), and the normalization method.

Recipes for phantom materials are readily available in the literature for different materials at a wide range of frequencies, e.g., agar (ISHIDA and KATO 1980), gels (BINI et al. 1984), or "superstuff" (CHOU et al. 1984).

For MW interstitial heating systems the SAR distributions of antenna arrays should be specified as a function of operation mode (either coherent or incoherent) and of the antenna insertion depth. For RF heating the electrode connection (or switching) patterns should be specified. Possible hot spots at entrance and exit points should be carefully observed.

Ferromagnetic seed techniques require specific assessment of the seed angle dependence, the operating Curie point, and the transition slope of each type of ferromagnetic seed used. For hot water circulation systems the range of cold and hot water flow rates needs to be checked prior to clinical application. Both hot water circulation systems and ferromagnetic seeds require characterization of temperature uniformity depending upon perfusion rates and applicator spacing.

As mentioned above, it may be recommended (e.g., for RF and MW heating techniques or for ferromagnetic seeds) that a calorimetric test of an applicator or a seed be performed prior to its actual application in a treatment. This can be done as a quick test to certify the overall functioning of all channels (generators + applicators) of the IHT equipment.

Forward and reflected power levels have to be documented regularly, preferably at short intervals at the start of a treatment session and with regular checks in the steady-state situation. For MW and RF techniques the reflective power should be kept below 10%–20% of the forward power.

38.4 Implant Geometry and Applicator Positioning

A number of considerations regarding the implant geometry and its consequences for applicator positioning and thermometry probe placement are summarized in Table 38.2, modified from the one given in the RTOG guidelines (EMAMI et al. 1991).

Ideally, the application of IHT should not require alteration of the established brachytherapy guidelines, with the exception that some additional probes might be required for invasive thermometry. The preferred geometry of brachytherapy implants has been defined in different brachytherapy "systems," e.g., the well-known Manchester system (or Paterson–Parker system), the Quimby system, and the more recently developed Paris system. These systems offer a set of rules for optimum source configurations and methods for specification of the treatment dose and the treatment volume. In general it is considered undesirable to deviate from these established guidelines for applicator positioning and, if possible, the interstitial

Table 38.2. Source and thermometry implant considerations (modified after EMAMI et al. 1991)

Factor	RF-LCF	RF-CC	MW antennas	Hot wire or hot water	Ferromagnetic seeds
1. Tumor coverage	← As for brachytherapy →				
2. Applicator spacing (mm)	10–15	10–15	12–20	< 10–13	< 10–13
3. Thermometry probes	← 2–6 additional catheters →				
4. Applicator orientation	Strictly parallel	Preferably parallel	Preferably parallel	Preferably parallel	≤ 30° of magnetic field
5. Other	1. Pairs same length and depth 2. Insulate normal tissues		1. Proper antenna length 2. Coherent dipoles, same depth		

heating technique should require no change in the common brachytherapy implant geometries.

However, in brachytherapy usually a range of applicator spacings is allowed, e.g., the Paris system allows (for wire sources of sufficient length) spacing of up to 20 mm. Clinical experience with IHT, although still limited, indicates that applicator spacings of more than 15 mm can result in inhomogeneous temperature distributions with cold spots in the regions of larger applicator spacings, e.g., in highly perfused regions like the base of tongue or the anal canal. Hot source methods seem to be most sensitive with respect to applicator spacing, as they rely only on thermal conduction, whereas MW IHT can be expected to allow larger spacings. The range of applicator spacings given in the table is somewhat intuitive: the actually allowed applicator spacing will be very much dependent on the tumor location, applicator geometry, and level of cooling through blood flow.

For all IHT techniques it appears valuable to attempt to obtain a parallel geometry and constant separation between neighboring applicators. For RF-LCF heating with single-segment electrodes strictly parallel geometries are needed because the current density will vary with electrode spacing. In addition, for RF-LCF heating it is recommended that equal-length segments be employed for all electrodes. MW antennas (at least coaxial dipole antennas) are dependent on the insertion depth and at least a minimum insertion depth corresponding to a quarter-wavelength (in tissue) at the applied frequency seems advisable. For ferromagnetic seeds the seed angle with respect to the axis of the externally applied field is of importance and deviations $\geq 30°$ from this axis should be avoided.

38.5 Special Problems of Measuring Inside Applicators

Typical examples of thermometry inside heating applicators are thermal measurements within RF needles or within or directly adjacent to MW antennas or RF-CC applicators. Generally this type of measurement is used to ascertain the temperatures obtained in tissue regions close to the applicators, often the maximum temperature regions within the implanted volume.

Advantages of this mode of thermometry are: (a) possibility of individual power control of all applicators and (b) indication of maximum temperature, possibly allowing prevention of treatment side-effects and toxicity. An important drawback of this type of thermometry is the possible presence of thermometry artifacts, e.g., due to self-heating in the case of MW antennas or RF-CC applicators and/or due to thermal resistance between the probe and the surrounding tissue. The accuracy of thermometry inside MW antennas has been discussed by Astrahan et al. (1988). Measured temperatures were found to differ from the estimated local tissue temperature by up to 8°C. In their design, self-heating distal to the antenna junction appeared to be the primary source of this error.

For CC (27-MHz) applicators the dielectric properties of the catheter material can be of importance: material with a relatively high loss factor can be expected to show significant heating of the catheter.

The magnitude of any possible thermometry artifact has to be known in order to be able to obtain meaningful data representing the actual local tissue temperatures. If either self-heating or electromagnetic interference is found to have an influence, measurements during power-off periods should be performed. If reliable temperatures can be obtained, this thermometry concerns only the regions close to the applicators, where generally significantly higher temperatures are procured in comparison to the tissue regions between the applicators. It is therefore recommended that thermometry inside heating applicators always be supplemented by measurements with probes in nonheated catheters.

Advantages of thermometry in nonheated catheters are: (a) assessment of actual tissue temperatures between the applicators, where temperature levels are generally lower, (b) minimal or no artifacts from the heating applicators, and therefore (c) reliable data for thermal dose–response evaluation. A drawback might be the possible underestimation of the high temperatures close to the heating applicators which might be relevant for treatment toxicity, especially when patients are treated under general anesthesia.

In order to obtain a full perception of the temperature distribution over the target volume, the application of thermal modeling using measured temperatures as input data is an interesting possibility. The principal advantage of IHT is the large number of invasive catheters and their small spacing relative to the size of the target volume. By using power-pulse measurement techniques with multipoint temperature probes in all catheters it should be possible to obtain small-scale data on the heat transport through blood flow over the whole target volume. These data can be used as input for thermal modeling. In combination with small-scale and sufficiently fast thermometry data, it should then be possible to obtain detailed information on the temperature distribution as a whole and to utilize this information for optimization.

38.6 Thermometry Requirements as a Function of Implant Geometry

In the RTOG guidelines a number of different locations for thermometry probe placement have been defined. It seems useful to summarize these definitions and the recommendations regarding the number of thermometry probes required as a function of implant geometry. In a given implant, for example a rectangular implant area treated with 16 applicators (arranged in four parallel planes of four applicators each), the following probe locations can be distinguished:

1. The center of the implant
2. The centers of subarrays [in general a subarray can consist of three applicators (triangle), four applicators (square), or more]
3. The tumor periphery
4. The surrounding normal tissue.

The preferred number of thermometry probes depends on the total number of heating applicators and the specific implant geometry. Global recommendations for the number of thermometry catheters as given in the RTOG guidelines are summarized in Table 38.3. Either thermometry catheters should be loaded with multipoint thermometry probes or thermal mapping with single probes along the catheter tracks should be performed.

Regarding the temperature monitoring during treatment, the RTOG recommends the following:

1. Multisensor probes or thermal mapping
2. Each sensor location measured at least every 15 min
3. Spacing between probe locations or map points:
   a) 5 mm for tumors less than 5 cm
   b) 10 mm for larger tumors.

Regarding the recommended minimum time interval between measurements at each probe location one may note that the requirement of measuring each location at least every 15 min is less strict than, for example, the quality assurance guidelines for ESHO protocols (HAND et al. 1989)

Table 38.3. Summary of the recommended number and location of thermometry probes as a function of the number of catheters in the implant (after EMAMI et al. 1991)

No. of heating appl.	Position A	Position B	Position C
	Center of implant	Centers of subarrays	Periphery
3–8	1	0	1
9–16	1	1	1
17–32	1	2	1
> 32	1	3	2

dealing with external, superficial hyperthermia. For reporting a summary of the treatment the latter guidelines recommend that the temperature at each sensor location must be recorded at 5-min intervals during the treatment; the data acquisition system should be able to scan all temperature sensors at 10- to 20-s intervals, while the data should be printed at 1-min intervals. Because there is no obvious reason to suppose that temperature distributions obtained with IHT will be more uniform and stable than those obtained with external heating methods, it seems prudent to set similar (strict) requirements for the frequency of temperature measurements.

References

AAPM Report 26 (1989) Performance evaluation of hyperthermia equipment (Report of AAPM Task Group No 1. Hyperthermia Committee). American Association of Physicists in Medicine

Astrahan MA, Luxton G, Sapozink MD, Petrovich Z (1988) The accuracy of temperature measurement from within an interstitial microwave antenna. Int J Hyperthermia 4: 593–607

Bini M, Ignesti A, Millanta L, Olmi R, Rubino N, Vanni R (1984) The polyacrylamide as a phantom material for electromagnetic hyperthemia studies. IEEE Trans Biomed Eng 31: 317–322

Chou CK, Chen GW, Guy AW, Luk KH (1984) Formulas for preparing phantom muscle tissue at various radiofrequencies. Bioelectromagnetics 5: 435–441

Emami B, Stauffer P, Dewhirst MW et al. (1991) RTOG quality assurance guidelines for interstitial hyperthermia. Int J Radiat Oncol Biol Phys 20: 1117–1124

Hand JW, Lagendijk JJW, Bach Andersen J, Bolomey JC (1989) Quality assurance guidelines for ESHO protocols. Int J Hyperthermia 5: 421–428

Ishida T, Kato H (1980) Muscle equivalent agar phantom for 13.56 MHz RF-induced hyperthermia. Shimane J Med Sci 4: 134–140

Seegenschmiedt MH, Visser AG (1991) Quality assurance for interstitial hyperthermia (summary of session in COMAC-BME workshop on Quality Assurance in Hyperthermia, Sabaudia, September 1990). COMAC-BME Hyperthermia Bulletin 5, January 1991, pp 85–91

39 The French Multicenter Trial: Results and Conclusions

C. MARCHAL, B. PREVOST, J.-M. ARDIET, J.-P. GERARD, and J.-M. COSSET

CONTENTS

39.1 Introduction

Investigations into the use of interstitial hyperthermia started in France in 1977 at the Institut Gustave Roussy, with the preliminary works of LEBOURGEOIS et al. (1978) followed by the physical works of DAMIA (1981) and the clinical experience of COSSET et al. (1982). This preliminary clinical experience was gained using parallel implanted needles and a home-made prototype built by the electronic laboratory of the Institut Gustave Roussy, and, later, using the first CGR Minerve system consisting of three generators of 25 W each operating at 0.5–1 MHz.

From 1981 to 1984, COSSET et al. (1985) carried out a pilot study on 23 patients (29 tumors) using tubes with flexible plastic ends attached to metallic central regions of different length in which the RF power was delivered to the central region by a single electrode equipped with a thermistor for continuous thermometry. After improving the technology in collaboration with Odam-Bruker Co., a clinical multicenter phase II evaluation of the Minerve hyperthermia system was commenced in 1985. By the time the trial was closed in 1989, 96 patients had been treated. GAUTHERIE (1988) reported the preliminary clinical results, and the last report is that by GERARD et al. (1991).

In Lille, the promising research of FABRE et al. (1989–1990) conducted by CHIVE et al. (1990), demonstrated the feasibility of combining interstitial microwave heating with microwave radiometry for temperature control (CHIVE and PREVOST 1991). A multicenter clinical phase II study coordinated by PREVOST (1991) was begun in Lille in 1989 and 27 patients have now been evaluated.

In Nancy, technical and physical research on a new capacitive interstitial heating technique operating at 27 MHz, conducted by MARCHAL et al. (1985) and NADI et al. (1988), led to the treatment of only five patients (MARCHAL et al. 1989, 1992).

More recently, interesting clinical applications of LCF hyperthermia in 11 patients with primary breast tumors were reported by FOURQUET et al. (1990) at the Institut Curie.

We have tried to summarize the French clinical experience with interstitial hyperthermia in Table 39.1. Unfortunately, only four French groups are still clinically using interstitial hyperthermia in combination with brachytherapy. A randomized phase II clinical study concerning large T2-T3 tumors of the mobile tongue and of the base of the tongue has just started.

C. MARCHAL, M.D., Ph.D., Unité d'Hyperthermie, Service de Radiothérapie, Centre Alexis Vautrin, Avenue de Bourgogne, F-54511 Vandoeuvre les Nancy, France
B. PREVOST, M.D., Centre de lutte contre le cancer Oscar Lambret, 1 rue Frédéric Combemale, BP 307, F-59020 Lille Cedex, France
J.-M. ARDIET, M.D., Service de Curiethérapie, Centre Léon Bérard, F-69003 Lyon, France
J.-P. GERARD, M.D., Professor, Service de Radiothérapie du Centre Hospitalier Lyon Sud, F-69310 Pierre Benite, France
J.-M. COSSET, M.D., Professor, Département de Radiothérapie, Institut Gustave Roussy, F-94800 Villejuif, and (current address) Département de Radiothérapie, Institut Curie, 26 rue d'Ulm, F-75231 Paris Cedex 05, France

Table 39.1. Summary of the different French clinical trials performed

Type of trial	Principal investigators	Material used	Tumors treated (total)	Complete response rate (%)	Toxicity (%)	Last report
Institut Gustave Roussy pilot study	J.M. Cosset	Minerve prototype (0.5–1 MHz)	29	66	25	1985
Multicenter phase II evaluation of the Minerve hyperthermia system (IGR, Lyon Cancer Center, Lyon Sud, Dijon)	J.M. Cosset J.P. Gerard J.M. Ardiet J.C. Horiot	Minerve apparatus (Bruker) (0.5–1 MHz)	96	61	26	1989
Phase II Multicenter study for interstitial microwave heating (Centre Oscar Lambret, Clinique Bourgogne, Lille)	B. Prevost S. De Cordoue--Rohart	HIMCAR prototype (915 MHz) HYLCAR apparatus (915 MHz (Brucker)	27	78	15	1992
Curie Institute pilot study (Paris)	A. Fourquet D. Pontvert G. Gaboriaud	Minerve apparatus (0.5–1 MHz)	11	82	27	1991
Centre Alexis Vautrin pilot study (Nancy)	C. Marchal M. Pernot S. Hoffstetter	Helyos prototype (27 MHz)	5	60	20	1992
Five clinical trials			168	69	23	

39.2 The Institut Gustave Roussy Pilot Study

In 1981, Cosset et al. (1985) initiated a pilot study at the Institut Gustave Roussy and between 1981 and 1984, 29 implantations were performed in 23 patients. All the lesions except three were located in previously irradiated sites (45–100 Gy). Fifteen lesions were cutaneous or subcutaneous metastases (11 from breast carcinoma, two from soft tissue sarcoma, one from uterine carcinoma, and one from a squamous cell carcinoma), six lesions were recurrent cervical lymph node metastases, six were recurrent squamous cell carcinomas of the skin, and two were recurrent tumors of the oral cavity. In the first 17 implantations of the series, a dose of brachytherapy of 30 Gy was applied, but after two local relapses, the dose was increased to 40 Gy and if the minimum temperature of 44°C was not reached during the hyperthermia session performed before brachytherapy, a second hyperthermia treatment was applied after the iridium had been unloaded.

During the hyperthermia session, the patients experienced minimal discomfort that was easily controlled with light sedation. Late effects could not be evaluated in six cases, but in eight cases small areas of necrosis were observed. In four other cases, large areas of necrosis occurred: two on the skin and two in the oral cavity.

After 2 months, 19 complete responses and four partial responses were observed among 23 evaluable tumors. Unfortunately six relapses occurred at between 5 and 13 months after a primary complete response. Four of them were located at the edge of the implantation and two were possibly due to a low radiation dose (30 Gy). Whereas the tumor response was near 83%, the local control was effectively lower at 56%.

The conclusions of this trial were that interstitial hyperthermia was technically satisfactory, that in most cases it yielded encouraging clinical responses with acceptable toxicity, and that further studies were therefore warranted.

39.3 The Multicentre Phase II Evaluation of the Minerve Hyperthermia System

From 1984 to 1989, a clinical phase II trial was performed in four French institutions – the Institut

Gustave Roussy, the "Lyon-Sud" hospital, and the Léon Bérard and Georges-François Leclerc centers – to evaluate the Minerve hyperthermia system. This multicenter study was carried out within the TVP (transfer and valuation of prototypes) process with the scientific and financial support of INSERM and of the French Ministry of Research and Technology. Its aims were:

1. To evaluate the efficiency of the system as an adjuvant to brachytherapy in the treatment of all types of cancers for which this therapeutic approach is appropriate. (The effectiveness of the technique used was assessed according to the tumor regression rate.)
2. To evaluate tolerance to the treatment and its effect on the adjacent normal tissues.

Ninety-six patients were eligible. Treatment was carried out on primary cancers of the tongue and the oral cavity, 23 gynecological tumors (of which only four were primary tumors), 16 rectal and anal cancers, 14 breast recurrences in a site previously irradiated, and 20 local recurrences or metastatic nodules of various origins. Interstitial hyperthermia was delivered by the Minerve machine with six heating lines, except for eight cases with 10 lines and three cases with 12 lines. In all cases hyperthermia was performed for 45 min before brachytherapy (20–60 Gy), usually under general anesthesia; in five cases a second hyperthermia session following prior brachytherapy was necessary.

As regards the thermal results, 43.5°C was reached in 96% of cases and homogeneous heating of the whole tumor volume could be achieved in almost 50% of the treatment sessions.

Immediate tolerance was good in 71 cases (74%), but eight patients had severe reactions such as burns, low hemorrhage, or cutaneous or mucosal necrosis. In 15 cases necrotic lesions required surgery, and four patients with extremely severe effects required a colostomy or an abdominoperineal resection. A complete tumor response was obtained in 59 cases (61%) and a partial response in 13 cases (14%).

A recent update of the data concerning 69 patients from this trial (30 with primary tumors and 39 with recurrences) found a complete response rate of 62% and a partial response rate of 17%. However, long-term local control fell to 43% (33% for primary tumors, 45% for recurrences not previously irradiated, and 54% for recurrences previously irradiated) (GERARD et al. 1991). Moreover, it was found that the local control rate was 52% when the minimum temperature reached was higher than 43°C and only 30% when it was lower than 43°C ($P < 0.05$). Toxicity also seems to be related to temperature since 30% of cases of necrosis were observed when the minimum temperature recorded was higher than 43°C and only 13% when it was lower (GERARD et al. 1991).

39.4 The Lille Hyperthermia Group Pilot Study

Since 1989, a pilot study has been conducted at two institutions in Lille on the use of a microwave interstitial system in patients with cancers of the mobile tongue or tumors of the base of the tongue in previously irradiated areas. In the Centre Oscar Lambret, the work is coordinated by B. Prevost; the patients are treated under general anesthesia. The interstitial microwave hyperthermia is delivered for 1 h at 42°–43°C (which is the radiometric temperature for monitoring the hyperthermia session) immediately before iridium-192 loading. At the Clinique Bourgogne, S. de Cordoue-Rohart is treating all her patients under neuroleptanalgesia and hyperthermia is performed before and/or after brachytherapy for 1 h at 42°C (radiometric temperature).

The HIMCAR system combining microwave (915 MHz) interstitial heating with multifrequency radiometry (3 and 5 GHz) seems of great interest (FABRE et al. 1990); the aim of this trial is not only evaluation of the method, but also appraisal of the efficiency of interstitial hyperthermia when treating primary tumors or performing salvage therapy in previously irradiated areas.

39.4.1 Primary Tumors of the Mobile Tongue

T2 and T3 N0 or N1 tumors were selected and treated either with brachytherapy (65 Gy) or with external beam radiotherapy (45 Gy) followed by brachytherapy 30–40 Gy. Nineteen cases were evaluated with a mean follow-up of 12 months (5–27 months); 15 (79%) complete responses were observed with three moderate complications such as intense mucositis and only one severe ulceration.

Of the four recurrences, which occurred after 3, 4, 8, and 13 months, three were locoregional.

39.4.2 Base of Tongue Tumors in Previously Irradiated Areas

The patients selected had a second cancer at the base of the tongue, which had previously been irradiated. This second localization was revealed between 5 and 96 months after treatment of the first primary tumor (mean: 48 months). In these cases, only salvage brachytherapy could be proposed. The usual dose was 55–60 Gy in combination with interstitial microwave hyperthermia for 1 h at 42°C delivered just before iridium-192 loading.

Eight patients were treated. Six (75%) responded completely with a mean follow-up of 11 months (range 6–27 months). No severe complication arose and the two local recurrences were observed after 10 and 14 months.

The conclusions of this pilot study are:

1. Microwave interstitial hyperthermia at 915 MHz may induce relatively good heating homogeneity in mobile tongue tumors and in tumors of the base of the tongue, which are known to be extremely difficult to heat correctly owing to the high blood flow rate of these tissues.
2. Multifrequency radiometry appears to be effective for temperature control of the tumor as compared with thermocouple and optic fiber sensor measurements and for driving the microwave power (Prevost et al. 1991; Fabre et al. 1990).
3. The complication rate is extremely low: there was only one severe complication in the 27 patients treated, even though some tumors were in previously irradiated areas.

39.5 The Institut Curie Pilot Study for Primary Breast Tumors

The preliminary clinical experience of the Institut Curie was reported by Fourquet et al. (1990). The data concern 11 women treated between November 1986 and October 1988, who had residual tumors after external beam irradiation (54 Gy in 6 weeks). Hyperthermia was delivered before iridium-192 loading, immediately following recovery from anesthesia for brachytherapy. The Minerve machine and metal–plastic catheters were used. Nine patients underwent only one hyperthermia session lasting 45 min at 41.5°–44.8°C and the iridium was then loaded within 1 h for a boost of 20 Gy. Two patients received two hyperthermia sessions, one before iridium loading and one after iridium removal.

No severe complications were observed, though there were three moderate burns (27%). The mean follow-up was 23 months and nine patients had a complete tumor response (82%) while two had tumor progression.

In conclusion, the study demonstrated that tumors of the breast can be safely heated without general anesthesia with a very good tumor response rate, thus suggesting that a prospective trial would be warranted to try to demonstrate that the combination of brachytherapy and hyperthermia is of benefit in patients with breast tumors that have partially responded to external beam radiotherapy.

39.6 The Centre Alexis Vautrin Pilot Study

In 1985, Marchal et al. proposed a new capacitive method of heating interstitially using flexible coated electrodes operating at 27.12 MHz. The advantages of such a method compared to classical ones are more uniform heating along a limited length, compatibility with conventional brachytherapy techniques, the simplicity, and the low cost (Nadi et al. 1988; Marchal et al. 1992). Experimental and clinical feasibility was demonstrated in a limited pilot study (Marchal et al. 1989). Five patients were treated with brachytherapy doses varying from 20 to 60 Gy. Three complete responses were observed, but pain induced during the treatment (even under light sedation) proved to be a limiting factor. The water circulation heating system was then preferred; however, the aforementioned method has been greatly improved by the Rotterdam group (Visser et al. 1991).

39.7 Interstitial Hyperthermia as Adjuvant Treatment to Brachytherapy for Advanced Cancers of the Base of the Tongue and of the Mobile Tongue: A Randomized Ongoing Phase II Study

39.7.1 Aims of the Study

1. To evaluate the reliability of the different methods of interstitial hyperthermia at a practical level.
2. To evaluate the short- and long-term tolerance of normal tissue that received irradiation only or in combination with interstitial hyperthermia.
3. To evaluate the efficiency of interstitial hyperthermia as an adjuvant treatment to brachytherapy

for primary tumors of the base of the tongue or of the mobile tongue.

4. To evaluate the rate of tumor regression, the local control, and survival with or without hyperthermia.

39.7.2 *Patient Eligibility*

1. All patients presenting with primary cancer of the base of the tongue or the mobile tongue can be recruited for the clinical study if they are treated with brachytherapy only or with brachytherapy in association with external beam radiotherapy.

2. All "large" (> 3 cm) infiltrating T2 and T3 tumors will be accepted for the study independent of their nodal status. The patients will be retrospectively classified according to their nodal status.

3. Patients with metastases will be excluded from the study.

4. All primary tumors will have been biopsied to prove that they are epidermoid carcinomas.

5. Patients will have a life expectancy in excess of 6 months.

6. Patients treated with first-line chemotherapy will be able to enter the study providing that the chemotherapy is not concomitant with the brachytherapy/external beam radiotherapy and that the patient has been examined by a specialist who has documented precisely the tumor limits and volume.

7. Patients with recurrences in preirradiated sites will be excluded.

8. Patients will have to be followed regularly in the center where the treatment has been performed.

9. The tumors selected will have to be technically accessible to the brachytherapy and thermotherapy treatments.

10. Only patients who have accepted the conditions of randomization enforced by the study and who have given their written consent will be entered in the study.

39.7.3 *Details of the Study*

Patients who meet the above-mentioned criteria will be randomized by center with or without hyperthermia, according to the drawing of lots.

Forty patients presenting with tumors of the base of the tongue and 40 patients with tumors of the mobile tongue will be included in the study over 2 years. In the event of a favorable response, these 80 patients will be included in a phase III study.

Patients will be randomized to receive either (a) radiotherapy alone, i.e., irradiation of the tumor and nodes according to the protocol in force at the center where the study is performed (generally 40–50 Gy to T and 50 Gy if N0 cases, and 65–70 Gy if a palpable node is present) followed by complementary brachytherapy to the tumor at a dose of 30–40 Gy, or (b) external beam radiotherapy and brachytherapy at the same doses, combined with interstitial hyperthermia in one 45-min session at 42°–45°C carried out after the unloading of the radioactive wires.

In the case of some T2 tumors, it would be possible to randomize patients to receive either brachytherapy alone (65–70 Gy) or brachytherapy at the same doses in combination with interstitial hyperthermia applied in only one session of 45 min at 42–45°C after the unloading of the radioactive wires.

Given the quality and number of the staff necessary to obtain results that may be exploited and are statistically significant, implementation of this protocol is feasible only within the framework of a multicenter study. To date the following centers have agreed to participate:

1. Centre Léon Berard in Lyon (Dr. J. M. Ardiet)
2. Centre Oscar Lambret in Lille (Dr. B. Prevost)
3. Clinique Bourgogne in Lille (Dr. S. de Cordoue-Rohart)
4. Centre Alexis Vautrin (Dr. C. Marchal).

We are now waiting for the end of this study to decide whether a further phase III randomized trial would be of interest.

References

Chive M, Prévost B (1991) Technical aspects and clinical evaluation of a microwave interstitial hyperthermia system using a multifrequency radiometric technique for temperature control and monitoring. Strahlenther Onkol 167: 51

Cosset JM (1990) Interstitial hyperthermia. In: Gautherie M (ed) Clinical thermology: interstitial, endocavitary and perfusional hyperthermia. Methods and clinical trials. Springer, Berlin Heidelberg New York, p 142

Cosset JM, Brule JM, Salama AM, Damia E, Dutreix J (1982) Low-frequency (0.5 MHz) contact and interstitial techniques for clinical hyperthermia. In: Gautherie M (ed) Biomedical thermology. Alan R. Liss, New York, pp 649–657

Cosset JM, Dutreix J, Dufour J, Janoray P, Damia E, Haie C, Clarke D (1984a) Combined interstitial hyperthermia and brachytherapy: the Institut Gustave Roussy experience. In: Jens Overgaard (ed) Hyperthermic oncology, vol 1. Taylor and Francis, London, pp 587–590
Cosset JM, Dutreix J, Dufour J, Janoray P, Damia E, Haie C, Clarke D (1984b) Combined interstitial hyperthermia and brachytherapy: Institut Gustave Roussy technique and preliminary results. Int J Radiat Oncol Biol Physics 10: 307–312
Cosset JM, Dutreix J, Haie C, Gerbaulet A, Janoray P, Dewars JA (1985) Interstitial thermoradiotherapy: a technical and clinical study of 29 implantations performed at the Institut Gustave Roussy. Int J Hyperthermia, 1: 3–13
Damia E (1981) Etude d'un système de chauffage à la fréquence de 0.5 MHz pour l'hyperthermie thérapeutique. Thèse Faculté des Sciences de Limoges N°381
Fabre JJ et al. (1990) Microwave interstitial hyperthermia controlled by multifrequency microwave radiometry: phase I trials. Innov Techn Biol Med 11: 236–248
Fabre JJ, Camart JC (1991) Microwave interstitial hyperthermia system monitored by microwave radiometry (HIMCAR) and dosimetry by heating pattern remote sensing. Proc Eur Microwave Conference, Stuttgart, pp 1409–1414
Fourquet A, Labib A, Campana F, Pontvert D, Gaboriaud G (1990) 192 Ir curietherapy and interstitial hyperthermia in primary breast cancer: preliminary results in 11 patients. Proc. ESTRO Meeting Sept 1990, p 257
Gautherie M (1988) Clinical evaluation of the Minerve hyperthermia system: synthesis, T.V.P process (Ministry of Research and Technology (MRT) report)
Gautherie M, Cosset JM, Gérard JP, Horiot JC, Ardiet JM, Akoun HEL, Alperovitch A (1988) Radiofrequency interstitial hyperthermia: A multicentre program of quality assessment and clinical trials. In: Sugahara J, Saito M (eds) In hyperthermic Oncology, vol 2. Taylor & Francis Publisher, pp 711–714
Gérard JP, Romestaing P, Ardiet JM, Delaroche G, Montbarbon X, Sentenac I, Cosset JM (1991) Interstitial hyperthermia: general overview and preliminary results. In: Urano F, Douple E (eds) Hyperthermia and oncology, vol 3. Springer, Berlin Heidelberg New York, pp 221–230
Le Bourgeois JP, Convert G, Dufour J (1978) An interstitial device for microwave hyperthermia of human tumors. In: Streffer C (ed) Cancer therapy by hyperthermia and radiation. Urban and Schwarzenberg, Baltimore, pp 122–124
Marchal C, Hoffstetter S, Bey P, Pernot M, Gaulard ML (1985) Development of a new interstitial method of heating which can be used with conventional afterloading brachytherapy techniques using Ir 192. Strahlentherapie 161: 523–557
Marchal C, Nadi M, Hoffstetter S, Bey P, Pernot M, Prieur G (1989) Practical interstitial method of heating operating at 27.12 MHz. Int J Hyperthermia 5: pp 451–466
Marchal C, Pernot M, Hoffstetter S, Bey P (1992) Clinical experience with different interstitial hyperthermia techniques. In: Handl-Zeller L (ed) Interstitial hyperthermia. Springer, Berlin Heidelberg New York, pp 207–228
Nadi M, Marchal C, Tosser A, Roussey C, Gaulard ML (1988) New interstitial hypertehrmia technique at 27 MHz. Innov Tech Biol Med 9: 105–115
Prévost B, Mirabel X, Chive M, Fabre JJ, Dubois L, Sozanski JP (1991a) Clinical evaluation of a microwave interstitial hyperthermia system with microwave radiometry. Strahlenther Onkol 167: 344
Prévost B, Mirabel X, Coche B, Chive M, Fabre JJ, Sozanski JP (1991b). Hyperthermie interstitielle microonde combinée à la curiethérapie dans le traitement des cancers de la langue. 2ème Congrès natl de la SFRO. Paris 12–13 Déc 1991. Bull Cancer (Paris) 78: 4–49
Prévost B et al. (to be published) 915 MHz microwave interstitial hyperthermia, part III Phase II clinical results. Int J Hyperthermia
Visser AG, Deurloo IKK, Van Rhoon GC, Levendag PC (1991) Evaluation of a capacitive coupling interstitial system. Selectron Brachytherapy J 5: 114–119

40 Clinical Considerations for the Design and Conduct of Hyperthermia Clinical Trials

M.H. SEEGENSCHMIEDT and C.C. VERNON

CONTENTS

40.1 Introduction

The biological and clinical rationale and the clinical use of hyperthermia (HT) in oncology have been extensively reviewed in recent literature (ARCANGELI et al. 1988; OVERGAARD 1989; SEEGENSCHMIEDT and SAUER 1992). In the past decade considerable progress has been made in several areas: (a) defining various molecular, cellular, and tissue effects of heat; (b) refining technical means of producing, measuring, and controlling therapeutic temperature distributions in vivo; (c) completing many phase 1–2 trials for a variety of tumor sites, HT techniques, and combinations of HT with radiotherapy (RT) and chemotherapy (ChT). Nevertheless, many phase 2 trials still have to be conducted to optimize the use of HT. Ideally, the increased understanding of basic biological effects and further technical improvement of HT equipment would guide researchers to modify future clinical applications of external and interstitial HT.

External and interstitial HT techniques have been used to treat various tumors in different combinations with other modalities; although the reported clinical results may strongly suggest a definitive place for HT, the final acceptance of HT must await the outcome of scientifically based controlled clinical trials with emphasis on technical and clinical quality assurance (QA) (HAND et al. 1989; EMAMI et al. 1991). Efforts are still required to determine the optimal treatment regimen. Clinicians and institutions intending to participate in HT trials should carefully reflect both their own experience and the positions of other involved investigators. Important clinical considerations with regard to the implementation of HT-RT in multicenter trials are summarized in this chapter with specific attention to combined interstitial HT-RT (IHT-IRT).

40.2 Institutional Requirements

If institutions intend to participate in clinical research into external and interstitial HT, they should comply with a variety of intra- and interinstitutional requirements.

Intrainstitutional requirements include:

1. General interest in and academic enthusiasm for investigating new treatment modalities and protocols using HT

M.H. SEEGENSCHMIEDT, M.D., Strahlentherapeutische Klinik der Universität Erlangen-Nürnberg, Universitätsstraße 27, W-8520 Erlangen, Germany

C.C. VERNON, M.A., FACR, MRC Hyperthermia Clinic, Hammersmith Hospital, Ducane Road, London W12 OHS, UK

2. Well established interventional RT experience when participating in interstitial HT protocols, which includes theoretical and practical aspects, clinical management, radiophysics, dosimetry, and radiobiology of brachytherapy
3. Well-defined in-house cooperation between radiation oncology, oncologic surgery or surgical specialities, anesthesiology, radiological physics, and nursery
4. Well-developed cooperation between clinical specialists and referring physicians
5. Sufficient patient load with a specific disease suitable for the investigative treatment protocol
6. HT equipment with appropriate performance characteristics to predict sufficient heating of the expected tumor types, locations, and target volumes
7. Sufficient support to cover expenses in terms of the time, material, and personnel involved in these investigations.

Interinstitutional cooperation between different groups of a multicenter trial has to be well structured, including the following features:

1. Full responsibility of an established study protocol office which involves a study chairman, clinical, technical, and statistical advisers, a protocol review board, established electronic data exchange, and continuous medical education and technical training for all study participants
2. Periodic study review strictly within the multicenter group prior to the final issue of a summary report
3. Identical technical and clinical QA standards, which includes site visits and equipment performance checks by an independent QA group
4. Equal ethical standards and clinical practice following the established legislation and guidelines of "good clinical practice" (GCP) and "good medical practice" (GMP).

Generally it is recommended that multicenter trials be organized within large national or international research groups, including major university clinics. An independent trial office should handle the eligibility check, randomization procedures, and data transfer; this controls uniform inclusion criteria, minimizes individual errors, and avoids criticism of bias.

40.3 Treatment Protocol Design

Multicenter clinical trials should follow a written protocol, which explicitly describes rationale, scientific background, and all objectives of the trials. The protocol design should avoid a broad variety of patient and tumor eligibility criteria together with different treatment techniques and poorly defined treatment endpoints. Instead, the following requirements are necessary:

1. Well-defined eligibility criteria
2. Careful patient (age, performance status, life expectancy) and tumor selection (anatomical site, tumor volume, tumor histology)
3. Precise description of RT (external/interstitial modality, dose/fractionation schedule, and total treatment time) and HT (external/interstitial technique, applicator description, treatment setup information
4. Defined treatment schedule (sequential or simultaneous HT and RT; HT prior to and/or after RT; short high temperature HT; continuous moderate temperature HT)
5. Precise thermometry technique (method of temperature monitoring, temperature–time parameters)
6. Defined treatment endpoints related to tumor (initial response, response at defined intervals, local control, overall and relapse-free survival) and normal tissue (acute and late toxicity)
7. Standardized data documentation and reporting
8. Description of implemented statistical methods (statistical tests, confidence intervals, etc.)
9. Methods of technical and clinical QA
10. Signed informed consent by each patient.

Specific aspects of trial design, performance rules, and data analysis have been published recently (Meinert and Tonascia 1986; Leventhal and Wittes 1988). Only with careful preplanning can a comprehensive design and successful conduct of HT trials be achieved. Important statistical aspects have been discussed in a previous chapter of this volume (Vernon and Seegenschmiedt, this volume, Chap. 36). As all HT trials should aim to improve unsatisfactory treatment approaches for human beings who suffer and may succumb to a malignancy, these studies must be performed in strict accordance with the ethics of the Helsinki Declaration, with approval by the institutional review board (IRB) or ethical committees and in adherence with the rules of GCP/GMP and existing (inter)national legislation. HT is only indicated when better treatment strategies have been ruled out and a possible benefit can be expected; only then does the HT procedure – which is costly in terms of both time and manpower and entails risk to the patient – appear to be justified.

40.4 Clinical Site Selection

Site-specific considerations, e.g., the implementation of interstitial HT for head and neck tumors or pelvic malignancies have been discussed in Chaps. 21 and 22. However, selection of sites for HT trials is not only dependent on what tumor sites could benefit from additional HT, but also on how safely and "effectively" and with which technique this specific site could be best heated. We can summarize the most important considerations for tumor and treatment site selection:

1. Selected primary tumors should be subjected to controlled trials, i.e., tumors in which initial and long-term tumor control are still disappointing using conventional treatment strategies (surgery with or without adjuvant therapy, ChT alone or combined with RT, etc.), e.g., advanced T3-4 head and neck tumors or advanced T3-4 N2-3 rectal cancer. With respect to any other tumor site, deviation from a conventional treatment strategy could in general be justified whenever the locoregional relapse rate exceeds 20%–25%.

2. Improvement of local control should be regarded as the major prerequisite in a specific tumor site for the achievement of an improved cure rate and survival. Recently tumor sites were reviewed in which local failure had a significant relative [11% for lung cancer, 95% for brain and CNS tumors (figures indicate percentage of annual deaths for which local failure was responsible)] or absolute (1700 deaths from corpus uteri cancer, 15600 deaths from prostate cancer) impact on survival based on figures of the American Cancer Society from 1985 (Kapp 1986). It was concluded that improved local control in 12 different tumor sites would have prevented about 82800 (35%) of all cancer deaths in the United States in 1985.

3. Retreatment of recurrences after previous RT usually involves many clinical problems; due to limited RT tolerance an indication is often given for combined HT-RT with reduced RT dose; only small lesions should be primarily treated with surgery.

4. Treatment of local metastases, e.g., metastatic N3 neck nodes, are an acceptable indication for combined HT-RT when used as a boost after external beam RT and when surgery is impossible; however, it should be assured that the patient's general condition and the tumor stage offer enough evidence to expect a survival of at least 6 months.

5. Reduction of high treatment toxicity (i.e., acute or chronic side-effects) provides another rationale to modify standard treatment; if toxicity exceeds 20%–25% with conventional therapy, a reduced RT dose combined with HT would be justified. Decreased morbidity should be possible when the differential response of normal and tumor tissues to heat exposure can be exploited. Clinical reports indicate that HT may enhance acute, but not long-term toxicity; even when HT was applied for heavily pretreated recurrences, the complications did not exceed 25%–30% (Seegenschmiedt and Sauer 1992).

A sufficient patient number should guarantee the projected accrual within a defined time period; any bias depending on time- or institutional-related factors should be avoided. One of the major limiting factors for accrual is other protocols competing for the same tumors. Statistical considerations should include the anticipated differences from alternative treatments, the projected level of statistical significance, the estimated chance of detecting this difference, and the statistical power and confidence limits of all specific results (Vernon and Seegenschmiedt, this volume, Chap. 36).

40.5 Technical Device Selection

Various technical devices which can be used to induce heat to a prescribed volume are available in the clinics or under evaluation in the laboratories. Specific details of interstitial HT devices have been discussed in previous chapters of this volume. However, all devices demonstrate specific shortcomings in their ability to apply sufficient heat to every part of the body.

The adequacy of a treatment should be evaluated with reference to the level (e.g., $T \geq 43$°C) and the thermal homogeneity achieved within the target volume [e.g., hyperthermia equipment performance (HEP) ≥ 75%). This depends not only on the applied HT device, but also on intrinsic tumor conditions (tissue perfusion, areas of tumor necrosis, physiological parameters pH and pO_2), and other treatment modifications (e.g., drugs). Hence superficial tumors have more often been represented in clinical trials than deep-seated malignancies, because only for those sites have appropriate HT devices been available in the past. Current recommendations promote the concept of 25% or 50% iso-SAR coverage (SAR = specific absorption rate) to fit the HT applicator properly to the prescribed target volume (HAND et al. 1989; DEWHIRST et al. 1990; EMAMI et al. 1991; MYERSON et al. 1992). Thus the HT technique should be chosen to achieve effective tumor heating but to avoid excessive normal tissue heating.

The impact of poor HT equipment and inadequate heating within a multicenter trial was well documented in the disappointing results of the randomized RTOG study 81-04; large tumors (> 3 cm diameter) were insufficiently heated and did not benefit from additional HT compared to small chest wall lesions (< 3 cm diameter), which were not only better heated but also yielded significantly better results with combined RT-HT versus RT alone (PEREZ et al. 1989, 1991). Thus in future trials QA procedures should be used which conform at least to international standards (HAND et al. 1989; DEWHIRST et al. 1990; EMAMI et al. 1991).

40.6 Assessment of "Thermal Dose"

Whereas the "radiation dose" is both physically and biologically reasonably defined, there is no convincing analogous concept available for a "thermal dose." The principal obstacle in prescribing a specific thermal dose to induce a specific effect is inability to acquire sufficient temporal and spatial thermal data within the target volume.

The concept of adequate heat distribution should be applied similarly to the RT dose distribution. Currently only an incompletely evolved radiobiology-based concept of thermal dose [thermal equivalent minutes (TEM) at 43°C] is available (SAPARETO and DEWEY 1984). Other thermal parameters were found to correlate with clinical response: initially parameters related to the minimal tumor temperature (DEWHIRST et al. 1984) and recently parameters related to a specified index temperature (CORRY et al. 1988) correlated best with initial and long-term tumor control. The impact of sufficient minimum thermal dose parameters is particularly important when only low and subcurative RT doses are applied. It is not clear whether relatively cool, randomly distributed tumor foci will be critical areas of possible tumor relapse, especially when tolerance-dose RT is used.

Practical constraints limit the number of thermometry positions in and around a specific tumor volume to be sampled. Efforts are underway to improve documentation of all temporal and spatial temperature variations within the heated target volume: (a) multipoint or scanning single point thermometry; (b) numerical models to calculate 2D and 3D SAR distributions (STROHBEHN 1984); (c) algorithms similar to the bioheat transfer equation (ROEMER and CETAS 1984) to predict isotherm distributions, which could eliminate invasive thermometry; and (d) special noninvasive thermometry techniques (BOLOMEY and HAWLEY 1990). A still suboptimal strategy of thermal data sampling was recently recommended by the RTOG QA committee (DEWHIRST et al. 1990; EMAMI et al. 1991).

Other obstacles prevent the uniform documentation and translation of thermal data into a retrospective, comparative, and prospective thermal dose prescription: (a) there is no way to determine a cumulative dose when more than one HT treatment is applied; (b) during fractionated RT and HT schedules there is no meaningful method available to account for sensitizing effects (e.g., step-down heating) and protective effects (e.g., step-up heating or thermotolerance) as well as physiological changes interacting with radiosensitization (e.g., tissue perfusion, cellular pH and oxygen level, nutritional status).

Nevertheless, a variety of thermal parameters have been established which have been derived as prognostic factors for tumor response, e.g., in treating soft tissue sarcomas with a combined HT-RT or HT-ChT schedule: (a) average Tmin, average Tmax, Tmean temperatures; (b) temperatures at the defined edge of the tumor (Tedge) and the temperature slope (dT/dr) across the outer tumor shell (OLESON et al. 1989); (c) intratumoral time-averaged temperatures calculated above specified index temperatures (Tindex), i.e., $T_{90}/T_{50}/T_{20}$ temperature values, where 90%/50%/20% of all sensors are above the index temperature (ISSELS et al. 1990). Also correlations between CT and MRI diagnostic parameters in conjunction with blood flow parameters, heating performance, and tumor regression have been examined (FELDMANN and MOLLS 1991).

In summary, optimal delivery of HT will ultimately depend on the ability to determine prospectively tumor control and treatment complications as a thermal dose–response function or biological isoeffect relationship. Only precisely quantified HT treatment parameters will allow evaluation of their relationship to the final treatment outcome.

40.7 Study Design Selection

The introduction and success of clinical concepts depend on stepwise achievement of four major components: biological and clinical plausibility, technical feasibility, clinical efficacy, and clinical impact on outcome. The increased sophistication of clinical trial design and analysis has changed clinical medicine. This is particularly true for drug development and testing: the terminology for clinical trials is mainly influenced by drug testing, but modifications are required to test new treatment modalities in oncology such as HT (PHILLIPS 1985). The present study designs used for clinical testing include: (a) *phase 1:* clinical feasibility and dose–response relationship; (b) *phase 2:* determination of suitability and treatment efficacy; (c) *phase 3:* randomized comparison between standard and new treatment. While the "gold standard" for drug evaluation is randomized clinical testing, the same sophisticated test tools have not yet been developed for new HT devices and clinical trials involving HT-RT.

The biological and clinical plausibility of using efficient HT devices which allow heating between 41° and 45°C throughout the tumor volume and over sufficient time is well established; rather the major challenge for all clinical HT-RT trials is still technical feasibility. This includes four different components: (a) practical use of an HT system in a clinical setting; (b) availability of reliable HT equipment; (c) technical features to produce internally consistent, repeatable, and reliable HT treatments; and (d) cost-effectiveness. Since we are still lacking HT equipment which meets all the above criteria, the clinical efficacy of HT currently may be difficult to prove. Therefore we recommend the following clinical approach, which includes four steps of testing.

40.7.1 Phase 0 Trial: Technical Feasibility

Although phase 0 trials are not defined in drug testing, we consider such trials to be an essential tool for pilot testing of new HT devices or new clinical approaches. During such a "laboratory testing phase" biological, technical, or clinical concepts can be investigated for their clinical potential. In the past these ideas have often been developed by one researcher within a single institution. To give a typical example: The initial development and testing of the Stanford scanning double spiral microwave applicator were conducted within a single laboratory using different static or dynamic phantoms for physical performance testing (KAPP et al. 1988). During further development, "signal" tumors in animals and humans underwent first clinical testing with the new HT devices; the optimized HT equipment was then implemented for intrainstitutional testing to treat large chest wall lesions with the special permission of the IRB. Today such HT equipment can be used at many other clinics.

In the past many trials have been exclusively designed to evaluate new HT devices and such studies will also play a decisive role in advanced clinical phase 2–3 testing; but we recommend deviating from drug testing and implementing a technically based phase 0 trial prior to any clinical study. Table 40.1 summarizes a stepwise phase 0 to phase 3 testing procedure to evaluate HT devices in a clinical setting. The initial technical testing is followed by initial and advanced clinical testing, which is performed on the basis of defined tumor, patient, and treatment characteristics. Evaluation criteria for phase 0 trials have already been proposed together with decision criteria for discontinuation of the trial unless specific thermal performance conditions are met: (a) the percentage of tumor temperature points $\geq 43°C$ for all treatments is $\geq 75\%$; (b) the percentage of treatments with $\geq 75\%$ of intratumoral temperature points $\geq 43°C$ is $\geq 50\%$; and (c) the percentage of treatments with an HEP rating $\geq 75\%$ is $\geq 20\%$ (STROHBEHN 1991).

After completion of a phase 0 trial one has to decide to continue with upgraded phase 1 testing. This decision is crucial to the success of further clinical trials and depends strongly on the above-outlined thermal parameters. If these criteria are not met, further phase 0 testing is necessary to redesign the HT device or improve clinical conditions to achieve an acceptable HT performance. Therefore phase 0 testing requires more precise eligibility criteria and extensive thermometry data sampling than one expects for a phase 1 trial. If, indeed, excellent thermal data indicate the technical feasibility of effectively heating a specific site, clinical questions can be posed in a phase 1 trial, and then less aggressive thermometry should be able to answer these questions. Table 40.2 summarizes the

Table 40.1. Evaluation of hyperthermia devices in clinical trials (modified from STROHBEHN 1991)

Phase 0: Equipment development and initial evaluation (20 subjects)

1. Equipment development for implementation in humans: Anatomical and technical specifications, design, and construction
2. Equipment – technical evaluation: Safety requirements, testing on phantoms and animals
3. Equipment – clinical evaluation: Clinical testing on selected and limited number of humans; specification of evaluation criteria and dose measures

Phase 1: Standardized equipment implementation (20–100 subjects)

1. Corresponding to clinical phase 1 study: Determination of toxicity and dose relationship
2. Improvement of technical equipment: Improvement of heating performance; reduction of treatment toxicity; improvement of user's device handling; improvement of data analysis package

Phase 2: Improved equipment implementation (100–200 subjects)

1. Corresponding to clinical phase 2 study: Evaluation of tumor suitability and effectiveness
2. Further optimization of technical equipment: Optimized heating performance; minimal treatment toxicity; optimized user's device handling; optimized data analysis

Phase 3: Optimized equipment implementation (100–200 subjects)

1. Corresponding to clinical phase 3 study: Comparison between standard and new treatment approach (randomized study design)
2. Achieving routine clinical handling with optimal technical equipment

Table 40.2. Eligibility and evaluation criteria in a phase 0 trial (modified from STROHBEHN 1991)

Eligibility criteria:

1. Selection of patients with *one* specific body site: e.g., intact breast, chest wall, neck
2. Selection of *one* specific heating technique: e.g., external microwave, interstitial radiofrequency
3. Use of *same* heat treatment conditions in all patients: e.g., same number, sequence, and fractionation of treatments, same treatment duration, same parallel treatment
4. High standard of invasive thermometry data sampling: e.g., ideal condition: "one measurement point per cm^3"

Evaluation criteria for each treatment:

1. Plot % temperature points $\geq T$index temperature, e.g., 43°C: assessment of specific Tindex values like T_{90}, T_{50}, and T_{20}
2. Calculate HEP rating: % volume with temperature $\geq$ 43°C: assessment of specific HEP rates, e.g., HEP $\geq$ 75% etc.
3. Record Tav, Tmin, Tmax, steady-state treatment time, and thermal dose in thermal equivalent minutes (TEM)

Evaluation criteria for all patients including all treatments:

1. Plot % of treatments with $P + \geq P$: P = % intratumoral temperature points $\geq$ 43°C
2. Plot % treatments with $P \geq$ HEP
3. Plot temperature points $\geq T$index for best 20% of patients and subsequently for next best 20%, etc.
4. Plot % temperature points $\geq T$index for Tav., Tmin, Tmax for all treatments
5. Plot % time interval at steady state with Tindex $\geq$ 43°C

essential evaluation criteria for phase 0 testing. Clinical researchers must agree on careful criteria to justify patient accrual for further phase 1–3 testing, which are similar to those for drug testing.

40.7.2 *Phase 1 Trial: Treatment Toxicity and Clinical Feasibility*

Phase 1 studies are designed to determine clinical feasibility with respect to toxicity and general mode of action induced by a specific treatment. The specific technical or clinical approach is tested under predefined protocol conditions. Similar to drug testing, phase 1 HT studies involve the use of heat in a time-temperature-dose escalation to determine the "dose"-dependent toxicity to critical organs and cytotoxic effects on malignant tissues. Side-effects are evaluated as heat damage and possible enhancement of toxicity, when combined with other modalities. Other than a small amount of information on the effect of time-temperature exposure on skin and brain matter, there is still a lack of genuine phase 1 trials, and in the past phase 1 trials have often been diluted by components of phase 2 testing. Usually phase 1 studies have been performed in patients with advanced disease outside the range of conventional therapy.

In most instances phase 1 trials have been conducted as intrainstitutional studies, but we recommend abandoning this policy and searching for fellow investigators from different institutions. Interinstitutional studies would help to avoid personal bias when analyzing initial results and ensure beneficial outside criticism; this in turn might speed up and broaden technical and clinical experience and prepare the scientific infrastructure to proceed to phase 2–3 trials. Essential features of cooperation between participating institutions are: identical technical and clinical standards, identical patient and tumor eligibility criteria, and a homogeneous treatment performance profile. Also standardized reporting should be implemented in all participating institutions (SAPARETO and CORRY 1989).

40.7.3 Phase 2 Trial: Tumor Suitability and Clinical Efficacy

Phase 2 trials aim to identify tumors suitable for the investigational treatment approach. With an optimized HT device (as a result of phase 0 testing) and known tissue toxicity limits (as a result of phase 1 testing), investigators have to identify therapeutic efficacy under predefined treatment conditions. Unfortunately in the past many phase 2 trials have applied fixed sequencing and time-temperature schedules without any prior attempt to define the optimal HT-RT regimen (in terms of sequencing and time-temperature schedule) or sufficient knowledge of the tolerated "maximum dose." As several parameters such as extent of prior treatment, anatomical site, histology, and volume of the tumor may all influence therapeutic efficacy, phase 2 trials have to be conducted in a precisely defined patient population using clinically relevant treatment endpoints and a standardized data reporting scheme.

Most former and current HT trials have been conducted on a so-called phase 2 level, but often they contained phase 1 study components; many of these trials have been severely flawed by insufficient heat application (PEREZ et al. 1989). Therefore we recommend that phase 2 studies be conducted only in a cooperative group with ongoing multicenter experience and institutionalized QA mechanism. Ongoing efforts are mandatory to optimize the safety and efficacy of a specific HT device and a specific clinical approach. Institutions which are new participants in multicenter studies need to be carefully monitored and have to adopt the same QA standards as all other institutions. We believe that this restriction is the only way to avoid a broad variety of treatment performance profiles. The ultimate goal of phase 2 testing is to show unequivocally positive results together with optimized technical and clinical performance to justify final phase 3 testing within an established cooperative group.

40.7.4 Phase 3 Trial: Randomized Comparison

Phase 3 studies are controlled clinical trials which are designed to ascertain improved efficacy of an investigational over the standard therapy. The new approach could result in a higher tumor response but equal morbidity or an equal tumor response but lower morbidity or both improved tumor response *and* reduced toxicity. The most comprehensive and clinically meaningful design for such a trial entails comparison of the best standard of RT for a tumor with combined HT-RT using the identical RT regimen. Patients are allocated to each treatment arm on a randomized basis. Strict technical and clinical QA criteria for the investigational HT treatment (HAND et al. 1989; EMAMI et al. 1991) and standardized data reporting (SAPARETO and CORRY 1989) are essential for phase 3 trials. This type of study also evaluates the outcome of the new treatment relative to the natural history of the disease, i.e., whether HT reduces treatment morbidity or improves local tumor control and subsequently long-term survival in patients with the specific tumor site and tumor type in question.

Phase 3 trials ultimately evaluate and summarize all biological technical, and preliminary clinical research in prior phase 0 to phase 2 testing. Therefore the design and conduct of these studies demand extreme care and include the following requirements:

1. Validity of the clinical question
2. Suitability of the HT device in terms of the desired performance characteristics
3. Sound biological basis for the chosen treatment regimen
4. Randomized or prospectively controlled trial design
5. Independent reference centers counseled for technical, clinical, and statistical study components
6. Periodic study review kept strictly within the multicenter group until a final group report has been issued
7. Definition of all exclusion criteria and reasons for premature termination of a phase 3 trial.

Obviously, only institutions which have already adopted equal treatment standards could scientifically conduct phase 3 testing.

Within the medical community flawed phase 3 trials have negative implications for further acceptance of a new treatment like HT. Hence efforts are necessary to initiate such a study only after stepwise phase 0 (equipment performance), phase 1 (treatment toxicity), and phase 2 (tumor suitability) testing with optimized technique and clinical approach. Prematurely initiated phase 3 trials conducted without technical sophistication and clinical optimization have failed to prove an advantage for combined HT-RT versus standard RT (PEREZ et al. 1989, 1991). This may be attributed to poor HT equipment, suboptimal clinical approach, and lack of QA, but lack of success cannot be simply related to thermal inefficacy; only if an *optimized investigative approach* fails to prove a significant difference compared to standard treatment would such a conclusion be justified.

40.8 Prognostic Parameters and Stratification

Several reviews have analyzed prognostic factors in trials involving external HT-RT (ARCANGELI et al. 1988; VALDAGNI et al. 1988; OVERGAARD 1989) and interstitial HT-RT (SEEGENSCHMIEDT and SAUER 1992). As pointed out earlier, in designing clinical HT-RT trials it is important first to identify all significant patient, tumor, and treatment parameters that may influence the outcome and secondly to stratify these parameters in phase 2–3 trials.

Stratification criteria are established prior to the enrollment of patients into a specific study: one also needs to adjust stratification to the specific study level and the scientific questions to be answered. The most decisive stratification needs to be made on the phase 0 level when inquiring into technical feasibility, i.e., differentiation between sufficient and insufficient heating of a specific tumor with a specific HT device. Previous phase 2–3 trials have randomized patients between standard RT and combined HT-RT without prior assessment of technical feasibility. As pointed out earlier, this approach may be completely flawed for HT. John Strohbehn, in his key address to the 9th ICRR in Toronto in 1991, proposed that *all* patients first be enrolled for a test heating of short duration to determine whether or not a satisfactory thermal performance can be produced based on HEP rating analysis; the results could be used to prospectively segregate patients who have an HEP rating $\geq 75\%$ as eligible for an HT-RT trial, whereas all other patients (i.e., those with an HEP rating $< 75\%$) would not qualify for the trial. To avoid ethical and clinical questions involved with such a study design, an alternative approach would be to prospectively divide the patients into three or more subgroups based on their initial HEP rating and to randomize between RT alone and RT-HT in each subgroup. This would help to determine the HEP rating required to produce a therapeutically significant difference.

In summary, we advocate that the technical feasibility of sufficiently heating a specific tumor volume (phase 0 testing) be considered the most important stratification criterion in all HT-RT trials (STROHBEHN 1991). Improved HT devices may not require this stratification in the future, so that one could directly start with phase 1–3 testing.

40.9 Evaluation of Results and Treatment Endpoints

In order to establish the credibility of HT-RT, investigators have to objectively demonstrate significant advances compared to the best standard RT. Therefore the endpoints of the study have to be prospectively defined. Radiobiological studies evaluate response to an experimental treatment by comparing the damage to the most resistant tumor cell population with that to the most sensitive (critical) normal tissues. In most clinical studies the WHO criteria (World Health Organization 1979) are used to determine tumor and normal tissue response. The same concept of complete disappearance (i.e., control) of tumors has been applied as an endpoint in most HT-RT studies dealing with palliation of locally advanced malignancies (KAPP 1986). Sufficient observation time allows the evaluation of response duration and likelihood of locoregional relapse. However, several additional aspects are involved in HT-RT trials which complicate the evaluation of treatment results, e.g., marked variations in respect of prior treatment, tumor volume, involved sites, and subjective impairment and reduced quality of life due to symptoms (pain, bleeding, infection, etc.). Important criteria for the evaluation of the objective and subjective response to curative/palliative HT-RT are summarized in Table 40.3.

40.9.1 Tumor Response and Local Control

Unfortunately, determination of tumor response to a specific treatment usually relies only upon assess-

Table 40.3. Criteria for evaluation of response in hyperthermia clinical trials (modified from NIELSEN et al. 1992)

Tumor response:
1. WHO criteria: complete response (CR), partial response (PR), no change (NC), progression of disease (PD), locoregional recurrence (REC)
2. Tumor growth delay, freedom from progression, time to relapse
3. Duration of local response; local tumor control

Normal tissue response:
1. General and organ-specific acute and late treatment toxicity
2. Radiation-induced toxicity versus hyperthermia-induced toxicity
3. Duration of recovery/healing

Survival analysis:
1. Overall (actuarial) survival, median survival
2. Disease-free survival and relapse-free survival
3. Symptom-free survival (palliative trials)

Assessment of symptoms:
1. Linear analogue self-assessment (LASA) using analogue scales
2. Scoring systems for different symptoms, like pain, hemorrhage, neurological deficit etc. using categorical scales
3. Change of analgesic drug medication or other medical requirements

Quality of life:
1. Karnofsky performance scale (KPS), WHO performance grading
2. Measures of functional and emotional status, e.g., EORTC scales for functional status/psychological distress, sickness impact profile (SIP)
3. Measures for general and treatment specific symptoms, e.g., functional living index cancer (FLIC), EORTC scale for lung and other sites

ment of tumor dimension changes, which are observed either clinically (superficial sites) or by means of imaging techniques (deep-seated sites). However, changes in tumor size may be misleading and unrepresentative for overall tumor control and individual therapeutic gain. This can be illustrated with three examples:

1. HT treatments can induce slow "persistent tumor regression" often leaving a small residual tumor mass which remains stable in size and appearance for months and sometimes years. If surgically excised, such a remaining mass often demonstrates no viable or encapsulated noninfiltrating tumor cells.

2. Clinical response may demonstrate "objective" tumor disappearance with respect to all radiological or clinical examinations. However, this finding is rarely confirmed by biopsies; subsequently such a lesion may develop a locoregional relapse within a short follow-up period.

3. Persistent tumor masses could be judged by their time interval to renewed progression (i.e., freedom from progression; growth delay); this measurement is not often used, but it could also provide useful information on local tumor control.

In all instances the questions to be considered are: What is the initial tumor response and at which level is it possible to define "local tumor control"?

Tumor growth delay may be a useful parameter when comparing different treatment schedules (e.g., one vs two HT treatments per week), but not when combining HT with RT due to the variety of additional normal and tumor tissue effects involved in the response pattern (TAIT and CARNOCHAN 1987).

Locoregional tumor control – the total and permanent disappearance of the disease from the primary site – is a major goal of many oncology strategies. This term, however, has been variably interpreted and differently formulated, such as "local control with a specific minimum follow-up," "nonfailure rate," or "initial local control rate." Perhaps the most acceptable methods of calculating local control rates are the Cutler–Ederer life-table and Kaplan–Meier product-limit methods, in which recurrence-free patients with short follow-up times are censored from the analysis at the date of last follow-up or intercurrent death (PARSONS et al. 1990). However, most patients who are submitted to HT-RT trials are treated for various palliative reasons and have only a limited survival probability; thus only the small subset of primary advanced tumors can be properly evaluated and compared to standard treatment results according to life-table analysis. For palliation evaluation of "local control" is somewhat questionable, and it would be better to introduce different palliative scores depending upon the scientific question and the specific response (NIELSEN et al. 1992).

40.9.2 Thermal Enhancement Ratio and Therapeutic Gain Factor

The efficacy of HT-RT can be reported as the thermal enhancement ratio (TER), which is defined as follows:

$$\text{TER} = \frac{\text{radiation dose alone to achieve a defined endpoint}}{\text{radiation dose with heat to achieve the same endpoint}}\,.$$

For example, one can compare the RT dose necessary to achieve a 50% response with the RT dose required in combination with HT to achieve the same endpoint. TER values are usually based on experiments and *isoeffect* calculation, but in most clinical studies they are reported on the basis of *isodose* levels, i.e., as the ratio of frequency of response after HT-RT to frequency of response after RT alone. However, it should be noted that isodose TER values are frequently greater than those obtained using isoeffect analysis (Overgaard 1989). In general, the isodose TER description is less useful because it depends on too many other tumor and treatment factors which are independent of the additional effect of HT, e.g., the steepness of the dose–response curve and the response to RT alone. Isoeffect TER data are normally used to analyze the mechanisms of combined HT-RT treatment, whereas isodose TER data can be applied to evaluate the clinical gain as long as no additional enhancement of normal tissue effects is observed in the combined HT-RT treatment schedule. Protocols designed to randomize to two or more radiation or thermal dose levels in two different arms of a study would allow estimation of both the tumor and the normal tissue isoeffect (Overgaard 1989).

In animal models and some clinical trials another parameter has been derived from tumor and normal tissue isoeffect TER values, which has been described as the therapeutic gain factor (TGF):

$$\text{TGF} = \frac{\text{isoeffect TER for tumor tissue}}{\text{isoeffect TER for normal tissue}}\,.$$

Therapeutic gain is measured by generating radiation dose–response curves with (HT-RT) and without (RT alone) heat for tumor and normal tissue. A $\text{TGF} > 1$ would imply that heat enhancement of radiation effect is greater in tumor than in normal tissue. One important aspect to be included in TGF analysis would be the time of response assessment, which could reveal different results reflective of either early or late effects. Future HT-RT studies will only demonstrate a therapeutic gain in potentially curable lesions if patients are randomized to receive the best conventional RT with or without HT. A therapeutic gain will be observed if increased tumor control occurs parallel with reduced normal tissue complications. Similarly, the relative increase in a specific tumor or normal tissue effect with constant RT dose and adjuvant HT has been described as the relative risk factor, the probability of a specific effect being evaluated by reference to the ratio of the incidence of the effect following HT-RT to its incidence following RT alone (Dewhirst et al. 1983). Hence all future HT-RT trials must generate as much normal tissue data as tumor data. This requires exact assessment and use of differentiated scoring systems for all relevant tumor and normal tissue types.

40.9.3 *Survival Analysis*

Improved local tumor control can result in prolonged survival. Survival is used as the treatment endpoint as long as a patient does not develop regional relapse or distant metastases; regional or distant failures necessitate modified reporting by use of the terms "duration of local control," "overall survival," and/or "relapse-free survival." Trials involving palliative patient care can use the description "symptom-free survival." Accepted methods of calculating survival plots are the Cutler–Ederer life-table and Kaplan–Meier product-limit methods in which, as mentioned above, patients with short follow-up are censored from the analysis at the last follow-up date or at intercurrent death (Parsons et al. 1990). Since in the past most patients have been treated for palliative reasons, survival data were never remarkable, and only patients with primary tumors can be expected to be properly evaluated.

40.9.4 *Palliative Response*

The use of "partial response" or "overall response" (complete plus partial response) is usually not recommended, because it has no radiobiological implication or may even inappropriately suggest "positive" results in a specific curative or palliative situation. Endpoints should be included that permit a more precise description and evaluation of palliative effects (Kaheki et al. 1990; Nielsen et al. 1992). A higher partial response rate using combined HT-RT compared to RT alone should never be extrapolated into the assumption that this approach may offer better palliation. The concept of palliative treatment implies alleviation of distress caused by a variety of symptoms; subjective impairment by symptoms may be completely unrelated to the actual tumor size or other objectively assessed parameters. Various potentially useful methods for the evaluation of palliative response have been described (DONOVAN et al. 1989), but so far no validated scoring systems have been applied in HT-RT clinical trials.

40.9.5 Normal Tissue Toxicity

Combined effects of HT-RT on normal tissue are assessed as early and late damage by using the WHO toxicity scores. If possible, RT-related and specific HT-induced complications are distinguished, such as burns or rapid necrosis. Heat- and radiation-induced damage cannot be described by the same toxicity parameters because they may occur at different intervals after treatment initiation and in different treatment areas or even outside them. Hence the conventional RT toxicity scoring system may not be applicable to HT-induced normal tissue damage.

Only a few studies have aimed to specifically address toxicity for different tissue types when comparing combined HT-RT and RT alone. In most studies, toxicity has just been mentioned as a percentage range without reflection on possible prerequisites or a specific description of the time and conditions of occurrence. So far maximum temperatures have been reported to correlate with heat-induced toxicity (VALDAGNI et al. 1988). Very few data are available on long-term toxicity and unusual side-effects, which should be more precisely monitored than in the past.

40.10 Clinical Trials Using Interstitial and Intracavitary Hyperthermia

40.10.1 Treatment Indications

The clinical rationale for present and future interstitial/intracavitary HT-RT (IHT-IRT) is based on the same principles as outlined previously for all other HT-RT trials, i.e., insufficiency of the results achieved with standard therapy. The four major indications for IHT-IRT are: (a) an improvement of local tumor control can be expected; (b) retreatment of recurrent and previously irradiated tumors becomes possible; (c) limited metastatic disease can be locally controlled; and (d) treatment toxicity can be reduced. Under the condition that the invasive nature of the planned brachytherapy procedure is appropriate to the nature and extent of the disease to be treated, improved locoregional therapy could increase relapse-free and disease-free survival and prevent a major portion of cancer deaths (KAPP 1986; OVERGAARD 1989). Lack of tumor control when using RT alone implies that complete tumor inactivation cannot be obtained without increasing the RT dose to a level which will damage normal structures in an unacceptable manner unless sensitizers like IHT are employed to enhance the response.

The use of IHT-IRT offers intrinsic advantages which allow application of this treatment combination for localized lesions not only as a "boost therapy" but also as the single treatment strategy. These advantages are: (a) deposition of a well-localized and high IRT-IHT tumor "dose"; (b) improved sparing of normal tissues and increased TGF; (c) individualized deposition of the RT dose, e.g., by differential unloading of radioactive sources, and of the HT "dose" by individual power steering of the heat sources; and (d) the possibility of extensive thermometry data sampling resulting in improved treatment performance. As a consequence, phase 1–2 clinical trials have already demonstrated a significant improvement in tumor response; thus not only recurrent or metastatic lesions but also advanced primary tumors can be considered for IHT-IRT trials.

Among patients with malignant tumors, locoregional relapse is just as predominant (68% dead with disease) as distant metastasis and a large proportion of the patients (50%) have *both* locoregional recurrence *and* distant metastasis (American Cancer Society 1991). Elimination of locoregional failure could increase survival in numerous malignancies, which can be approached by either interstitial or intracavitary methods. Long-term disease-free survival after locoregional salvage or improved primary therapy can be regarded as proof that better management of the primary lesions results in higher survival rates, because in various of these tumors a correlation can be found between incidence of local failure and distant metastases (SUIT and WESTGATE 1986).

40.10.2 Tumors and Treatment Sites

Present limitations on effective heating of deep-seated tumors leave us with two options for IHT-IRT trials. Patients with accessible and confined medium depth or superficial tumors (ARCANGELI et al. 1988); for which IHT-IRT can be used either (a) as an adjuvant treatment to standard RT management in the primary treatment of advanced or persistent tumors, or (b) in the palliative management of recurrent and metastatic tumors.

There are numerous malignancies which can be approached either by interstitial (tumors of the brain and CNS, oral cavity and oropharynx, breast, skin, lung, ovaries, uterine corpus and cervix, prostate) or intracavitary methods (esophageal, bronchial, bile duct, deep colorectal, cervical, urethral, vaginal, and prostate tumors). For trials involving IHT-IRT in the past, the preferred sites have been located in the head and neck, intact breast, chest wall, and pelvic region, largely owing to the longstanding clinical tradition of brachytherapy in these sites. A literature review demonstrates that 36% of all interstitial HT-RT applications have been performed in the head and neck region for base of tongue, floor of mouth, and oropharyngeal carcinomas, and that, likewise, 36% have been carried out in the pelvis for various gynecological (cervix and corpus uteri, vagina, ovaries) and colorectal tumors. Together with chest wall and breast (14%), these sites account for about 85% of all treatment sites (Table 40.4).

As shown in Chaps. 23 and 24 of this volume, the results obtained in historical trials have been remarkable despite the fact that they have been achieved with large variations among the treated lesions and applied HT-RT schedules and with nonoptimized heating technologies. Trials in which site-specific results have been summarized are presented in a literature review (Table 40.5). Obviously, in previous studies breast and chest wall lesions (72% CR rate) and head and neck lesions (69%) achieved better response rates than pelvic and other lesions. As pelvic lesions are more difficult to reach and implant, these results may reflect the technical inability of the applied HT technology to achieve a satisfactory heating performance. Moreover, these high CR rates have to be treated with caution, as similar response rates have been reported with interstitial RT alone. To prove that therapeutic enhancement is brought about by the addition of interstitial HT, the results need to be confirmed in future prospectively randomized phase 2–phase 3 trials, controlling and stratifying all previously established prognostic pretreatment and treatment parameters.

40.10.3 Treatment Stratification

As pointed out earlier, the technical feasibility of adequately heating a specific tumor volume (phase 0 testing) is currently the most important stratification criterion required for all future HT-RT trials (STROHBEHN 1991) including internal heating technologies, although improved HT devices may render this stratification unnecessary in the future. Moreover, all patient- and tumor-related prognostic factors which have been determined in early clinical phase 1–2 testing have to be considered for stratification in controlled phase 3 trials. A brief overview of the prognostic factors identified in previously conducted trials is given in Table 40.6.

Depending upon the specific tumor site, tumor type, treatment technique, and IHT-IRT treatment

Table 40.4. Survey on body sites treated in trials using interstitial thermo-radiotherapy (HT-RT) (modified from SEEGENSCHMIEDT and SAUER 1992)

Authors	Year	Breast	Head and neck	Pelvis, gynecological	Pelvis, colorectal	Skin	Other sites	Total
SURWIT et al.	1983	–	–	21	–	–	–	21
ARISTIZABAL and OLESON	1984	2	9	36	9	–	8	64
COSSET et al.	1985	11	9	1	–	6	2	29
PUTHAWALA et al.	1985	8	20	9	4	–	2	43
EMAMI et al.	1987	6	29	4	3	–	6	48
RAFLA et al.	1989	6	15	8	6	–	–	35
PETROVICH et al.	1989	9	23	4	–	4	4	44
GAUTHERIE et al.	1989	14	35	23	16	–	8	96
VORA et al.	1989	24	9	20	18	5	5	81
COUGHLIN et al.	1991	–	9	12	–	6	41	68
SEEGENSCHMIEDT et al.	1992	2	62	14	9	–	3	90
Total experience		82 (14%)	220 (36%)	152 (25%)	65 (11%)	21 (3%)	79 (13%)	619 (100%)

Table 40.5. Site-specific results in trials using interstitial thermo-radiotherapy (HT-RT)

Author, year	HT technique (type/frequency)	Total no. of patients	Tumor site (no. of CRs/total pts.)			
			Head and neck	Pelvis	Breast and chest wall	Others
SURWIT et al. 1983	RF – 0.5 MHz	21	–	7/21 (33%)	–	–
PUTHAWALA et al. 1985	MW – 915 MHz	43	15/20 (75%)	10/13 (77%)	5/8 (63%)	2/2 (100%)
VORA et al. 1989	RF – 0.5 MHz	19	–	10/19 (53%)	–	–
GAUTHERIE et al. 1989	MW – 915 MHz	96	24/35 (69%)	23/39 (59%)	11/14 (79%)	3/8 (39%)
RAFLA et al. 1989	MW – 915 MHz	35	8/15 (53%)	8/14 (57%)	3/6 (50%)	–
PETROVICH et al. 1989	MW – 915, 630 MHz	44	16/23 (70%)	3/4 (75%)	7/9 (78%)	2/8 (25%)
GOFFINET et al. 1990	RF – 0.5 MHz	10	5/5 (100%)	3/5 (60%)	–	–
SEEGENSCHMIEDT et al. 1992	MW – 915 MHz	90	39/62 (63%)	17/26 (65%)	2/2 (100%)	–
Summary results[a]		358	107/160 (69%)	81/141 (57%)	28/39 (72%)	7/18 (39%)

MW, microwave; RF, radiofrequency; CR, complete response
[a] Data from ARISTIZABAL and OLESON 1984, COSSET et al. 1985, EMAMI et al. 1987, VORA et al. 1989, and COUGLIN et al. 1991 provide no site specific results and have not been included in this summary

Table 40.6. Survey on prognostic parameters in trials using interstitial thermo-radiotherapy (HT-RT)

Authors	Year	Tumor class	Radiation dose	Tumor volume	Minimum temperature	Other thermal factors	Others
ARISTIZABAL and OLESON	1984	NA	+	+	+	*T*max+	NA
COSSET et al.	1985	NA	+	+	+	Satisfactory "heating"	Relapse+
PUTHAWALA et al.	1985	NA	NA	NA	NA	NA	Site–
EMAMI et al.	1987	NA	NA	+	+	% > 42°c	CR+
PETROVICH et al.	1989	NA	–	+	–	TEM– *T*max+	Site– CR–
GAUTHERIE et al.	1989	NA	NA	NA	NA	% > 42°C	Burns–
VORA et al.	1989	+	–	NA	–	NA	NA
COUGHLIN et al.	1991	NA	+	+	+	HEP rating	–
SEEGENSCHMIEDT et al.	1992	+	+	+	+	% TQ 41°C+ *T*max+	CR+ Relapse+

NA, not available; TEM, thermal equivalent minutes; HEP, hyperthermia equipment performance; CR, complete response
+ = prognostic impact of parameter; – = no prognostic impact of parameter

schedule, the following prognostic factors have been identified in previously conducted IHT-IRT studies:

1. Tumor histology, localization, and volume
2. Tumor type or classification, such as primary advanced, primary persistent, recurrent, or metastatic lesion
3. General patient performance criteria such as Karnofsky Performance Score and extent of metastatic burden
4. Previous disease history and extent of previous treatment approaches
5. RT dose treatment parameters
6. HT thermal performance characteristics such as minimum tumor temperature, % temperatures ≥ index temperature, thermal quality (TQ), and thermal equivalent minutes (TEM)

To answer the scientific questions posed by clinical HT-RT trials precisely and rigorously, on the one hand a sufficient number of patients and tumors need to be entered, but on the other hand sufficient homogeneity in as many aspects as possible is required, with only a few factors to be stratified; this can be achieved by applying tight eligibility criteria.

40.10.4 Treatment Techniques

Clinical data using interstitial HT-RT have shown excellent results compared to trials which have employed external HT techniques; besides different modes of heat induction, several interstitial and intracavitary HT technologies have to be distinguished: the available HT technologies which have been broadly applied in clinical practice have been extensively reviewed in previous chapters of this volume (Chaps. 23–26). As previously shown, differences in tumor response depend strongly on the ability to sufficiently heat a specified target volume, but may also be attributed to radiobiological differences of thermal radiosensitization induced by the different treatment schemes: short-term or long-duration continuous HT applied in conjunction with fractionated external beam RT, or short-term high dose rate (HDR), long-term low dose rate (LDR), or pulsed HDR brachytherapy. The chosen or institutionally established brachytherapy technique will always limit the range of available IHT technologies, as none of the IHT technologies can be combined with all of the IRT techniques.

Moreover, the choice of an adequate heating device for a particular lesion must be based on several factors, including tumor dimension and location, specific tissue properties and perfusion characteristics, and possible implant configurations (spacing between heating sources, template versus free-hand implant, flexible plastic versus rigid metal implants, etc.). Although further technical progress can be expected, the current clinical and technical ITH practice can be summarized as follows:

1. *Radiofrequency (RF) techniques* are useful for tumors which are implanted with an array of parallel, equidistant needles that are of equal active heating length (template technique). Applications in the pelvis for gynecological and colorectal tumors are most appropriate. RF techniques can also be used for certain breast and chest wall, head and neck, and extremity tumors as well as intraoperatively for abdominal and pelvic tumors.

2. *Mircrowave (MW) techniques* are mandatory for applications which require nonparallel or flexible implants (free-hand implants, looping tech-

Table 40.7. Survey on potential clinical trials using interstitial thermoradiotherapy (HT-RT)

Tumor site	Tumor type	Trial design	RT prescription	HT technique[a]
Base of tongue Floor of mouth	T3-T4 advanced primary/persistent	Randomized Phase 2–phase 3	Full dose external plus "interstitial RT boost"	(1) MW - 915 MHz [2] RF - 27 MHz [3] HS - HWP/FMS
Base of tongue Floor of mouth	Any T with prior RT recurrent/metastatic	Nonrandomized Phase 0–phase 1	Interstitial RT alone up to tolerance level	(1) New technologies: HS-HWP/FMS; US [2] New fractinations[b]
Brain	Grade 3-4 primary astrocytoma	Randomized Phase 2–phase 3	Full dose external plus "interstitial RT boost"	(1) MW - 915 MHz [2] HS–HWP/FMS resistive wires [3] RF - 27 MHz
Brain	Any grade/prior RT recurrent astrocytoma	Nonrandomized Phase 0–phase 1	Interstitial RT alone up to tolerance level	(1) New technologies [2] New fractionations[b]
Cervix/corpus uteri	T2-T3 advanced primary/persistent	Randomized Phase 2–phase 3	Full dose external plus "interstitial RT boost"	(1) RF–LCF 0.5 MHz RF - 27 MHz (2) HS–HWP/FMS [3] MW - 915/434 MHz
	Any T/prior RT recurrent/metastatic	Nonrandomized Phase 0–phase 1	Interstitial RT alone up to tolerance level	(1) New technologies (2) New fractionations[b]
Prostate	Large B2/C advanced primary/persistent	Randomized Phase 1–phase 3	Full dose external plus "Interstitial RT boost"	(1) RF–LCF 0.5 MHz RF - 27 MHz (2) HS–HWP/FMS [3] MW - 915/434 MHz
	Any localized tumor recurrent/metastatic	Nonradomized Phase 0–phase 1	Interstitial RT alone up to tolerance level	(1) New technologies (2) New fractionations[b]

MW, microwave; RF, radiofrequency; HS, hot source; HWP, hot water perfusion; FMS, ferromagnetic seeds; US, ultrasound; RT, radiotherapy; HT, hyperthermia

[a] Techniques of choice are indicated by parentheses, and other available techniques by brackets

[b] Simultaneous high temperature HT and/or continuous moderate temperature

niques, etc.) and in tissues with high blood perfusion. This includes head and neck, brain, and some pelvic and extremity lesions. For lesions which require heat localization at depth only those antennas should be employed which prevent energy deposition along the feeding line and overheating of the surface (e.g., choke design).

3. *Ferromagnetic seed (FMS) techniques* allow clinical treatments with few or no invasive thermometry measurements. They are recommended for lesions which need a high degree of localization and few externalized connections. This is useful in situations where high precision implants can be achieved during surgery, as for thoracic, abdominal, and intracranial tumors. Applications in the brain or prostate now appear clinically feasible. However, for this technique very close spacing and parallel orientation of FMS are mandatory.

4. *Hot water perfusion (HWP) techniques* can be applied similarly to FMS techniques, but they are more restricted owing to the external connection requirements; thus localized deep heating may not be possible. Although applications in many body sites, including the brain and eye, have been reported, no exclusive applications of these thermal conduction techniques have been demonstrated.

5. *New heating technologies (e.g., ultrasound and laser HT)* have to be tested in phase 0–phase 1 trials to demonstrate technical feasibility. It should be possible to use multielement ultrasound tubular transducers to heat esophageal, bronchial, vaginal, and colorectal tumors in conjunction with intracavitary radiotherapy.

In summary, some investigators favor interstitial MW techniques owing to their radiative features, while others prefer interstitial RF techniques owing to the smaller variability of heating along applicators and in complex implants. The specific advantages and disadvantages of each interstitial HT technique have been summarized previously (SEEGENSCHMIEDT and SAUER 1992). In addition, the principal technical data have been compiled and matched with potential clinical trials using interstitial (Table 40.7) or intracavitary HT techniques (Table 40.8). This overview can be used as an agenda and general guide for future clinical trials.

Table 40.8. Survey on potential clinical trials using intracavitary thermoradiotherapy (HT-RT)

Tumor site	Tumor type	Trial design	RT prescription	HT technique[a]
Esophagus	T2-T3 advanced Primary/persistent Nonresectable	Randomized Phase 2–phase 3	Full dose external plus intracavitary RT (± chemotherapy)	(1) MW – 915 MHz (2) RF – 27 MHz [3] US–0.5–5.0 MHz
	Any T with prior RT recurrent/metastatic	Nonrandomized Phase 0–phase 1	Intracavitary RT alone (± chemotherapy)	(1) New technologies: US, laser, HWP (2) New fractionations[b]
Bronchus	T2-T3 advanced Primary/persistent Nonresectable	Nonrandomized Phase 0–phase 1	Full dose external plus intracavitary RT (± chemotherapy)	*New technologies:* (1) MW – 915 MHz (2) RF – 27 MHz
Bile duct	T2-T3 advanced Primary/persistent Nonresectable	Nonrandomized Phase 0–phase 1	Full dose external plus intracavitary RT	[3] US–0.5–5.0 MHz [4] Laser HT [5] HS–HWP
Vagina	T2-T3 advanced Primary/persistent Nonresectable	Nonrandomized Phase 0–phase 1	Full dose external plus intracavitary RT	*New fractionations:* (1) Simultaneous high temperature HT
Urethra	T2-T3 advanced Primary/persistent Nonresectable	Nonrandomized Phase 0–phase 1	Full dose external plus intracavitary RT	(2) Continuous moderate temperature HT
Anal canal Lower colorectum	T2-T3 advanced Primary/persistent Nonresectable	Nonrandomized Phase 0–phase 1	Full dose external plus intracavitary RT	

MW, microwave; RF, radiofrequency; HS, hot source; HWP, hot water perfusion; FMS, ferromagnetic seeds; US, ultrasound; RT, radiotherapy; HT, hyperthermia

[a] Techniques of choice are indicated by parentheses, and other techniques by brackets

[b] Simultaneous high temperature HT and/or continuous moderate temperature HT

Two other new internal HT approaches have not been addressed in the aforementioned tables: (a) intraoperative HT techniques combined with intraoperative RT for a variety of abdominal tumors, and (b) perfusional HT techniques in conjunction with radio-chemotherapy for tumors of the extremities, localized single liver metastases, or other well-localized organ metastases which can be reached by intra-arterial infusion. With respect to intraoperative interstitial HT-RT (IOHT-RT), two different approaches can be chosen: (a) implementation of IOHT-RT directly during the surgical procedure using different interstitial or external HT techniques, or (b) operative implantation of various materials (e.g., plastic tubes for afterloading, ferromagnetic seeds etc.) to be secondarily activated with radioactive sources and heating devices. The first clinical experience, using the second approach was reported in a small series of 12 patients presenting with thoracic or abdominal tumors which were found to be unresectable at surgery (Frazier and Corry 1984). Other preliminary results of phase 1 clinical studies from Dartmouth and Washington DC have applied various interstitial and external HT techniques with microwave and ultrasound devices and have yielded quite encouraging results (Goldson et al. 1987; Colacchio et al. 1990). In summary, by using an intraoperative approach, various abdominal tumors, including pancreatic, gastric, and small and large bowel malignancies, can be added to the broad spectrum of clinical sites for potential future studies.

40.10.5 Treatment Schedule

In past trials involving IHT-IRT the most significant differences have been related to the "treatment schedule," which comprises all details of the two involved treatment modalities, namely RT and HT. Obviously there has been a lot more information provided for the HT treatment regimen than for the RT regimen. The available data on treatment schedules are very confusing and have differed from institution to institution and even within the same clinic. Thus the following aspects have to be precisely defined in future trials: (a) accepted "treatment temperature," (b) optimal duration of the HT treatment, (c) optimal number of heat treatments, (d) use of external or interstitial HT techniques, (e) sequencing of HT and RT, and (f) optimal RT treatment including single and total RT dose, RT fractionation scheme, and external or interstitial mode of RT application. Most of these factors are not independent variables of a specific treatment schedule.

Treatment Temperature. General agreement exists that the whole time-temperature matrix has to be documented during HT, including definition of the spatial distribution of all assessed thermometry points. In sect. 40.7.1 we have already defined the initial goals of a phase 0 trial and the specific thermal performance conditions which should be attained in further phase 1–3 studies: (a) the percentage of tumor temperature points $\geq 43°C$ for all treatments is $\geq 75\%$; (b) the percentage of treatments with $\geq 75\%$ of intratumoral temperature points $\geq 43°C$ is $\geq 50\%$; and (c) the percentage of treatments with an HEP rating $> 75\%$ is $\geq 20\%$ (Strohbehn 1991) (Table 40.1). In addition, acceptable minimum, "mean" and maximum temperatures should be described in the protocol definition of "thermal dose." Most likely the minimum temperatures will correlate with tumor response and the maximum temperatures with normal tissue toxicity. Thus the potential cold and hot spots of the treatment volume need to be controlled with optimized invasive thermometry.

Duration of Treatments. In most studies IHT treatments have been applied for approximately 1 h at steady-state temperatures of 41°–44°C. This treatment duration was chosen for practical reasons of subjective tolerance. However, interesting new treatment concepts propose the use not of high temperature 43°–44°C IHT sessions sequentially to IRT, but rather of moderate temperature 41°C IHT continuously during LDR-IRT (Garcia et al. 1992), chemotherapy (Marchosky et al. 1992), or pulsed HDR-IRT (Armour et al. 1992; Handl-Zeller and Handl 1992) in order to increase the TER and possibly also the TGF despite a considerably reduced "therapeutic temperature level." Thus in the future a variety of trials will be devoted solely to establishing the possible additional gain of long-duration IHT compared to short-term IHT.

Optimal Number of HT Treatments. At present no optimal number of IHT sessions can be cited, and the necessary number may in fact depend strongly on the quality of the IHT treatments. In many previous trials just one IHT session reaching 43°–44°C for 45–60 min prior to IRT was effective and practical, because it was closely connected to general anesthesia and the implantation procedure and not complicated by thermotolerance, as it is recommended that a second IHT should not be applied within 72 h after a prior IHT treatment. It is worthwhile to note that trials applying two IHT sessions yield no better results than those with just one IHT session. In the future the application of long-duration IHT concomitant with LDR-IRT or pulsed HDR-IRT may overcome the whole problem of sequencing and optimal number of IHT treatments.

External or Interstitial HT Combined with IRT. In the past, several approaches have been reported. The scheme "external beam RT plus interstitial HT-RT or interstitial HT alone" has been applied for primary advanced tumors which had not previously received RT. The intention was to improve conventional standard therapy with an enhanced tumor boost. On the other hand, the scheme "interstitial HT-RT without external beam RT" has been used for recurrent tumors which had already received full-dose RT, in order to improve normal tissue tolerance for a second RT course. However, for future trials the mode of HT application will be less important than the optimal thermal performance of the chosen HT technique adapted to a specific tumor and site.

Sequencing of IHT and IRT. Previous IHT-IRT trials have used different *sequential* schedules: (a) IHT plus IRT with one IHT session either before or after IRT, (b) two IHT sessions before and after IRT, (c) IHT combined with external beam RT, or (d) interstitial and external HT combined with external beam RT. However, biological data strongly suggest that sequential HT and RT act as independent modalities affecting different tumor cell populations. Therefore these schedules require a sufficient thermal performance of IHT, and the efficacy is dominated by hyperthermic cytotoxicity, although some thermal radiosensitizating activity may still persist. In vivo and in vitro studies also emphasize that simultaneous application of HT and RT maximizes the TER, whereas sequential application with an interval of more than 30 min before or after RT is much less effective (SAPARETO et al. 1978; OVERGAARD 1980, 1989). The highest TER has been observed when HT was applied during or in the middle of an IRT session; HT before IRT was less effective, but HT after IRT provided the least benefit (JONES et al. 1989). Only a few data exist on the combination of brachytherapy with long-duration moderate HT in the range of 40°–41°C (ARMOUR et al. 1992). Chapter 4 of this volume presents the initial results of in vitro experiments on the effects of long-duration moderate HT alone on the cell cycle; these results are very promising and suggest a potential benefit of such HT in combination with LDR-IRT. Very recently IHT techniques have been developed which allow delivery of truly *simultaneous* HT-RT such as hot water perfusion techniques in conjunction with HDR-IRT (HANDL-ZELLER and HANDL 1992) and a template technique with multiplexed multisegment radiofrequency HT in conjunction with LDR-IRT (CORRY et al., this volume, Chap. 41).

Optimal RT Treatment Schedule. In past IHT-IRT trials the variation in the RT doses and RT treatment schedules have been striking and confusing. However, the reasons for this variation can be better understood when consideration is given to the types of lesion being treated: (a) previously irradiated lesions could not be treated with full-dose RT and in these instances the RT dose was usually limited to 20–40 Gy applied with IRT; (b) primary advanced lesions which had not received previous RT could be treated with 50–70 Gy, with the boost dose being delivered by interstitial IHT-IRT. For future trials it is important to separate these different tumor types in precisely described RT protocols. In all of these trials RT should be carefully prescribed and the best standard of RT treatment should be chosen with or without additional IHT.

The excellent results obtained with IHT-IRT suggest the latter's potential value in the management of implantable malignancies. However, these results have to be treated with caution as almost equally good results have been achieved in similar tumor and patient groups treated with IRT alone (KAPP 1986). The potential differences need to be confirmed in randomized phase 3 trials which carefully control for pretreatment prognostic factors, conduct technical and clinical QA protocols, and adequately record thermal performance. Two randomized studies comparing IRT alone and combined IHT-IRT have already been initiated and await evaluation: the American RTOG 84-19 study and the ESHO 4-86 protocol. Further trials are mandatory, as these early studies have been performed with a lower standard of technical and clinical QA than has recently been recommended (Dewhirst et al. 1990; Emami et al. 1991).

40.11 Future Perspectives

In conclusion, although technical problems currently limit our ability to achieve optimal thermal performance in implantable tumors, many technical innovations can be expected in the near future to meet the challenges. The specific advantages and disadvantages of current IHT techniques demand careful selection of the specific technique in clinical practice. We believe that IHT-IRT is already a versatile and safe treatment modality which can be adapted to a variety of tumor sites; it is easily compatible with any standard free-hand or template or intracavitary brachytherapy technique and can be reasonably applied to nearly all malignant lesions that have been suboptimally treated in the past by standard treatment strategies: implantable locally recurrent, locally metastatic, and selected primary advanced and persistent tumors of the brain, head and neck, chest wall, abdomen, pelvis, and many other sites. Although presently the only established place for IHT-IRT is in palliative treatment of recurrent or metastatic tumors in previously irradiated areas, adjuvant implementations seem to be well justified.

Based on all the foregoing considerations, four areas of future research need to be distinguished in which clinical studies will have to focus on various technical, biological, clinical, and quality control aspects of IHT-IRT. The targets of future research include:

1. Further improvement of current interstitial and intracavitary HT techniques (e.g., individual power steering, phase shifting, or multisegment applicator design)
2. Analysis of various biological, biomolecular, and physiological effects and mechanisms involved in thermal cytotoxicity and radiosensitization of LDR-IRT versus HDR-IRT or pulsed HDR-IRT
3. Systematic assessment of TER and TGF for different treatment schedules, different metabolic situations, and different perfusion characteristics in both tumor and normal tissue
4. Improvement of invasive thermometry techniques (e.g., automatic thermal mapping) and further development of noninvasive thermometry methods (impedance tomography, microwave radiometry, nuclear magnetic resonance)
5. Clinical implementation of prospective treatment planning and thermal modelling
6. Computer software upgrading of screen and mouse-controlled menus and implementation of other user-friendly software components, e.g., integrated thermal performance analysis by various algorithms
7. Improved compatibility of treatment documentation to the HDS format (Sapareto and Corry 1989)
8. International exchange and evaluation of thermal performance data for different techniques and treatment sites, leading to the design and conduct of prospective randomized trials for specific tumor types and sites (Tables 40.7, 40.8).

Ongoing clinical research will still have to be conducted on two different levels: phase 0–1 trials will be required to test all new technical, biological, and clinical concepts, whereas phase 2–3 trials will need to be carried out to examine the possible clinical benefit of IHT in combination with the best conventional treatment strategy. All previous "phase 1–phase 2 trials" (according to drug testing definition) will either have to be terminated, when not conducted in the outlined manner, or have to be advanced to phase 2–3 trials as long as the heating performance is sufficient. Multicenter trials are an essential step towards the acceptance of IHT-IRT. Clinical issues of optimization to be resolved include:

1. Establishing dose–response curves for tumor and normal tissues
2. Optimal selection of appropriate IHT techniques for individual tumor sites
3. Optimal implantation and spacing of heating applicators
4. Possible limitation of target or tumor volume for effective IHT performance
5. Risks and benefits of additional analgesia or even general anesthesia during IHT treatments
6. Optimization of IHT-IRT treatment schedule with respect to IHT frequency (including the use of long-duration IHT) and sequencing of IHT-IRT
7. Selection of appropriate study concepts to be applied for specific tumor sites.

In the future strong emphasis will also have to be placed on QA guidelines to control the broad spectrum of possible critical treatment parameters. All these studies will provide more conclusive answers and even further ideas for broad adjuvant and palliative clinical use of IHT-IRT.

When considering the sometimes questionable efficacy and tremendous costs involved with other "new cancer drugs" and the ongoing diversification of oncological management of cancer, it can be anticipated that within the next decade further biological and physiological research, improved heating technology, and routine clinical practice will establish a clinically convincing role for IHT-IRT, at a reasonable financial cost, in the adjuvant and palliative treatment of various confined malignancies.

References

American Cancer Society (1991) American Cancer Society, Cancer facts and figures 1991

Arcangeli G, Overgaard J, Gonzalez-Gonzalez D, Shrivastava PN (1988) Hyperthermia trials. Int J Radiat Oncol Biol Phys 14: S93–S109

Aristizabal SA, Oleson JR (1984) Combined interstitial irradiation and localized current field hyperthermia: results and conclusions from clinical studies: Cancer Res [Suppl] 44: 4757s–4760s

Armour E, Wang Z, Corry PM, Martinez A (1992) Equivalence of continuous and pulse simulated low dose rate irradiation in 9L gliosarcoma cells at 37°C and 41°C. Int J Radiat Oncol Biol Phys 22: 109–114

Au KS, Cetas TC, Shimm DS et al. (1989) Interstitial ferromagnetic hyperthermia and brachytherapy: preliminary report of a phase I clinical trial. Endocurietherapy/Hyperthermia Oncol 5: 127–136

Bolomey JC, Hawley MS (1990) Noninvasive control of hyperthermia. In: Gautherie M (ed) Methods of hyperthermia control. Springer, Berlin Heidelberg New York, pp 35–111

Colacchio TA, Coughlin CT, Taylor J, Douple E, Ryan T, Crichlow RW (1990) Intraoperative radiation therapy and hyperthermia. Arch Surg 125: 370–375

Corry PM, Jabboury K, Kong JS, Armour EP, McCraw FJ, LeDuc T (1988) Evaluation of equipment for hyperthermia treatment of cancer. Int J Hyperthermia 4: 53–74

Cosset JM, Dutreix J, Haie C, Gerbaulet A, Janoray P, Dewars JA (1985) Interstitial thermoradiotherapy: a technical and clinical study of 29 implantations performed at the Institute Gustave Roussy. Int J Hyperthermia 1: 3–13

Coughlin CT, Ryan TP, Stafford JH et al. (1991) Interstitial thermoradiotherapy: the Dartmouth experience 1981–1990. In: Chapman JD, Dewey WC, Whitmore GF (eds). Radiation research: a twentieth-century perspective, vol 1. Academic, San Diego CA P31 02 WP: 386 (abstract)

Dewhirst MW, Sim DA, Wilson S, DeYoung D, Parsells JL (1983) The correlation between initial and long-term responses of pet animal tumors to heat and radiation or radiation alone. Cancer Res 43: 5735–5741

Dewhirst MW, Sim DA, Sapareto S, Connor WG (1984) Importance of minimum temperature in determining early and long-term responses of spontaneous canine and feline tumors to heat and radiation. Cancer Res 44: 43–50

Dewhirst MW, Phillips TL, Samulski TV et al. (1990) RTOG quality assurance guidelines for clinical trials using hyperthermia. Int J Radiat Oncol Biol Phys 18: 1249–1259

Donovan K, Sanson-Fisher RW, Redmans S (1989) Measuring quality of life in cancer patients. J Clin Oncol 7: 30–35

Emami B, Perez CA, Konefal J et al. (1987) Interstitial thermoradiotherapy in treatment of malignant tumors. Int J Hyperthermia 3: 107–118

Emami B, Stauffer P, Dewhirst MW et al. (1991) Quality assurancce guidelines for interstitial hyperthermia. Int J Radiat Oncol Biol Phys 20: 1117–1124

Feldmann HJ, Molls M (1991) Clinical investigations on blood flow in malignant tumors of the pelvis and the abdomen. In: Vaupel P, Jain RK (eds) Tumor blood supply and metabolic microenvironment: characterization and implications for therapy. Fischer, Stuttgart (Funktionsanalyse biologischer Systeme 20: 143–153

Frazier OH, Corry PM (1984) Induction of hyperthermia using implanted electrodes. Cancer Res [Suppl] 44: 4864s–4866s

Garcia DM, Nussbaum GH, Fathman AE, Drzymala RE, Bleyer M, DeFord JA, Welsh DM (1992) Simultaneous chronic LDR interstitial radiotherapy and conductive interstitial hyperthermia in treatment of recurrent prostatic tumors. In: Gerner EW (ed) Hyperthermic oncology, vol 1. Summary papers. Taylor & Francis, London, p 386

Gautherie M, Cosset JM, Gerard JP et al. (1989) Radiofrequency interstitial hyperthermia: a multicentric program of quality assessement and clinical trials. In: Sugahara T, Saito M (eds) Hyperthermic oncology 1988, vol 2. Taylor & Francis, London pp 711–714

Goffinet DR, Prionas SD, Kapp DS et al. (1990) Interstitial 192 iridium flexible catheter radiofrequency hyperthermia treatments of head and neck and recurrent pelvic carcinomas. Int J Radiat Oncol Biol Phys 18: 199–210

Goldson AL, Smyles JM, Ashayeri E, DeWitty R, Nibhanupudy JR, King G (1987) Simultaneous intraoperative radiation therapy and intraoperative interstitial hyperthermia for unresectable adenocarcinoma of the pancreas. Endocurietherapy/Hyperthermia Oncol 3: 201–208

Hand JW, Lagendijk JW, Bach Andersen J, Bolomey JC (1989) Quality assurance guidelines for ESHO protocols. Int J Hyperthermia 5: 421–428

Handl-Zeller L, Handl O (1992) Simultaneous application of combined interstitial high- or low-dose rate irradiation with hot water hyperthermia. In: Handl-Zeller L (ed) Interstitial hyperthermia. Springer, Wien New York, pp 165–170

Issels RD, Prenninger SW, Nagele A et al. (1990) Ifosfamide plus etoposide combined with regional hyperthermia in patients with locally advanced sarcomas: a phase II study. J Clin Oncol 8: 1818–1829

Jones EL, Lyons BE, Douple EB, Dain BJ (1989) Thermal enhancement of low dose rate irradiation in a murine tumour system. Int J Hyperthermia 5: 509–523

Kaheki M, Ueda K, Mukojima T, Hiraoka M, Seto O, Akanuma A, Nakatsugawa S (1990) Multiinstitutional clinical studies on hyperthermia combined with radiotherapy or chemotherapy in advanced cancer of deep-seated organs. Int J Hyperthermia 6: 719–740

Kapp DS (1986) Site and disease selection for hyperthermia clinical trials. Int J Hyperthermia 2: 139–156

Kapp DS, Fessenden P, Samulski TV et al. (1988) Stanford University institutional report. Phase I evaluation of equipment for hyperthermia treatment of cancer. Int J Hyperthermia 4: 75–115

Leventhal BG, Wittes RE (1988) Research methods in clinical oncology. Raven, New York

Marchosky JA, Welsh DM, Horn BA, Van Amburg AL (1992) Experience with long-duration interstitial hyperthermia and systemic BCNU in the treatment of recurrent malignant brain tumors. In: Gerner EW (ed) Hyperthermic oncology, vol 1. Summary papers. Taylor & Francis, London, p 387

Meinert CL, Tonascia S (1986) Clinical trials. Design, conduct and analysis. Monographs in epidemiology and biostatistics, vol 8. Oxford University Press, New York

Myerson RJ, Emami B, Perez CA, Straube W, Leybovich L, von Gerichten D (1992) Equilibrium temperature distributions in uniform phantoms for superficial microwave applicator: implications for temperature-based standards of applicator adequacy. Int J Hyperthermia 8: 11–21

Nielsen OS, Munro AJ, Warde PR (1992) Assessment of palliative response in hyperthermia. Int J Hyperthermia 8: 1–10

Oleson JR, Manning MR, Sim DA et al. (1984) A review of the University of Arizona human clinical hyperthermia experience. Front Radiat Ther Oncol 18: 136–143

Oleson JR, Dewhirst MW, Harrelson JM, Leopold KA, Samulski TV, Tso CY (1989) Tumor temperature distributions predict hyperthermia effect. Int J Radiat Oncol Biol Phys 10: 559–570

Overgaard J (1980) Simultaneous and sequential hyperthermia and radiation treatment of an experimental tumor and its surrounding normal tissue in vivo. Int J Radiat Oncol Biol Phys 11: 1507–1517

Overgaard J (1989) The current and potential role of hyperthermia in radiotherapy. Int J Radiat Oncol Biol Phys 16: 535–549

Parsons JT, McCarty PJ, Rao PV, Mendenhall WM, Million RR (1990) On the definition of local control. Int J Radiat Oncol Biol Phys 18: 705–706

Perez CA, Gillespie B, Pajak T, Hornback NB, Emami B, Rubin P (1989) Quality assurance problems in clinical hyperthermia and their impact on therapeutic outcome: a report by the Radiation Therapy Oncology Group. Int J Radiat Oncol Biol Phys 16: 551–558

Perez CA, Pajak T, Emami B, Hornback NB, Tupchong L, Rubin P (1991) Randomized phase III study comparing irradiation and hyperthermia with irradiation alone in superficial measurable tumors. Am J Clin Oncol 14: 133–141

Petrovich Z, Langholz B, Lam K et al. (1989) Interstitial microwave hyperthermia combined with iridium-192 radiotherapy for recurrent tumours. Am J Clin Oncol 12: 264–268

Phillips TL (1985) Clinical trials of new developments in radiation oncology. In: Veronesi U, Bonadonna G (eds) Clinical trials in cancer medicine. Academic, New York, pp 173–199

Puthawala AA, Syed AMN, Khalid MA, Rafie S, McNamara CS (1985) Interstitial hyperthermia for recurrent malignancies. Endocurietherapy/Hyperthermia Oncol 1: 125–131

Rafla S, Parikh K, Tchelebi M, Youssef E, Selim H, Bishay S (1989) Recurrent tumors of the head and neck, pelvis and chest wall: treatment with hyperthermia and brachytherapy. Radiology 172: 845–850

Roemer RB, Cetas TC (1984) Applications of bioheat transfer simulations in hyperthermia. Cancer Res [Suppl] 44: 4788s–4798s

Sapareto SA, Corry PM (1989) A proposed standard data file format for hyperthermia treatments. Int J Radiat Oncol Biol Phys 16: 613–627

Sapareto SA, Dewey WC (1984) Thermal dose determination in cancer therapy. Int J Radiat Oncol Biol Phys 10: 787–800

Sapareto SA, Hopwood LE, Dewey WC (1978) Combined effects of X-ray irradiation and hyperthermia on CHO cells for various temperatures and orders of application. Radiat Res 73: 221–233

Sapozink MD, Cetas T, Corry PM, Egger MJ, Fessenden P (1988) Introduction to hyperthermia device evaluation. Int J Hyperthermia 4: 1–17

Seegenschmiedt MH, Sauer R (1992) The current role of interstitial thermo-radiotherapy. Strahlenther Onkol 168: 119–140

Seegenschmiedt MH, Sauer R, Fietkau R, Iro H, Chalal JA, Brady LW (1992) Five year experience with interstitial thermal radiation therapy for head and neck tumors. Radiology 184: 795–804

Strohbehn JW (1984) Calculations of absorbed power in tissues for various hyperthermia devices. Cancer Res [Suppl] 44: 4781s–4787s

Strohbehn JW (1991) An engineer looks at hyperthermia. In: Dewey WC, Edington M, Fry RJM, Hall EJ, Whitmore GF (eds) Radiation research: a twentieth-century perspective, vol 2. Academic, San Diego, pp 14–25

Suit HD, Westgate SJ (1986) Impact of improved local tumor control on survival. Int J Radiat Oncol Biol Phys 12: 453–458

Surwit EA, Manning MR, Aristizabal SA, Oleson JR, Cetas TC (1983) Interstitial thermoradiotherapy in recurrent gynecological malignancies. Gynecol Oncol 15: 95–102

Tait DM, Carnochan P (1987) Thermal enhancement of radiation response: a growth delay study on superficial human tumour metastasis. Radiother Oncol 9: 231–240

Valdagni R, Liu FF, Kapp DS (1988) Important prognostic factors influencing outcome of combined radiation and hyperthermia. Int J Radiat Oncol Biol Phys 15: 13–24

Vora NL, Forell B, Luk KH et al. (1989) Interstitial thermoradiotherapy in recurrent and advanced carcinoma of malignant tumors: seven years experience. In: Sugahara T, Saito M (eds) Hyperthermic oncology 1988, vol 1. Taylor & Francis, London, pp 588–590

World Health Organization (WHO) Handbook for reporting results of cancer treatment. World Health Organization, Geneva

41 Thermobrachytherapy: Requirements for the Future

P.M. Corry, D. Gersten, S. Langer, and A. Martinez

CONTENTS

41.1 Introduction

Brachytherapy provides an obvious and sometimes ideal setting for combining hyperthermia with radiation therapy. Such combination therapy has been done in the past primarily using microwave technology where multiple antennae are placed intratumorally into plastic catheters previously inserted for this purpose (e.g., Perez and Emami 1985; Couglin and Strohbehn 1989). There are a number of situations, particularly in the head and neck region, where this methodology is useful but does not lend itself easily to automation and does not adapt well to the simultaneous application of afterloaders. Another situation where hyperthermia can and has been applied (e.g., Aristizabal and Oleson 1984; Kong et al. 1986; Vora et al. 1987) is for implants that involve stainless steel needles to contain the radioactive materials which are usually done in conjunction with a cutaneously attached template guidance apparatus (e.g., Martinez et al. 1984). Other approaches include needles heated with electrical heating elements (Garcia et al. 1992) or hot water, ferromagnetic seeds contained within plastic catheters, and RF-driven capacitively coupled plastic-coated electrodes. Ultrasonic interstitial and intracavitary applicators promise more functionality and versatility but are not yet in clinical use.

Irrespective of the heating methodology, acute pain associated with power application has been reported as the primary limiting factor in achieving acceptable temperature distributions for sufficiently long periods (Corry et al. 1988; Kapp et al. 1988; Sapozink et al. 1988; Shimm et al. 1988). This pain is often associated with elevated temperatures themselves as well as direct power deposition interactions with the involved tissues. This has been found to be the case for tumors with nerves encased by the tumor and is a particularly significant factor for advanced malignancies in the pelvis and abdomen. Fortunately, recent work (e.g., Ling and Robinson 1988; Armour et al. 1991, 1992; Wang et al. 1992) has demonstrated that mild hyperthermia (40°–41°C for long durations) can yield thermal enhancement ratios (TER) between 2 and 3 and the elimination of dose rate effects. These temperatures are more often than not the maximum achievable clinically. Additionally most of the clinical studies referenced above applied hyperthermia for 1 h prior to the low dose rate radiation and for 1 h after completion of the radiation therapy course, usually 48–72 h. This was done *not* because those regimens have been demonstrated to be optimal but was dictated *solely* by the practical limitations of the systems used for tumor temperature elevation. The rather rudimentary nature of currently available commercial systems poses other practical problems. At the present time the administration of hyperthermia is a labor-intensive and time-consuming exercise, often requiring several hours for physicians, physicists, nurses, and technologists. This is particularly true for interstitial hyperthermia administration.

Future systems must be designed to permit clinical protocols which can test for optimal heat administration regimens which must include simultaneous heat and radiation for protracted time

P.M. Corry, Ph.D; D. Gersten, B.S.; S. Langer, M.S.; A. Martinez, M.D., FACR; Department of Radiation Oncology, Division of Brachytherapy and Research, William Beaumont Hospital, 3601 West Thirteen Mile Road, Royal Oak, MI 48072, USA intervals. They should incorporate adequate hardware and software capabilities to accommodate unattended operation for prolonged periods (16–24 h per day). Setup complexity must be reduced and technology applied to reduce the labor intensiveness. Unless these steps are taken, we risk abandoning this potentially very effective addition to the cancer treatment armamentarium either because we find it to be to cumbersome and time consuming or because we apply only suboptimal treatment regimens and experience equivocal results.

In considering the desirable design characteristics of interstitial and intracavitary hyperthermia systems we have broken them down into three areas. First are the hardware features central to the overall system. The second section deals with the characteristics of the programs that must drive the computer systems controlling the power deposition. Finally we have outlined the thermometry requirements to satisfy quality assurance issues, minimize toxicities, and permit efficacy assessment of treatment as a function of thermal dose.

41.2 Hardware Requirements

Table 41.1 outlines the principal design features of systems that would satisfy the primary goals discussed above. If all of these features could be included, such a system would approach what might be defined as an ideal system. The order of importance of the various factors will depend a great deal on the physical setup in any given treating institution and upon the treatment philosophy of the physicians involved in the program. For this reason, it is difficult to define the most important factor(s) and all should be given equal weight in the design process.

The requirement for compatibility with automatic afterloaders is a result of our desire to apply simultaneous heat and radiation over a protracted period of time (48–72 h). From the points of view of personnel safety, ease of nursing care, and the need to minimize the effort of other professionals, this feature is essential. While there are no reports of combining hyperthermia with high dose rate brachytherapy in the literature as yet, the biological rationale to do so is strong and we and others plan to implement such programs in the near future. To implement these regimens, both the hyperthermia and the afterloading systems must operate compatibly. Depending upon the fractionation scheme, each will have to be set up 6–10 times over a 2 to 4-day period directly impacting the issue of setup and patient–machine interface complexity. Interface versatility is also affected by the fact that the precise nature of the implant (number and pattern of electrodes) is rarely predetermined, requiring flexibility. Furthermore, blood perfusion can only be estimated in advance, is known to vary between tumors and between treatments, and can be altered by a variety of common medications. These factors require that power deposition be dynamically controlled throughout the treatment volume continuously. To gain some understanding of the potential magnitude of this problem, consider Table 41.2, which presents the number of electrical connections necessary for various system designs and implant sizes using RF local current field (LCF) hyperthermia systems.

The "ideal paired" case is for a design where all electrodes can be connected arbitrarily as pairs, permitting any electrode to be connected with any other electrode dynamically. In real situations this level of flexibility is unnecessary; however, the capability of switching power between one electrode and each of its neighboring electrodes (paired neighbors) is a real requirement. For a common size implant, with 36 needles, this requires that 220 wires be connected to the 36 needles. Experience with the Oncotherm system, which is capable of

Table 41.1. Interstitial hyperthermia systems: hardware design criteria

- Compatible with simultaneous automatic afterloaders, including both high and low dose rate systems
- Dynamic alteration of the power deposition pattern in three dimensions at all times during therapy
- Fully automated control and data acquisition
- Minimum setup complexity
- Portable and usable in the patient's hospital room

Table 41.2. Interstitial RF hyperthermia: electrode requirements

System design	Implant size (electrodes)				
	2×2	3×3	4×4	6×6	6×10
	Electrical connections required				
Ideal paired	12	72	240	1260	3540
Paired neighbors	12	40	84	220	388
Unpaired	4	9	16	36	60
Oncotherm	12	40	40	40	40

exciting 20 needle pairs through 40 wire connections, convinced us that some other solution had to be found if the patient–machine interface were to be sufficiently simplified while satisfying all of the other design requirements.

To this end a new system was designed which satisfied the "unpaired" connection requirements given in Table 41.2. Although there are only 60 wire connections, all connections for the ideal paired and paired neighbor configurations are satisfied. This was achieved first by redesigning the MUPIT template used to guide the implant to incorporate printed circuit boards as integral components to effect all electrical connections to the needles. This HUPIT template is shown in Fig. 41.1. There are 59 positions, at 11-mm separations (9 × 7 array, corners missing), for stainless steel needles the ends of which connect to the afterloaders for the radioactive isotope. The power-generating circuitry connects as the needle traverses the template to induce hyperthermia. There are 48 positions between these needles for dedicated thermometry catheters. Connection to the power generator is via two snap-on connectors at opposite ends of the template. The microprocessor-controlled power generator has the capability of applying RF power between any two needles in the implant at any instant in time. After each programmed time period (usually 20 ms) the power is multiplexed to two other needles until the entire implant is scanned. This process is repeated ad infinitum until the control algorithms determine that the desired temperature distribution has been achieved. The inherent flexibility minimizes the information necessary prior to doing the implant and reduces setup time to a few minutes once the technical staff are trained in the use of the system.

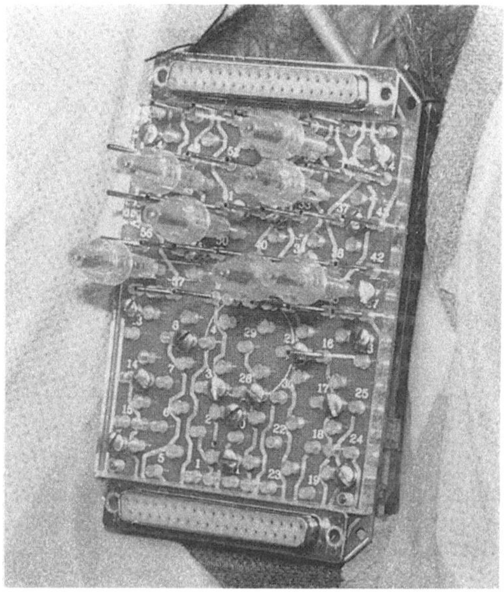

Fig. 41.1. Photograph of a HUPIT template placed intraoperatively during an implant procedure for a recurrent gynecological cancer. Thirty-three stainless steel needles were placed during the procedure. The electronic portion of the template is incorporated into the cover section and is added near the end of the procedure. The connectors at the top and bottom are for power introduction. Seven dedicated thermometry catheters were placed as the last step prior to the patient leaving the operating room. The plastic hubs are the removable obturators for the thermometry catheters. Afterloader connections are made to the end of each needle in a conventional manner. It was necessary to have the manufacturer (Nucletron) modify the afterloader connector tubes to be electrically nonconducting

Treatment planning software is used after the implant is done to determine the initial power deposition patterns. However, all parameters are under operator control at all times during therapy to

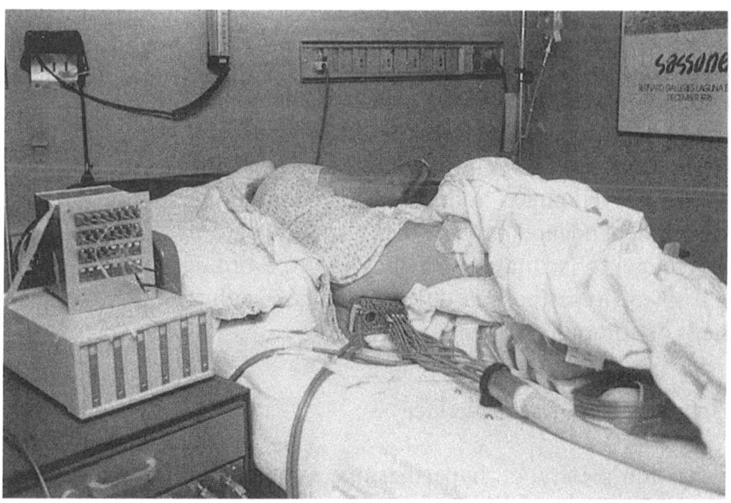

Fig. 41.2. A photograph of a patient undergoing combined treatment for a recurrent prostate carcinoma. The patient lies on his left side. Connection to the 18 afterloader positions is shown at the *lower right*. Thirty-two thermometry sensor connections are shown at the *far left* with the thermometry electronics directly below, which in turn rest on top of the power generation computer. Cables connecting the power generating computer at each end of the template are also shown

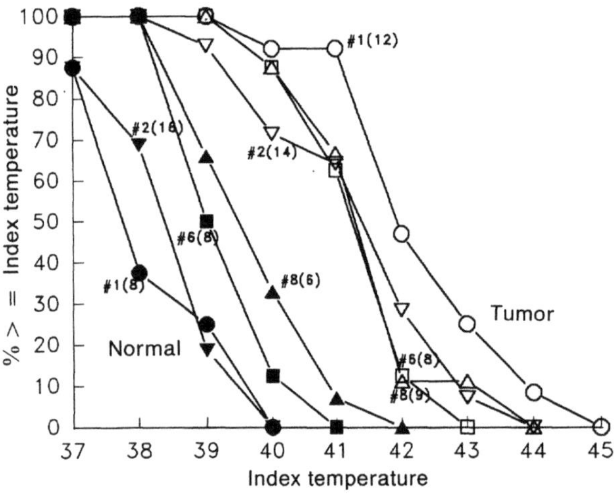

Fig. 41.3. Index temperature distributions for four patients treated with simultaneous long duration moderate temperature hyperthermia continuously for 48–72 h

account for factors such as varying blood flow and patient tolerance which cannot be accurately determined in advance. This system satisfies all of the design criteria save one: Since the stainless steel needles are not segmented, power is controlled only in two dimensions rather than the more ideal situation where it would be controlled in three dimensions. To achieve this it will be necessary to develop needles that are segmented along their length. This system is shown diagrammatically in Fig. 41.2 and the full setup treating a patient with an anorectal recurrence is shown in Fig. 41.2. Temperature distributions for four patients are given in Fig. 41.3.

41.3 Software Requirements

As with all contemporary systems of this type we have relied heavily on the use of microprocessor and computer technology to achieve the desired functionality and versatility. In the development of the system we have arrived at a set of desirable characteristics for the software which, while applicable to interstitial applications, in fact apply to any hyperthermia system. A principal objective in the software development effort was maintaining device independence in the high level program (C language) to facilitate its application to a broad spectrum of hyperthermia devices and use with a variety of computer systems.

41.3.1 Graphical User Interface

As the complexity of hyperthermia systems increases, the reliability and responsiveness of software controlling these systems becomes critical. For example, with the interstitial unit described above, 64 thermometry points are sampled every 15 s and potentially up to 194 heating entities are controlled with this limited data input. Added complexity of scanned and phased array ultrasound systems as well as scanned or segmented microwave antenna arrays require virtually instantaneous responses to assure patient safety. Loss of control by the program or failure to respond to interrupts within 100 ms are considered unacceptable. Additionally it was clear that a modern graphical user interface (GUI) was essential since the amount of data under consideration has escalated far beyond what treatment technologists are accustomed to ($\approx 10^5$ bytes/h). After attempting the use of commercial GUI software, such as Microsoft Windows, we found that their response characteristics, even on newer Intel 80486 based computers, were unacceptably slow. None of these interfaces were designed for an intensely interrupt-driven real-time environment. To circumvent these limitations, we developed a real-time GUI designed specifically for this type of application. The desirable software design features were found to be:

1. A graphical presentation screen with at least 800×600 spatial resolution in 256 colors. 1024×768 resolution is preferable.
2. Capability of managing 256 thermometry data input points every 15 s.
3. Capability for management of a large number of heating "entities" (256). A "heating entity" is defined as any physical element or logical combination thereof capable of elevating tumor temperature. Examples are needles, needle pairs, microwave antennae, ultrasound transducers, etc.
4. A "friendly," intuitive user interface which is the same for all hyperthermia systems. Manipulation of the displays must be intuitive and easy to use. Menus, windows, icons, dialogue boxes, and a standard pointing device (e.g., mouse) provide the user direct interaction with the operating program. The software must present an accurate representation of temperature distributions throughout the tumor volume in a well-organized, easily understood format. Several (five to ten) temperature and analysis display windows must be available simultaneously and all updated in real time.
5. Device independence. The high level software (C language) must be usable on many machines with minimal modification.
6. Response time to hardware interrupts less than 10 ms.

7. Response time to operator intervention less than 100 ms.
8. Unattended operation for indefinite periods of time.

A GUI satisfying all of the design criteria described has been implemented and is now in use for the interstitial and magnetic induction systems which we have developed. Other salient features of this software are:

1. The program provides the treatment technician with all the information necessary to make intelligent treatment decisions.
2. All entity heating parameters can be dynamically altered and/or displayed.
3. All temperature regulation, power control, and data logging is automatic and can operate without user interaction for indefinite periods of time.
4. Fail-safe provisions effect a complete system shutdown (line power off) in the event of loss of program control within 100 ms.

4.1.3.2 Representative Displays

41.3.2.1 Bargraph

The Bargraph display presents the instantaneous temperatures of the selected group or level of sensors. Each bar displays the temperature numerically, the sensor number, and an indicator of the temperature trend.

41.3.2.2 History

The History display draws a line graph showing temperature versus time. Any arbitrary start and end time may be entered by the user. The temperature range can also be interactively set.

41.3.2.3 Entity

The Entity display allows the user direct access to parameters which control power regulation. A mix of display only and changeable parameters is presented. Temperature regulation information is also displayed in the Entity window. Regulation points may be added or deleted at any time during the treatment.

41.3.2.4 Index

The Index display presents the user with a global perspective of the temperature distribution within a treatment volume. The percentage of temperature points at or above index temperature are plotted against the index temperature. This display provides the clinician with visible evidence of the efficacy of the therapy. This window can also display temperature distribution parameters such as T_{90}, T_{75}, etc.

41.3.3 Treatment Device Control

To achieve the flexibility necessary for device-independent hardware control, a modular software design is essential. We have divided the functions required in a real-time clinical system into the following two categories:

1. *High level user interactive software*
   a) High level control
   b) Displays
   c) Patient data logging

2. *Low level operating system resident device drivers*
   a) Temperature acquisition
   b) Hyperthermia device control
   c) Motion control.

All high level functions communicate to the thermometry and heating hardware through the low level device drivers. They, in turn, provide the necessary control over the particular thermometry and heating devices being used. The low level drivers effectively hide the actual mechanics of the underlying hardware from the high level functions. At no time do the high level functions need to know the identity of the hardware they are controlling. If a high level display function needs to know how many thermometry sensors are available for display, it simply "asks" the appropriate low level temperature device driver. Similarly, when a high level function creates a display which allows control of the heating unit, it "asks" the hyperthermia control driver which parameters are valid to display and edit, allowing all high level functions to be reused and provide a consistent interface to the user. This software has been implemented on heating systems by Labthermics Technologies and two in-house devices and with thermometry systems from Omega, Metrabyte, and Labthermics.

41.4 Thermometry Requirements

Thermometry requirements are dictated primarily by quality assurance criteria and the need to control temperatures in three dimensions at some prescribed level. The prescription should be expressed in terms of the temperature distribution throughout the treatment volume and not in terms of a given temperature at any given point within the volume. A convenient way of describing the distribution is the percentage of intratumoral temperature points at or above a given index temperature (Corry et al. 1988). For example, in Fig. 41.3 the T_{90} was approximately 40°C and the T_{75} 41°C, which was the prescribed level. The software described above has the capability of computing and displaying this type of information in real time, providing the technologist operator with the ability to assess compliance with the prescription continuously. This type of real-time analysis also permits alteration of the power deposition pattern to comply with the prescription if necessary. The Radiation Therapy Oncology Group (RTOG) in the United States has developed comprehensive quality assurance guidelines for interstitial hyperthermia which are sufficiently extensive to permit this form of analysis and control (Emami et al. 1991). Table 41.3 summarizes the approximate recommended number of sensors as a function of tumor volume.

These guidelines also outline recommended placement of the sensors. Catheters containing multiple sensors or a single scanned sensor must be placed to accurately represent the central and peripheral aspects of the tumor. Temperatures in tumor tissue central to the arrays of heating entities must also be monitored. For adequate control and patient safety, normal tissue temperatures must also be determined but specific recommendations are not described. It must be emphasized that these numbers are recommended minima for quality assurance purposes. For many systems additional sensors will be necessary to achieve adequate three-dimensional power deposition control. Clearly, future systems will require expanded data acquisition capabilities over those of the past. Thirty-two point measurement capability appears to be the minimum required number and for versatility sixty-four is highly desirable.

Table 41.3. Recommended implanted sensors

Tumor volume (ml)	Minimum number of sensors
5	12
10	15
50	18
100	24
200	30
500	48

41.5 Discussion

In this chapter we have attempted to outline what we believe are the requirements for future interstitial hyperthermia systems to achieve several essential goals.

1. Possess sufficient versatility that any desired heat/radiation treatment regimen can be tested for efficacy.
2. Automate and simplify the operator–machine and machine–patient interfaces to the point that they can be used in any treatment setting while minimizing the involvement of physicians and physicists. An additional benefit here is a substantial reduction in cost.
3. Provide fully automatic data acquisition and control which guarantee treatment prescription compliance. If, due to factors such as patient tolerance, it cannot be achieved, involved personnel must be informed and make appropriate decisions and/or adjustments.
4. Provide adequate quality assurance and data interchange capability to permit multi-institution clinical trials for efficacy.

An important factor in achieving these goals over the past few years has been the realization that extensive thermometry is essential to the assessment of the adequacy of tumor temperature distributions. Corry et al. (1988) demonstrated that as the number of intratumoral temperature sensors increases, our estimation of the heating adequacy decreases. This observation has been confirmed in two other institutions (B.A. Emami at Washington University and M.W. Dewhirst at Duke University, personal communications), and it has been established that the true assessment of the temperature distribution requires 10–15 sensors. Using less than this number invariably results in false confidence and has been the critical factor in the failure of some clinical trials to demonstrate efficacy in the past (e.g., Perez et al. 1989). Equally important for the success of clinical trials is treatment documentation. Due to the sheer volume of data produced, the necessity for standardized data reduction and analysis is obvious. In the system described here we have complied with a published data recording and reporting standard (SAPARETO and CORRY 1989). While it would certainly be possible to develop other (perhaps better) methods, to the best of our knowledge this is the sole published standard and it has been adopted by the RTOG for all clinical trials involving hyperthermia in the United States. Whatever system is developed, some reporting standard is essential if data from multi-institutional trials are to be interpreted and compared accurately.

The interstitial hyperthermia system that we have presented as representative of future requirements, while meeting most of them, is not the only way of accomplishing these ends. Hot source technology (electrically heated implant needles, GARCIA et al. 1992), while lacking some versatility in control, could be modified to meet most of the outlined criteria. Microwave technology may well be more difficult to adapt if the requirements for simultaneous radiation and compatibility with afterloading equipment are adhered to. One possibility is the incorporation of motor-driven scanning antennae. Another is plastic catheters with segmented helical antennae embedded in the catheter wall (Satoh et al. 1988; ASTRAHAN et al. 1991) for three-dimensional power deposition control. This latter approach would permit the simultaneous use of the catheters for heating and irradiation and they could be connected to afterloaders. Interstitial ultrasound is another method with great, but as yet undeveloped, promise. Irrespective of the methodology used, it is essential that equipment be developed along the general lines described here if the full potential of interstitial hyperthermia is to be realized.

Acknowledgment. This work was supported in part by grant CA-44550 from the U.S. National Cancer Institute.

References

Armour EP, Wang Z, Corry PM, Martinez A (1991) Sensitization of rat 9L gliosarcoma cells to low dose rate irradiation by long duration 41° hyperthermia. Cancer Res 51: 3088–3095

Armour EP, Wang Z, Corry PM, Martinez A (1992) Equivalence of continuous and pulse simulated low dose rate irradiation in 9L gliosarcoma cells at 37° and 41°. Int J Radiat Oncol Biol Phys 22: 109–114

Aristizabal S, Oleson J (1984) Combined interstitial irradiation and localized current field hyperthermia: results and conclusions from clinical studies. Cancer Res 44 (Suppl) : 4754s–4760s

Astrahan MA, Imanaka K, Josef G et al. (1991) Heating characteristics of a helical coil microwave applicator for transurethral hyperthermia of benign prostatic hyperplasia. Int J Hyperthermia 7: 141–155

Corry PM, Jabboury K, Kong JS, Armour EP, McCraw JF, Leduc T (1988) Phase I evaluation of equipment for hyperthermic treatment of cancer. Int J Hyperthermia 4: 53–74

Couglin CT, Strohbehn JW (1989) Interstitial thermoradiotherapy. Radiol Clin North Am 27: 577–588

Emami B, Stauffer P, Dewhirst MW et al. (1991) RTOG quality assurance guidelines for interstitial hyperthermia. Int J Radiat Oncol Biol Phys 20: 1117–1124

Garcia DM, Nussbaum GH, Fathman AE, Drzymala RE, Bleyer M, DeFord JA and Welsh D (1992) Concurrent Ir-192 brachytherapy and long duration conductive interstitial hyperthermia for the treatment of recurrent carcinoma of the prostate. Endocurie/Hyperthermia Oncol 8: 151–158

Kapp DS, Fessenden P, Samulski TV, Bagshaw MA, Cox RS, Lee ER (1988) Stanford University institutional report: phase I evaluation of equipment for hyperthermic treatment of cancer. Int J Hyperthermia 4: 75–116

Kong JS, Corry PM, Saul PB (1986) Hyperthermia in the treatment of gynecologic cancers. In: Freedman R, Gershenson (eds) Diagnosis and treatment strategies for gynecologic cancers. The University of Texas Press, Austin, Texas

Ling CC, Robinson E (1988) Moderate hyperthermia and low dose rate radiation. Radiation Res 114: 379–384

Martinez AM, Cox RS, Mundson E (1984) A multiple site perineal applicator (MUPIT) for treatment of prostatic, anorectal and gynecological malignancies. Int J Radiat Oncol Biol Phys 10: 297

Perez CA, Emami BA (1985) A review of current clinical experience with irradiation and hyperthermia. Endocurietherapy/Hyperthermia Oncol 1: 257–277

Perez CA, Gillespie B, Pajak T, Hornback NB, Emami BA, Rubin P (1989) quality assurance problems in clinical hyperthermia and its impact on therapeutic outcome. Int J Radiat Oncol Biol Phys 16: 1989

Sapareto SA, Corry PM (1989) A proposed standard format for hyperthermia treatment data. Int J Radiat Oncol Biol Phys 16: 613–627

Sapozink MD, Gibbs FA, Gibbs P, Stewart JR (1988) Phase I evaluation of hyperthermia equipment: University of Utah institutional report. Int J Hyperthermia 4: 117–132

Satoh T, Stauffer PR, Fike JR (1988) Thermal distribution studies of helical coil microwave antennae for interstitial hyperthermia. Int J Radiat Oncol Biol Phys 15: 1209–1218

Shimm DS, Cetas TC, Oleson JR, Cassady JR, Sim DA (1988) Clinical evaluation of hyperthermia equipment: the University of Arizona institutional report for the NCI hyperthermia equipment evaluation contract. Int J Hyperthermia 4: 39–52

Vora N, Forrel B, Cappil J, Lipsett J, Archambeau JO (1987) Interstitial implant with interstitial hyperthermia. Cancer 50: 2518–2523

Wang Z, Armour EP, Corry PM, Martinez A (1992) Elimination of dose rate effects by mild hyperthermia. Int J Radiat Oncol Biol Phys 24: 965–973

Subject Index

List of Contributors

Jean-Michel Ardiet, M.D.
Service de Curiethérapie
Centre Léon Bérard
F-69003 Lyon
France

L.V. Baert, M.D.
Professor, Department of Urology
University Hospital K.U.L.
Brusselsestraat 69
B-3000 Leuven
Belgium

Luther W. Brady, M.D.
Department of Radiation Oncology
and Nuclear Medicine
Hahnemann University
Broad & Vine Streets, MS 200
Philadelphia, PA 19102-1198
USA

J.C. Camart, M.S.
IEMN CHS UMR 9929
CNRS Université des Sciences et
Technologies de Lille
Bât 94
F-59655 Villeneuve d'Ascq Cédex
France

Thomas C. Cetas, Ph.D.
Department of Radiation Oncology
University of Arizona
1501 North Campbell Avenue
Tucson, AZ 85724
USA

Maurice Chive, Ph.D.
IEMN CHS UMR 9929
CNRS Université des Sciences et
Technologies de Lille
Bât 94
F-59655 Villeneuve d'Ascq Cédex
France

K.L. Clibbon, Ph.D.
Department of Electrical and Electronic
Engineering
University College of Swansea
Singleton Park
Swansea SA2 8PP
UK

T.A. Colacchio, M.D.
Section of General Surgery
Department of Surgery
Dartmouth-Hitchcock Medical Center
Lebanon, NH 03756
USA

Peter M. Corry, Ph.D.
Department of Radiation Oncology
Division of Brachytherapy and Research
William Beaumont Hospital
3601 W. 13 Mile Road
Royal Oak, MI 48072
USA

Jean-Marc Cosset, M.D.
Professeur
Département de Radiothérapie
Institut Gustave Roussy
F-94800 Villejuif
France
and current address:
Département de Radiothérapie
Institut Curie
26 rue d'Ulm
F-75231 Paris Cédex 05
France

Christopher T. Coughlin, M.D.
Section of Radiation Oncology
Department of Medicine
Dartmouth-Hitchcock Medical Center
Lebanon, NH 03756
USA

J. Crezee, Ph.D.
Department of Radiotherapy
University Hospital Utrecht
Heidelberglaan 100
NL-3584 CX Utrecht
The Netherlands

Chris J. Diederich, Ph.D.
University of California San Francisco
Radiation Oncology Department
San Francisco, CA 94143-0226
USA

Ralph R. Dobelbower, Jr., M.D., Ph.D.
Department of Radiation Therapy
Medical College of Ohio
C.S. #10008
Toledo, OH 43699
USA

E.B. Douple, M.D.
Section of Radiation Oncology
Department of Medicine
Dartmouth-Hitchcock Medical Center
Lebanon, NH 03756
USA

Bahman Emami, M.D.
Radiation Oncology Center
Mallinckrodt Institute of Radiology
Washington University School of Medicine
510 S. Kingshighway, Box 8224
St. Louis, MO 63110
USA

Jean-Jacques Fabre, Ph.D.
IEMN CHS UMRE 9929
CNRS Université des Sciences et
Technologies de Lille
Bât 94
F-59655 Villeneuve d'Ascq Cédex
France

Rainer Fietkau, M.D.
Strahlentherapeutische Klinik
Universität Erlangen-Nürnberg
Universitätsstraße 27
W-8520 Erlangen
Germany

B. Frankendal, M.D., Ph.D.
Department of Gynecologic Oncology
Örebro Medical Center Hospital
S-701 85 Örebro
Sweden

Peter Fritz, M.D.
Radiologische Universitätsklinik
Abteilung Strahlentherapie
Im Neuenheimer Feld 400
W-6900 Heidelberg
Germany

Jean-Pierre Gerard, M.D.
Professeur
Service de Radiothérapie du Centre
Hospitalier Lyon Sud
F-69310 Pierre Benite
France

David Gersten, B.S.
Department of Radiation Oncology
Division of Brachytherapy and Research
William Beaumont Hospital
3601 W. 13 Mile Road
Royal Oak, MI 48072
USA

G.G. Grabenbauer, M.D.
Strahlentherapeutische Klinik
Universität Erlangen-Nürnberg
Universitätsstraße 27
W-8520 Erlangen
Germany

Perry W. Grigsby, M.D.
Associate Professor, Radiation Oncology Center
Mallinckrodt Institute of Radiology
Washington University School of Medicine
510 S. Kingshighway, Box 8224
St. Louis, MO 63110
USA

Eric W. Hahn, Ph.D.
Forschungsschwerpunkt Radiologische
Diagnostik und Therapie
Deutsches Krebsforschungszentrum
Im Neuenheimer Feld 280
W-6900 Heidelberg
Germany

Jeffrey W. Hand, Ph.D.
Hyperthermia Clinic
MRC Cyclotron Unit
Hammersmith Hospital
Du Cane Road
London W12 OHS
UK

Leonore Handl-Zeller, M.D.
Universitätsklinik für Strahlentherapie und -biologie
Alserstraße 4
A-1090 Wien
Austria

W. Hürter, Ph.D.
Deutsches Krebsforschungszentrum
Im Neuenheimer Feld 280
W-6900 Heidelberg
Germany

Kullervo H. Hynynen, Ph.D.
University of Arizona Health Sciences Center
Radiation Oncology Department
1501 North Campbell Avenue
Tucson, AZ 85724
USA

Heinrich Iro, M.D.
Hals-Nasen-Ohren-Klinik der Universität Erlangen-Nürnberg
Waldstraße 1
W-8520 Erlangen
Germany

Ellen L. Jones, M.D., Ph.D.
Harvard Joint Center for Radiation Therapy
50 Binney Street
Boston, MA 02215
USA

R.S.J.P. Kaatee, M.Sc.
Department of Clinical Physics
Dr. Daniel den Hoed Cancer Center
Groene Hilledijk 301, P.O. Box 5201
NL-3008 AE Rotterdam
The Netherlands

C. Koedooder, Ph.D.
Department of Radiotherapy
Amsterdam University Hospital
Academisch Medisch Centrum
Meibergdreef 9
NL-1105 AZ Amsterdam Zuidoost
The Netherlands

F. Koenis, M.Sc.
Department of Radiotherapy
Amsterdam University Hospital
Academisch Medisch Centrum
Meibergdreef 9
NL-1105 AZ Amsterdam Zuidoost
The Netherlands

I.K.K. Kolkman-Deurloo, M.Sc.
Department of Clinical Physics
Dr. Daniel den Hoed Cancer Center
Groene Hilledijk 301, P.O. Box 5201
NL-3008 AE Rotterdam
The Netherlands

Jan J.W. Lagendijk, Ph.D.
Department of Radiotherapy
University Hospital Utrecht
Heidelberglaan 100
NL-3584 CX Utrecht
The Netherlands

Steve Langer
Department of Radiation Oncology
Division of Brachytherapy and Research
William Beaumont Hospital
3601 W. 13 Mile Road
Royal Oak, MI 48072
USA

Peter C. Levendag, M.D., Ph.D.
Department of Radiotherapy
Dr. Daniel den Hoed Cancer Center
Groene Hilledijk 301, P.O. Box 5201
NL-3008 AE Rotterdam
The Netherlands

W.J. Lorenz, M.D.
Deutsches Krebsforschungszentrum
Im Neuenheimer Feld 280
W-6900 Heidelberg
Germany

Kenneth H. Luk, M.D., FACR
Department of Radiation Oncology
Good Samaritan Regional Medical Center
1111 E. McDowell Road
Phoenix, AZ 85006
USA

Michael A. Mackey, Ph.D.
Section of Cancer Biology
Division of Radiation Oncology
Mallinckrodt Institute of Radiology
Washington University School of Medicine
4511 Forest Park Blvd.
St. Louis, MO 63108
USA

Christian Marchal, M.D., Ph.D.
Unité d'Hyperthermie
Service de Radiothérapie
Centre Alexis Vautrin
Avenue de Bourgogne
F-54511 Vandoeuvre les Nancy
France

Alvaro Martinez, M.D., FACR
Department of Radiation Oncology
Division of Brachytherapy and Research
William Beaumont Hospital
3601 West Thirteen Mile Road
Royal Oak, MI 48072
USA

Andrew McCowen, B.Sc., M.Sc., Ph.D.
Department of Electrical and
Electronic Engineering
University College of Swansea
Singleton Park
Swansea SA2 8PP
UK

C.A. Meeuwis, M.D., Ph.D.
Department of ENT Surgery
Dr. Daniel den Hoed Cancer Center
Groene Hilledijk 301, P.O. Box 5201
NL-3008 AE Rotterdam
The Netherlands

Hollis W. Merrick, M.D.
Department of Surgery
Medical College of Ohio
C.S. #10008
Toledo, OH 43699
USA

Andrew J. Milligan, Ph.D.
Department of Radiation Therapy and
Nuclear Medicine
Thomas Jefferson University
11th and Walnut Sts.
Philadelphia, PA 19107
USA

Curtis Miyamoto, M.D.
Department of Radiation Oncology
and Nuclear Medicine
Hahnemann University
Broad & Vine Sts., MS 200
Philadelphia, PA 19102-1198
USA

Jaap Mooibroek, M.Sc.
Department of Radiotherapy
University Hospital Utrecht
Heidelberglaan 100
NL-3584 CX Utrecht
The Netherlands

F. Morganti, Ph.D.
IEMN, UMR CNRS 9929
Département Hyperfréquence et
Semiconducteurs
Bât. 94
Université des Sciences et Technologies de Lille
F-59655 Villeneuve d'Ascq Cédex
France

J. Nadobny, Ph.D.
Klinikum Rudolf Virchow
Freie Universität Berlin
Strahlenklinik und Poliklinik
Augustenburger Platz 1
W-1000 Berlin 65
Germany

G.J. Nieuwenhuys, Ph.D.
Kamerlingh Onnes Laboratory
Leiden State University
Nieuwsteeg 18
NL-2311 SB Leiden
The Netherlands

Konstantina S. Nikita, Ph.D.
Department of Electrical and
Computer Engineering
National Technical University of Athens
42 Patison Street
GR-10682 Athens
Greece

PETER PESCHKE, M.D.
Forschungsschwerpunkt Radiologische Diagnostik und Therapie
Deutsches Krebsforschungszentrum
Im Neuenheimer Feld 280
W-6900 Heidelberg
Germany

ZBIGNIEW PETROVICH, M.D.
Professor and Chairman,
Department of Radiation Oncology
University of Southern California,
School of Medicine
1441 Eastlake Avenue, Room 34
Los Angeles, CA 90033-0804
USA

BERNARD PREVOST, M.D.
Centre de lutte contre le Cancer
Oscar Lambret
1 rue Frédéric Combemale, BP 307
F-59020 Lille Cédex
France

F. REINBOLD, M.D.
Deutsches Krebsforschungszentrum
Im Neuenheimer Feld 280
W-6900 Heidelberg
Germany

DAN ROOS, Ph.D.
Department of Gynecologic Oncology
Örebro Medical Center Hospital
S-701 85 Örebro
Sweden

THOMAS P. RYAN, M.S.
Section of Radiation Oncology
Dartmouth-Hitchcock Medical Center
Lebanon, NH 03756
USA
and
Thayer School of Engineering
Dartmouth College
Hanover, NH 03755
USA

ROLF SAUER, M.D.
Professor and Chairman
Strahlentherapeutische Klinik der
Universität Erlangen-Nürnberg
Universitätsstraße 27
W-8520 Erlangen
Germany

W. SCHLEGEL, M.D., Ph.D.
Deutsches Krebsforschungszentrum
Abteilung Biophysik und
Medizinische Strahlenphysik
Im Neuenheimer Feld 280
W-6900 Heidelberg
Germany

P. SCHRAUBE, M.D.
Radiologische Universitätsklinik
Abteilung Strahlentherapie
Im Neuenheimer Feld 400
W-6900 Heidelberg
Germany

MARTIN SEEBASS, Ph.D.
Konrad-Zuse-Zentrum für
Informationstechnik Berlin
Abteilung Numerische Software-Entwicklung
Heilbronner Straße 10
W-1000 Berlin 31
Germany

M. HEINRICH SEEGENSCHMIEDT, M.D.
Strahlentherapeutische Klinik der
Universität Erlangen-Nürnberg
Universitätsstraße 27
W-8520 Erlangen
Germany

DAVID S. SHIMM, M.D.
Department of Radiation Oncology
University of Arizona
1501 North Campbell Avenue
Tucson, AZ 85724
USA

C. SMED-SÖRENSEN, M.D.
Department of Gynecologic Oncology
Örebro Medical Center Hospital
S-701 85 Örebro
Sweden

PENNY K. SNEED, M.D.
Assistant Professor
Department of Radiation Oncology
Room L-75 (Box 0226)
University of California San Francisco
505 Parnassus Avenue
San Francisco, CA 94143-0226
USA

Bengt Sorbe, M.D., Ph.D.
Department of Gynecologic Oncology
Örebro Medical Center Hospital
S-701 85 Örebro
Sweden

Baldassarre Stea, M.D., Ph.D.
Department of Radiation Oncology
University of Arizona
1501 North Campbell Avenue
Tucson, AZ 85724
USA

Adrian C. Steger, M.S., F.R.C.S.
Department of Surgery
King's College School of Medicine and Dentistry
The Rayne Institute
123 Coldharbour Lane
London SE5 9NU
UK

John W. Strohbehn, Ph.D.
Thayer School of Engineering
Dartmouth-Hitchcock Medical Center
Hanover, NH 03755
USA

N.K. Uzunoglu, Ph.D.
Department of Electrical and Computer Engineering
National Technical University of Athens
42 Patison Street
GR-10682 Athens
Greece

Jan D.P. van Dijk, Ph.D.
Department of Radiotherapy
Amsterdam University Hospital
Academisch Medisch Centrum
Meibergdreef 9
NL-1105 AZ Amsterdam Zuidoost
The Netherlands

C.A.J.F. van Geel, B.Sc.
Department of Radiotherapy
Dr. Daniel den Hoed Cancer Center
Groene Hilledijk 301, P.O. Box 5201
NL-3008 AE Rotterdam
The Netherlands

C.M.C. van Hooye, B.Sc.
Department of Radiotherapy
Dr. Daniel den Hoed Cancer Center
Groene Hilledijk 301, P.O. Box 5201
NL-3008 AE Rotterdam
The Netherlands

G.C. van Rhoon, B.Sc.
Department of Radiotherapy
Dr. Daniel den Hoed Cancer Center
Groene Hilledijk 301, P.O. Box 5201
NL-3008 AE Rotterdam
The Netherlands

N. van Wieringen, M.Sc.
Department of Radiotherapy
Amsterdam University Hospital
Academisch Medisch Centrum
Meibergdreef 9
NL-1105 AZ Amsterdam Zuidoost
The Netherlands

Clare C. Vernon, M.A., FRCR
MRC Hyperthermia Clinic
Hammersmith Hospital
Ducane Road
London W12 OHS
UK

Andries G. Visser, Ph.D.
Department of Clinical Physics
Dr. Daniel den Hoed Cancer Center
P.O. Box 5201
Groene Hilledijk 301
NL-3008 AE Rotterdam
The Netherlands

Nayana L. Vora, M.D.
Division of Radiation Oncology
City of Hope National Medical Center
1500 E. Duarte Road
Duarte, CA 91010
USA

Michael Wannenmacher, M.D.
Professor and Chairman
Radiologische Universitätsklinik
Abteilung Strahlentherapie
Im Neuenheimer Feld 400
W-6900 Heidelberg
Germany

Gerd Wolber, Ph.D.
Forschungsschwerpunkt Radiologische
Diagnostik und Therapie
Deutsches Krebsforschungszentrum
Im Neuenheimer Feld 280
W-6900 Heidelberg
Germany

P. Wust, M.D.
Klinikum Rudolf Virchow
Freie Universität Berlin
Strahlenklinik und Poliklinik
Augustenburger Platz 1
W-1000 Berlin 65
Germany

Springer-Verlag and the Environment

We at Springer-Verlag firmly believe that an international science publisher has a special obligation to the environment, and our corporate policies consistently reflect this conviction.

We also expect our business partners – paper mills, printers, packaging manufacturers, etc. – to commit themselves to using environmentally friendly materials and production processes.

The paper in this book is made from low- or no-chlorine pulp and is acid free, in conformance with international standards for paper permanency.

MIX
Papier aus verantwortungsvollen Quellen
Paper from responsible sources
FSC® C105338

If you have any concerns about our products,
you can contact us on
ProductSafety@springernature.com

In case Publisher is established outside the EU,
the EU authorized representative is:
Springer Nature Customer Service Center GmbH
Europaplatz 3, 69115 Heidelberg, Germany

Printed by Libri Plureos GmbH
in Hamburg, Germany